Essential Guide to Calving

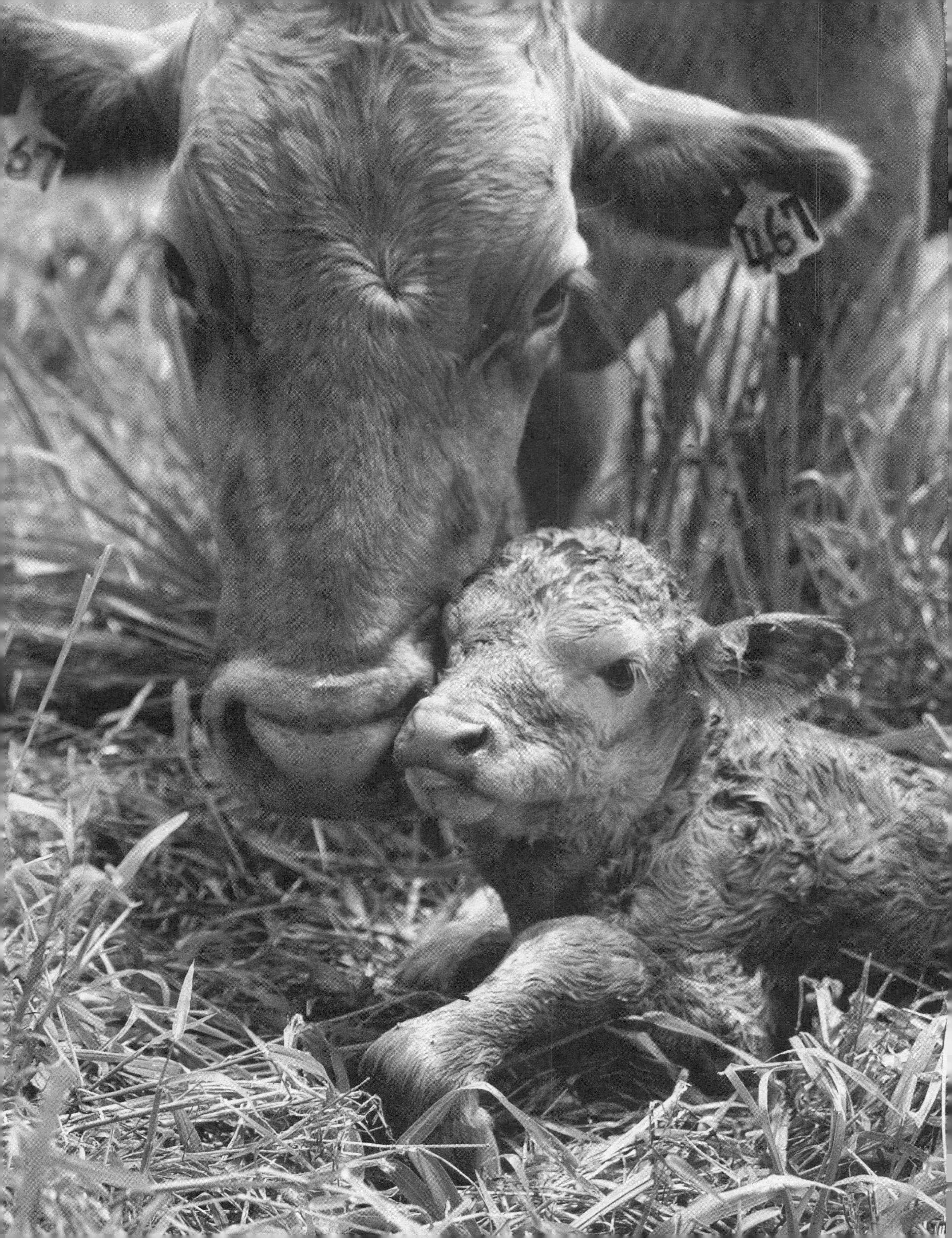

467

Essential Guide to CALVING

Giving Your Beef or Dairy Herd a Healthy Start

HEATHER SMITH THOMAS

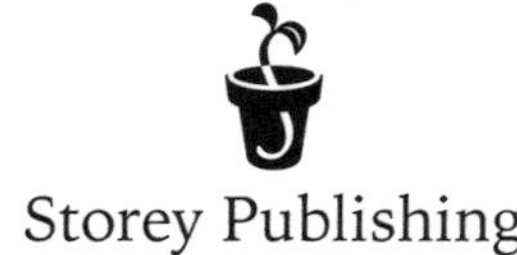

Storey Publishing

The mission of Storey Publishing is to serve our customers by publishing practical information that encourages personal independence in harmony with the environment.

Edited by Sarah Guare and Rebekah-Boyd Owens
Art direction and book design by Jessica Armstrong

Cover photographs by © blickwinkel/Alamy Images: front and spine, and © Andrea Hansen: back
Interior photographs by © Heather Smith Thomas, except for © Fotosearch: page ii, and © Andrea Hansen: pages viii and ix
Illustrations by © Elara Tanguy, except for © Elayne Sears: pages 20, 32, 80, 82 top right, 157, 274

Indexed by Susan Olason, Indexes and Knowledge Maps

Printed in United States by Versa Press
10 9 8 7 6 5 4 3 2 1

LIBRARY OF CONGRESS CATALOGING-IN-PUBLICATION DATA

Thomas, Heather Smith, 1944–
Essential guide to calving / by Heather Smith Thomas.
p. cm.
Includes index.
ISBN 978-1-58017-706-1 (pbk. : alk. paper)
ISBN 978-1-58017-707-8 (hardcover : alk. paper)
1. Calves. 2. Cattle—Parturition. I. Title.
SF205.T47 2008
636.2'089892—dc22

2007049726

DEDICATION

This book is dedicated to my husband, Lynn,
who has been my partner and teammate through 40 years
of delivering calves and keeping them healthy.

Contents

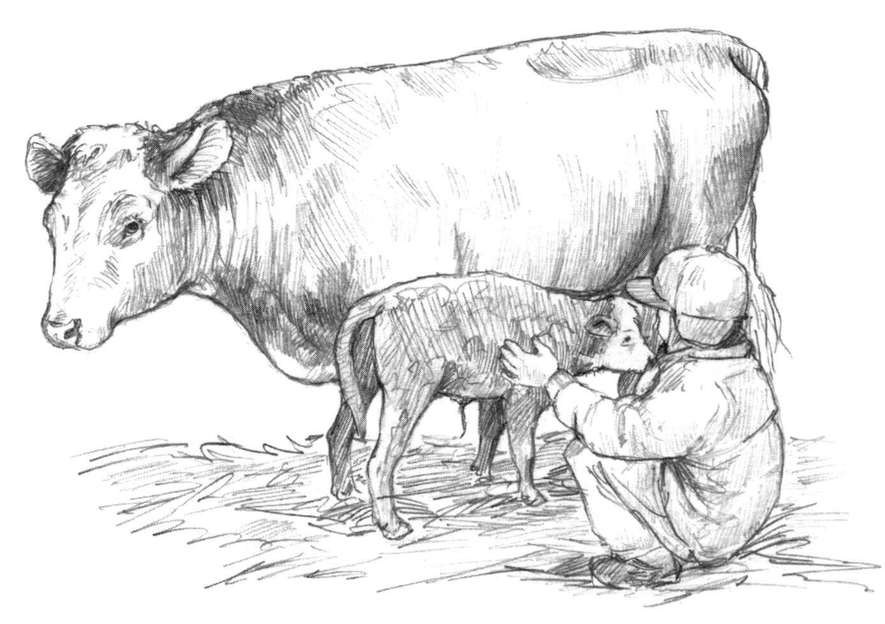

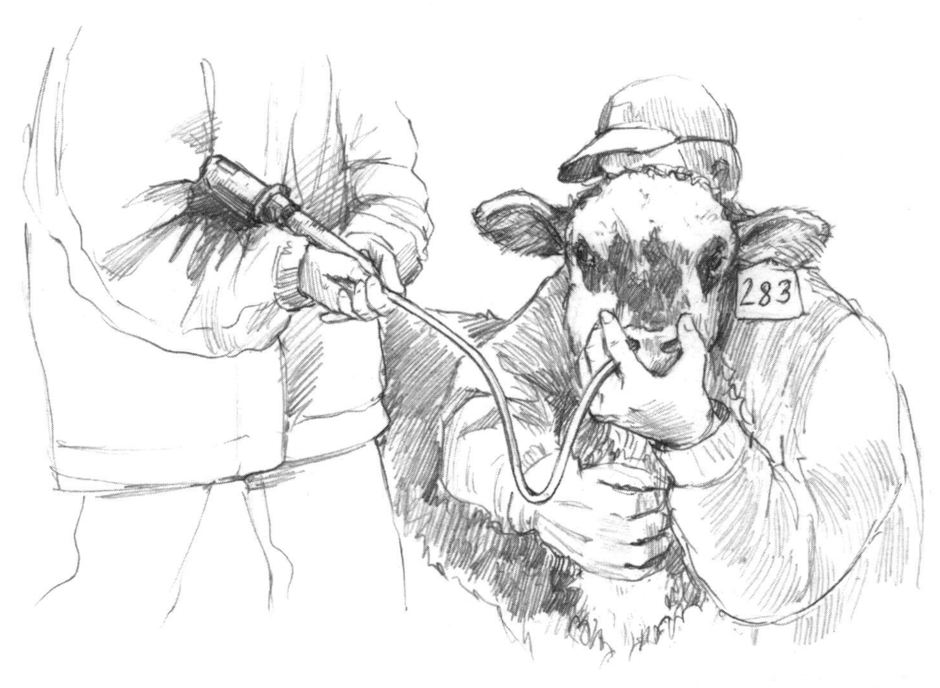
283

Preface

THIS BOOK FOCUSES on the most important aspect of raising cattle: calving. Crucial to anyone who breeds cattle is helping a cow have a successful pregnancy, getting the calf born safely, and making sure the calf gets off to a good start and stays healthy during the first weeks of life. This handbook is meant to become a bible for anyone who wants to start raising cattle and a helpful reference for stockmen who already have cow/calf operations, large or small. It's a book you'll most likely refer to again and again — the kind of reference I wish I'd had when I was starting out.

People who raise livestock, including small farmers who are going "back to the land" to have a more satisfying life and hobby farmers who keep livestock, are choosing to do so because they like animals and want to learn to care for them. Those who raise sheep and goats, for instance, do so because they want a hands-on animal experience; they want to do it all — including learning how to assist in the birthing of the young. People who raise cattle are no different. They want to be able to take care of their animals on their own instead of having to rely on the vet for every little problem. Many people who choose to raise livestock today are doing it to get back in tune with Nature, to fully interact with their animals, and to be true herdsmen. (*Note:* Many women who raise cattle refer to themselves in traditional terms such as "stockmen" and "herdsmen." Therefore, this sort of gender-inclusive usage has been borrowed for the writing of this book.)

Folks who pursue a dream of raising livestock may know nothing about cattle reproduction and calving, yet they are serious in their intentions and want to obtain the best, most in-depth information available. The purpose of this book is to help them accomplish the goal of providing better care to their animals. Why not learn all we can about proper care during calving time? Learning about the animals is part of why we raise cattle (or any other livestock) — and making a living raising cattle is quite achievable if you learn to take care of them properly and minimize losses.

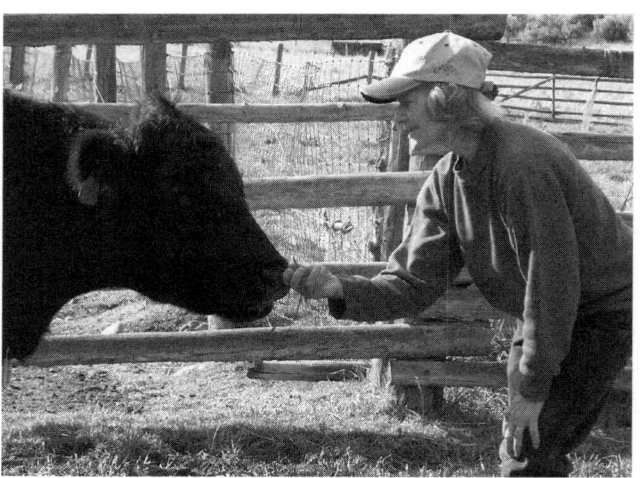

Why not learn all we can about proper care during calving time? Learning about the animals is part of why we raise cattle (or any other livestock) — and making a living raising cattle is quite achievable if you learn to take care of them properly and minimize losses.

This book will be helpful whether you have a family milk cow, only a few cows, or a big herd of beef cows. In these pages, you can look up whatever you need to know about a calving problem or a critical situation with a newborn calf. If you're a small producer, you may never encounter a set of twins, a breech presentation, or a calf born prematurely — or you might have to handle these challenging births tomorrow. Knowing about some of the situations that may occur and having a good idea about what will be done in the event of difficulties will give you more confidence and an ability to determine whether the problem is something you can handle yourself or one for your veterinarian.

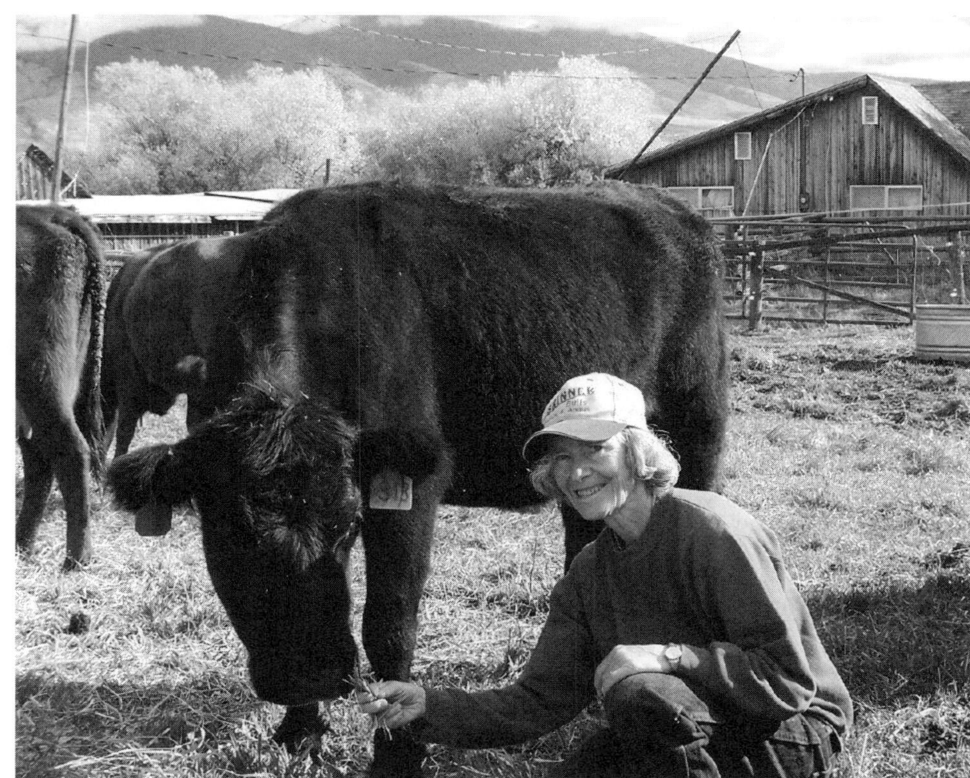

Heather Smith Thomas and Buffalo Girl — one of the young cows in the Thomas herd.

The small farmer with a few cows and the family with one milk cow have one advantage over a rancher with a large herd: frequent cow handling opportunities. Rather than being wild, these animals are manageable and are often pets. This can make it easier to diagnose, check, or treat a problem.

On our ranch, my husband and I have dealt with thousands of births over the years and have been fanatical about saving every calf, regardless of the circumstances. The small farmer doesn't have the opportunity to experience all the possible calf-birthing challenges of a rancher, but he or she still needs to know how to handle all kinds of situations. There isn't always time to call a vet and still end up with a live calf. In a calving emergency, very often the future health of a calf (or cow) will be in your hands. This book is a resource that helps you know the right questions to ask your veterinarian. But more importantly, perhaps, it is a guide that provides diagrams and information that will help prepare you to plunge in and do what needs to be done — at least until the vet arrives. It is a tool that enables the livestock breeder to become a more proficient bovine midwife and caretaker. While there is no substitute for hands-on experience, this book can give you an excellent starting point.

No matter what your livestock situation, it's important to remember that calving, calfhood care, and aftercare of a cow that has given birth are not mysterious. Although your vet can help with problems that arise and can manage difficult situations, it's also quite possible that you, the livestock raiser, can address many of these issues and unexpected events skillfully. This book tells you how.

Acknowledgments

Most of the information in this book comes from decades of experience raising cattle — calving them and caring for them in health and illness. My husband and I continue to learn all we can about taking the best care of our cows and calves. This education has included advice and help from a number of veterinarians over the years with regard to calving problems and treating sick calves, and I wish to thank them — especially Dr. Peter J. South, Dr. Ron Skinner, Dr. Dick Rath, "Doc" Hatfield, Dr. Robert Cope, Dr. Jeff Hoffmann, and Dr. Todd Tibbitts.

I also want to thank the many people I have interviewed for articles on cattle reproduction/calving/calf health for various ranch and livestock publications. Their input has also added to my education: Bruce Anderson, DVM, PhD (Caine Veterinary Teaching and Research Center, University of Idaho, Caldwell); Louis Archbald, DVM, PhD (University of Florida); Tom Besser, DVM, PhD (veterinary bacteriologist, Washington State University); George Barrington, DVM (Washington State University); Keith Bramwell (University of Idaho Extension); Ellen Belknap, DVM (Auburn University); Anthony Blikslager, DVM, PhD (North Carolina State University); Marie Bulgin, DVM (Caine Veterinary Teaching and Research Center, University of Idaho, Caldwell); Stuart Burns, DVM (private practice, Paris, Kentucky); Dr. Peter Chenoweth (Kansas State University); Dr. Glenn Coulter (Lethbridge Research Centre, Alberta, Canada); Dr. Joe Diedrickson; Bob Douglas, PhD (BET Reproductive Laboratories, Lexington, Kentucky); Ed Duran (Idaho State University Extension animal scientist); Clive Gay, DVM (Washington State University); Mike Gaylean, DVM (Department of Animal Science, Texas Tech University); Don Hansen, DVM (Oregon State University Extension veterinarian); Dr. Elaine Hunt (North Carolina State University, College of Veterinary Medicine); Ray Kaplan, DVM, PhD (University of Georgia veterinary parasitologist); John Kastelic, DVM, PhD (Lethbridge Research Centre, Alberta, Canada, reproductive physiologist); Dennis Maxwell (McNay Research Farm, Iowa State University); Duane McCartney (Agriculture and Agri-Food Canada Research Station, Lacombe, Alberta); Duane Mickelson, DVM (Washington State University); Bob Mortimer, DVM (Colorado State University); Geoff Smith, DVM, PhD (North Carolina State University, College of Veterinary Medicine); Don Spiers, PhD (University of Missouri, Department of Animal Science); Patricia Talcott, DVM (Idaho State University); Gary Williams, DVM, PhD (Texas A&M University, reproductive physiologist); Milo Wiltbank, PhD (University of Wisconsin); and Curtis Youngs, PhD (Iowa State University).

There have also been a number of veterinary textbooks that have been useful to us over the years, including *Veterinary Medicine: A Textbook of the Diseases of Cattle, Sheep, Pigs, Goats and Horses,* 7th ed., by D. C. Blood and O. M. Radostits (London: Bailliere Tindall, 1989); *Veterinary Medicine*, 9th ed., by O. M. Radostits, et al. (New York: Elsevier Saunders, 2000); *Veterinary Obstetrics and Genital Diseases*, 2nd ed., by Stephen J. Roberts (Ithaca, NY: published by author, 1971); *Veterinary Reproduction and Obstetrics,* 4th ed., by Geoffrey H. Arthur (London: Bailliere Tindall, 1975); and *Arthur's Veterinary Reproduction and Obstetrics,* 8th ed., by David E. Noakes, et al. (Philadelphia: Saunders, 2001).

Introduction

Some of us are destined to be nurturers of life. We express and perform this basic role in many different ways. Some people become nurses or doctors or veterinarians; others grow crops or beautiful gardens or flowers or livestock. I became a cow mother, a bovine midwife.

As a small child, I loved animals and felt my dreams had come true when we moved to a ranch and I had a horse of my own and my father's cattle to help care for. But keeping animals alive and healthy is sometimes a challenge; it takes a great deal of commitment to care for them properly and always do your best for them.

Looking back at my growing-up years, I realize I made a lifelong commitment very early on that resulted not only from the joys of working with animals but also from the frustration and anguish when things didn't go right. I'll never forget the time my young foal slipped into a coma after a serious injury and died in my arms, or the time I sat helplessly beside a little calf we had treated for diarrhea and pneumonia but could not save. I suppose it was then that I vowed to become an animal caretaker, a nurse who would try to relieve their pain and keep them alive and healthy.

Since then, I have grown up, married, and brought up two children, and my husband and I have raised a lot of cattle. For us, ranching is a way of life, not just an occupation. It makes demands upon us and requires commitment beyond any nine-to-five job. Calving time was, for many years, a hectic season that demanded a 24-hour-a-day effort. Because our cows had to be bred in April, before they went to summer range, we calved in January, when the weather was bitterly cold and the cows needed very close observation and assistance. Yet it was, and always will be, my favorite time of year. The miracle of birth and new life never grows old.

I remain enthusiastic even when I've been up all night shuttling cows into the barn to calve; or I'm up to my armpits inside a heifer helping to correct a malpresented calf or pull a calf too large to be born easily; or I'm spattered in cow manure, drenched in amniotic fluids, and kicked and stomped by an uncooperative mama-cow-to-be. Somehow, it all becomes worthwhile and very satisfying as I sit back afterward and watch the results.

It's very rewarding to see a wet and shivering and very-much-alive new baby calf, which might not have survived without my efforts, looking around bright-eyed and wondering. Meanwhile, the new mother gives a few tentative licks and then wholeheartedly plunges into motherhood, mooing and talking to the calf and shaking her head at me protectively, as if to say, "Stay away now. He's mine."

Calving time was, for many years, a hectic season that demanded a 24-hour-a-day effort. Yet it was, and always will be, my favorite time of year. The miracle of birth and new life never grows old.

I remember my first difficult calf birth as if it were yesterday, even though I was very young at the time. My parents were gone one evening, attending a meeting downtown. I was alone at the ranch. We had a young heifer that was due to calve, and after dark, I went down to the corral to check on her. She was in hard labor, lying flat on her side, straining and groaning. The amnion sac had appeared with two little hooves in it, but the heifer made no progress. I sat beside her, watching her labor, agonizing and suffering with her, the pale moonlight glistening on the amnion sac as the little feet tentatively entered the world but could come no farther.

I realized she needed help, so I ran to the house and tried, without luck, to phone my parents. I hurried back down to the corral by the creek and sat by the heifer awhile but didn't know how to help her. Finally, in desperation I ran back to the house and phoned a neighboring rancher. I was very young and shy, so it took a lot of courage to ask him to help —

but the heifer's plight made me brave. The rancher came and helped me pull the calf. That baby survived because of the intervention of a timid child. I was so proud and happy; I felt as though I was a fairy godmother to that calf.

I suppose that night decisively set the course of my life. I knew what I wanted to do. I was destined to become a cow midwife.

This book is the culmination of 50 years of interaction with calving cows and their babies and the quest for ways to handle the various problems that arose. Our local veterinarians helped my husband and me in that quest by assisting us in difficult situations and teaching us many things about bovine obstetrics, reproduction, and calf health care. I've also been able to interview dozens of veterinarians and professors at universities over the years while writing articles for livestock publications on various aspects of cattle care and reproduction.

This calving handbook is an attempt to put practical and essential information into simple terms for those who raise cattle. In it I use some examples from our own herd to help make this information real. Part 1 deals with pregnancy and calving. Part 2 discusses care of the recently calved cow and her newborn calf. Part 3 gives advice on the handling of situations and problems you might encounter during a calf's first weeks or months of life.

It is my hope that these chapters will be much easier to read than any veterinary textbook, yet will be of value to anyone who wants to learn more about the miracle of calving and what to do to prevent or resolve some of the problems that might come along. If you have only a few cows, you may never experience some of the problems described in this book. But if or when you encounter something you've never seen before, the chapters here can be a handy reference to find out more about a challenging or mystifying problem. Knowing more about these situations may also help you determine what you can handle by yourself and when you need to call a vet.

Every difficult case can be a valuable learning experience. It's my hope that this book will be a guide along the way.

PART 1

Pregnancy and Calving

Chapter 1

How It All Begins

The Cows and the Bulls

CALVING IS THE END PHASE OF A MIRACLE that begins nine months earlier, when a *cow* (a bovine female that has had a calf) or *heifer* (a young female bovine before she has a calf) is bred and conceives and starts the pregnancy. A good stockman must know the basics of bovine reproduction to ensure that all the cows and heifers in the herd become pregnant and have a safe pregnancy. This means you must become familiar with some of the more technical aspects of reproduction.

Reproductive-Tract Anatomy and Function

Understanding the basic workings of the cow's reproductive tract is helpful, especially if you use artificial insemination (AI). But even if your cows are bred by a bull, knowledge of the reproductive tract is essential for a better understanding of calving and any problems associated with it.

The cow's reproductive tract includes the *vagina,* which leads from the external opening (the *vulva*), through the *pelvis* to the *cervix,* which serves as a doorway into the *uterus* and the *uterine horns.* Each uterine horn tapers to a tiny tube (the *oviduct*) that leads to an *ovary,* an oval-shaped organ 1 to 1½ inches (2.5 to 3.8 cm) long. The ovaries produce eggs that have the potential to be fertilized and become calves. The ovaries also produce hormones, primarily estrogen and progesterone, that play an important role in reproduction.

The vagina (or *birth canal*) is the passageway between the uterus and the vulva. During mating, the bull deposits *semen* or *seminal fluid,* a secretion containing sperm, via the penis into the vagina, near the cervix. These sperm travel directly through the cervix into the uterus. When a cow is bred by *artificial insemination* (*AI*), semen is deposited (using a long *pipette*) directly through the open cervix.

The cow's urinary bladder is situated beneath the vagina, which is used not only for reproduction but for ridding the cow's body of urine as well. The

How the Tract Works

The ovary's eggs travel through the oviduct to the uterus, which is divided into two horns that are joined for a short distance in the body of the uterus.

The cervix, between the body of the uterus and the vagina, has thick walls and a small opening with overlapping folds. During pregnancy, the opening is filled with a thick plug of mucus that seals the uterus and protects it from contamination. The rings that usually keep the cervix tightly closed relax during estrus and during calving; the opening enlarges to allow passage of sperm into the uterus when the cow is bred and during labor at the end of pregnancy to allow passage of the calf.

REPRODUCTIVE TRACT OF THE COW

When planning to breed your cattle and assist cows, heifers, and their calves in the birthing process, it's a good idea to familiarize yourself with the life-giving reproductive system involved.

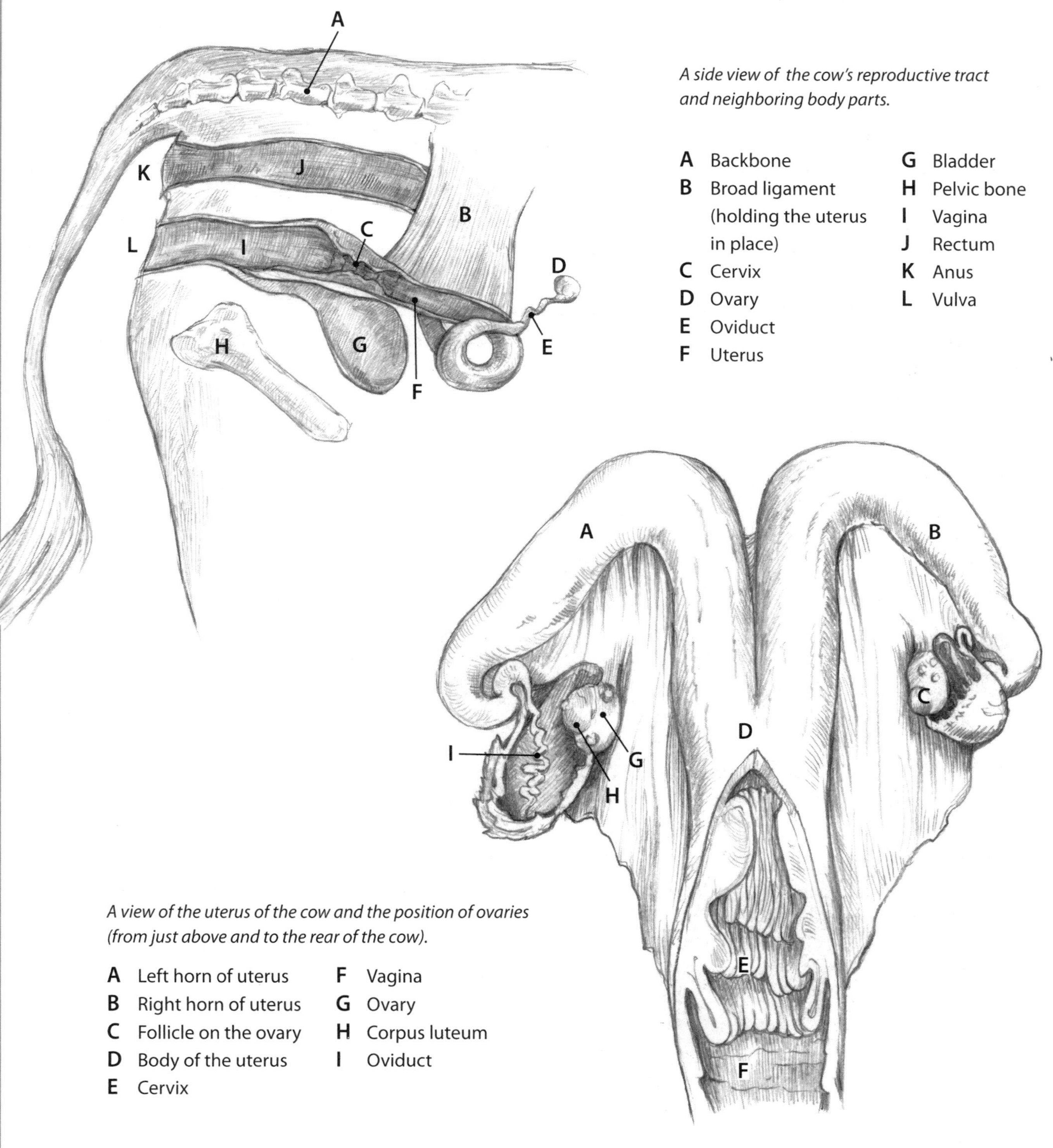

A side view of the cow's reproductive tract and neighboring body parts.

- **A** Backbone
- **B** Broad ligament (holding the uterus in place)
- **C** Cervix
- **D** Ovary
- **E** Oviduct
- **F** Uterus
- **G** Bladder
- **H** Pelvic bone
- **I** Vagina
- **J** Rectum
- **K** Anus
- **L** Vulva

A view of the uterus of the cow and the position of ovaries (from just above and to the rear of the cow).

- **A** Left horn of uterus
- **B** Right horn of uterus
- **C** Follicle on the ovary
- **D** Body of the uterus
- **E** Cervix
- **F** Vagina
- **G** Ovary
- **H** Corpus luteum
- **I** Oviduct

urethra also empties the bladder into the portion of the vagina nearest the vulva — a part that's restricted in diameter by sphincter muscles near the urethral opening. When the cow urinates, she squats with her back arched and empties the bladder; urine rushes directly out of the rear portion of the vagina through the vulva.

The Estrous Cycle

A cow's ovaries emit eggs in a cyclic process called the *estrous cycle,* which, with its characteristic length and sequence of events, enables the cow to be bred at a certain time and to conceive.

A cow's ovary contains thousands of tiny *follicles,* each of which holds a *germ cell* that contains half the chromosomes a calf requires (the other half is supplied by the bull's sperm). Each of these germ cells has the potential to mature and become an egg if that follicle completes its development. Most of these cells never develop, however, and are absorbed by the ovary, usurped by the follicles that do develop and enlarge.

Follicles that enlarge go through a series of phases in which more layers of cells are added to the single layer surrounding the egg. This creates a cavity in the center of the follicle. Secretion of *estrogen* in the developing follicle causes it to enlarge further and produce the mature egg. Estrogen is also the hormone that brings the cow into *heat* — the period of time in which she is receptive to a bull. When the follicle matures, the side opposite the egg bulges and becomes thin. During *ovulation,* this thin part ruptures to release the egg, which then moves into the oviduct.

After ovulation, cells in the follicle that has just erupted change to create the *corpus luteum* (*CL*), which starts producing *progesterone.* This hormone suppresses further development of estrogen and follicles. Progesterone levels rise as the cow shows signs of heat. A high level of progesterone is necessary to prepare the uterus to receive a fertilized egg and maintain a proper environment for pregnancy.

If the egg that was released is fertilized and eventually attaches to the uterine lining, it then sends a message to the ovary signaling the ovary to retain the CL it has produced and create more. This high level of progesterone ensures that the pregnancy will continue. If the egg is not fertilized and therefore does not attach to the uterine lining, this message is never sent and the CL on the ovary soon recedes. As a result, this allows a new crop of follicles to start growing and producing estrogen and maturing their eggs. As before, one of the follicles eventually creates enough estrogen to bring the cow back into heat — giving her another chance to become pregnant if she's bred.

Twins

Usually just one follicle in the ovary becomes dominant and enlarges enough to ovulate, and as a result just one egg is released after each heat period. Sometimes, though (in about 13 percent of cows), twin ovulations take place, though not all resulting pregnancies are carried to term. Twins occur in 1 to 7 percent of all births. About 94 percent of these are fraternal twins (that is, from two eggs that erupt and are fertilized at the same time) and 6 percent are identical twins (two embryos form from a single fertilized egg). Triplets are rare, occurring once in every 7,500 births.

Some herds have a higher or lower incidence of twins, depending on the cows' breed and family lines. Twinning is hereditary, and some families of cows have a much higher rate of twinning than the average.

Fertilization

When a mature egg is released during ovulation, it enters the funnel-shaped opening of the oviduct, which carries it to the uterus. Since ovulation takes place about 12 hours after a cow goes out of heat, there should be sperm waiting for the egg if the cow was bred during her heat period. The sperm enter the uterus through the cervix (which opens when the cow is in heat) and swim through the uterus into each of its horns — traveling toward the oviducts at the same time the mature egg enters an oviduct. On occasion, both ovaries release eggs, resulting in an egg in each oviduct and the possibility of twins.

An egg remains viable for only a few hours, so it's important that sperm have been introduced in the cow and are ready and waiting before ovulation. Sperm swim up the oviduct to meet the egg as it starts its journey down this tube. If the egg is fertilized, it becomes a *conceptus* and continues traveling down the oviduct toward the uterus, which it reaches within the next three or four days. If the egg is not fertilized, it dies along the way and degenerates.

The Role of Hormones

Normal reproduction depends on the interaction of several *hormones,* chemical substances produced by the cow that regulate certain organ functions. Estrogen and progesterone are produced in the ovaries and play major roles in reproduction. These hormones work as a team. Estrogen brings the cow into heat and prepares the reproductive tract for receiving the sperm, and progesterone calms things down and creates the environment for a steady, stable pregnancy or the interlude between heat periods if the cow does not become pregnant. Development of the *udder* also depends on both hormones. Estrogen stimulates the growth of milk ducts and progesterone triggers development of clusters of tiny milk-secreting glands on the ducts.

A QUIRK OF HORMONES

IT'S AMAZING what the influence of hormones can do to cows. About 20 years ago we had a yearling heifer named Tevya who suddenly thought she was a mother after being bred. The act of breeding may have triggered production of extra hormones, which affected the behavior of this heifer, just as the manual stimulation of the birth canal can sometimes make a cow think she's had a calf. Tevya took quite a shine to one of the calves in her pasture. She "adopted" him and followed him around, mooing at him, licking him, and loving him. When the cattle went to the open range later that spring, Tevya stayed with that calf and his real mother all summer, and she worried over him and babied him from sunup to sundown, just as if he were her own.

Estrogen

The hormone estrogen is created in the ovaries by maturing follicles. It regulates development and functioning of the reproductive tract and initial development of the uterus. Estrogen triggers the onset of heat or estrus, the period in which the cow is receptive to breeding; plays a role in the growth of the animal and where fat is deposited in the body; and prepares and triggers onset of sexual activity in the young heifer or in a cow by bringing on her first heat cycle after calving.

Progesterone

Progesterone is the predominant hormone between heat cycles and during pregnancy. It is responsible for, and necessary to, the continuation of pregnancy once the embryo establishes itself in the uterus, because it suppresses further development of follicles in the ovaries and thwarts production of estrogen. Progesterone levels rise while the cow is still in heat, because this hormone is crucial for preparing the uterus to receive a fertilized egg and provide an environment in which the egg can grow. Once pregnancy is established, high levels of progesterone are necessary to make sure there are no changes in the uterus that might terminate pregnancy. Progesterone also keeps the cow from coming back into heat after she has been impregnated.

Other Hormones

There are other hormones necessary in the pregnancy of a cow. The *pituitary gland,* in the cow's brain, produces *follicle stimulating hormone* (*FSH*) and *luteinizing hormone* (*LH*), which directly influence production of the main ovarian hormones. FSH triggers the growth, development, and function of the follicle in the ovary, which creates estrogen, and LH causes the follicle to rupture (ovulation) and subsequently causes the development of the CL.

Several other hormones play a significant role in regulating the cow's reproductive system. *Prostaglandins* secreted by the uterus affect the estrous cycle by causing the CL to regress so that follicles can develop and create the estrogen necessary to trigger a new heat cycle. If an embryo has attached to the uterine wall, however, it sends a signal to the uterus that the cow or heifer is pregnant and to prevent prostaglandin release. Without prostaglandins, the CL remains in place on the ovary, where it continues to produce progesterone and keeps the cow from coming back into heat. This protects the pregnancy from the contractions and secretions of the uterus during heat, which aid passage of sperm but are dangerous to a developing embryo.

Some of these hormones are produced commercially and are useful in manipulating heat cycles in cattle. For instance, they may be used for heat synchronization in a group of cows or heifers to get them all bred at about the same time by AI.

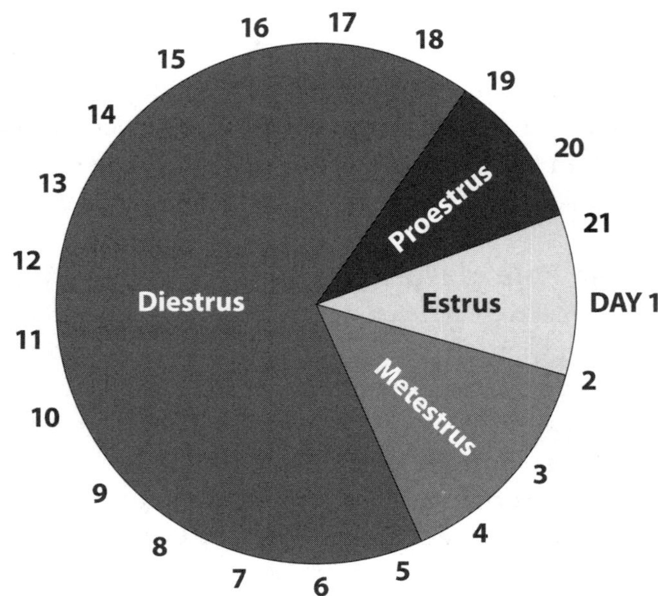

The stages of an estrous cycle in cattle.

The Estrous Cycle in Greater Depth

The estrous cycle in cows consists of a series of events that recur in definite order. A complete cycle averages 20 days in heifers and 21 days in cows, ranging from 17 to 24 days from the start of one heat period to the start of the next, if the cow doesn't become pregnant. During the last part of the cycle, the reproductive tract prepares for the next estrus and ovulation.

Stages of the Estrous Cycle

The estrous cycle can be broken into four stages: *proestrus, estrus, metestrus,* and *diestrus* (see chart, page 6).

1. ***Proestrus.*** The follicles attain final growth and secrete estrogen, which causes the cow to come into *standing heat* (estrus).
2. ***Estrus.*** Also known as heat — the period of time in which the cow is receptive to breeding with a bull.
3. ***Metestrus.*** About 12 hours after the end of standing heat, ovulation occurs, and the CL forms and secretes progesterone.
4. ***Diestrus.*** The CL continues to secrete progesterone. If the cow does not become pregnant, the CL regresses at the end of diestrus and the cycle begins again.

SYNCHRONIZING ESTRUS

Under normal circumstances, about 5 percent of the cow herd will be in heat on any given day during breeding season. Breeding by AI requires observing the cows for heat several times a day for three to four weeks, and daily work for the person inseminating the cows. Heat cycles in a group can be manipulated, however, with the use of hormones, so they all come into heat about the same time. Heat detection and insemination can be diligently done for just three or four days instead of a whole month. Commercial hormone products, such as Prostaglandin, can be given to all the females to regulate the cycle.

Daily Cycling through Estrus

In general, the following timetable is accurate for most cows. Keep in mind, however, that these time frames are averages; some cows have a slightly longer or shorter sequence of events. If the cow is bred and *settles* (becomes impregnated), the CL that forms in the ovaries when she goes out of heat will persist and keep the cow from coming back into heat.

Day 0 — standing heat

This results from increased levels of estrogen produced by a maturing follicle. Secretions from the reproductive tract act as a lubricant for breeding and aid the travel of sperm through the uterus. At the end of this period, which usually lasts from 12 to 24 hours, the mature follicle ruptures and ovulates in response to a surge of luteinizing hormone (LH) from the pituitary gland. Ovulation usually takes place 12 hours after the cow goes out of heat.

Days 1 and 2 — alteration of cells that line the follicle

These cells change and create the CL in the area where ovulation occurred.

Days 2 to 5 — growth of the CL

The growing CL produces high levels of progesterone, which causes the regression of any other follicles that were maturing. During the early part of this phase, a portion of the lining over the *caruncles* (small protuberances on the uterus upon which the placenta attaches during pregnancy) becomes engorged with blood, and bleeding from the smaller capillaries may occur. This postestrual bleeding, caused by withdrawal of estrogen, may create a hint of bloody discharge by day 2 or 3 after the cow or heifer goes out of heat. If you didn't see her in heat, this is evidence that she was in heat a few days earlier.

Days 5 to 16 — continued development of the CL

The CL usually reaches its maximum growth and production of progesterone by day 15 or 16. Called diestrus ("between estrus"), this is the longest phase of the estrous cycle. Progesterone secreted by the CL blocks any LH release from the pituitary, so the ovaries are relatively inactive. No follicles can mature or ovulate. The cervix is tightly closed, and there are no secretions from the reproductive tract.

Days 16 to 18 — follicles on the ovaries begin growing again

The resulting estrogen secretion stimulates the uterus to secrete prostaglandins, which cause rapid regression of the CL.

Days 18 and 19 — the CL becomes nonfunctional

As a consequence, very little progesterone is released, so progesterone and other hormones perform no more blocking action. Several follicles on the ovaries grow and one becomes dominant, secreting increasing amounts of estrogen.

Days 19 and 20 — heat again

This results from an increase in estrogen and the corresponding decrease in progesterone. The cycle has now returned to day 0.

Behavioral Signs of Heat

There are several behavioral signs of estrus. These are often more pronounced in heifers than in cows.

As the cow or heifer comes into heat:

- She may be restless and bawling.
- She wanders in search of a male, sniffing other cattle.
- She may do three or four times as much traveling as she does on a day when she's not in heat.
- She may sniff the vulva of other cows, or they may sniff her vulva, sensing that she somehow smells different.
- She may interact more with herd mates, licking them or fighting with them. If there are several cows in heat, they will gather together and ride each other or a bull. Cows coming into heat or going out of heat all will be part of the group engaging in mounting or fighting activity.
- She may start to ride other cattle and stand for them to mount her. She may put her chin on the back or rump of another cow to test whether that cow will stand to be mounted. If the cow to be mounted is also in heat, she will stand still; if not, she will move away or turn around to *bunt* the mounting cow with her head.
- During early heat, a cow will usually stand and let another cow or heifer mount her before she'll stand for the bull, and she'll also try to mount the bull before she'll stand still for him to breed her. The bull will often rest his chin on the cow's rump or loin area to test whether she will stand before he tries to mount her.

NO DOUBT ABOUT IT

In a group of cattle, a cow in heat is very obvious in her actions and mounting activity. In large pastures or range conditions, this behavior can be seen from a distance and will attract a bull.

Cows or heifers in heat spend most of their time in these activities and spend less time eating or lying down, chewing the cud. Milk production drops temporarily. In dairy cows this sudden drop in milk is a clue that a cow is coming into heat. In beef cattle there is also less milk production in a cow in heat, but she may have a full udder due to her calf not having a chance to nurse because of all the disruptions; his mother may not stand still long enough for him to nurse while she is interacting with other cattle.

The duration of standing heat varies among individuals, ranging from 6 to 24 hours (12 to 16 hours is average), and may also vary from one heat cycle to the next.

As a cow goes out of heat, for a few hours she may continue to stand for other cows to mount her but will no longer accept the bull.

As a cow goes out of heat, for a few hours she may continue to stand for other cows to mount her but will no longer accept the bull.

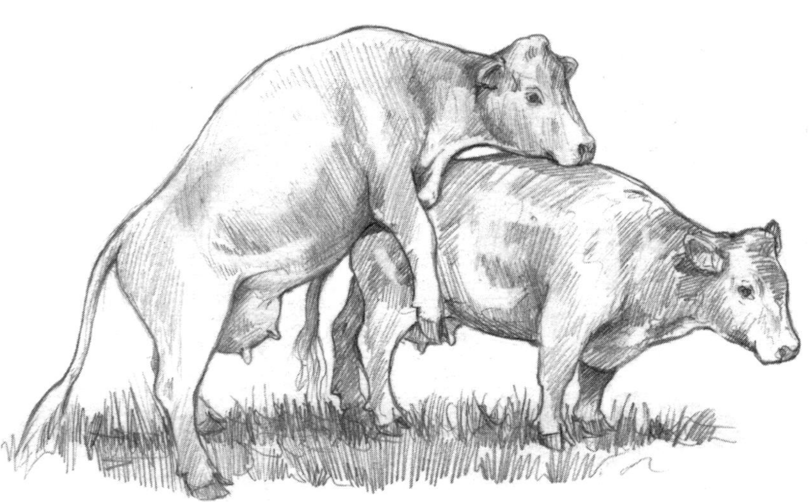

A cow in heat will usually stand still and let other cows mount her.

Physical Signs of Heat

The following are some of the physical signs of heat:

- A cow in heat secretes *mucus* from glands in the uterus, cervix, and vagina to allow the sperm to swim to the oviducts.
- The cervix is relaxed and open, to enable sperm from the bull to enter the uterus.
- There may be discharge from the vulva, a transparent mucus that has the consistency of egg white and is so viscous that it holds together in a long string. This mucus may be smeared over the cow's buttocks and flanks from tail swishing.
- The cow's tail may be slightly raised and her vulva may be a bit enlarged (swollen) and reddened.
- If the cow is with other cattle, she will usually have a ruffling of hair over her tailhead and hip bones from mounting activity.
- The evidence of heat, visible for a few hours or days afterward, may include mud on the cow's hips and flanks from the feet of animals that mounted her, or in spring, when the cow is shedding, the hair will be rubbed off over her tailhead and hip bones by other mounting cattle. In some cases there are abrasions and raw areas on her hips or tailhead if she was mounted frequently, especially if there's more than one bull in the herd and the bulls competed for her.
- If the cow was actually bred, she will hold her tail out afterward for several hours or days because of vaginal irritation. Many cows will hold their tails out for 24 hours or more after being bred, especially if they're bred repeatedly and the vagina is quite irritated. Even after the cow no longer holds her tail out, it may kink out a bit when she travels, especially if she trots. The "tail out" position is a sure sign that a cow has been bred, even if the actual breeding was not observed.

- The bull makes a leap and a thrust when he ejaculates. Sometimes he will mount and enter the cow but not ejaculate, especially if he's tired. This won't cause much irritation and the cow won't become pregnant.
- The thrusting of the bull during breeding and irritation of the vagina will cause her to stand with her back arched, straining as soon as he dismounts. A small yearling bull may not irritate her vagina as much as a larger bull, but she will still stand with her back arched briefly after being bred.
- There may be discharge of the bull's seminal fluid from the cow's vulva. There also may be a whitish yellow discharge from a cow's vulva a day or two after she's been bred. Though it may look like pus, it's usually nothing to worry about unless the cow has a uterine infection (see chapter 6). Typically, the uterus efficiently will clean out the extra debris from breeding (seminal fluid, dead sperm, etc.), flushing it out while the newly created conceptus, the fertilized egg, is safe in the oviduct.
- There may be a bright red, bloody tinge to otherwise clear mucous discharge about 48 hours after a cow has gone out of heat (see Days 2 to 5 in the estrous cycle, on page 9). This bloody discharge is observed more often in heifers that were recently in heat than in cows and can be seen even if the female was not bred. If you notice this discharge, you can make a good estimate that the cow will be back in heat again in 17 to 19 days.

Short Estrous Cycles

Though a cow usually returns to heat 18 to 24 days after her last heat, if she's not bred and settled, short estrous cycles sometimes occur in which she returns to heat 7 to 12 days after her last heat. This may be caused by a nonfunctional CL or by a CL that doesn't form after ovulation or that died prematurely, and by progesterone levels that remain too low to keep the cow from coming back into heat.

Heat Is Hard on a Calf

The hours when a calf's mother is in heat can be stressful for the young animal. He tries to travel with her during the mounting and chasing activity but is often bunted away by other cows or the bull. If the weather is hot, cold, or stormy, this exertion and stress make the calf susceptible to illness.

He's also vulnerable to digestive upset because he may not be able to nurse for much of the day if other cattle involved in mating activities shove him away from Mama. Sometimes the milk tastes different while she is in heat and the calf may not want to drink it. After the heat has passed, when the calf is hungry he will load up on milk, which can lead to problems. Indeed, any time a calf skips a meal and then overloads on milk, he is at risk for enterotoxemia (see chapter 11).

Short cycles are common, especially when a cow starts cycling again after calving. Her first heat after calving, usually a few weeks to two months after calving, may be followed by another just 7 to 12 days later. Immediately after calving, follicles in the cow's ovaries begin to grow again but may take longer to ovulate because she is nursing a calf. It takes a while for the cycle to normalize after calving, though if a cow loses her calf and dries up her milk, she'll return to heat sooner.

Short estrous cycles are common, especially when a cow starts cycling again after calving.

Even if a cow comes into heat soon after calving, you don't want her bred that early; the uterus is not yet ready for another pregnancy. Complete *involution* (shrinking back to normal size) of the uterus takes some time. Wait at least 45 days before rebreeding the cow.

False Pregnancy

On rare occasions the CL does not regress even though the cow has not become pregnant. It continues to secrete progesterone, and the cow does not return to heat — and you might assume she is pregnant. In other instances the cow develops a cystic ovary and does not show heat. In these cases, you might also assume she is pregnant, unless she's checked by a veterinarian to determine her true status.

Anestrus

This term means "no estrus" and refers to a period in which the cow does not cycle. Most cows experience *anestrus* after calving — when it may last from three weeks to three months, depending on the cow's age and nutritional factors — because the uterus and reproductive tract need time to recover fully from calving. In some instances, however, cows ovulate 14 to 16 days after calving.

If the cow is milking heavily or is underfed, a period of anestrus may last longer. As a rule, young cows that have had their first calves and are nursing calves generally take longer than older cows to return to estrus after calving. A two-year-old cow is under more nutritional stress than an older cow because she's still growing herself as well as trying to feed her calf.

Does Estrus Always Follow Ovulation?

A cow in *anovulatory heat* (heat without ovulation) may be in standing heat and may allow a bull to breed her, but she will not become pregnant. The opposite situation can also occur: A cow may ovulate but show no signs of heat, and a bull will not mount her. This is often called *silent heat* or *quiet heat* and is not uncommon during the first weeks after calving. Many cows have a silent heat during the first and second ovulation after calving.

In domestic cows, the period after calving is generally the only time anestrus occurs. Healthy, well-fed cows will cycle year-round otherwise and can usually be bred any time of year. They are not seasonal breeders, like mares and ewes.

If the cow is milking heavily or is underfed, a period of anestrus may last longer.

Heat Cycles after a Cow Becomes Pregnant

On rare occasions a cow may experience one or two heat cycles after becoming pregnant. Coming into heat after becoming pregnant or being rebred may or may not cause her to lose the pregnancy. This is why a breeding date may not correspond with her calving date; she may have become pregnant during an earlier breeding and will calve ahead of when you expect.

Sexual Maturity in the Heifer

At birth each individual ovary in a heifer calf may contain as many as 150,000 tiny follicles, each consisting of an *oocyte* (egg cell) surrounded by a layer of *epithelial* cells (covering cells). Soon after the cow is born, the ovaries start to develop and the follicles begin to grow.

In domestic cattle, *puberty,* the time of development of reproductive capabilities, followed directly by *fertile* heat cycles, often occurs before the heifer is physically mature enough to become a mother. Puberty may occur in a heifer anywhere from 5 to 18 months of age, with 10 months being average, depending on the breed and individual and her nutritional status. A well-fed, fast-growing heifer calf of an early-maturing breed may start having heat cycles before she is weaned off her mother and may reach puberty at five to eight months of age. This is a good reason to remove bulls from the herd after breeding season is over, rather than leave them with the cows all year. Even bull calves have been known to impregnate young heifers before the heifers' weaning time.

TOO YOUNG TO BE A MOTHER

OUR FIRST EXPERIENCE with early-onset puberty happened when, unbeknownst to us, Prue's seven-month-old calf Prunella was bred. Prue was a pet, born with a cleft palate and raised on a nipple bucket because she couldn't nurse on her mama. She never went to the range with the other cows in summer, but instead stayed home with our milk cow, Liza.

That summer a bull of ours broke his foot. After he recovered enough to start walking again, we turned him out on pasture with Prue and Liza because we didn't want him to be knocked around by the other bulls while he was healing. Our bulls were in a confinement pasture by then, since our breeding season was over. We didn't worry about Prue or Liza because they were already bred, and we didn't worry at all about Prue's calf, Prunella. She was big for her age, having a mama who milked well and plenty of good, green pasture.

Though she got pregnant by our injured bull, she was too immature to calve successfully the next May, and her calf had to be delivered by cesarean section (see chapter 5). We raised the calf on a bottle because Prunella didn't mother him.

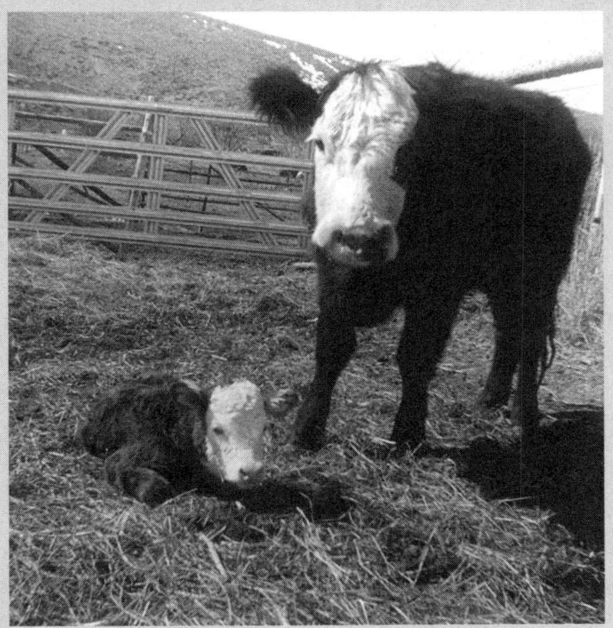

In this old photo, Prunella is just a few hours old and has been licked dry by Prue, her mama. Prunella was bred at seven months by our injured bull and had to have her baby delivered by c-section.

The first heat cycles of a maturing heifer may not be obvious. Some heifers have silent heat, which a bull won't recognize and during which they aren't sexually receptive. A small percentage of heifers show heat but do not ovulate; these allow other heifers to ride them, and they may stand to be mounted and bred, but they do not become pregnant. In other words, a heifer's first heat cycles may not be fertile.

The age at which a heifer shows heat depends on the breed (smaller, earlier-maturing cattle tend to show heat several months sooner than cattle of larger breeds that grow for a longer period of time), her season of birth, nutrition, and health (an animal stunted by illness may take longer to reach puberty). Well-fed heifers grow faster and reach mature weight sooner than do thin heifers. Body size, rather than age, is the main factor that triggers puberty in a heifer. Most stockmen feed heifers well enough so that the heifers will reach 65 to 70 percent of mature weight a month before breeding season. This ensures that they'll have fertile heat cycles.

A well-fed, fast-growing heifer calf of an early-maturing breed may start having heat cycles before she is weaned off her mother and may reach puberty at five to eight months of age. This is a good reason to remove bulls from the herd after breeding season is over, rather than leave them with the cows all year.

Factors That Affect Fertility in the Cow

There are a number of factors that may hinder or prevent reproduction. Some are herd problems (infectious diseases spread through the herd from animal to animal or from wildlife to cattle) and others are problems specific to an individual cow or heifer.

Physical Abnormalities of the Reproductive Tract

On rare occasions, a heifer has an abnormality — such as small, inactive ovaries or an improperly formed vagina, cervix, or uterus — that interferes with normal reproductive ability. Other abnormalities that may occur are a lack of continuation between uterus and vagina caused by an obstruction or a *blind tube vagina* (where the vagina is not connected to the uterus) and an absence of one of the uterine horns.

If the ovaries are normal, the affected heifer may have regular heat cycles but cannot become pregnant. On occasion, uterine secretions collect in the segmented uterus and cause the uterus to become so large that it could be mistaken for an early pregnancy if the heifer is examined rectally.

A common abnormality is a *persistent hymen,* which creates constriction of the vagina. This may consist of a tight ring of tissue just inside the vulva or a complete partition between vulva and vagina. If the persistent hymen is caused by a constricting ring, the heifer can be bred but will need help during calving (see chapter 3). A complete blockage, however, will interfere with reproduction and will result in fluid buildup in the vagina.

A cow may develop a tumor on the ovary that interferes with proper hormone production. Some types of tumors secrete estrogen, causing the cow to appear to be in heat all the time, whereas other tumors secrete masculine hormones, which result in the cow's not coming into heat at all. Tumors can generally be detected by your veterinarian. Some tumors can be treated or removed, while others cannot, and the cow must be sold or butchered.

Some abnormalities of the genital tract occur following a difficult birth or a cesarean-section birth. A difficult birth may cause inflammation of the cervix or vagina due to injury or adhesions. Following a cow's surgery, part of the uterus may adhere to an adjacent stomach or to the intestines or abdominal wall. These problems usually prevent conception, and the cow will not have any more calves.

Freemartins

A heifer that was born twin to a bull is called a *freemartin* and is usually not fertile. While the two developed in the uterus, there was some fusion of placental blood vessels between the fetuses. The *testosterone,* or male hormone, from the male twin affects the female's development. Likewise, there is the mixing of certain cells that leads to the establishment of male and female cells in the blood of each twin. In many of these cases, the female reproductive tract does not develop properly. The vagina often ends in a short, closed tube and has no cervix. Though external reproductive parts may look normal, internal reproductive organs are not.

Similarly, in the female twin, the ovaries are usually undeveloped. The newborn freemartin twin also often has an enlarged *clitoris* (the small organ located at the external lower portion of the vulva) with a tuft of hair at the vulva. Because about 92 percent of heifers that are twins to bulls are sterile freemartins, they should not be kept for breeding purposes; they'll probably never be able to reproduce.

It's also possible to have a freemartin that is not known to have been a twin. Because some freemartin reproductive problems occur as early as 30 days after conception, a heifer fetus may have some of these alterations in her body that persist even if her male twin dies early in the uterus and is resorbed and she is carried full term. Such a heifer may have normal-looking external genitalia but has abnormalities in her sex chromosomes that make her infertile.

Infections

A common cause of infertility in cows is uterine infection. Some degree of infection is inevitable after calving; bacterial contamination can occur during or immediately after birth due to open access to the uterus. Contamination of the uterus can also occur during breeding. Usually this infection is temporary, however, unless the level of contamination is too great, or the cow's natural defenses are not strong enough to throw it off, or injury to the reproductive tract gives bacteria more opportunity to become well established.

In some instances, bacteria overcome the cow's natural defenses, such as in the case of a difficult birth, when tissues are damaged, or in the case of a retained placenta. If bacteria become established in the uterine tissues and produce toxins that are absorbed into the bloodstream, the cow may become very sick.

Under normal conditions, the reproductive tract is resistant to bacterial proliferation because when the tract is open (during breeding and calving), it is under the influence of estrogen, which aids greatly in this defense. During breeding and calving, there is also an increased blood supply, which brings more white blood cells to the area to combat infection.

In some instances, however, bacteria overcome the cow's natural defenses, such as in the case of a difficult birth, when tissues are damaged, or in the case of a retained placenta. If bacteria become established in the uterine tissues and produce toxins that are absorbed into the bloodstream, the cow may become very sick (see chapter 6). In other instances, bacteria simply cause inflammation of the uterine lining and do not affect the general health of the cow, but can make an unhealthy environment in the uterus. This means an attaching embryo will have a more difficult time. The cow may cycle and conceive, but when the embryo comes out of the fallopian tube a few days later, it can't successfully attach to the uterine lining and therefore dies. The cow returns to heat, but unless the infection clears up (which may require several weeks or months after calving or even treatment), the cow will never be able to carry a pregnancy.

Nutritional Stress or Heavy Milking after Calving

Some cows that milk heavily but aren't fed enough to meet their demands for lactation may lose weight and won't start cycling soon after calving. In fact, they may not cycle again until they are past the peak of lactation or after their calves are weaned and they regain weight.

Research has shown that heavy-milking cows that eat adequately (due to their nutritional demands during lactation) tend to have lower progesterone levels. If progesterone is low, a cow may develop cystic ovaries and won't cycle (see page 16). This may be one reason that higher-producing cows are more prone to cystic ovaries.

Interestingly, dairy cows return to heat sooner than most beef cows even though they are producing more milk, in part because the suckling action of a calf seems to inhibit ovulation. If calves are taken off their dams early (30 to 60 days after calving), the mama cows almost always resume cycling much more quickly than they do when they are raising a calf. In fact, a cow that aborts or loses her calf early will return to heat even sooner. The return to cycling is due partly to not being suckled and partly to dry-up of milk and the consequent decreased drain on the cow's body.

Nutritional Deficiencies

In order to cycle, a cow must be adequately fed. Mother Nature wants to make sure the female's body is capable of maintaining pregnancy. If her body is barely able to maintain itself, the cow won't cycle.

A thin cow will take longer to resume cycling after calving than will a well-fed cow. If the situation is borderline, a cow may go into silent heat or start cycling but won't be able to maintain her pregnancy if bred.

A cow needs adequate nutrition, especially energy and protein. She also needs certain vitamins and minerals to maintain a healthy reproductive tract. If she's short on vitamin A, copper, selenium, or some other important nutrient, she may be less fertile or may not cycle.

For instance, fertility in heifers is frequently impaired if their copper utilization is affected by too much *molybdenum,* a naturally occurring mineral

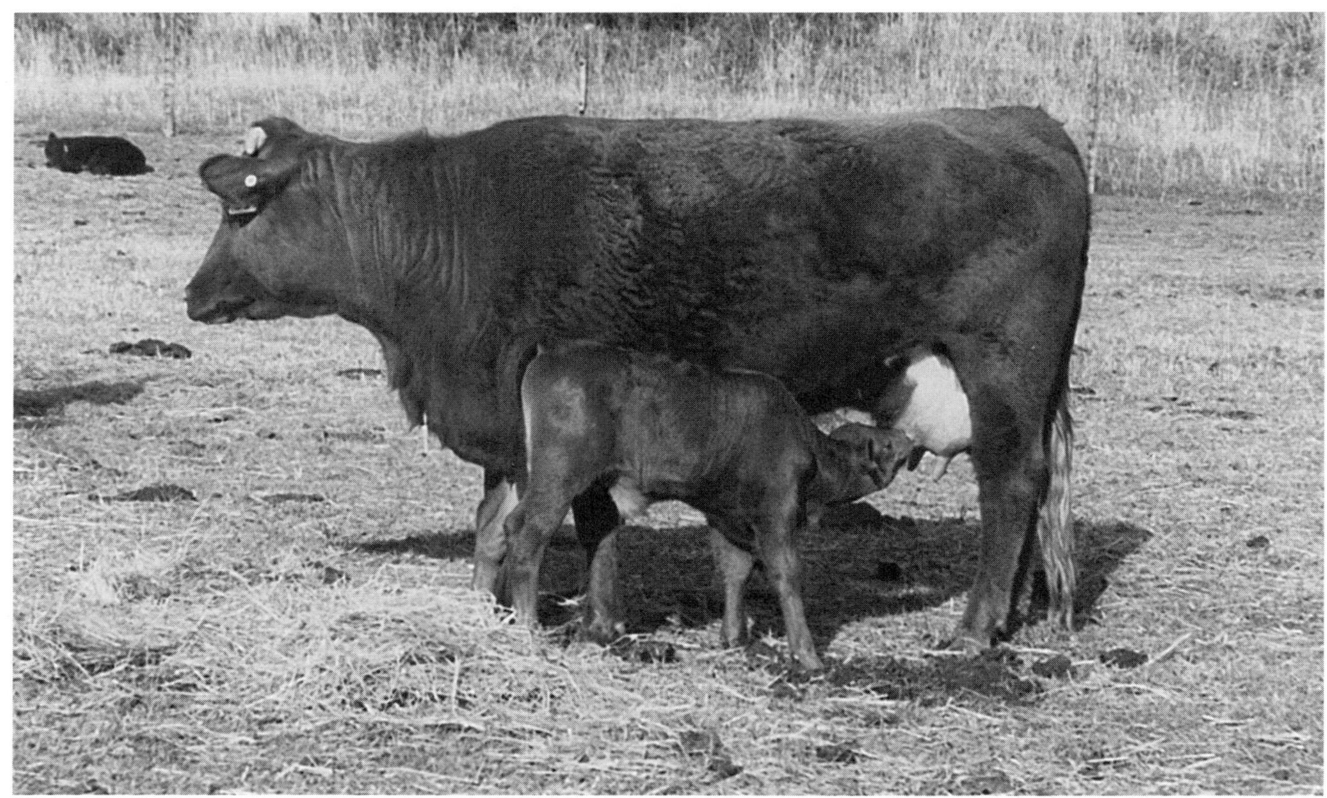

Cows that produce an abundance of milk may not cycle as quickly after calving as will cows with average milk production.

found in the soil and often located in low-lying places after millions of years of runoff from higher elevations. In fact, the resulting copper deficiency can delay puberty in heifers by 8 to 12 weeks and can greatly reduce the conception rate in cows. Indeed, copper deficiency can reduce the conception rate after calving, lead to early embryo loss, and cause a reduction in pregnancy rates. Copper-deficient cows may show normal estrous behavior but do not ovulate (and will not become pregnant) and may eventually stop cycling. If your herd is experiencing less than optimal pregnancy rates, check individual cows' copper levels. It's not very expensive to correct a copper or selenium deficiency, and supplementation often leads to higher conception rates, healthier calves, and less disease.

Iodine deficiency is another nutritional problem that can interfere with optimum reproduction by causing embryonic death, abortion, stillbirths, or weak calves. If you live in an iodine-deficient region, this can be corrected by feeding a salt-and-mineral mix containing iodine.

Cystic Ovaries

A *cystic ovary* is an occasional cause of infertility in beef cows and a common cause of infertility in dairy cows; it is more often found in older cows than in first-time calvers. It also occurs more frequently in high-producing cows that milk the most and raise the biggest calves and tends to occur fairly soon after calving rather than later in lactation.

Cows that "go cystic" may show estrus once after calving, but heat cycles after that are erratic. Some of these cows seem to be in heat all the time and some do not show heat at all. For cows that do show a heat cycle, the first heat after calving may or may not be fertile. Within the first month or so after calving, some follicles grow and then die; the cow may become cystic for a while and then normalize. If the condition is going to correct itself, it usually does soon after calving, but if a cow reaches 100 days or more (more than three months) after calving, the likelihood of spontaneous resolution is reduced substantially. In such cases, your vet can treat the cow with a hormone injection that causes one of the ovary's follicles to ovulate.

In a herd where hormones are given to cows or heifers ahead of breeding to synchronize them for a timed AI program, these hormones (such as progesterone) will generally jump-start cows that are cystic and will eliminate the problem.

There are actually two types of ovarian cysts, follicular cysts and luteal cysts. With a luteal cyst, a follicle tries to ovulate but can't because of the mixed message it's receiving from the pituitary gland, due to the high blood levels of progesterone. As the follicle grows older, it may secrete an abnormal mix of hormones. The cow may exhibit abnormal sexual behavior, but most cows with luteal cysts don't show heat. In fact, you might assume these cows are pregnant.

About 40 percent of cows with cystic ovaries eventually resolve without treatment, but some continue in this condition for months or years.

With follicular cysts, a follicle grows to regular size and becomes dominant but doesn't get a message to ovulate, so all follicles keep producing estrogen. As a result, the cow may be in heat constantly or in a strong standing heat about every three days, but because she doesn't ovulate, even if she's bred repeatedly, the cow can't become pregnant.

To determine if the cow has a cystic ovary, your vet can check her, palpating the ovaries to determine whether they are normal. You might also notice that after a while the cow with a cystic ovary develops changes in her body that make her look more masculine.

About 40 percent of cows with cystic ovaries eventually resolve without treatment, but some continue in this condition for months or years. Chances for success are better if the treatment is administered before the cow begins taking on more masculine characteristics. Often, a cow with a cystic ovary is sold because she is an *open cow* (a cow not impregnated). It is more logical to sell her than treat her, since she'll miss a year of producing a calf.

Heat Stress

If cows are bred in summer, hot weather and humidity can sometimes be a cause of infertility or embryo loss. A common time for heat stress to cause embryonic loss is in the first week after mating, when the embryo fails to attach to the uterus. In extremely hot, humid weather, however, a cow may lose a pregnancy any time in the first month. Rarely, heat stress is the cause of pregnancy loss in late gestation, when anything that stresses the cow or fetus can trigger a premature birth, which usually results in death of the calf.

Cattle on fungus-infected fescue pastures have poor heat tolerance and will more readily suffer reproductive problems.

In climates with hot summers, it's best to select a later-in-the-year or earlier breeding/calving season or cattle with more heat tolerance. British and European breeds don't handle heat as well as zebu (such as Brahmans) or zebu crosses or Senepol. Likewise, dark-colored cattle are more stressed by heat than light-colored ones because dark colors absorb more heat. In fact, black cattle tend to have higher body temperatures — up to 104°F in hot weather — than light-colored cattle, which have a body temperature of 102°F.

Weather stress, resulting from either extreme heat or extreme cold, also affects breeding behavior. Cows are generally in heat for a much shorter length of time during adverse weather conditions of any kind, and some cows go into silent heat during hot or cold weather.

Other Stressors

As stated earlier, stress of any kind may affect a cow's reproduction ability. If a cow is ill, in pain, or lame, she may not cycle as normally as a healthy, comfortable cow. For example, a lame cow won't travel to graze or may be intimidated at the feeding area by cows that take advantage of her disability. As a result, she may not eat enough feed. Likewise, the stress of a long transport or an episode of extreme physical exertion during early gestation may result in early embryo loss.

For more information on diseases that can cause infertility or conditions that lead to loss of pregnancy in cows, see chapter 2.

Factors That Affect Fertility in the Bull

A bull must be sexually mature in order to breed cows. Some are mature enough to breed as yearlings, while others are more fertile by the time they are 1½ to 2 years old. To learn if a young bull is mature or if any bull is fertile, it's important to have him examined by a veterinarian, who can check the bull's reproductive organs and do a semen check and sperm count.

Scrotal Shape and Circumference

The shape and size of the *scrotum* can often give a clue as to whether a bull is sexually mature or fertile. Indeed, measuring the scrotum is one of the ways to evaluate yearling bulls, along with a semen check and physical examination of the reproductive tract. Bulls with inadequate testicular size do not produce as much sperm and are less fertile than bulls with larger *testicles*.

Scrotal Size

Scrotal size correlates to puberty: The young bull's testicles enlarge as he goes through puberty, which occurs at different ages in various breeds and individuals. Bulls of smaller, faster-maturing breeds reach puberty more quickly (accompanied by a slowing of their growth) and have larger scrotal size as yearlings than big-framed animals that mature later and grow for a longer time. Some bulls in breeds that grow to be very large have barely reached puberty at one year of age.

To be fertile as a yearling, a bull should have a minimum scrotal circumference of 12.2 to 13 inches (31 to 33 centimeters), depending on breed, whereas 14 inches (35.6 centimeters) is average. Most stockmen prefer to use bulls whose yearling measurements are more than 14.2 inches (36 centimeters) for optimal fertility.

Scrotal circumference gives not only a clue about a bull's fertility but also an indication of how early his daughters will reach puberty. Bulls with a large scrotum at an early age will mature quickly, and so will their daughters. If you plan to keep heifers for future

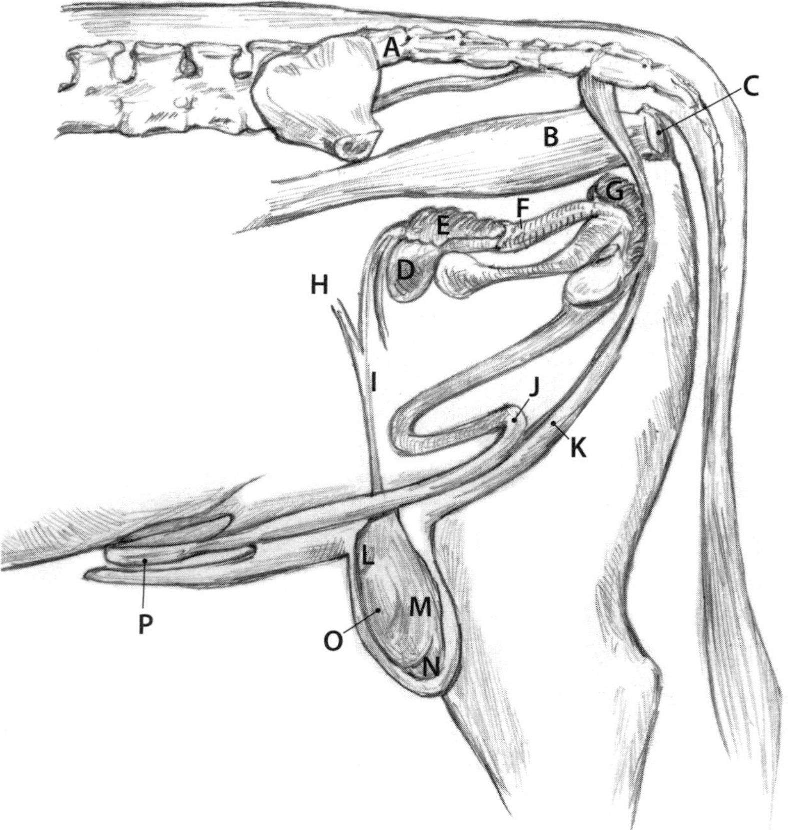

BULL REPRODUCTIVE TRACT

- **A** Backbone
- **B** Rectum
- **C** Anus
- **D** Urinary bladder
- **E** Seminal vesicular gland
- **F** Prostate
- **G** Balbo cavernosus muscle
- **H** Spermatic cord
- **I** Vas deferens
- **J** Distal sigmoid flexure of penis
- **K** Retractor penis muscle
- **L** Head of epididymis
- **M** Body of epididymis
- **N** Tail of epididymis
- **O** Testis (testacle)
- **P** Glans penis

Measuring a Bull's Scrotum

For nature to take its course, you'll want your cows and heifers bred by a bull whose yearling scrotal circumference was at least 12.2 to 13 inches (31 to 33 centimeters). For optimal fertility, however, use mature bulls whose yearling measurements were more than 14.2 inches (36 centimeters).

Take the following steps to measure a bull's scrotum and see if he's ready for action:

1. Restrain the bull in a chute with a pole behind him so he can't kick.
2. Before applying the measuring tape, make sure the testes are pressed firmly into the lower part of the scrotal sac so they are side by side and all skin wrinkles that might interfere with accurate measurement are eliminated.
3. Place the thumb and fingers of one hand on the sides of the scrotum.
4. Slip up over the scrotum the looped tape measure made especially for this purpose and pull it tight, with moderate tension around the largest portion.
5. If you don't have a special looped tape measure, you can improvise by using a loop of string and marking it, then measuring the string afterward.
6. Make note of the scrotal measurements in your records book for future reference.

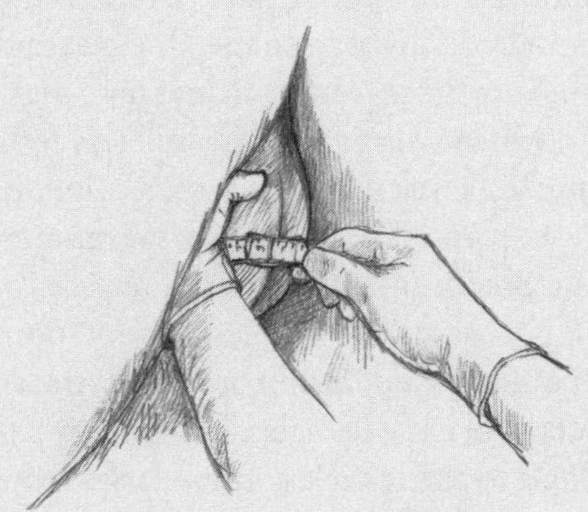

To measure scrotal circumference, the bull is restrained in a chute and the scrotum is measured around its largest area, where the testicles are widest.

cows, make sure they were sired by a bull that had a larger-than-average scrotum at an early age. A late-maturing bull will sire heifers that are also late maturing. Consequently, be aware that these heifers may not breed in time to calve on schedule for their first calf. Remember: Fertility is an inherited trait; keep daughters of a very fertile bull when selecting replacement females for your cow herd. Daughters of a subfertile or late-maturing bull will not be as productive.

BIGGER'S NOT ALWAYS BETTER

Be cautious about using a bull with huge testicles (more than 15.5 inches or about 40 centimeters at one year of age). Some of these bulls are more inclined to suffer testicular degeneration. Testicles this large at this age are not normal.

Scrotal Shape

A normal, fertile bull has a pear-shaped scrotum with an obvious neck at the top. A fat bull may have a straight-sided scrotum with no narrowing at the top, indicating too much fat deposited in the neck of the scrotum, thus, generally, poor fertility resulting from the insulating effects of the fat, which inhibits heat loss and proper cooling of the testes in warm weather.

Another undesirable characteristic is the V-shaped scrotum; that is, it tapers to a pointed tip at the bottom. Bulls with such scrotums often are not as fertile as bulls with a normal, pear-shaped scrotum. A V-shaped scrotum holds testicles up, closer to the body. Bulls with this scrotal shape usually have undersized testicles that don't produce semen of adequate quality.

Remember, when examining a bull's scrotum, the testicles must be able to move freely up and down for proper temperature regulation. The bull draws them closer to his body in cold weather and lowers them at other times to keep them cooler than body temperature, which is necessary for sperm production and viability. When a veterinarian checks a bull for breeding soundness, he or she will feel the testicles to make sure they can move freely and that there are no adhesions between them and the scrotal wall. Adhesions may result from injury or from frostbite the previous winter.

Testicles should be uniform in size. If one is larger than the other or is different in shape, this may indicate a problem. Sometimes one testicle is held higher than the other, which won't make the bull less fertile unless it is quite high; in such instances, it might not be able to move up and down properly for temperature regulation. Sometimes one or both testicles are rotated, which is not a problem unless the rotation is extreme; this could cause a *torsion* or twist in the coil of blood vessels above the testicles and thereby slow the flow of blood to the testicles. These large vessels are very important for temperature regulation and heat exchange, and a severe twist may impair this mechanism.

EVALUATING SCROTAL SHAPE

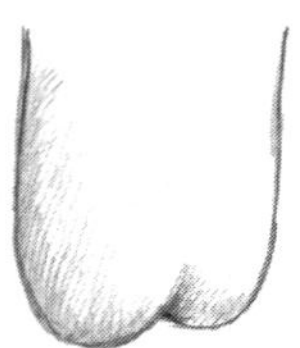

Undesirable: straight sides (no neck)

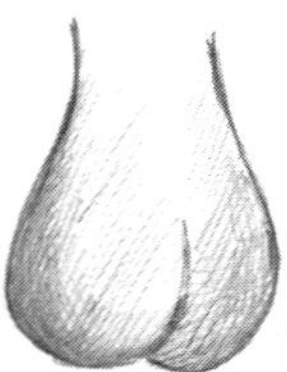

Normal: pear-shaped scrotum

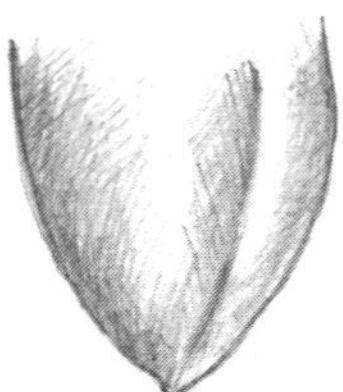

Undesirable: tapered (V-shape)

The Reproductive Tract

When the vet collects semen to count and evaluate sperm, he or she will also check the functioning of reproductive organs and whether there is evidence of previous injuries that could interfere with the bull's fertility or ability to service cows.

One common cause of trouble is abnormality of the *foreskin,* the fold of skin over the penis. Some problems are inherited and others are due to injury. Some injuries are obvious, showing excessive swelling or inability to retract the penis, but others can't be seen until the bull tries to extend his penis to breed a cow. Bulls with a loose *sheath* and foreskin (a genetic trait that often correlates with being naturally hornless) are more prone to injury, such as tearing of the sheath.

Another reproductive-organ difficulty leading to the inability to breed is penile deviation: The penis is not straight when the bull extends it. It may drop down or have an S-curve or a rainbow deviation; that is, it bends in a semicircle. A corkscrew or rainbow deviation may not be apparent with conventional fertility testing; the ejaculator device used by the vet won't create a full extension of the penis. You must see the bull attempt to breed a cow in order to detect this problem.

Other possible problems are a bruised or swollen penis, nerve damage, hair rings that restrict circulation, a prolapse of the foreskin, and even warts on the penis. Most of these problems can be diagnosed and treated by a vet if the damage is not too great, but the affected bull will be unable to breed for a while and should be removed from the herd until he recovers so that the injury doesn't become worse when he tries to breed.

General Soundness

If a bull becomes tired or injured, he may not do his job. A bull must be physically fit and adequately fed for athletic ability and energy; he must be neither too thin nor too fat. If he's too thin, he may run out of gas before the breeding season is over. If he's too fat, he may tire easily and lose his desire to breed or travel if the cows are in a big pasture. A large belly may also interfere with the athletic act of breeding.

Even if he is fertile, a bull won't settle cows if he's lame or ill or has some other problem that interferes

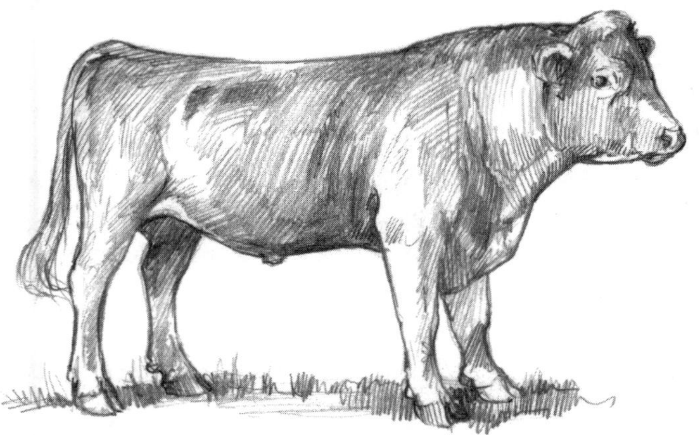

If bulls become thin, they may have impaired fertility and low energy levels during the breeding season.

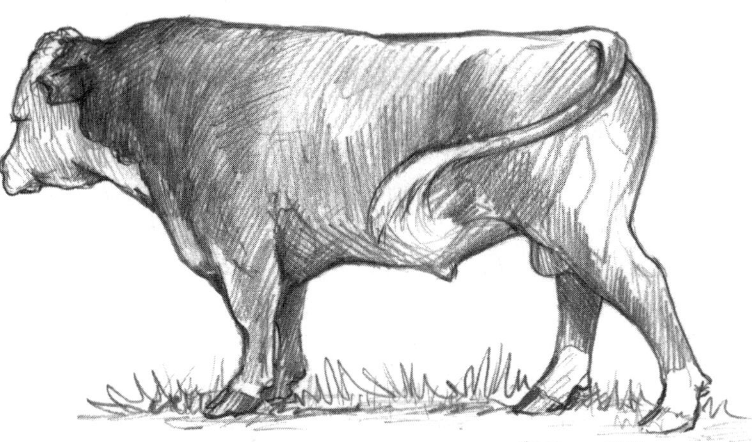

Bulls need to be well fed, healthy, and in good condition for optimal fertility and energy during the breeding season.

with his ability or desire to breed them. A physical problem may cause him discomfort when he mounts a cow, so he may not try. For instance, *foot rot* (an acute infection) can make him too lame and sore to try to breed cows.

If the bull has poor conformation, he may strain his hind leg joints. A bull that is *sickle hocked* (that is, he has too much angle in the hock joints) or *post-legged* (he is too straight in stifles and hocks) may suffer injuries that can hinder his mating ability. If he was overfed on grain while growing up, he may have foot problems due to *founder* (inflammation of the hoof-secreting part of the foot) or joint problems and damage resulting from rapid growth and excess weight that cause him to go lame. Likewise, back problems, commonly seen in older bulls and in bulls with too much calcium in their diet from alfalfa or feed *supplements,* may cause a bull to stop breeding cows.

Health, Nutrition, and Environment

A bull that's severely underfed or suffering from a nutritional deficiency will not be as fertile as a sound, well-fed bull. He may not have the endurance to keep up with breeding, and he won't settle many cows. Similarly, an overweight bull will not perform and may not be fertile.

Also, illness can reduce a bull's ability to breed cows. If a bull is sick, he won't feel like expending effort, and if he's been ill with fever, he'll have a period of infertility for 60 to 90 days after the fever passes. Sperm that are forming during the time the bull has a fever will die or be abnormal because of the bull's higher body temperature. In fact, any illness that raises a bull's temperature very high for very long (even an acute case of foot rot) can make him temporarily infertile.

Hot, humid weather can actually make bulls temporarily infertile. Sperm production is optimum when the temperature of the scrotum is kept a few degrees cooler than the bull's normal body temperature of 101 to 102°F. If the environmental temperature is 100°F or higher (especially with high humidity, which thwarts sweat evaporation), the bull is unable to keep his testes cool enough for healthy sperm production.

Semen quality also declines dramatically during hot weather, with effects that show up later. The *spermatogenic* (sperm production) *cycle* is about 60 days from the time the sperm cell is produced until it is mature and *ejaculated.* Semen quality is directly impaired, however, during a period of high heat and for up to 60 days after this time. The problem may be mild — the bull has a normal sex drive and mates with cows, but more cows than usual come back into heat because they did not settle — or severe, resulting in a complete wipeout of all the sperm stored in the testes.

To avoid the adverse effects of hot, humid weather, don't schedule the breeding season during the hottest part of the year. If you have a heat wave in a moderate climate, make sure cattle have adequate shade during the daylight hours and plenty of water. If you have a small herd and a well-ventilated barn, keep your bull in the barn during the heat of the day and turn him out in the evening for breeding at night. You can easily lure him back into the barn in late morning with a bucket of grain. Although this arrangement is labor intensive, it may keep the bull from becoming infertile.

Severely cold, windy weather can also affect a bull's fertility. Scrotal frostbite creates damage that can be either temporary or permanent. The resulting scar tissue may make it impossible for the bull to raise and lower his testicles. If there is a scabby area at the lower portion of the back of the scrotum, have your veterinarian check the bull before the next breeding season. To prevent scrotal frostbite, in cold weather provide adequate windbreaks for bulls and plenty of bedding so the animals don't have to lie on frozen ground.

Libido

Bulls must have the desire to breed cows — but fertility and sex drive are not necessarily related. A fertile bull can't get cows pregnant unless he actually breeds them.

The largest, fastest-growing bulls may not have the best sex drive. Some bulls are lazy or slow about breeding or are more interested in fighting other bulls than in looking for cows in heat. Individual bulls have varying degrees of sex drive. Detecting these differences may be difficult at first; almost every bull will get excited and breed a cow when first turned in with females (though some are slow and blundering even then), but you won't be able to tell whether a bull will keep up his efforts through an entire breeding season.

In a small pasture and with a long breeding season, you might get by with a bull that's not a very aggressive breeder. In these circumstances, he'll eventually get the cows bred. In range areas, however, where a bull must travel long distances to seek out all the cows in heat, his sex drive becomes very important.

Sperm Count

The bull must have an adequate number of sperm to settle cows. Even though only one live sperm is needed to fertilize an egg, it takes large numbers of sperm swimming up the oviduct to create a proper environment — the perfect chemical composition of fluid — for fertilization to occur.

It's wise to have your bull's semen production and viability checked before each breeding season, even if it was fine the year before. Injury or infection or weather stress in the bull may interfere with proper semen production. Your veterinarian can take a semen sample and perform a sperm count using a microscope. This count checks not only the total number of sperm but also the number of normal, abnormal, and dead sperm.

Experience

Some young bulls are not as dependable as older bulls in getting all their cows bred, especially when they're confronted with the prospect of several cows in heat at once. They may spend all their time with one cow and ignore the others. Older, more experienced bulls are more likely to distribute their services more efficiently. They'll breed a cow once and go on to the next.

Psychological Factors

Many psychological factors are at play if you have more than one bull breeding your cows.

The general rule of thumb is one bull for every 25 to 30 cows. Many stockmen, however, think that if four bulls are turned out with 100 cows, each bull will sire about 25 calves — but it doesn't work this way. The pecking order and psychological factors determine what happens. A socially dominant and aggressive bull may sire most of the calves or keep other bulls from breeding cows even if he himself doesn't get the job done — which means you'll end up with some open cows. A dominant bull may dissuade younger bulls from breeding cows. Older bulls often intimidate younger ones, and horned bulls intimidate *polled bulls.* Some bulls have more sex drive and try to do most of the breeding; others

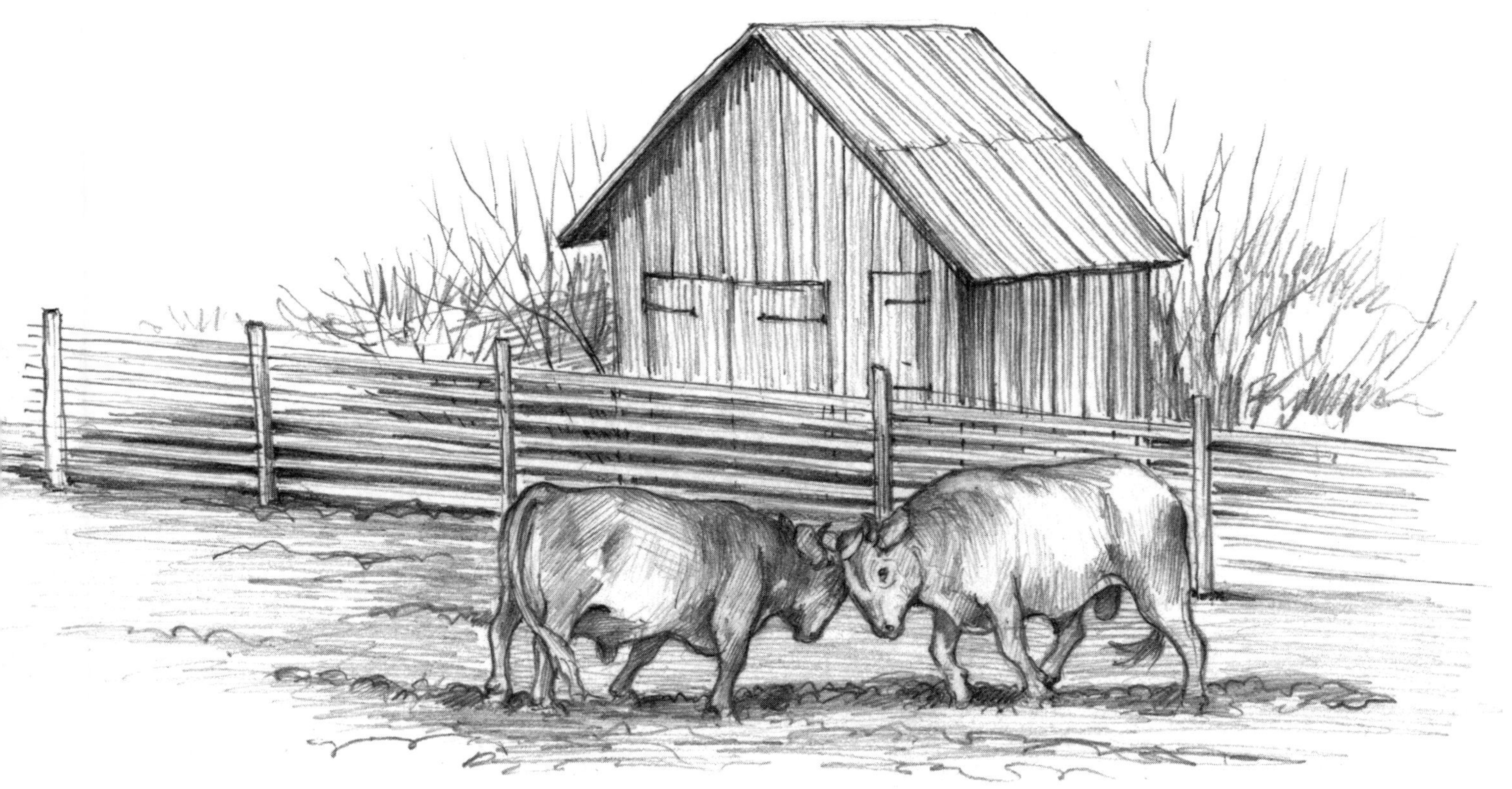

Some bulls spend all their time fighting.

do more fighting than breeding. A bull may take his harem to a corner of the pasture to keep them away from other bulls, even from a bull in the next pasture. He may spend more time jealously herding and guarding these cows than breeding them.

It's important to remember that every bull is an individual and that cattle are very social animals. Both pecking order and individual attitudes can have an impact on what happens with bulls in the breeding herd.

Social dominance in bulls should be taken into consideration when you are determining breeding groups, pastures, and placement of bulls. Psychological factors can alter the balance of power in multibull breeding groups if you add a bull or take one out — which in turn can influence whether all the cows get bred.

A variety of changes can occur. Bulls that got along reasonably well may no longer be compatible after a newcomer is introduced. Subordinate bulls may spend all their time fighting for top position after a dominant bull is removed. Often there are fewer problems in a breeding group if you leave the same bulls with the same cows all breeding season rather than upsetting the social order by adding or switching bulls. It should be said that in some instances, a lazy bull will try to breed more cows if another bull is put with him. The additional bull spurs the lazy bull into competition.

How Many Cows per Bull?

The answer to this question depends on the size and terrain of your pastures and the length of the breeding season.

> **BULLIES MAY NOT BE TOP BREEDERS**
>
> Just because a bull is aggressive doesn't mean he'll be a good breeder. Sometimes a quiet, mild-mannered bull will stick to business and breed cows while the aggressive ones spend all their time fighting.

If you leave cows with a bull for 45 to 60 days or longer and have small pastures, you can usually get by with one bull for every 30 to 50 cows — if the bulls are good breeders. In a season this long, a cow has more than one or two chances to get pregnant. If a bull can't get the job done on the cow's first cycle, there'll be another chance later. If you have fewer bulls in a breeding group, there are fewer risks of injuries due to fighting or cows getting hurt by being chased and repeatedly bred by too many bulls.

For a short breeding season (45 days or fewer), you need to make sure no cows get missed. It helps to have several small breeding pastures if you have more than just a few cows. Divide them into small groups of 25 to 50 cows per pasture, selecting one to three bulls for each group. With this arrangement, there's a greater chance of getting every cow bred because though on some days there will be many cows in heat at once, there will be only a few in heat in each group. Remember that with larger groups, there's an increased risk of bulls fighting for cows in heat and of cows being chased or repeatedly bred.

Even in a small group, however, pay close attention to what's going on. If there are two bulls in a group, they may fight and keep each other from breeding; using one or three bulls per group may be a better choice. If there are three bulls, one may be able to breed the cow in heat while the other two are busy fighting. If there's just one bull in a group, however, he'd better be one you can depend on. You should watch to make sure he's getting his cows bred, especially if there are several in heat at once. Remember the differences between yearling bulls and older bulls. If you're paying attention, you'll know if a bull is able to do his job.

BULLS SOMETIMES HERD COWS

LITTLE JOHN, a horned Hereford bull, provided our first experience with a bull herding his cows. Little John had a mellow nature, but when he was with cows, he tried to keep them away from any other bulls. Whenever we moved his cows from one pasture to another or tried to bring them into the corral, he'd run in front of them and stop them or keep them from going to the gate. To move the cows, we had to get the bull out of the way.

One day he ran to the front of the herd to stop his cows, and I galloped after him on my horse to shoo him out of the way. I was surprised: He turned to swat at my horse with his horns. My horse surprised me even more: Instead of being intimidated by the bull, he reared up and struck Little John in the face with his shod front feet. This startled the bull, and when he backed off, I was able to get the cows through the gate.

In the years since Little John, we've had a number of bulls, of various breeds and crosses, that have jealously herded their cows. This herding nature may hark back to when cattle were wild and bulls tried to keep their harems from getting close to another bull's territory.

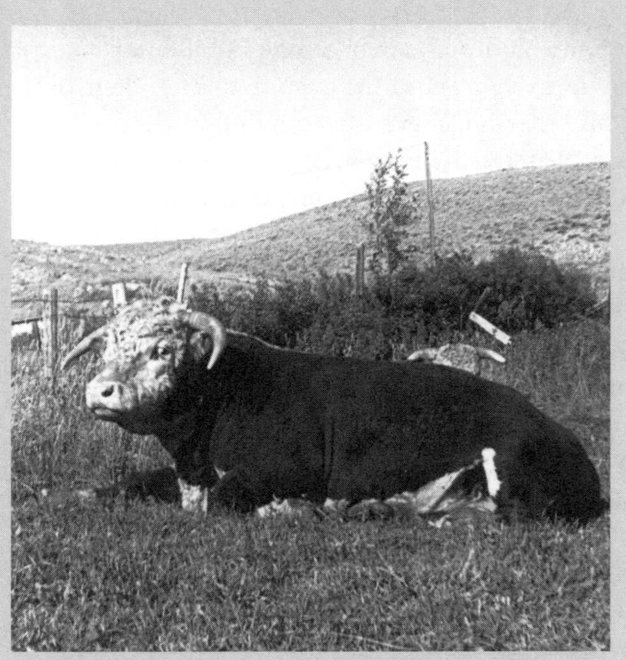

Although Little John was usually a laid-back bull, he'd herd cows to keep them from other bulls in the pasture at breeding time.

A Word About Bulls

Unless you are breeding all your cows by artificial insemination (AI), as some dairies do, you need a good bull, or several, relative to the number of cows (see above). And unless you calve year-round (an impractical way to manage cows — except in some dairies — and impossible to market calves at uniform size), bulls should be kept separate from other cattle when not being used for breeding. You don't want cows bred out of season or heifers bred too young. A young bull will also do much better if kept separate from cows, especially after breeding season is over. He's still growing and needs time off from chasing after cows so he can regain lost weight and grow better — and be in better condition for next year.

Thus you need a separate pen or pasture for bulls, with good fences. It's always healthier for bulls to have room to exercise (and to be out of the mud in wet seasons) so, if you have the room, a pasture is usually better than a small corral. Electric wire (if it's always working) can augment a pasture fence to ensure that bulls don't try to go through it, and it also helps to have a buffer field or pen between them and any females. If they can't get nose-to-nose with females, they're not as tempted to crash the fence.

Bulls Are Bulls

Handle bulls with firmness and respect and never forget that they are bulls; their instinct is to dominate other animals. Don't make a pet of any bull. If he looks upon you as an equal and has no fear/respect, he will eventually become dangerous as he gets older and more aggressive. In his mind you must always be the dominant member of the team, never to be challenged.

Carry a weapon (stick, whip) but also keep a very confident attitude. If a bull respects you, you generally don't need to use your weapon; it's enough to just have it with you and to dominate him with your confidence. If he knows you are afraid, you should not be handling him.

Some bulls, especially dairy bulls, become aggressive at a very early age, and others become more so as they get older (usually age four or five). A few remain mellow and manageable longer. If a bull starts challenging you, get rid of him.

Feed and Nutrition

Bulls need good feed, but this doesn't mean grain. If a bull needs grain to stay in good body condition, he's not going to sire feed-efficient offspring and thus is not the kind of animal you want. Since most bulls are now sold as yearlings rather than as two-year-olds, many seedstock producers overfeed young beef bulls to get them big enough fast enough to look good by sale time. Fat young bulls often "fall apart" when turned out with cows; they are not in strong athletic condition and tire more readily. They may lose weight rapidly due to the sudden drop in nutrition levels coupled with the drastic increase in exertion. Overfeeding leads to fertility problems (see above) and founder and other feet and leg problems.

Adequate nutrition for a yearling bull's growth can be provided with good pasture or good-quality hay with high protein level. Mature bulls should do fine on pasture or good grass hay or a grass-alfalfa mix. Watch body condition closely and adjust the feed accordingly. If older bulls get too fat, this not only hinders fertility but can also impair athletic ability, stamina, and sex drive.

If bulls start losing weight, increase the quantity or quality of feed. A good mineral supplement is also important for optimal fertility if your feeds are deficient.

Selecting a Bull

A bull provides half the genetics for any calves you sell or keep as future cows, so you want a good one that suits your goals. If he's a purebred, check his performance records, and those of sire and dam, to learn what to expect from his calves regarding birth weight, weaning weight, and so on. If he'll be breeding heifers, make sure he isn't too large and heavy (or he may injure them during breeding), and check his projected birth weights to make sure he'll sire small calves that are easy-born but grow quickly.

Conformation Pointers

Evaluate him visually to make sure he has good conformation, will stay sound, and will sire daughters with good conformation. He should have strong feet and legs (good bones and strong hoofs), not crooked or weak, and should travel well — with legs moving straight forward instead of crookedly. If he has too much angle in his hind legs or not enough angle in his hocks and stifles (called *post-legged*), he may suffer strain and injury when trying to breed cows. He should have a strong back (not be swaybacked or humped up) and be long in body and not pot-bellied.

If you'll be keeping daughters as future cows, always look at the bull's mother, especially her udder shape and milking ability. His daughters will be a lot like his mother, and if she has a serious fault (such as big teats at calving time, fertility problems, or bad disposition), they likely will too.

Temperament

Make sure he has a good disposition and is easy to handle. Temperament is partly inherited. You want a bull that not only sires easy-born, fast-growing calves and good-milking daughters, but also passes on calm, intelligent behavior. How you handle and train your cattle can make a big difference in tractability, but it helps if they have good intelligence and an easygoing nature to begin with. An aggressive/mean or wild/flighty bull will sire calves with the same bad attitude. They will be difficult to handle, more easily stressed, and won't gain weight as readily as calmer individuals. Never use a bull that has traits you wouldn't want to see in your calves.

Before the Breeding Season

Vaccinate bulls annually (or semiannually, for some diseases) and make sure vaccinations are current ahead of breeding season (at least three weeks ahead). Have your vet do a breeding soundness exam and semen check, even if the bull was fine last year. The bull may have suffered injury or infection between then and now; you want to make sure he'll be fertile and able to breed cows. Some states require a test for trichomoniasis before breeding.

Vet Check

Before you buy or borrow a bull, always have a breeding soundness exam (see above) to check his semen and any other factors that could affect his fertility or breeding ability.

Reproductive Behavior

When a cow comes into heat, she will seek a bull and start mounting him and other cows, but it may still be a few hours before she will stand for the bull to mount and breed her (see above). Bulls are continually traveling through the herd, checking cows to detect the ones that are in heat or coming into heat. He smells the vulva of a cow and also smells her urine. During heat, a cow urinates frequently and the bull samples the odor and taste of her urine. The in-heat cow releases pheromones in body fluids (especially urine and sweat glands in the flank area), and he can detect those. He may be able to smell an in-heat cow some distance away if a breeze brings odors in his direction. Able to identify a cow in pre-heat up to two days before she comes into heat, a bull may keep close track of her (staying near and guarding her from other bulls) until she does.

He makes tentative attempts to mount the cow, but if it's still early in her heat period, she may not stand. He keeps checking her by resting his chin on her back or rump, and he mounts and breeds her only when she is ready and holds her back rigid.

When the bull mounts the cow to breed, he finds his proper position to enter the vulva with his penis (which may take a few seconds or may be immediate), then gives a strong thrust as he ejaculates. This is usually a leap, with hind legs leaving the ground. If he actually breeds her, the cow will stand humped up, with her tail raised, after he dismounts. If the bull did not thrust (merely mounting and dismounting without giving his leap) and the cow does not hold her tail out afterward, he did not ejaculate; she was not bred.

Breeding by Artificial Insemination (AI)

There are many pluses to artificial insemination (AI) and many reasons to consider it for your cows.

Why AI?

A farmer with only a few cows may not want to invest in a bull or have the nuisance of keeping a bull. Many dairymen don't bother with a bull, especially because dairy bulls are notorious for bad disposition and dangerous aggression.

Use of AI is also a way to use superior genetics to improve your herd at much less expense than buying a top-quality bull. You can select from any breed and purchase semen from several bulls that might complement or improve your herd.

Use of AI is also a way to use superior genetics to improve your herd at much less expense than buying a top-quality bull.

AI also has benefits with regard to herd size. If you have a small herd that might not justify having more than one bull, you can breed your cows and heifers to any number of good bulls by using AI, selecting certain sires for certain cows or a different sire with calving ease for heifers. In a large herd, you can save money by not having to buy a lot of bulls.

No matter the number, there is a great deal of management and expense involved in keeping bulls, there's a big investment in purchasing good bulls, and there's always a risk that a bull will get injured and will be unable to sire calves. In addition, bulls are hard on fences and devour quite a bit of feed that cows could eat. Selective breeding requires several pastures for different breeding groups. Use of AI allows you to keep cows in more convenient groups for pasture rotation without having to keep breeding groups separate.

Because AI doesn't settle 100 percent of cows, however, most stockmen use a *cleanup bull* afterward to breed any cows that did not become pregnant with artificial insemination. Keeping one cleanup bull, is less trouble than keeping a group of bulls for breeding.

ARTIFICIAL INSEMINATION

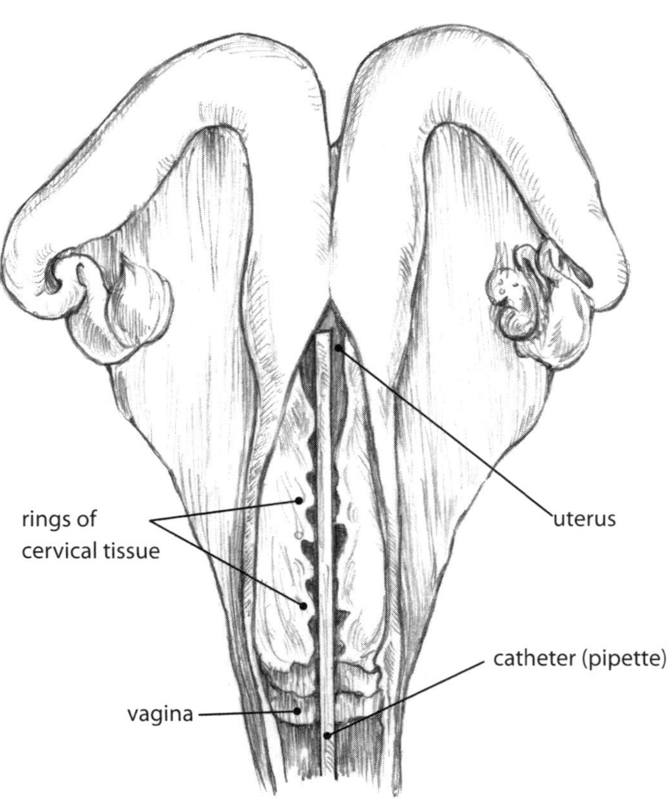

The folds and blind endings in overlapping rings of tissue in the cervix can make it difficult to pass the catheter through the cervix when depositing the semen into the uterus with a catheter (pipette).

A Successful AI Program

If you opt for AI, work with a technician who does the procedure all the time. This will result in a high success rate; that is, a high percentage of cows will become pregnant. You may eventually want to learn to do AI yourself, but remember that it's a skill that takes some basic instruction and a great deal of practice; someone who does it all the time has a higher success rate than a beginner.

For a successful AI program, your cows and heifers should be individually identified with ear tags, brisket tags, a freeze brand, or some other system that enables you to see an animal's number from a distance. Accurate records (heat cycles, breeding dates, etc.) are crucial. Adequate facilities are also important: You'll need a good corral and chute that allow you to get a cow in and restrain her for insemination without stressing her. Remember: If the cow is upset and excited, your success rate will drop. Stress is detrimental to conception.

Watching Cows for Optimal Insemination Times

You may choose to watch cows and heifers closely during the season in which you want them bred to determine when each one is in heat so that the technician can inseminate them at the optimal time. You could also synchronize the herd with the use of hormones so that they'll all come into heat in a two- to three-day period, enabling them to be inseminated at the same time. You can discuss these options with a bovine vet or an AI technician to determine what will work best for your situation.

The best times to observe cows are at dawn and dusk, during the cooler parts of the day or night in summer, and during the warmer parts of the day in cold weather.

Heat detection is the most time-consuming and also the most imporant aspect of AI. At a minimum, you must carefully observe the cows for at least 30 minutes twice a day, in early morning and late evening, to recognize and interpret their signs of heat. If you see them only once a day, you'll certainly miss the signs in a lot of cows. Studies have shown that about 22 percent of cows show signs of heat between 6 AM and noon, about 10 percent between noon and 6 PM, about 25 percent between 6 PM and midnight, and 43 percent between midnight and 6 AM.

The best times to observe cows, then, are at dawn and dusk and also during the cooler parts of the day or night in summer or the warmer parts of the day in cold weather. The most inconclusive times are when cattle are inactive due to adverse weather conditions and when they are distracted by food or a stressful condition. Hot, cold, or stormy weather will diminish estrous activity. Feeding time is not a good time to watch for signs of heat because the cows are more interested in coming to the feed and eating than in breeding. The best times to observe are quiet times when nothing else is going on to disturb or distract the cows.

Follow the general AI rule of thumb and inseminate a cow within 24 hours of the first observation of heat, preferably late in the heat period. You'll want to do this because ovulation takes place after the cow is no longer in standing heat and because the egg lives only 6 to 10 hours.

Gestation: Development of Embryo and Fetus

After the cow or heifer is bred and settled, pregnancy lasts roughly nine months and a week, give or take a few days. *Gestation* (length of pregnancy) generally takes 283 days in cattle, but this is an average; it will vary among breeds and individuals. Gestation length is an inherited trait, and you can select for cattle with longer or shorter gestation periods.

There is a correlation between length of gestation and calf size at birth because the fetus grows fastest toward the end of gestation. Some breeds are known for having a long gestation and larger calves at birth (which can lead to difficult deliveries), whereas others are known for smaller calves at birth due to a shorter gestation length.

The Effects of Gestation Length

Because gestation length is directly related to calf size at birth, a pregnancy that lasts longer than average usually results in a bigger calf at birth. If you want easy-calving cows, select cows and bulls that produce low-birth-weight calves, which generally means shorter gestation lengths.

Shorter gestation is also an advantage in getting cows rebred on time. A cow with a long gestation doesn't have as many days to recover from pregnancy and start cycling before the next breeding season. The larger calf may also have an impact on her recovery time: If it was a difficult birth, the cow's reproductive tract may take longer to recover from delivery.

The Embryo

After fertilization, the egg begins to divide as it moves down the oviduct by contractions of that tiny tube. By the time it reaches the uterine horn, three to four days later, the egg contains 16 to 32 cells.

For a while, it floats in the uterus, nourished by uterine milk (see Development of the Placenta, page 31). At about 12 days of age, it attaches to the lining in the uterine horn and continues to grow. The membranes that develop around it enlarge swiftly and fill with the same fluid that surrounds the embryo. The larger external membrane, the *chorion* (water bag), is a long balloon filled with *allantoic fluid* that encloses the smaller, rounder *amnion sac.* The amnion sac, filled with *amniotic fluid,* encases the embryo itself. By the time the embryo is 35 days old, the growing chorion and its allantoic fluid distend the horn of the uterus, and has expanded into the second uterine horn.

The Conceptus Develops

The developing bovine conceptus is termed an *embryo* from the period between about day 12 until about day 45 of gestation.

During this period, major tissues, organs, and systems of the body are formed; by the end of this time, the embryo is readily recognizable as a calf (as opposed to a foal, lamb, piglet, or puppy). At this stage the eyelids develop. By 22 days of gestation, the tiny heart has formed and is beating, and by 25 days the buds that will become front legs have appeared and the development of eyes and brain is well advanced.

It is during this early embryonic period (12 to 45 days) that many severe birth defects or developmental abnormalities occur (see chapter 2). It's also during this period that many pregnancies are lost. A tiny embryo may die and be expelled unnoticed during the cow's next heat or may disintegrate and be absorbed by the cow's body.

The Fetus

At about day 45, the embryo becomes a *fetus.* The various organs, tissues, and systems continue to differentiate and become more recognizable. By day 70 the organs and body systems of the developing calf are all working.

From this point on there are no radical changes in the fetus aside from its growth and maturation. Increase in size and weight is a geometric curve, increasing very rapidly in the last two to three months of gestation. From day 210 to day 270, the fetus's increase in weight is equal to three times the increase that took place from the time of fertilization up to day 210.

By the fifth month, you can often see movement on the cow's right side, as the fetus kicks and squirms. If you press your hand on the cow's right flank, you might feel the bulge and push of the calf's foot as it shoves against you.

What changes are going on in the pregnant cow? The uterus distends and drops farther into the abdomen as the fetus grows. The increasing weight of the fetus and fluids draws it forward and downward, and after about the fourth or fifth month of gestation, the uterus rests on the floor of the abdomen, beneath the intestines. (The uterus is usually located on the right side of a cow because the left side of the abdomen contains the large rumen.) By the fifth month, you can often see movement on the cow's right side, as the growing fetus kicks and squirms and moves about. If you press your hand on the cow's right flank, you might feel the bulge and push of the calf's foot as it shoves against your hand.

During the first half of gestation, the fetus can be in any position in the uterus; it moves around a great deal. In late gestation, however, it has no room to turn around. In early gestation, about half of all fetuses are facing forward or backward, but by late gestation, about 95 percent are facing the pelvis, in proper position for birth. At some point between five and six months, the body length of the fetus exceeds the width of the amnion sac, and it is at this stage that the final birth position is decided.

By the last month of gestation, the fetus may be so large that its length exceeds the distance from the cow's diaphragm to her pelvis; the front legs and

DEVELOPMENT OF THE BOVINE CONCEPTUS

During the embryo stage — the first 45 days — all the major organs and parts of the body are formed. After that, the conceptus is called a fetus and is recognizable as a tiny calf. Also by then, the fetal membranes have attached to the uterine lining in the caruncle areas, and cotyledons have begun to form.

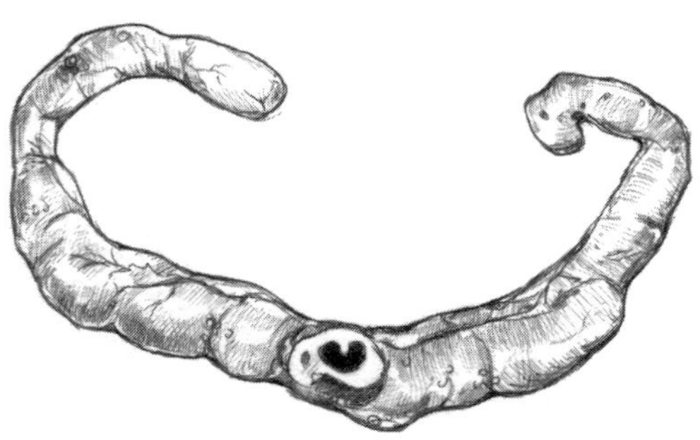

Conceptus at 30 days of gestation in the embryo stage. *The spherical amnion sac contains the embryo and is surrounded by the elongated allantochorion sac, which extends into both uterine horns.*

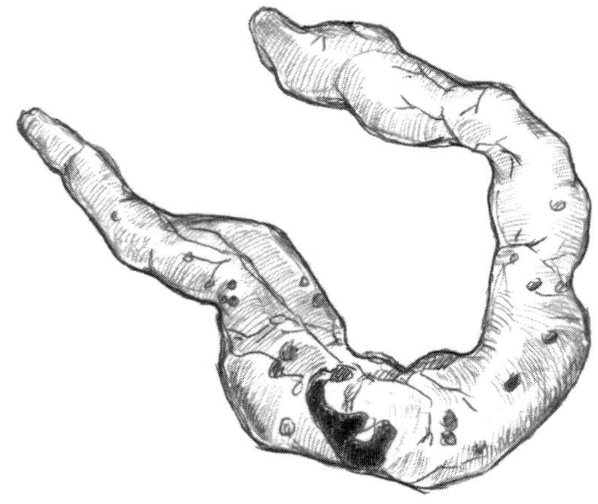

Conceptus at 60 days of gestation. *This is the early fetal stage.*

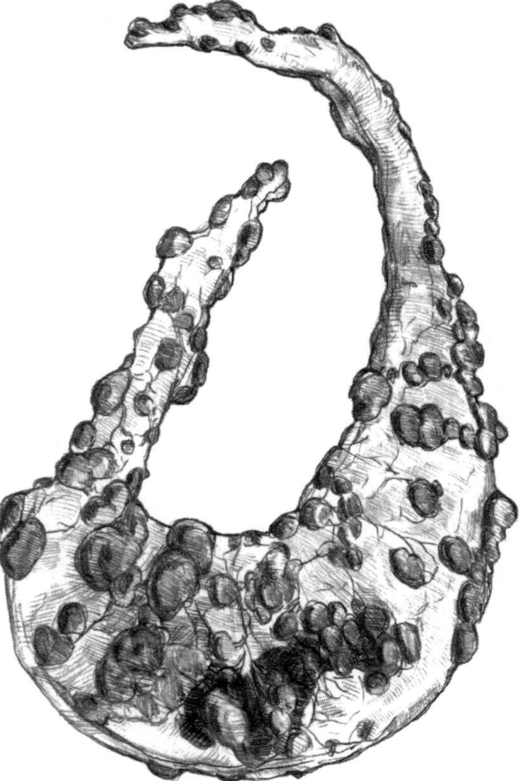

Conceptus at 90 days of gestation. *The fetus is surrounded by the placenta, and the cotyledons are becoming larger.*

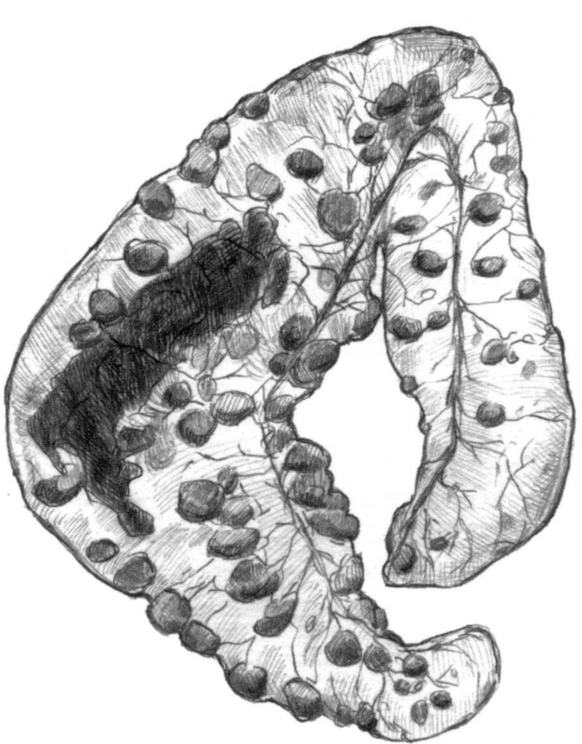

Conceptus at 115 days of gestation. *By this stage, the fetus itself can sometimes be felt by rectal palpation, floating in fluid in the enlarging uterus.*

nose of the fetus may push the uterine wall into the pelvis a little, extending the uterus and its contents back over the top of the cervix.

Development of the Placenta

By days 40 to 60, the allantochorion sac attaches to the uterine lining, forming the *placenta*. Until then the embryo is nourished by *uterine milk* that seeps through the chorion and amnion. This thick, yellow-white fluid is secreted by uterine glands.

By Day 35 the allantochorion has many fingerlike protrusions, which contain capillary tufts that grow into corresponding tiny pits in the *caruncles* (little bumps) on the uterine lining.

Thus are formed the *cotyledons* (lumpy, dark red "buttons") that attach the placenta to the uterine lining. These are the many little doorways through which nutrients and gases (oxygen, carbon dioxide) are exchanged between fetus and mother cow: The cow's blood brings nutrients and oxygen and takes away waste products and carbon dioxide. There is no direct blood flow between mother and fetus; everything is filtered through the placenta.

There are about 120 cotyledons in the cow, arranged in four rows along each uterine horn. Since membranes surrounding the fetus extend into the nonpregnant horn, there are some cotyledons in that horn, too, providing more attachment for adequate exchange and nourishment for the growing fetus. Most of the allantoic fluid (the water in the *water bag*) is on either side of the fetus, with one end of the sac in the nonpregnant horn of the uterus. The fetus floats in the middle of this outer water bag, in its inner bubble of amniotic fluid, attached only by the *umbilical cord*.

The fluid within these membranes around the fetus increases throughout pregnancy (five quarts at five months and more than five gallons at term). The allantoic fluid is watery in contrast to the amniotic fluid in the sac directly surrounding the calf, which, by the final third of gestation, becomes thicker and more mucuslike. This gives the amniotic fluid more lubricating ability, which is helpful during birth. Further, while the outer water-bag membrane is thin and transparent, the inner amnion sac is thicker and tougher.

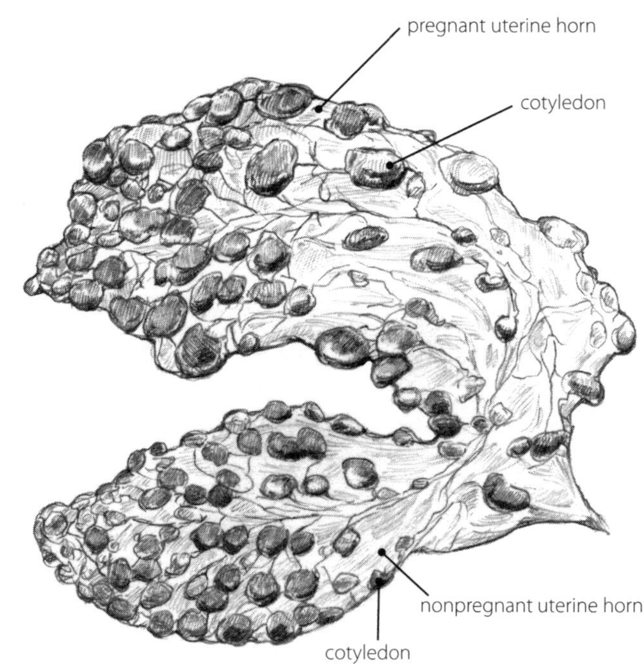

The placenta of the cow; cotyledons in the nonpregnant horn of the uterus are smaller.

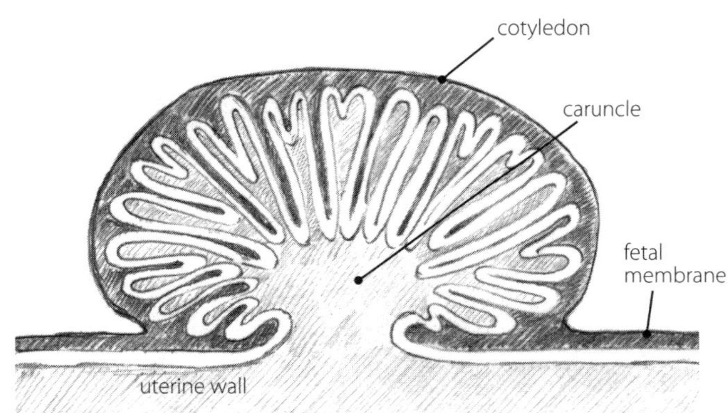

Placentome of the cow showing the cotyledon and the maternal caruncle.

The cow's blood brings nutrients and oxygen and takes away waste products and carbon dioxide. There is no direct blood flow between mother and fetus; everything is filtered through the placenta.

Selecting a Vet

If you don't already have a veterinarian who does your cattle work, find one before your cows start calving — and don't wait until you have an emergency. A vet who does only small-animal work won't be the best one to help with a fetal or calving problem or pregnancy detection. A vet who does a lot of bovine pregnancy checking will be much more accurate than a vet who does this only occasionally.

Also keep in mind that large-animal work sometimes requires long arms and a lot of strength. A difficult calving, for example, is easier for a vet to resolve if he/she is not only well practiced in bovine obstetrics but also able to manipulate a calf whose turned-back head or breech-presented legs are out of reach for a short-armed person.

If you are new to the area, ask around. Check with your neighbors or ask at the local feed store or county agent's office for names of stockmen to query. Those who have been in business a long time will have experience with the various vets in the area and some definite opinions about which ones are the best for cattle work.

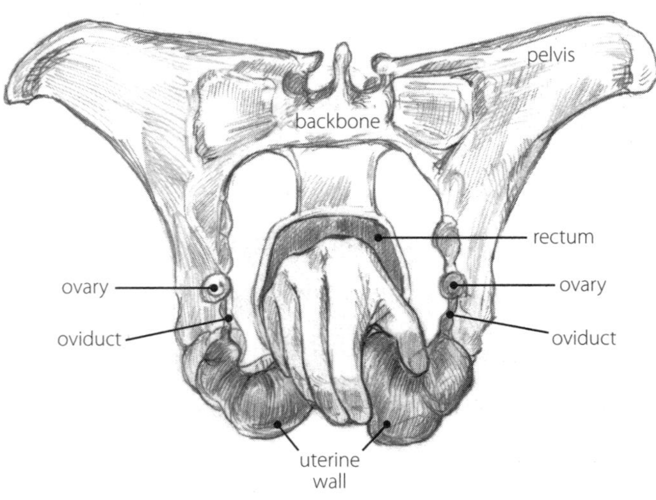

A view of the uterus in a cow that's not pregnant (lookingfrom inside the cow, toward her rear end). The reproductive tract can be easily palpated via the rectum (situated directly above it) for pregnancy checking or to determine the health and status of the ovaries.

Pregnancy Diagnosis

It's helpful to check your cows a few months after breeding season to determine if there are any that didn't become pregnant.

Some of these will be obvious; you'll see them continue to cycle, being ridden by other cattle. If a bull is still with the herd, these cows may be *repeat breeders,* breeding again late in the season. If they have a problem that interferes with fertility, they may not settle, though, no matter how many times they are bred. You should cull open cows or late calvers.

An open cow is a freeloader, robbing profit from the rest of the herd. A cow that calves late in the year may have a problem that makes her less fertile, and she may be open or late again the next year. Calves born later than the rest won't be large enough to sell with the group. In a spring-calving herd, a late calf must be kept through winter, at greater expense.

Veterinary Examination

Pregnancy and stage of gestation can be definitively determined using ultrasound or rectal palpation.

Ultrasound can detect pregnancy earlier than palpation, sometimes as early as 13 days after breeding, but is more expensive. Most stockmen have their veterinarian check cows via rectal examination when cows are put through the chute for their semiannual vaccinations in the fall. If cows are bred in spring or early summer, the pregnancy can readily be detected during a fall working. Clues as to whether a cow is pregnant can be detected via rectal palpation as early as 35 days and definitely by 45 days of gestation.

The veterinarian can *palpate* (feel with her fingers) the reproductive tract (ovaries, uterus, uterine arteries) through the rectal wall. For instance, the position of the ovaries will change as pregnancy advances; the increased weight of the uterus pulls them deeper into the abdominal cavity. Similarly, as we've discovered, after the fifth month of gestation, the weight and size of the uterus cause it to sink down to rest on the abdominal floor.

The increased size of the uterus (if it can still be reached and felt via the rectum) is a clue that the cow is pregnant; in most cases this enlargement can be easily determined within 90 days of pregnancy, and

PREGNANCY DETERMINATION BY RECTAL PALPATION

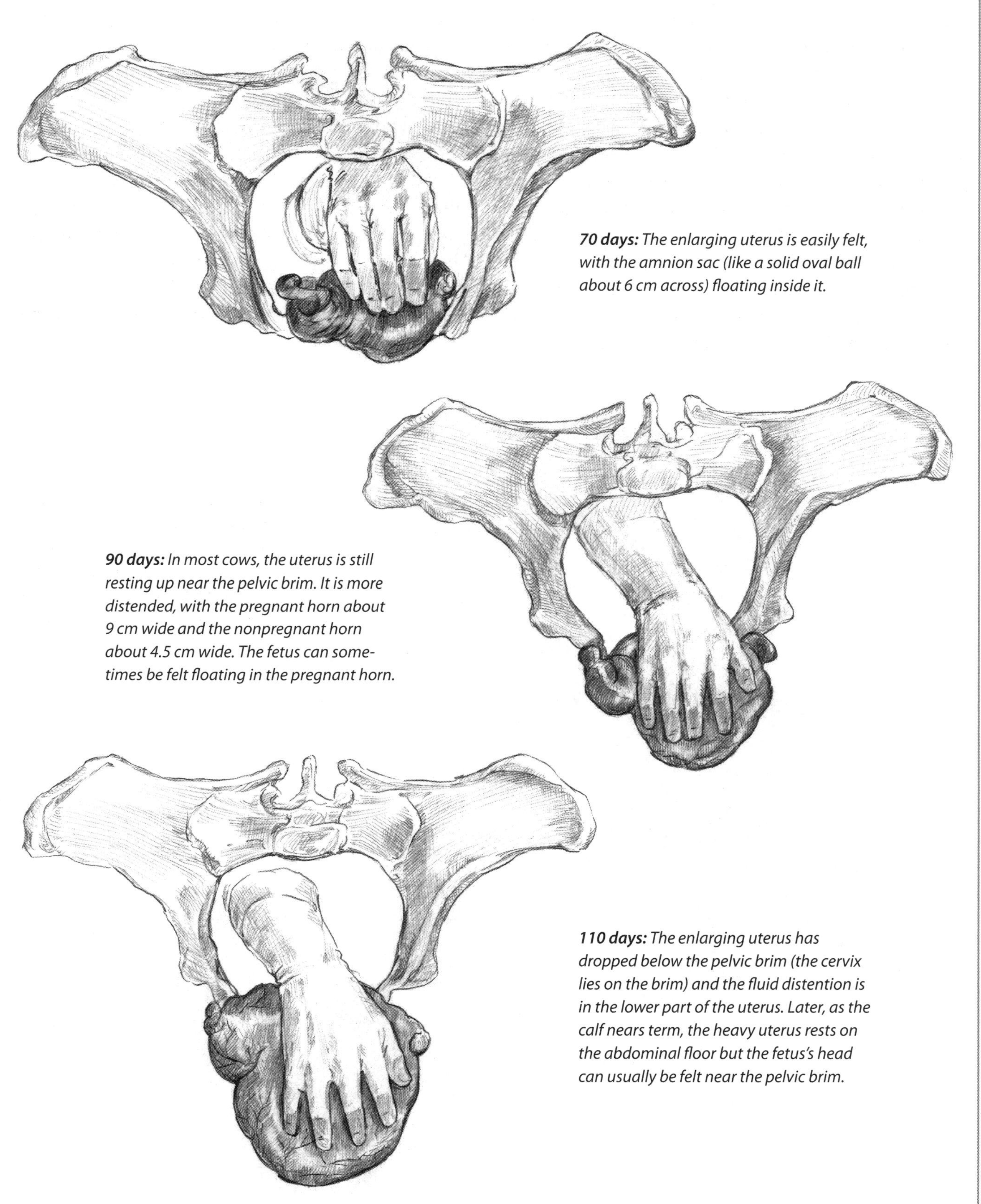

70 days: *The enlarging uterus is easily felt, with the amnion sac (like a solid oval ball about 6 cm across) floating inside it.*

90 days: *In most cows, the uterus is still resting up near the pelvic brim. It is more distended, with the pregnant horn about 9 cm wide and the nonpregnant horn about 4.5 cm wide. The fetus can sometimes be felt floating in the pregnant horn.*

110 days: *The enlarging uterus has dropped below the pelvic brim (the cervix lies on the brim) and the fluid distention is in the lower part of the uterus. Later, as the calf nears term, the heavy uterus rests on the abdominal floor but the fetus's head can usually be felt near the pelvic brim.*

sometimes it is even possible to palpate the tiny fetus within the uterus.

From 4 to 5½ months of gestation, it's possible to feel the fetus about half the time. Between 5½ and 7½ months, however, it becomes more difficult to reach the uterus. If the veterinarian can reach far enough, he or she may be able to touch the fetus's head or flexed limbs that lie just beyond the pelvic brim. If touched, the fetus will usually move.

From 7½ months until the end of gestation, it's easier to feel the fetus. It has grown so much in size that the front legs are closer to the pelvis, unless the cow is deep-bodied and has had many calves and her uterus is way down in her abdomen. If the pregnant uterus cannot be reached, there are other indications that the cow is pregnant. The vet can feel some of the cotyledons attaching the placenta to the uterus. In addition, the uterine arteries become larger and have a strong vibrating pulse.

A vet who palpates many cows is generally fairly accurate in the diagnosis of a pregnancy, whereas a vet who is not experienced may misjudge a few cows. He or she may call an open cow pregnant or vice versa. An experienced bovine practitioner can also tell you the stage of gestation with fair accuracy in most cases. The best determination of a cow's due date, however, is good breeding records. If you know when a cow was actually bred (if she did, indeed, become pregnant), you'll know just when to expect her to calve.

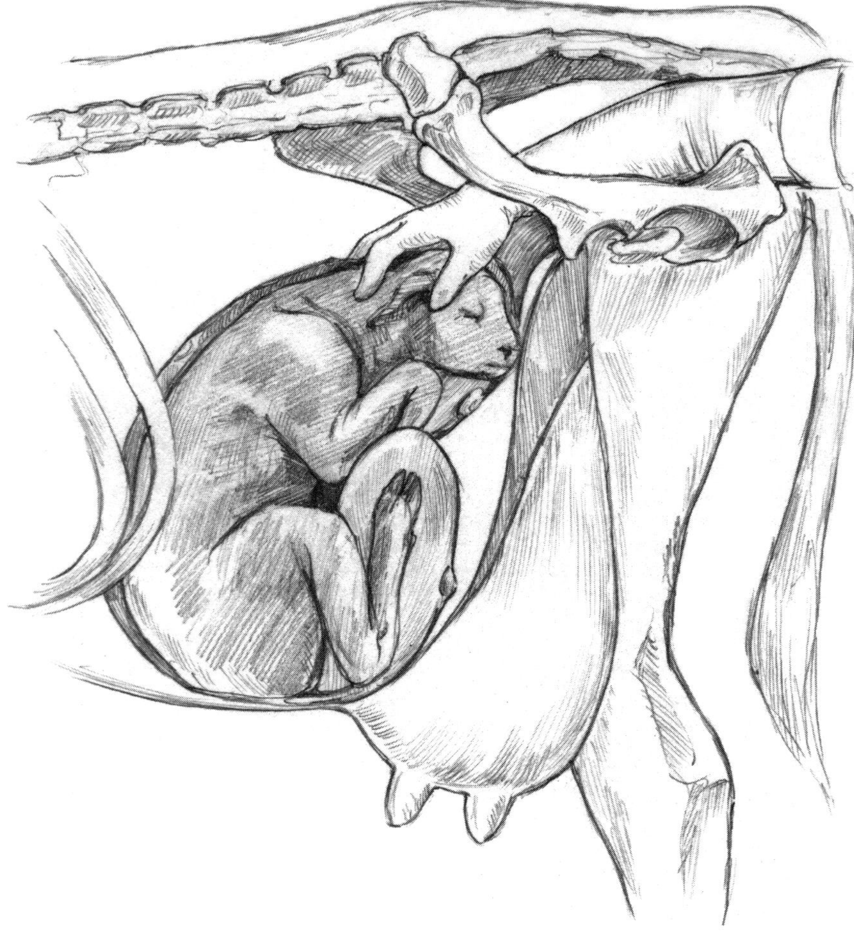

Palpating the uterus via the rectum; size and position of the uterus and fetus approaching full term. *The fetus and uterus have enlarged to the point where the fetus is in easy reach. If the fetus is in proper position, its head can be easily felt.*

Observation

You might find clues to indicate that the cow or heifer is pregnant, such as increase in belly size during late gestation. Some cows or heifers, however, will not look very pregnant and can fool you.

Changes in the udder can also be seen, especially in heifers. Teats begin to enlarge in about the fourth month of gestation in many heifers, and in the sixth month, the udder begins to develop. This swelling is progressive, and many heifers have a large udder for at least a month before calving. They may also develop swelling along the belly just in front of the udder. As with belly size, however, a few heifers may not have much udder development until the end of gestation.

The Blood Test

A simple way to check for pregnancy involves taking a blood sample from a vein under the cow's or heifer's tail. Fill a small (3 to 5 ml) vial with the blood following your vet's instructions. Send the samples to a lab, where they will use the BioPRYN test to detect the presence of a pregnancy-specific protein secreted by the placenta. The results of this accurate test are often ready within 48 hours.

The advantages to the blood test are convenience and lower expense, especially when checking only a few cows. Drawing the blood yourself saves you the cost of a veterinarian's visit and the blood test can be performed at 30 days after breeding, compared to the 45- to 90-day wait before a palpation can be performed. Blood tests are actually safer for the cow and the embryo or fetus than rectal examination. For more information regarding the blood test, check the company's website at *www.biotracking.com.*

Care of the Bred Heifer or Cow

To ensure a safe and healthy pregnancy, a bred heifer or cow needs proper care.

- Make sure pregnant cattle have an adequate and well-balanced diet with no vitamin or mineral deficiencies. Your local Extension service, feed companies, or private consultants can answer questions about nutrition. If the pregnant cow is nursing a calf, the cow needs adequate feed or good pasture to provide her nutrient needs. Even though her need for extra feed for the fetus will be minimal until the last trimester, her demands will be great if she is feeding her present calf.
- Heifers bred for their first calf need excellent nutrition because they're still growing. The demands of pregnancy are not as great as the needs of their own body to reach adequate size and maturity before calving. The heifer especially needs protein and energy for growth between weaning and calving so that she'll reach at least 80 to 85 percent of her mature size and weight by the time she calves as a two-year-old. Heifers should reach 65 percent of their mature weight by breeding time (at about 15 months of age) and 85 percent by calving (at 24 months). If a heifer will mature at 1,100 to 1,200 pounds, she should weigh at least 715 to 780 pounds when she's bred and 935 to 1,020 when she calves. A heifer that is well grown (but not fat) will be better able to give birth without difficulty than a heifer that's undernourished and too small for her age.
- Control *parasites,* and vaccinate at the appropriate stages of pregnancy. If vaccinations are up to date, a cow is less likely to suffer loss of pregnancy from infectious disease and will be able later to create for her just-born calf the antibodies that accumulate in her *colostrum* at the end of gestation. Ask your veterinarian to help you create an appropriate vaccination and parasite-control program.
- If the cow is feeding a calf, he should be weaned before the cow reaches the final stages of gestation. For example, if her present calf was born in February and she was rebred in May, her calf should be weaned by November at the latest to make sure the cow has a chance to recover body condition and to provide adequately for her growing fetus.

Chapter 2

Problems That May Occur during Pregnancy

When a cow or heifer is bred and settled, sometimes pregnancy is terminated early due to the death of the conceptus. In other instances, a cow may give birth to a fetus that is not mature or healthy enough to be viable or she may calve prematurely, making it necessary for the calf to have intensive care to survive. This chapter discusses what can go wrong during gestation and why.

Abnormalities of Gestation

Many factors influence embryonic and fetal development. Vulnerability of the developing conceptus and certain developmental problems vary at different stages of pregnancy.

While the embryo travels down the fallopian tube to the uterus, it is safe from harmful influences. When it reaches the uterus, however, it's more exposed, and also susceptible to problems because it's growing so rapidly, with differentiation of various tissues and systems.

Each organ has a critical period of development during which it can be altered by harmful external influences. Many organs can be damaged early (in the embryonic stage) whereas others — such as parts of the heart, brain, and urinary/genital tract that develop later in gestation — are more vulnerable in these later fetal stages.

Abnormal Development

Some *congenital* defects (those that exist at birth) in calves are due to accidents in development caused by *teratogens* (any factor that causes an abnormality in a developing embryo or fetus). The teratonic agent may produce abnormalities that make it impossible for the calf to survive after birth. Teratogens, introduced by the herdsman or other cattle or found in the surrounding environment, include drugs, hormones, chemicals, viruses, toxic plants, and high temperature.

Some abnormalities cause birthing problems if the fetus is deformed. Joints may be fused in a *lupine* deformity (see chapter 15), meaning the calf's legs can't be straightened enough to come through the birth canal. In a defect called *schistosoma reflexus,* a fetus's backbone bends (with the tail close to the head) and the chest and abdomen are incompletely formed, exposing internal organs.

Sometimes a normal fetus has an abnormal twin attached to the fetal membranes. Because this *fetal mole* or *acardiac monster,* a mass of connective tissue (often with skin and hair) has no sex organs, it doesn't pose the threat of freemartin development of the normal calf. Other examples of abnormalities in calves that may hinder birth are cases of a *double monster* (two-headed calf), a hydrocephalic calf (one with an enlarged forehead), and a calf with extra legs.

MISCELLANEOUS BIRTH DEFECTS

Congenital abnormalities may be caused by hormone imbalance in the dam, genetics (inherited defects), nutritional deficiencies, or overdoses of certain elements of diet. Teratogens, agents such as chemicals, drugs, infections, and plant poisons that affect the normal growth of the embryo or fetus when encountered by the dam at certain stages of development, may cause problems when the various organs and body parts are forming.

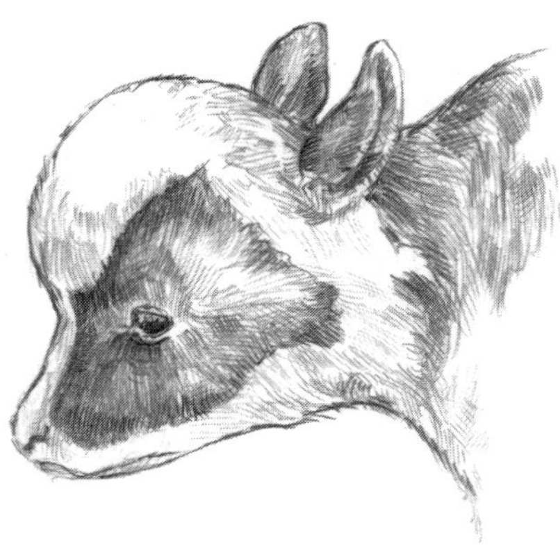

Hydrocephalus. *A hydrocephalic calf is a calf born with too much fluid inside the skull. A calf that can still fit through the pelvis has a very mild case.*

Double monster. *The birth of a rare two-headed calf is an abnormality with an unknown cause.*

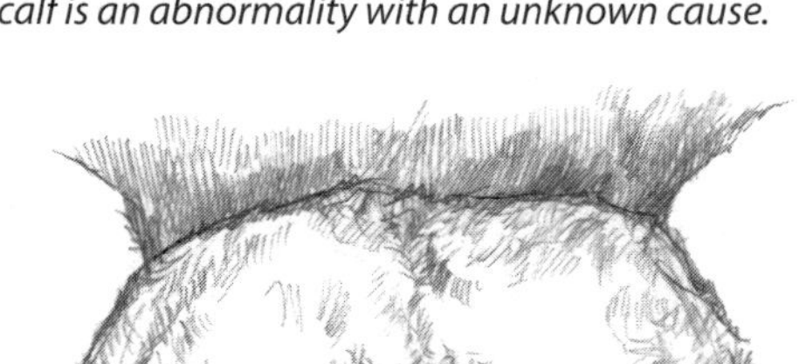

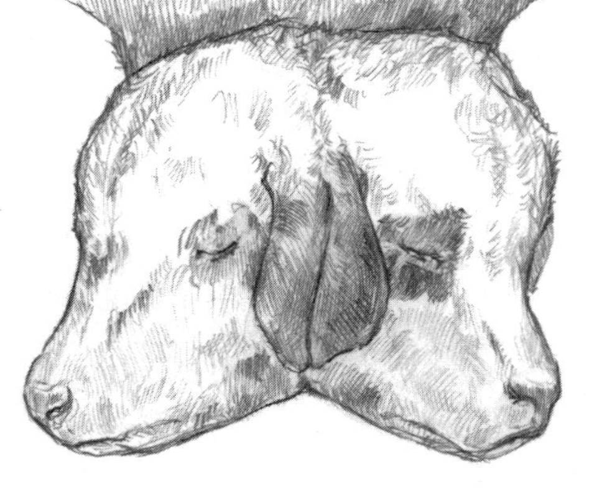

Otter calf. *Holsteins sometimes inherit the congenital defect that results in the birth of calves with no legs.*

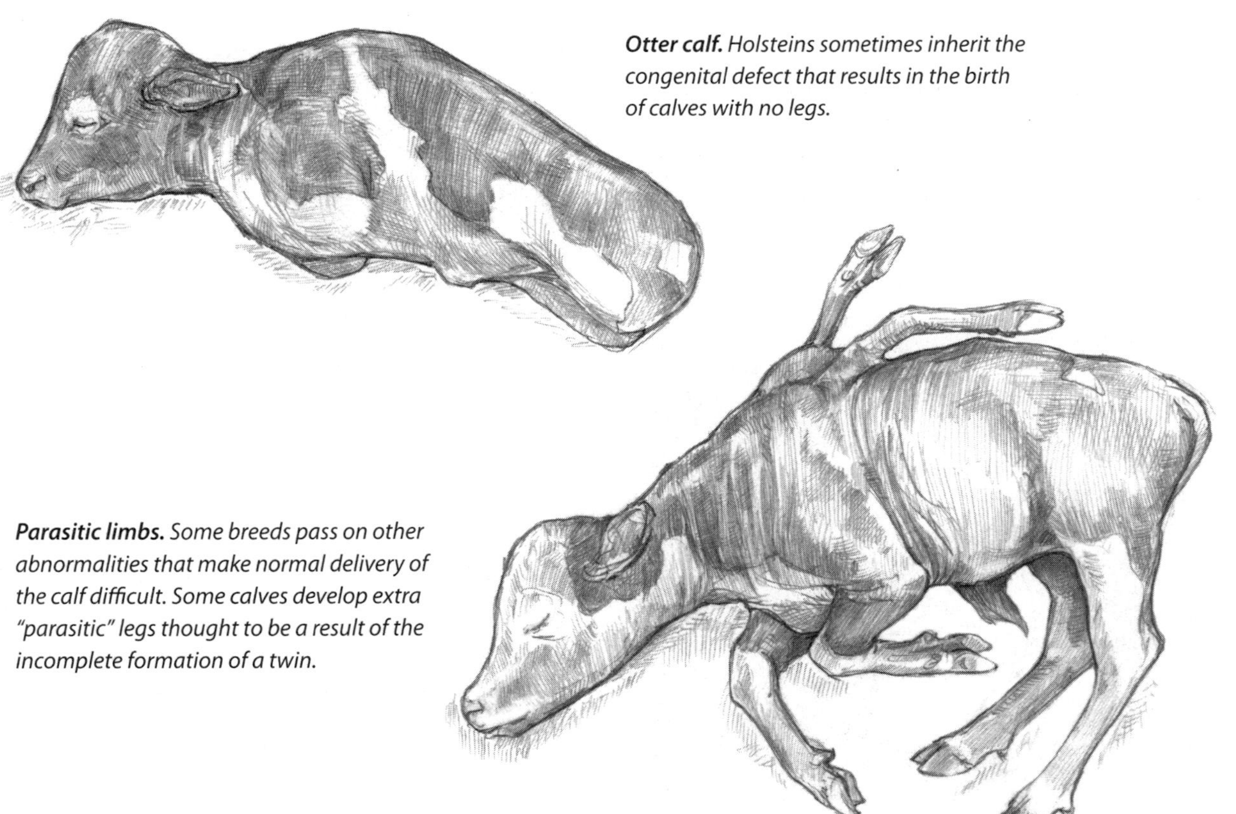

Parasitic limbs. *Some breeds pass on other abnormalities that make normal delivery of the calf difficult. Some calves develop extra "parasitic" legs thought to be a result of the incomplete formation of a twin.*

OUR EXPERIENCE WITH HYDROCEPHALUS

THE FIRST HYDROCEPHALIC CALF from our herd was aborted at 7½ months of gestation. When we were hiking in our mountain pasture to check cattle, we discovered the aborted fetus, and its young mama, Salud, standing beside her dead baby, licking it. Due to the small size of the calf at that stage of her third pregnancy, Salud was able to pass the enlarged head through the birth canal without help, which was fortunate, since we were not expecting any calves yet and were not checking the cows very closely.

The only other case of hydrocephalus we've had was E.T., born in 2003 to Alvina, one of our son's cows. This calf was full term but small, and Alvina had him without assistance. His was a very mild case with only a slightly domed forehead, but he was not quite normal. He had trouble walking; he sometimes staggered sideways. He was able to live a relatively normal life, growing large enough to butcher. We kept him and his mother at home, off the range, in a small, flat pasture so E.T. wouldn't fall down the steep hillsides on our range pastures.

A calf with a forehead so large that he can't be born without assistance usually has so much fluid around the brain that he won't live very long. E.T. was not this bad, but he would never have made it to adulthood with his impairments. He survived the five months until butchering with very careful management.

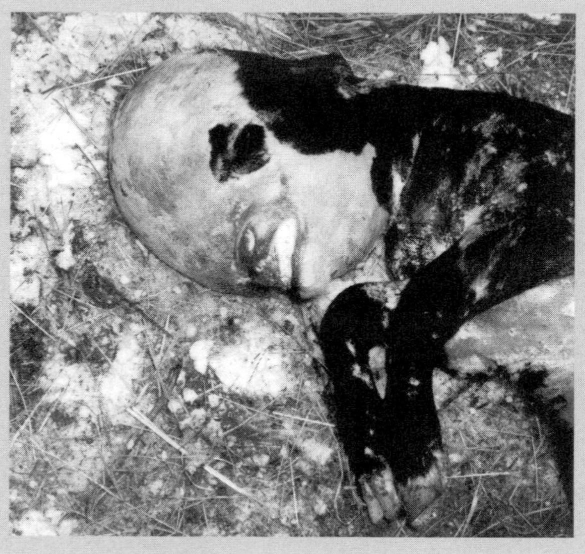

Some congenital defects are inherited: For example, *dwarfism* is seen in Angus and Hereford breeds, *otter calves* (calves with no legs) in Holsteins, double muscling in Charolais, and calves with *edema* (swelling) in the legs and head in Ayrshires.

Hydrocephalus

A fetus may develop a large forehead due to accumulation of fluid there (water on the brain). If the calf goes full term, the front of the head is usually too big to fit through the cow's pelvis. Your vet may deliver him by cesarean section (see chapter 5) or by making a hole in the forehead of the calf and compressing the skull to make it smaller (in extreme cases, the skull is very thin and easy to crush) to facilitate delivery through the birth canal. It's important to note that a hydrocephalic calf can't survive after he's born.

Excessive Fluid Surrounding the Fetus

On rare occasions either the amnion sac, surrounding the fetus, or the allantoic sac, the outer water bag, produces too much fluid.

Extra fluid in the amnion sac (a condition called *hydramnios*) is more rare and generally occurs only in Dexter cattle that have abnormal, "bulldog" calves (a hereditary condition that may produce the extra fluid as early as the third or fourth month of gestation).

She may become so weak or impaired by her large belly that she has trouble getting up and down. If she does survive to term, she generally needs help to calve.

Most instances of excess fluid in the outer water sac (*hydroallantois*) occur in the last trimester. The fetus is often small for this stage of gestation, and the condition is characterized by a sudden increase of fluid, which becomes noticeable when the cow develops a huge belly. The later this happens, the better chance of the cow surviving until the end of pregnancy. If her belly is

OUR EXPERIENCE WITH HYDROALLANTOIS

IN 1971, one of our Hereford cows, Red Cheeks, developed a large belly two months before she was due. We asked our vet if she might have twins. He told us it was more likely that she had excess fluid around the calf.

As her belly grew larger and it became harder for her to get up and down, the vet said she needed to have the calf early, and he gave her an injection to induce labor, telling us she'd need help to calve and that we should watch her and break her water to let fluid out.

We checked on her through the night, the next day, and the following night but saw no signs of labor — we didn't know that when the uterus is so distended, it can't contract strongly, and the cow might not show evidence of labor. After checking her the next day, we found that her cervix still was not dilated much; we could not yet reach a hand through it to break her water sac. The following day and night I kept looking at her — still no sign of labor — but at some point that night her uterus ruptured. The next time I looked out the window, she was lying dead in the calving pen.

When we talked with our vet later, he told us we could have reached through the small opening of the cervix with something to poke the water bag. If we had known what to do, we might have been able to save the cow.

distended as early as six to seven months of gestation, the cow's chances of survival are reduced because the large volume of fluid puts pressure on her lungs and digestive tract; she doesn't have room to breathe or eat much and, as a result, she loses weight. She may become so weak or impaired by her large belly that she has trouble getting up and down. If she does survive to term, she generally needs help to calve. Not only is she is weak, but also her uterus may not be able to contract properly because it is so distended, and the cervix may not dilate fully.

If it becomes obvious the cow is not going to make it to term, she should be humanely slaughtered. Your vet may choose to do a cesarean section (chapter 5) to save the cow and possibly the calf, if he is far enough along in gestation to survive, but the surgery must be performed carefully; the excess fluid must be allowed to escape slowly. If fluid rushes out of the uterus too fast, the cow may go into shock.

After the calf is removed by c-section or traction, the veterinarian should check to make sure there is not a second calf; twins are common in cases of hydroallantois, and the second calf is sometimes missed, particularly if traction is used.

Sometimes the calf in this situation is abnormal. Often he is undersize for his stage of gestation, as there may be a correlation between the extra fluid in the uterus and fewer numbers of cotyledons (attachments for the placenta), which means fewer nutrients coming to the calf via the bloodstream of the *dam* (the mother).

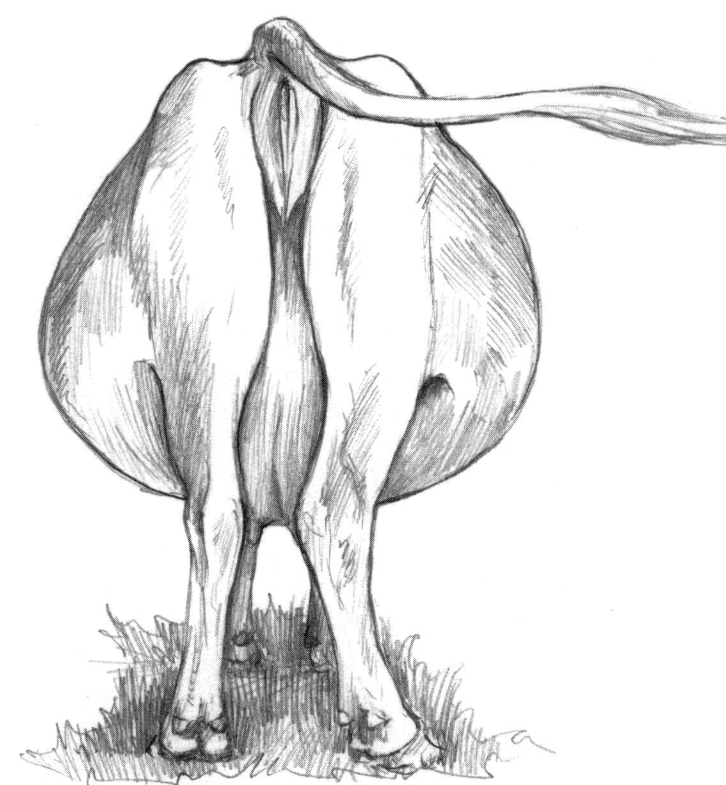

A cow with hydroallantois has too much fluid around the fetus and a distended uterus. This is a life-threatening condition.

Mummified Fetus

On occasion, death of a fetus does not result in abortion; the dead fetus remains in the uterus, but its mass can't be resorbed once it has developed bones. Sometimes, however, the fetal fluids are totally resorbed. The fetal membranes become dry and shriveled, and the uterus contracts around the dead fetus, which may become twisted and contorted.

In other instances the fetal membranes become surrounded by a thick, gummy, chocolate-colored material like dehydrated, coagulated blood. The longer the fetus has been dead, the less fluid there will be around it and its membranes. The tissues may become dry and leatherlike as a result of the lack of fluid.

Mummification, as described above, may occur any time between three and eight months of gestation. The CL in the ovary persists, and the cow's body still thinks and acts as if she's pregnant. The dead fetus remains in the uterus, and because it is no longer capable of sending hormone signals that trigger the beginning of labor, the cow may remain pregnant past her predicted calving date. This condition may be discovered only if you begin to wonder if the cow is really pregnant and you have her examined by a veterinarian.

After the condition is diagnosed, the vet can give the cow an injection of hormones to induce labor so she'll abort the dead fetus. This usually happens within two to four days after the injection. You must watch the cow, however, to make sure she does expel the fetus; otherwise, she may develop an infection in the uterus because her cervix is open to disease as a result of induced labor (see Fetal Maceration, page 41).

Sometimes a mummified fetus is expelled spontaneously close to what would be the end of gestation (you may see the dark red-brown membranes hanging from the vulva), but often the cow does not go into labor to abort the mummy, and labor must be induced.

On occasion, when a cow or heifer is carrying twins, one fetus will come to term normally while the second fetus will die and mummify. If this happens, the mummy is expelled along with the live twin when he's born.

Because there is no uterine infection associated with a mummified fetus, the cow generally comes back into heat after getting rid of the mummy, with good chances of successful pregnancy.

OUR EXPERIENCE WITH MUMMIFICATION

OUR FIRST EXPERIENCE with a mummified fetus occurred when our Holstein milk cow Baby Doll approached her due date, but her udder didn't fill and she didn't look pregnant. Our vet checked her and said she had a mummy and that the fetus had probably died more than four months earlier, at about 4½ months of gestation.

He gave her an injection to induce labor, and several days later we helped her deliver the tiny mummy.

Another time, a rattlesnake bit our cow Jana on the side of the face. The snakebite resulted in an infection and a high fever. Because she was so ill, I brought her three miles from our mountain pasture to the corral, where we took her temperature, which was 107°F (41.6°C). I gave her antibiotics, and also treated her with Banamine to reduce inflammation and fever. She would not eat or drink.

Three times a day we put a nasogastric tube into her stomach (via the nostril) so we could feed her a slurry of several gallons of water mixed with grain pellets we'd soaked up and mashed in the blender. This "soup" could be poured down the stomach tube with a big funnel. We fed her this way for six days, until she started eating and drinking again. We feared she would abort after such a high fever, but a few months later, she went into labor very near her due date. What emerged, however, was the mummified fetus that had died during her life-threatening septicemia and fever.

Prolonged Gestation

This can be caused by fetal mummification or by a live fetus that has an abnormality — part of the calf's brain is missing, for example, or the fetus has no pituitary gland to send a signal to the cow to begin the birth process. These fetal abnormalities interfere with the onset of labor. If a cow's labor is long overdue, she should be checked by a veterinarian.

Fetal Maceration

If a cow loses her pregnancy (the fetus dies, and she goes into labor to abort it) but she cannot expel the dead fetus, *maceration* occurs, meaning the soft tissue rots and is digested by bacteria.

Whenever the cervix opens, bacteria can enter the uterus. If during an abortion the uterus fails to push out the fetus because of the lack of uterine contractions, or because the cervix fails to dilate enough for the fetus to pass through, or because the fetus is in an abnormal position for birth through the cervix and vagina, bacteria that enter the uterus while the cervix is open become established in the fetal tissues and digest them, leaving only the bones.

If the infection is treated with antibiotics, the cow will usually recover, but you should allow plenty of time (three to four months) before she is rebred.

The result is swelling and rapid putrification of soft fetal tissues. The cow may strain or have a foul, reddish-gray discharge from the vulva. She may experience a fever and loss of appetite. Examination of her reproductive tract will reveal a distended, swollen fetus with tissues full of gas. The vet will have to remove the rotten fetus, which can be accomplished with careful, gentle traction and lots of lubrication if the cervix is still dilated. This can be a life-threatening condition. The cow must have antibiotics immediately after the fetus is removed.

If the cervix is not dilated enough to remove the dead fetus, the vet may give the cow hormones to relax the cervix so that the fetus can be removed in its entirety or in pieces without much danger of injury to the cow. If the infection is treated with antibiotics, the cow will usually recover, but you should allow plenty of time (three to four months) before she is rebred.

On occasion, you may not notice that the cow has attempted to abort a dead fetus, and in a long-standing case there may be no signs of illness if the infection remains contained within the uterus and does not seriously affect the cow herself. There may not be discharge from the vulva. In such instances, if the cow is examined rectally, the vet may feel the fetal bones floating freely in the uterus in pus or moving against each other. In these cases, there's little hope for recovery of the reproductive tract; the uterine lining becomes thick with degenerative changes and scar tissue. If a lot of pus is present, the cow can be treated with antibiotics and administered hormones to try to induce labor to expel the pus and bones, which may pass through the cervix with the pus.

Often in such cases, however, the amount of pus is small if the condition is long-standing, and the bones may be embedded in the uterine lining. The cervix may be very hard and will not dilate even when hormones are given to the cow. The longer the condition has existed, the greater the damage to the uterus and the poorer the chance for recovery. The cow will probably never be able to have another calf and should be culled to slaughter.

Becoming Pregnant

When a fertile bull is left with a cow herd for several months, there's a greater chance that nearly all the cows will be impregnated — even late calvers, slow breeders, and cows that suffer early embryo loss. Yet most stockmen don't want a long calving season, because often a late cow has a fertility problem. Even if she eventually settles, her calf next year will be born late, and may be too small to sell with the group. She will probably breed late again or come up open. It's best to cull her and replace her with a more fertile individual.

For a short calving season and a more uniform calf crop — and to weed out subfertile cows — many stockmen leave a bull with cows for only 45 days. This gives most cows an opportunity for two estrous cycles in case they don't settle on the first breeding or if they experience early embryo loss. With two chances, the fertile cows will be pregnant, and by culling the cows that are open after a 45-day breeding season, you can get rid of cows that always calve late. Since fertility is heritable, culling slow breeders and late calvers ensures that you keep only the heifers born of fertile cows.

Causes of Abortion

Pregnancy loss (early loss or resorption of an embryo or abortion of a fetus in later stages of gestation) can be triggered by many causes. *Abortion* is the expulsion of a premature, live fetus before it reaches a viable stage or expulsion of a dead fetus at any stage of gestation. If the loss occurs before 45 days of gestation, it's called *early embryonic death.*

Under normal conditions, one or two out of every 100 cows will abort for one reason or another, and these miscellaneous abortions are generally no cause for alarm regarding herd health. A single abortion is usually an isolated incident and represents something that went wrong with that cow. To play it safe with a cow that's had an abortion, however, quarantine her for a while in case she has a disease, and dispose of the aborted fetus properly — if you find it.

SIZE AND CHARACTERISTICS OF ABORTED FETUSES

Gestation Length	Description of Fetus
2 months	Size of a mouse
3 months	Size of a rat
4 months	Size of a small cat
5 months	Size of a large cat
6 months	Size of a small dog; hair around eyes, tail
7 months	Size of a beagle; fine hair on body and legs
8 months	Full hair coat; teeth slightly erupted
9 months	Full-size; incisors fully erupted

Many pregnancy losses in early gestation take place without being noticed; the embryo or fetus is not large enough to be observed. In very early gestation, the dead embryo may be resorbed by the cow's body rather than expelled or may come out with uterine fluid. Any time after two months of gestation, the fetus and placental tissues are usually expelled, but if a cow is at pasture and isn't closely observed, you may not notice.

Pregnancy Loss at Different Stages of Gestation

Many pregnancy losses occur early, and a cow returns to heat on schedule. If the embryo dies after it has attached to the uterine lining, however, and the cow's body has recognized the pregnancy, it may be longer before she comes back in heat. If embryo death is due to uterine infection, it's usually followed by *pyometra* (pus in the uterus). The cow has a closed cervix (no discharge), the CL on the ovary persists, she does not come back into heat, and you'll assume she's pregnant.

A single abortion is usually an isolated incident and represents something that went wrong with that cow. To play it safe with a cow that's had an abortion, however, quarantine her for a while in case she has a disease, and dispose of the aborted fetus properly — if you find it.

Early Losses

Early losses may be caused by a variety of factors, and sometimes the causes of these losses are never identified.

Defective embryos, genetic or otherwise. Embryos may be genetically defective or defective for some other reason and may not survive. In fertile cows the conception rate is greater than 90 percent when bred by a fertile bull, but by the time the cows are far enough along in gestation to detect pregnancy (any time after 45 days when palpated rectally or after 13 to 28 days when checked with ultrasound), there may be only 70 to 80 percent that are actually pregnant from any single service. The other 20 to 30 percent may have had defective embryos, or some other factor (such as heat stress) influenced the loss.

If cows are with a bull long enough to have a chance to rebreed, those that experienced early embryo loss have another opportunity for a viable pregnancy. In a herd of healthy, fertile cows, more than 90 percent of them should be safely pregnant after 45 days if they have two chances to breed.

Heat stress. This may cause early pregnancy loss in a hot, humid climate. To avoid this stress, acquire heat-resistant breeds (see chapter 1, page 18).

Malnourishment. In a drought or any instance when cows are severely undernourished, conception rates are reduced, and cows already pregnant are at a higher risk for early embryonic loss.

Miscommunicating hormones. Pregnancy loss can also be due to miscommunicated hormonal signals between the growing embryo and the tissue that becomes the placenta, especially if the CL on the ovary isn't maintained. As shown in chapter 1 (page 6), the CL is an important key to continuation of pregnancy because it produces progesterone. If the level of progesterone in the cow's body drops too low, she will come back into heat and lose the pregnancy.

Once the pregnancy has passed 60 days, it is usually considered safe from hormonal changes, because the CL remains on the ovary and keeps progesterone levels high. Nevertheless, the cow is vulnerable to other causes of pregnancy loss for a variety of reasons, the most common being some type of infection.

Multiple Births a Few Weeks or Months Apart

In some instances, a pregnant cow comes back in heat, producing yet another egg that's capable of being fertilized, and is rebred. If this happens, the embryo or fetus she is already carrying may be lost.

Changes in the uterus during this heat period endanger the already growing embryo or fetus, though in some cases it survives and the later conceptus does not, and you wonder why the cow calves so early when you saw her rebred later.

More rarely, cows have given birth to another healthy calf a month or more after the original one! Instead of being aborted, the first one continues to grow and the second conceptus is successfully implanted in the uterus, probably in the other horn. The cow thus carries two calves at different stages of development. Usually birth of the first calf would terminate the gestation of the second, younger one, because labor affects both fetuses. But if the second is in the other horn of the uterus, there's a chance it might not be kicked out when the full-term calf is born. It may continue to grow and develop and be born at a later date.

Though very rare, a double pregnancy can confound the cow's owner when the cow suddenly gives birth to another calf a few weeks or months after the arrival of the first.

Noninfectious Causes of Abortion

Noninfectious factors that can cause a cow to lose her pregnancy range from genetic abnormalities (see page 36) to malnutrition.

Malnutrition

If cows are underfed during early pregnancy, they may abort. Being undernourished can also make a cow more susceptible to other problems, including infectious disease, which may cause death of the embryo or fetus.

Injury or Stress

Some abortions in late pregnancy are due to injury or stress. Severe stress triggers production of hormones, including *cortisol,* a natural *steroid* that helps an animal cope with the short-term effects of stress but also may cause the cow to go into labor and calve prematurely.

Some people worry that an injury, such as falling on ice or being jabbed in the belly by another cow while fighting, might hurt the fetus and cause abortion, but the fetus is well protected. It floats in fluid in the uterus, buffered from severe bumps and jolts. Usually, when a cow aborts following injury, she does so from the flood of cortisol in her body triggered by the stress of pain, inflammation, and blood loss, rather than from the injury itself.

Avoid using steroids such as dexamethasone because they can cause a cow to go into labor and deliver her calf prematurely. Dexamethasone is sometimes given to cattle to help reduce swelling, inflammation, and pain from injury or disease, but it should not be given to pregnant cows.

Fever

Fever from any cause, including heat stress or inflammation, can make a cow abort. If she has fever higher than 106°F (41°C) for any length of time, the uterine environment grows too hot for the developing embryo or fetus. If a cow is sick, she might abort from stress, but it is always worth treating the pain and fever with an eye to saving the pregnancy. Treatment with Banamine, harmless to the fetus, can help reduce pain, fever, and inflammation and thus reduce stress and the risk of abortion.

Poisons and Toxins

Poisons such as iodine found in the environment or introduced by the herdsman can cause pregnancy loss. Sodium iodide is given *intravenously* (IV) to treat *bony lump jaw,* an infection that settles in the bone, creating enlargement and drainage that is difficult to clear up, but there is risk of abortion when a pregnant cow receives this treatment.

Locoweed

Toxins in certain plants can also cause abortion. *Locoweed* (a leguminous plant of western North America) may cause abortion at any stage of gestation. Small amounts of this plant may cause deformities in the calf, but large amounts generally result in abortion. Cattle eat locoweed when other, more palatable plants are scarce, such as in the early spring. Although the evidence is not conclusive, some scientists believe that once cattle start eating the toxic plant, they become addicted and seek it out, even when good forage is available.

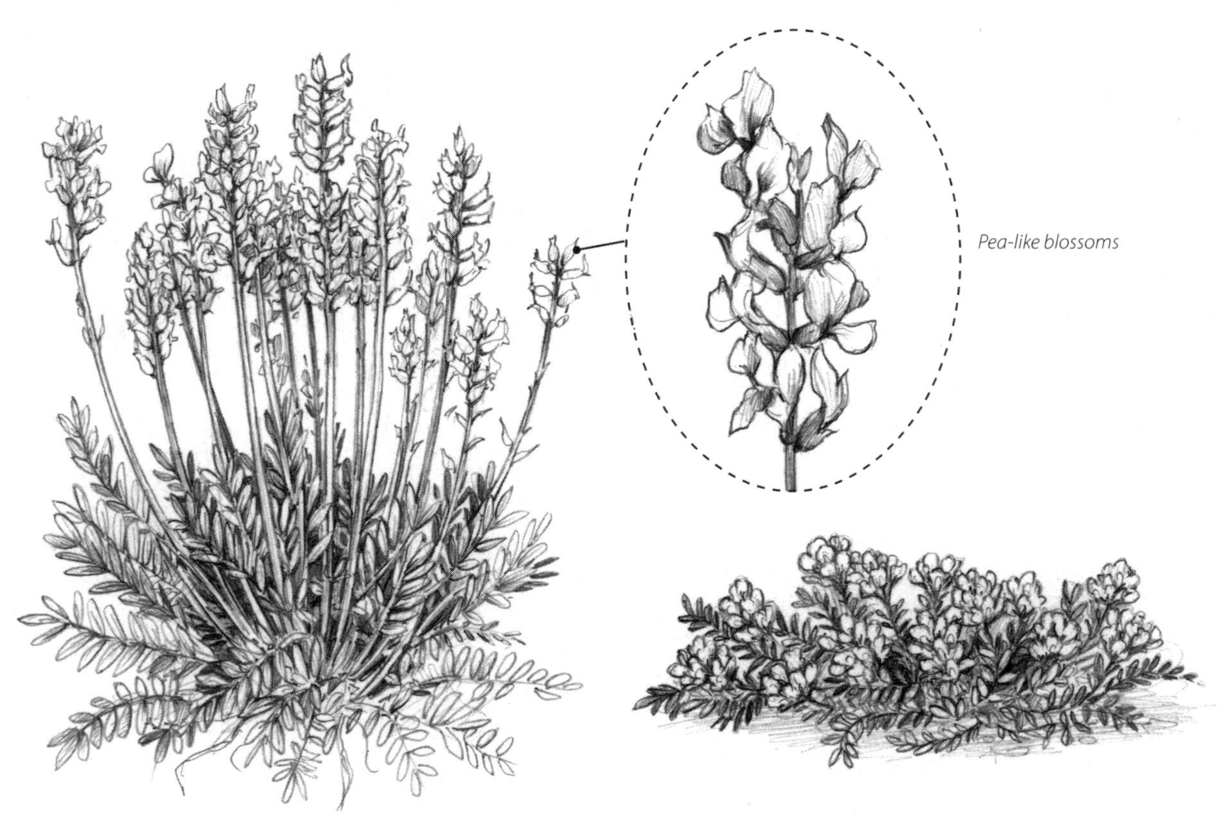

Wild-growing locoweed varies greatly in height and color, but all species are toxic and can cause birth defects and even abortion if ingested by pregnant cows and heifers.

Ponderosa Pine

Abortion may occur in the last trimester if a pregnant cow eats Ponderosa pine needles during that period. She may abort a few days after ingestion or up to two weeks later. If the calf is born alive, he's usually premature, weak, and small, and may die soon after birth. *Retained placenta* (failure to shed fetal membranes after birth) is quite common as a result of a pregnant cow or heifer eating Ponderosa pine needles. Be aware that it may take the cow two to three weeks to *clean* (shed the placenta; see chapter 6).

Because Ponderosa pine trees grow in every western state, with stands stretching from Canada to Mexico and with greater distribution than any other native tree except Douglas fir, this type of abortion is common. Cattle usually don't eat the needles in summer but may during winter, when the weather is cold, either directly from low branches or felled trees or by ingesting dried needles on the ground. Don't be fooled into thinking that brown and brittle needles are harmless to the cow herd. They are just as toxic as green ones.

A pregnant cow that has eaten these needles may have excessive vaginal discharge or bleeding, very little mammary development, incomplete dilation of the cervix and birth canal, weak uterine contractions, and a difficult birth. Because of these complications, she may develop serious infection and thus need antibiotics along with hormones to help her shed the placenta. If the cow's calf is born alive, he may need colostrum from a source other than his sick mama, antibiotics, and intensive supportive care.

Because Ponderosa pine trees grow in every western state, with stands stretching from Canada to Mexico, and with greater distribution than any other native tree except Douglas fir, retained placenta abortion is common.

To prevent problems, keep pregnant cattle (especially those in late gestation) out of pastures that contain Pondorosa pine trees.

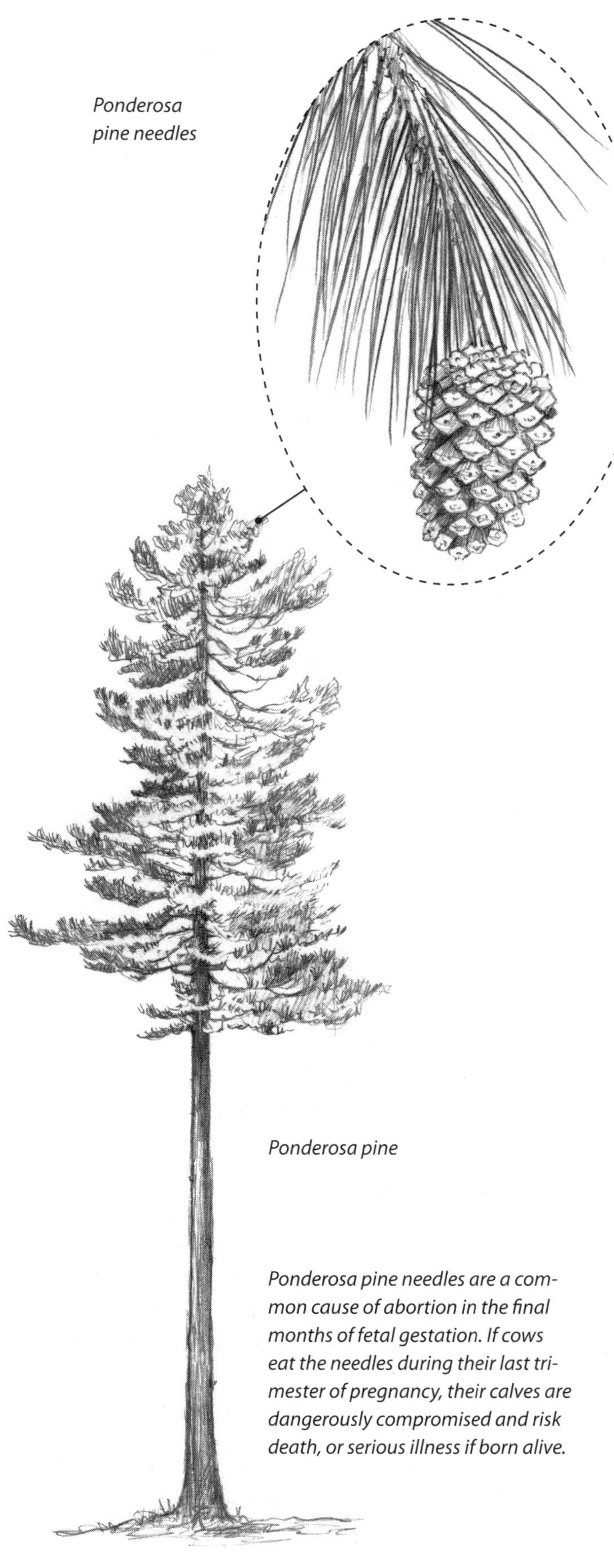

Ponderosa pine needles are a common cause of abortion in the final months of fetal gestation. If cows eat the needles during their last trimester of pregnancy, their calves are dangerously compromised and risk death, or serious illness if born alive.

Broom Snakeweed

Broom snakeweed may also cause abortion. It is a low-growing, sticky-leaved shrub that grows in great abundance in the southwestern United States and Mexico and on the prairies of Canada. Cattle consume the brush when forage is scarce in winter.

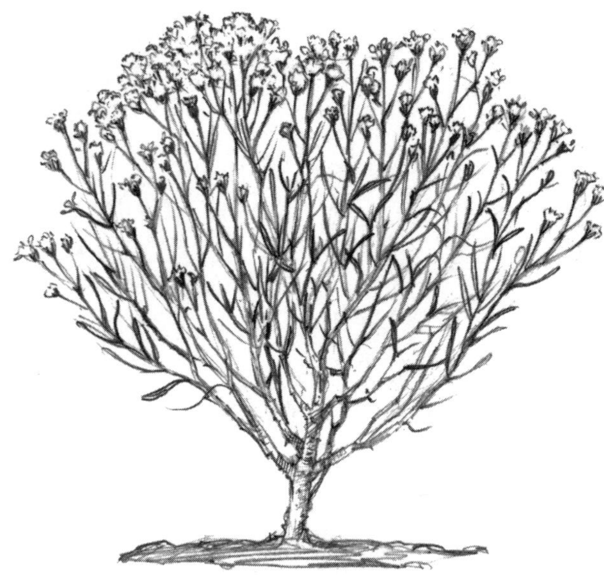

Broom snakeweed

> ## Collecting Abortion Samples
>
> Because it should be done as soon after the abortion as possible, collect samples from an aborting cow yourself if your vet isn't available.
>
> Find the aborted fetus if you can, and collect at least part of the placenta, using sterile gloves. Don't wash the tissues. Put them in plastic bags and refrigerate but don't freeze them.
>
> Make a note of the cow or cows that aborted. Contact your vet to find out where the samples should be sent for testing and how to do it, or take them to your vet's in a cooler so that he or she can send them for you.

Mold

Sweet clover is often blamed for abortion, but the culprit is actually a mold on the clover. In fact, moldy sweet clover hay or silage causes more abortions than does actually eating the growing plant.

Some molds are dangerous to the fetus during the third through seventh months of gestation, whereas *Aspergillus* causes abortion in the last trimester. Molds are thought to cause between 3 and 10 percent of abortions in cattle.

The signs of the mother cow's mold ingestion may include lesions on the aborted fetus (gray-white, thickened patches that look like ringworm) and on the placenta, a discolored placenta (gray, yellow, or red-brown), and abnormal cotyledons (which may be thick, wrinkled, or leathery). The only abortion we've had from mold occurred when we were feeding silage we'd purchased from another farm because we'd run short on hay that year. Some of it was quite moldy, and as a result, one of our cows aborted a seven-month-old fetus.

Infectious Causes of Abortion

The most common cause of pregnancy loss at any stage of gestation is infection from contamination of the uterus. A viral or bacterial disease in the cow at certain stages of pregnancy when the embryo or fetus is vulnerable to that particular disease is also a likely cause of abortion. The cow may not be very sick with the disease herself — sometimes, for instance, *leptospirosis* (see page 50) is very mild — but if it affects her unborn calf, she may abort.

Infection within the Reproductive Tract

Cows are hardy — compared to mares, for instance — and generally throw off infection introduced at calving time, but occasionally an infection becomes well established (chapter 6) and terminates a cow's next pregnancy early or causes infertility. There is also the risk that an infection following calving will be severe enough to kill the cow if it gains access to the circulatory system.

Placentitis. Premature separation of the placenta from the uterus is sometimes caused by inflammation, or *placentitis,* which may be due to viral or bacterial infection. Sometimes, however, the cause of the separation is never determined.

Injury during calving. A cow may develop an infection in the vagina or uterus, perhaps from injury to the tissues during a difficult birth.

Introduction of contamination. Dirty hands may introduce infection at calving if anyone has to reach into the uterus to reposition the calf.

Cervical-plug failure. Infection may terminate a pregnancy if the cervical seal is broken for any reason. The cervical plug, created by high progesterone levels early on, is responsible for sealing off the uterus from the vagina. If the cervical seal is compromised, bacteria from the vagina may contaminate the uterus. If bacteria gain access to the vulnerable uterus, this generally causes death of the fetus, and it will be aborted.

DANGERS OF DEXAMETHASONE

ONE SEPTEMBER, VERONICA, A 13-YEAR-old cow became ill on our summer range. When we discovered her, she was breathing fast, with her head and neck outstretched. We slowly eased her down the canyon two miles, but she could go no farther, so we rode home and borrowed a stock trailer, put a halter on her, and pulled her into the trailer so that we could haul her the seven miles home. We took her temperature, which was very high, and called our vet to describe her symptoms.

He advised us to treat her with antibiotics and anti-inflammatory drugs to try to ease her pain and fever. She had swelling in her neck and throat; it wasn't a typical pneumonia. Our vet suggested giving dexamethasone to help reduce the swelling. We also sprayed her with water several times a day because the weather was hot and she was panting and struggling to breathe. We thought about giving her fluids by stomach tube but were afraid the passage of a tube into either her throat or nose would impair her breathing and stress her even more. So we restricted our supportive care to trying to keep her cool.

Several days later, she felt better, enough to eat and drink, but she also aborted her 4½-month-old fetus. The dexamethasone had possibly helped save the cow but caused her to abort her baby.

Diseases That May Cause Pregnancy Loss or Abortion

If the abortion rate in a herd exceeds 1 or 2 percent, there's the likelihood that an infectious disease is involved, and you should get help from your vet to try to determine the cause. The vet can aid you in taking samples of aborted tissues and sending them to a diagnostic lab.

Several common diseases that cause abortion can be prevented by vaccination, but if your herd has not been vaccinated against a certain disease before, and has no immunity, vaccination may not be very effective in the short term and in the face of an outbreak. In this situation, enlist the help of your veterinarian for ways to minimize your losses, and begin a vaccination program to prevent future outbreaks and losses. These diseases may be bacterial, viral, or protozoan.

Bovine Virus Diarrhea (BVD)

Bovine virus diarrhea (BVD) is caused by a virus that has several strains and types, some of which are *cytopathic,* which means they are able to alter tissue cells, causing death of an embryo or fetus or birth defects, and some of which are *noncytopathic*, or unable to alter the tissue cells.

How it's spread. BVD is spread via contact with an infected animal's secretions or discharges, including saliva, nasal discharge, urine, semen, and discharge from coughing, or from a persistently infected carrier animal that acquired the virus before birth when its mother came in contact with the virus.

In an infected cow, the virus crosses the placental barrier to infect the fetus. Even if the dam does not show illness herself or gets over it quickly, the unborn calf will be infected. The outcome of fetal infection depends on the stage of gestation (age of the embryo or fetus at the time it is infected) and the strain of the virus. *Persistently infected* (PI) *animals,* calves that were infected in utero during the first three to four months of gestation, serve as a continual source of BVD infection for the herd, and if they live long enough to become cows, they give birth to PI calves.

Result of infection. BVD can cause mild or serious, sometimes fatal, illness in cattle, depending on the type or strain, and may cause abortion at the time of infection or up to several months later. It may also cause mummification of the fetus, which sometimes happens in an early-gestation infection when the dead fetus is retained rather than aborted, or birth defects, such as eye lesions, partial hairlessness, and other abnormalities, if the infection occurs between 50 and 100 days of gestation.

A BVD abortion is rarely noticed because the fetus is small. Infection of the dam during the first month of gestation usually results in death and resorption of the embryo and the cow's return to heat.

Often this disease causes abortion indirectly: It inhibits the cow's *immune system* and makes her susceptible to other types of infection, including leptospirosis (see page 50) and infectious bovine rhinotracheitis (see page 50). Even if a cow is vaccinated against these diseases, she may not build immunity to them if she has BVD. Vaccination of infected calves will not protect them against other diseases, either, because they cannot mount an immune response. A fetus infected during the third trimester (after 150 days of gestation) may be normal at birth but test positive for BVD virus. The fetus's immune system was mature enough at the time of infection to develop an immune response and create antibodies; these calves usually survive and get over the disease. In contrast, a fetus infected by a noncytopathic strain of BVD (one that does not kill the fetus or create birth defects) before it develops a competent immune system at 100 to 125 days of gestation may end up persistently infected because the fetus's immature immune system cannot fight it. At that early stage, the fetus does not recognize the virus as foreign and therefore tolerates it and remains infected for the rest of its life — carrying the virus in its body fluids and serving as a continual source of infection for other cattle.

Treatment. There is no treatment.

Prevention. The best protection is to eliminate all sources of infection within the herd. Your vet can help you with a testing program to identify PI animals. Keep up a vaccination program using *modified live-virus vaccine* ahead of breeding to ensure that cows have the strongest possible protection in early pregnancy, and never let cattle become exposed to infected animals or to any cattle with unknown history. Any purchased animals should be tested to make sure they are not PI before they're added to your herd.

A herd-health program should include annual vaccination against BVD for cows using modified live-virus vaccine between calving and rebreeding. Calves should be vaccinated at weaning time, and heifers should be revaccinated as yearlings before they're bred for the first time. *Note:* If cows must be vaccinated during pregnancy or their calves must be vaccinated before weaning, it is safest to use *killed-virus vaccines* to avoid risk of abortion or birth defects in the fetus, though the modified live-virus vaccines give longer-lasting immunity. Consult your vet for help in designing the most appropriate, safe, and effective vaccination program and schedule for your particular herd.

Brucellosis (Bang's Disease)

Infection with the bacterium *Brucella abortus* is the most common cause of abortion in cattle worldwide. In the United States and Canada, however, *brucellosis*, or *Bang's disease*, has been almost eliminated. An extensive control program was started several decades ago that involved testing herds, slaughtering all carrier cows, and vaccinating all heifer calves kept for breeding. The incentive to eradicate this disease was primarily the fact that humans can acquire it as *undulant fever.* It can be spread to anyone who drinks milk from infected cows and to those who handle infected, especially aborting, cows.

Almost all states are now free of brucellosis, but it is still present in bison and elk in a few areas, such as Yellowstone National Park, in Wyoming. These infected animals continue to be a very real threat to cattle that come in contact with them or when elk or bison come onto the same feeding areas and bed grounds as cattle. Thus, vaccination of heifer calves is still required in states surrounding Yellowstone Park.

How it's spread. Brucellosis is spread through contact with aborted fetuses, tissues, and fluids; it is further spread by dogs, coyotes, wolves, and scavenger birds that carry these tissues away from the immediate area. Ingestion by cattle of bacteria from contaminated pasture, feed, or water is a common route of infection.

■ **Result of infection.** Brucellosis causes abortion in the second half of gestation and retention of the placenta.

Note: Any suspected or positive diagnosis of brucellosis must be reported to your state veterinarian.

■ **Treatment.** Cattle with brucellosis are typically sent to slaughter rather than treated because the disease is so dangerous to humans and the aim is to eradicate it.

■ **Prevention.** If you are in a state or province of Canada that's free of brucellosis, you don't need to worry about this disease, unless you take a risk and buy cattle from another state with questionable status. If you live in a state that still has a control program, you are required to have a vet vaccinate your heifer calves between four and ten months of age (before puberty) and have a metal ear clip and a tattoo in a heifer's ear as proof of the vaccination.

Chlamydia

The *chlamydia* organism, neither bacterium nor virus, is similar to a virus. *Chlamydia psittaci* occasionally infects cattle and is closely related to a strain that infects sheep and humans.

■ **How it's spread.** Chlamydia is spread by direct contact between animals and by the ingestion of feed and pasture grasses and forage contaminated by aborting animals.

■ **Result of infection.** This pathogen can inhabit the reproductive tract of bulls and cows and may cause sporadic abortions at seven to nine months of gestation. In some herds, abortion loss is as high as 10 percent in the last trimester. If an infected calf is born alive, he may be dull and lethargic and may die soon after birth or fail to grow well.

■ **Treatment.** Tetracyclines are sometimes used to treat pregnant cows that have been exposed to this infection, but this is not very practical because the animals must continue to be treated until they calve.

■ **Prevention.** There is a vaccine for sheep but none for cattle. The best prevention is to isolate aborting animals and destroy any aborted tissues or fetuses.

Note: Pregnant women should not handle these tissues or fetuses, as the organism could cause them to abort their child.

Enzootic Bovine Abortion (Foothill Abortion)

Foothill abortion occurs in the central and eastern foothills of California, western Nevada, and southern Oregon. The causative agent has not yet been identified, though some researchers believe it to be the spirochete *Borrelia,* which also causes Lyme disease, a problem in the northeastern United States.

■ **How it's spread.** It seems to be spread by a certain type of tick that is always present in areas where these abortions occur.

■ **Result of infection.** Abortions occur three to four months after exposure to the tick. (Pregnant cows between 35 days and six months of gestation when exposed to the tick tend to abort.)

■ **Treatment.** There is no treatment.

■ **Prevention.** There are no vaccines, but cattle exposed to the causative organism, either before becoming pregnant or if they've experienced abortion from this infection, have immunity for several years. Cattle at greatest risk are those that have never been previously exposed and are brought into these areas when they are one to six months' pregnant. If you live in an area known for this problem, the best prevention is to breed only cattle that are native to the area or to bring in open cows (such as cows with young calves that are not yet rebred) or young heifers.

Haemophilus somnus

Many healthy cattle, both male and female, have the *Haemophilus somnus* bacteria in their urinary and genital tracts without evidence of illness.

How it's spread. Since the organism often lives in the semen and genital tract of the bull, it may be spread to cows and heifers via breeding.

Result of infection. Occasional cases of septicemia, pneumonia, and infection of the brain and spinal cord. It can also cause abortion and inflammation of the uterine lining and vagina (though it's not a common cause) and may be a factor in infertility if cows have a uterine infection.

Treatment. Haemophilus somnus is treated with antibiotics.

Prevention. There are vaccines for preventing respiratory diseases caused by *Haemophilus somnus,* but the pathogens responsible for reproductive disease are often considered to be a different strain; vaccination is generally not effective.

Infectious Bovine Rhinotracheitis (IBR)

Infectious bovine rhinotracheitis (IBR), a very contagious viral disease, is common in feedlots and groups of weaned calves and wherever many unvaccinated cattle are confined together.

How it's spread. The virus is readily spread by direct contact or coughing. If a cow is pregnant when she contracts the virus, the fetus may be infected.

Result of infection. This disease causes upper respiratory illness and a condition called red nose. IBR is also a common cause of late-term abortion and is often mistaken for leptospirosis. Abortions from IBR may occur any time during gestation but are most common during the second half. Some full-term fetuses are stillborn, and a few are born alive but soon die. In a herd outbreak, more than half the cows may abort, though cows infected in early pregnancy are less likely to do so.

Treatment. There is no treatment.

Prevention. Routinely vaccinate for IBR with modified live-virus vaccine once a year, just before breeding, when cows are not yet pregnant. All heifers should be vaccinated at least a month before their first breeding, and all cattle need a booster shot each year. Combination vaccines give protection against IBR and bovine virus diarrhea (BVD; see page 47). Give modified live-virus vaccines at least three weeks before breeding during the period after calving. Killed vaccines can be given to pregnant cows or to calves nursing from pregnant cows to protect the calves from the respiratory form of the disease.

Note: There is always some risk of abortion when using modified live-virus vaccines on calves nursing from pregnant cows. The calves may shed the virus and infect their mothers unless the cows already have good immunity from previous vaccination.

Leptospirosis

This disease (sometimes referred to as lepto) is probably the most common cause of infectious abortion in the United States, now that brucellosis is fairly well controlled. There are many types of *leptospirosis* bacteria but only five that generally cause abortion in cattle: *Leptospira canicola, L. pomona, L. icterohaemorrhagica, L. grippotyphosa,* and *L. hardjo.* There are vaccines for these, and combination vaccines that take care of all of them.

How it's spread. Lepto is spread by contact with the urine of sick and carrier animals (including rodents, pigs, cats, canines, deer, elk, and antelope). Urine may contaminate feed and water: Wildlife may urinate in a water source or a cattle feed ground, and rodents sometimes urinate in a haystack. Bacteria enter the cow through breaks in the skin on her feet and legs when she's walking in contaminated water or through her nose, mouth, or eyes if she has contact with contaminated feed, water, or urine. Bacteria can also be transmitted by semen from an infected bull. Outbreaks sometimes follow the congregating of cattle for feeding, vaccinating, and so forth.

Result of infection. Abortion can occur at any stage of pregnancy, even in cows that do not appear sick. Cows in the second half of pregnancy will usually abort one to three weeks after recovery from an acute case of lepto. Not all affected cows abort; some give birth to weak calves that die within a few days. Abortions from lepto often result in a retained placenta and infection of the uterus, but cows usually recover and conceive again. It's easiest to *culture* (grow the microorganisms in the laboratory) lepto from urine of the aborting cow rather than from the fetus or placenta.

Treatment. Lepto is treated with antibiotics. Some lepto infections require treatment so the cow won't continue to spread the bacteria for several months or years.

Prevention. Vaccination bolsters a cow's immunity for about six months. Since lepto can cause problems at any time during the cow's pregnancy, many veterinarians recommend vaccinating cows twice a year: prior to breeding, such as during springtime vaccinations, and again with a booster five or six months later, such as during fall pregnancy checks.

Listeriosis

This bacterial disease affects the nervous system in cattle and sheep, causing *encephalitis* (inflammation and infection in the brain), but *listeriosis* can also cause abortion.

How it's spread. The bacteria are often present in the environment (in soil, bedding, feed) and gain entry to the body by ingestion (eating poor-quality or contaminated silage) or via the nervous or respiratory system. Some cows do not become ill but are carriers, shedding bacteria in their feces and milk.

Result of infection. The organism may settle in the placenta, causing abortion in late pregnancy, which can be accompanied by fever before, during, or after. The placenta may have yellow or gray spots, and the aborted fetus often has spots on its liver.

Treatment. Antibiotics are effective if given early, before symptoms of illness are severe. Usually, though, by the time you know an animal is sick, it's too late for treatment that can prevent abortion.

Prevention. Don't feed spoiled silage or silage that's contaminated with soil. There is a vaccine, but its effectiveness is questionable.

Neosporosis

This disease is caused by the protozoan *Neospora caninum*.

How it's spread. *Neosporosis* is spread when infected canines or cats contaminate feed and pastures with fecal material. An infected cow can spread protozoa to her fetus. If the infected calf is a heifer, she may infect her own fetus when she matures and becomes pregnant.

Result of infection. Once inside the cow's body, the organism creates cysts. The predator (for example, coyote, fox, dog) then eats the grazing animal or her aborted fetus, ingests the cysts, and starts the life cycle all over again in its digestive tract. If the protozoa in the cow affect the heart and brain of her fetus, it dies and is aborted, usually at four to six months of gestation. Sometimes the calf is normal but carries the protozoa in its body forever.

Treatment. There is no treatment.

Prevention. There are no vaccines. It helps, however, to keep dogs from eating aborted fetuses and other dead tissues and to keep them from contaminating feed supplies with feces.

Salmonellosis

See chapter 11 for an extensive overview of the effects of salmonella on calves.

How it's spread. A cow with diarrhea will spread *salmonellosis* to other cattle via contamination of feed, water, and pasture.

Result of infection. Infection with salmonella can cause severe diarrhea, fever, and abortion; sometimes a cow will abort late in pregnancy with no sign of illness. Salmonella can be deadly to young calves.

Treatment. Your vet can prescribe the most appropriate oral antibiotic for each situation. Salmonella is resistant to some of the commonly used antibiotics.

Prevention. The best protection against salmonellosis is not to bring infected animals onto your farm. Once the disease is there control consists of diligent efforts to prevent contamination by isolating sick animals from the rest of the herd and the use of vaccination.

Sarcocystosis

Sarcocystosis, a protozoan disease caused by various species of *Sarcocystis,* is fairly common in cattle but only rarely causes abortion, which can occur if a cow has a massive infection.

How it's spread. Like *Neospora* infections, the protozoa can be spread to cattle from predatory animals (e.g., dogs, coyotes, foxes, wolves, raccoons, and cats) that shed *oocysts* (protozoan "eggs") in their feces. These can survive in the environment a long time and may be ingested by cattle.

Result of infection. Cattle generally don't show much sign of illness, but if a cow eats many oocysts, she may abort during the last trimester of gestation.

Treatment. There is no effective treatment.

Prevention. The only ways to prevent this disease are to be sure that you do not feed uncooked meat or offal to pets and to make sure no infected canines or cats defecate on pastures or hay. There is no vaccine.

Trichomoniasis

Trichomoniasis is caused by the protozoan *Trichomonas fetus;* some areas of North America, particularly the western United States, where cattle from a number of ranches may run in common on public rangelands, have a mandatory testing program for bulls to control this disease. Often stockmen don't know they have it in their herd, but they may have an abnormally high number of open cows after the breeding season.

How it's spread. The protozoan is spread to cows via infected bulls.

Result of infection. The disease usually results in early embryonic death, with the cow soon returning to heat, but if she's rebred, she again loses the embryo. The infection is a common cause of repeat breeders and infertility. Most cows abort before five months of gestation.

Treatment. Cows generally clear themselves of infection after several heat cycles and finally become pregnant, but bulls remain infected, with the protozoa living in the bulls' reproductive tracts. In states with mandatory testing programs, every bull must be "trich" tested before breeding season, and any carrier bulls must be culled.

Prevention. Protection consists of buying only *virgin bulls* (bulls that have never bred a cow), testing bulls every year and culling any that test positive, and making sure no cows are bred by a questionable bull.

There's a vaccine for cows, but it isn't always effective if they are bred by infected bulls, nor will it guard bulls against becoming infected. Keeping a closed herd is the best prevention.

Tuberculosis

This bacterial disease was once eradicated in the United States, but in recent years *tuberculosis* (TB) has been reintroduced to cattle in Michigan, Texas, and California from infected wildlife or by cattle from Mexico. As of 2006, California and Texas were again free of TB. Michigan is still fighting it because the disease became established in the deer population.

■ **How it's spread.** TB is spread through contact with infected animals.

■ **Result of infection.** Cows infected with TB may have damaging changes to the uterus and fallopian tubes and may have an obvious, thick discharge from the vulva. They may abort or give birth to a premature calf.

■ **Treatment.** Treatment is not an option; infected animals must be culled.

■ **Prevention.** Purchase only animals that are proved free of TB where necessary. Slaughter all animals that test positive for tuberculosis. Disinfect or destroy any feed and water troughs, bedding, and so on that were used by infected animals.

Vibriosis (Campylobacteriosis)

Vibriosis is a venereal disease (sometimes referred to as *vibrio*) caused by the bacterium *Campylobacterfetus venerealis;* it results in early embryonic death and abortion. There are three strains of the disease.

■ **How it's spread.** One strain is transmitted to a cow at time of service from an infected bull, and bulls become infected by breeding an infected cow. The strain that causes abortion in sheep and the strain found in dogs' intestines are spread to cattle through ingestion of contaminated hay or pasture.

■ **Result of infection.** The cow conceives, but the infection causes inflammation of the uterus. Often the embryo dies so early that the cow returns to heat soon, leaving you to assume she didn't settle. In some cases the embryo survives to become a fetus, lives a few months, and is then aborted.

■ **Treatment.** There is no benefit to treating cows; they become immune three to six months after the infection. Antibiotics can be used to clear the infection in bulls.

■ **Prevention.** Use artificial insemination or vaccinate cows each year before breeding, and don't use infected bulls.

Note: Cows can be protected from only one strain by vaccination. Bulls can be carriers of the bacteria for several years unless treated. If you never introduce an infected animal into your herd, vibrio will not be a concern. If you use community pastures or pasture next to other cattle, it's safest to vaccinate your cows.

Management to Prevent Abortions

If your herd experiences an abortion rate higher than 1 percent, talk with your vet to try to determine the cause and develop a vaccination or management program to prevent losses. Often, the cause can be determined if your vet sends a freshly aborted fetus or some of the placental membranes to a diagnostic lab or takes blood samples from the aborting cow or the fresh placenta.

Unnoticed and Undiagnosed Abortions

Many abortions aren't noticed; a cow simply turns up open later. In the second half of gestation, you may see some abortions (the placenta is hanging from the cow's vagina for a few days, or you find the aborted fetus), but these may not be diagnosed. The cow may be healthy, and an examination of the fetus or fetal membranes by a diagnostic lab may not determine the cause.

Precalving Problems

Occasionally, a cow will develop a problem in late pregnancy before calving time that becomes life-threatening unless it's resolved. These include vaginal prolapse, uterine torsion, abdominal hernia, swelling, paralysis, ingestion of hardware, and premature calving.

Vaginal Prolapse

Occasionally, a nonpregnant cow suffering from irritation and inflammation of the vaginal tissues (*vaginitis*) during a heat cycle or following breeding will strain until she pushes the rearmost portion of her vagina out of her vulva. More often, a cow does this in late pregnancy, but sometimes a *prolapse* happens in earlier stages of pregnancy.

Some cows have a structural weakness of the reproductive tract that allows part of the vagina to prolapse. Most common in Herefords, Simmental, and Charolais, this is an inherited problem that's passed from mother to daughter, or from sire to daughter if the bull's mother had this weakness. Alternatively, too much fat in the connective tissue around the vagina may predispose a cow to this problem; it happens more often in cows that have skipped a calving year or have lost a calf and have become fat as a result of not *lactating* (producing milk). Cows on legume pastures and that are otherwise fat are at higher risk. Prolapses are also more common in older cows.

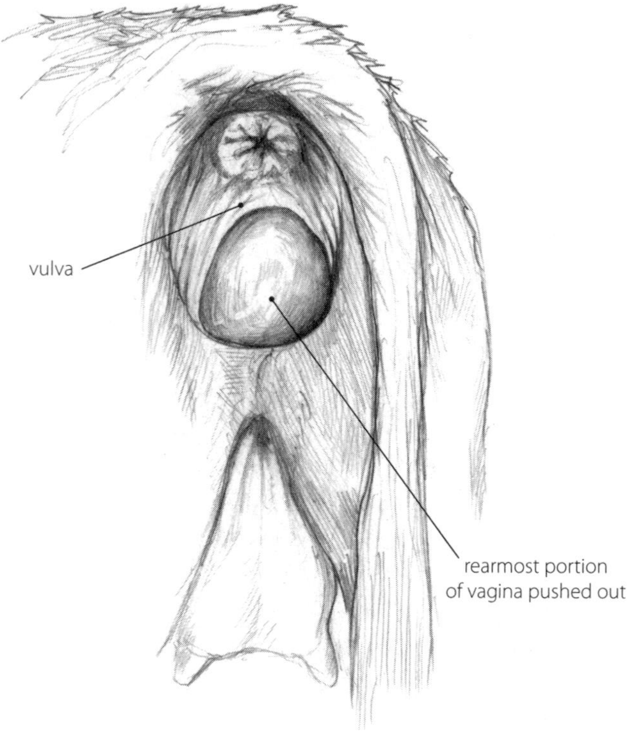

A prolapsed vagina.

Prolapse in Late Pregnancy

The pressure and weight of the large uterus in late pregnancy causes the vaginal tissue to protrude from the vulva when the cow is lying down — especially if her hind end is slightly downhill. In addition, the tissues around the birth canal in late pregnancy have become relaxed and there is increased pressure in the abdominal cavity that pushes out the vagina when the cow is lying down.

If the cow is still several weeks away from calving when she starts prolapsing, the condition will get worse before she calves; advancing pregnancy puts more pressure on the vagina.

Signs of Prolapse

At first, the bulge is the size of an orange or grapefruit and resembles a pink ball protruding from the vulva. The bulge usually retracts when the cow gets up and pressure is relieved. If the cow prolapses every time she lies down, however, the condition worsens, especially if she strains. Sometimes just the presence of the bulging tissue stimulates the cow to strain, which forces more tissue to protrude. The exposed vaginal tissue becomes dirty and manure flows over it when the cow defecates. This causes irritation and more straining. A heavily pregnant cow will often strain when she passes manure while lying down or will strain from irritation of a mild prolapse, which makes the prolapse worse.

Eventually, the tissue grows to the size of a volleyball and can't go back in, even when the cow gets up and walks around. The prolapsed tissue becomes dirtier, dries out, and becomes damaged and infected. Because blood circulation to these tissues is impaired, they become swollen and vulnerable to injury. Infection, though it may be present, is not a major concern; the vaginal lining is not a sterile environment and can recover from an infection once the tissues are pushed back inside to their normal position.

OUR EXPERIENCE WITH PROLAPSES

A FEW WEEKS BEFORE Button Bottom (one of a group of cows we leased in 1972) calved, we saw the grapefruit-sized ball protruding from her vulva. Never having seen this before, we called our vet, who put the prolapse back in and stitched the cow, winding umbilical tape around leather buttons that were anchored to her skin with suture material. We didn't keep that cow another year.

A few years later, our cow Jillie prolapsed before calving, but we didn't have to stitch her. She was gentle enough to let me walk up behind her and push the prolapse back into her vagina. Because we were calving in January and watching cows closely, each time I'd see her prolapse, I'd push it back. We kept her many more years but had to do this every year during the last week before she calved.

By contrast, Chamelean was nine years old when she first prolapsed, after having many calves and a set of twins — and she was not gentle enough to let us push it back. The first few days, we'd get her up and run her around and the prolapse would go back, but finally it reached the point where it wouldn't, so we put her in the chute to stitch her up. We kept Chamelean for two more years and went through the ordeal of stitching her before she calved and removing the stitches at calving time, then we sold her.

The worst case was Cammie, who prolapsed in late summer, when she was four months pregnant. She was a fat three-year-old that skipped a year. (She was pregnant with her second calf but was not lactating that summer.) Riding out to check the cows, we found her on the range with a prolapsed vagina that was dirty, hard, and dry and covered with flies. The tissues had been out several days, and she would have died if we hadn't been able to bring her home to wash up the prolapse and replace it.

After all this, we had learned the hard way that the bull we bought several years earlier sired daughters with this problem.

The biggest problem is swelling. The longer the inverted tissue is left outside the cow's body, the more swelling occurs and the harder it is to replace the prolapse. Swelling also restricts the passage from the bladder. In some cases, the bladder is part of the prolapse; it's trapped within the inverted tissues so that the cow can't urinate until the prolapse is resolved. Her straining while trying to urinate will aggravate the problem.

If the prolapse must be corrected by stitching, cull the cow, and if you are unlucky enough to have a bull that sires daughters with this problem, don't keep any more heifers from him.

In addition, if she starts calving, the bulge of tissue impedes the birth of the calf and may result in death of the calf and more damage to the cow. Thus, it is imperative to replace the prolapsed tissues.

If a cow prolapses in late pregnancy, watch her closely. You won't have to intervene if the bulge of pink tissue remains small and always retracts. If the tissues grow larger and won't go back in, you must correct the problem. Some cows have a mild prolapse every time they approach calving and it never gets worse, but others get worse each year. If you gamble and keep a prolapsed cow for another pregnancy, be prepared for a greater problem the next year. If the prolapse must be corrected by stitching, cull the cow, and if you are unlucky enough to have a bull that sires daughters with this problem, don't keep any more heifers from him.

Replacing the Prolapse

- Restrain the cow in a chute with a pole behind her to prevent her from kicking. Clean off the ball of tissues before pushing it back (to prevent irritation from contamination and potential inflammation and infection): Wash the tissues gently with warm water and a mild disinfectant such as Nolvasan diluted with water to remove

HOW TO STITCH THE VULVA TO PREVENT RECURRING VAGINAL PROLAPSE

To prevent recurring prolapse of the vagina, stitch the vulva with umbilical tape. Follow the instructions below.

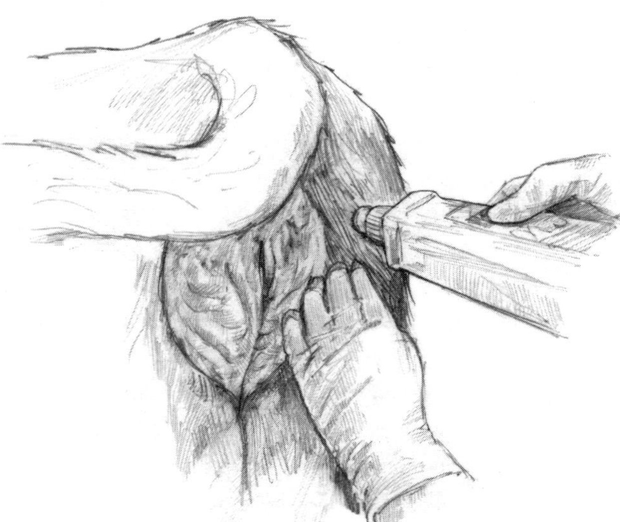

After replacing the prolapse, *clean and scrub the vulva and the area around it with a warm-water bottle and mild soap in preparation for stitching.*

The first stitch *anchors the umbilical tape in the tough, haired skin next to the vulva.*

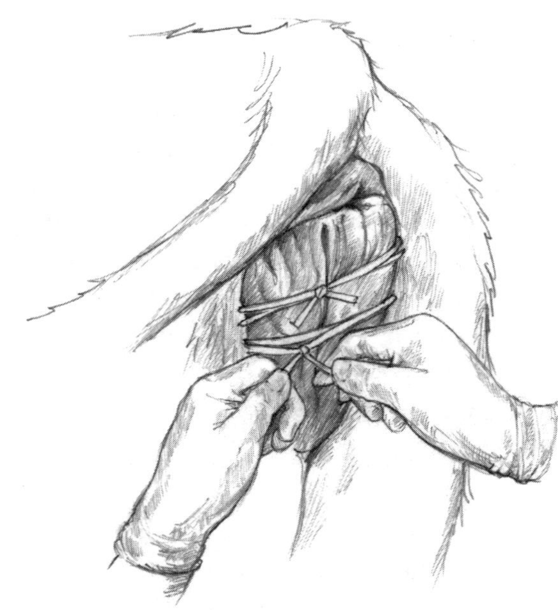

Tie off each stitch *as you complete it.*

manure and dirt. Use clean hands or clean rubber gloves while working. *Note:* If the prolapse has been out for several days, the tissues may be dry and damaged and harder to clean up and push back in.

- Often the full urinary bladder is trapped in the prolapsed tissue and makes the prolapse larger. Lift up the ball of tissue to enable the bladder to empty, so it can be replaced.
- When you replace the tissues, the cow will strain as you try to push the inverted vagina back in; thus, replacing it may be difficult.
- Stitch the prolapse. This is necessary because the cow will prolapse every time she lies down until she calves and relieves the pressure. You or your vet can perform this procedure. Use a large, curved surgical needle or a needle used for sewing up a stuffed turkey and *umbilical tape* (a strong, wide cotton strip that usually comes on a spool). The tape is less apt to pull out than suture thread and is not abrasive. The stitches should be anchored in the tough, haired skin at the sides of the vulva. They won't easily tear out of this area, and the haired skin is also less sensitive than the skin of the vulva itself. It takes at least three cross-stitches to keep the vulva safely closed so the inner tissues can't push out if the cow strains. She can urinate through the stitches, but the vulva cannot open enough for prolapse.
- Once the cow is stitched, watch her closely as she approaches calving. Unless the stitches are removed when she starts to calve, the cow will tear them out or have difficulty calving. During early labor, monitor her continuously. As soon as she starts active labor, straining to expel the calf, cut and pull out the stitches, using scissors, tin snips, or a sharp knife.

After Calving

After the cow has calved, the pressure that caused the prolapse will no longer exist. She generally won't have any more problems until the next pregnancy. Rarely, a cow has a structural weakness that causes prolapse of the uterus after calving (see chapter 6), but this is usually not related to the tendency for a vaginal prolapse.

Uterine Torsion

On occasion the pregnant uterus rotates, twisting in the part next to the cervix. This sometimes occurs during gestation but occurs more frequently at calving time during early labor (see chapter 4).

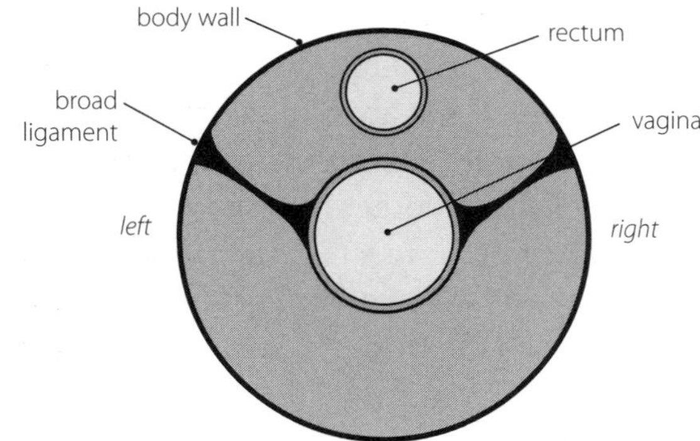

A normal uterus and vagina, *suspended by the broad ligament.*

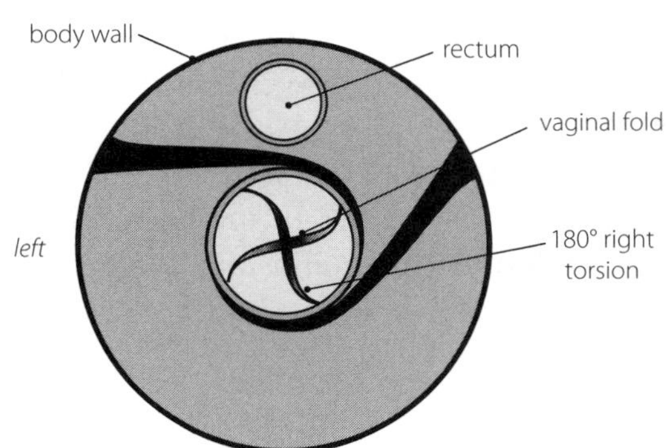

A 180-degree right (clockwise) torsion of the uterus, *with a twist in the vagina.*

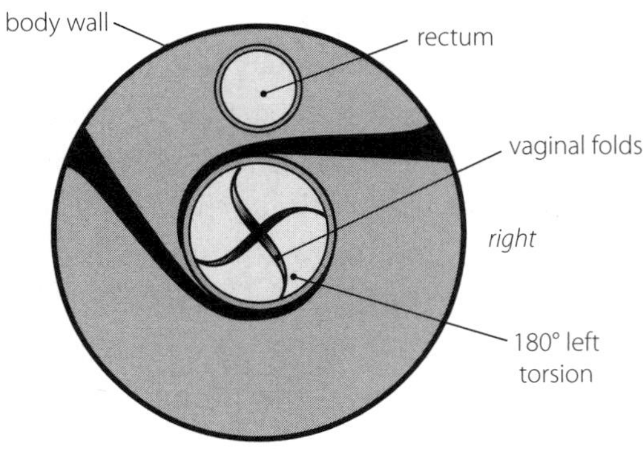

A 180-degree left (counterclockwise) torsion of the uterus, *putting a twist in the vagina in the opposite direction.*

The lower, larger part of the uterus is supported by the floor of the abdomen in late pregnancy and may swing when the cow is getting up and down. Any sudden shift, whether from slipping or falling or being knocked by another cow, could cause the uterus to swing so much that it turns over. Sometimes, even a very active fetus moves enough to cause the uterus to rotate.

Torsion is rare in heifers; it's seen more frequently in cows that have calved before, especially those with deep, spacious abdomens. Cows with twins seldom have torsions because two calves more completely fill the abdominal space and create a broader base for the uterus as it rests on the muscle floor of the abdomen.

Some torsions occur in late gestation and may be present for days or weeks without signs, becoming obvious only when the cow goes into labor and can't deliver the calf.

If a torsion is minor (only 45 to 90 degrees), it may correct during labor. Torsions greater than 180 degrees completely obstruct the birth canal; the calf cannot be born until it's corrected. Torsions that are this significant and that occur during gestation may create swelling and obstruction of blood vessels, which interferes with blood supply to the uterus and eventually causes death of the fetus. The cow may show abdominal pain and may go into shock and die. In other cases the fetus mummifies, and the cow shows few symptoms.

Correcting a Uterine Torsion

See chapter 4 for approaches to returning the uterus to its normal position.

Abdominal Hernia

A cow in late pregnancy may suffer rupture or muscle separation in the lower part of the abdominal wall, due perhaps to a severe blow, such as being horned in the belly, or to a weakness in the abdominal muscles, which allows the heavy uterus to drop through it; this is referred to as an *abdominal hernia.* The separation is generally in the rear part of the belly, a little to the right of the midline and behind the navel. You may first notice the problem as swelling about the size of a football, but quickly this swelling becomes larger, drooping down to hock level. The heavy uterus and the fetus within it then drop completely out of the abdomen, so that nothing protects the uterus from the outside world except the cow's skin and a great deal of swelling.

An abdominal hernia is a serious condition. A cow that develops one should be kept in a safe place where she won't be jostled by other cows and should be closely watched. She will usually give birth to a live calf but may have difficulty calving and need the assistance of you and the vet. At the time of calving, your vet will determine whether the hernia can be repaired after removal of the calf or the cow should be butchered.

Swelling under the Belly

Some cows, especially heifers, suffer from a great deal of swelling as they approach calving due to the distended uterus's pressure on the mammary glands and veins. The swelling may become so great that it extends forward almost to the elbow and droops quite low under the belly. At first it may be mistaken for a hernia, but it is usually nothing to worry about; it resolves after the cow calves.

Paralysis

On rare occasions, a heavily pregnant cow becomes weak due to mineral deficiencies or dietary problems that interfere with proper metabolism and is unable to rise after she lies down.

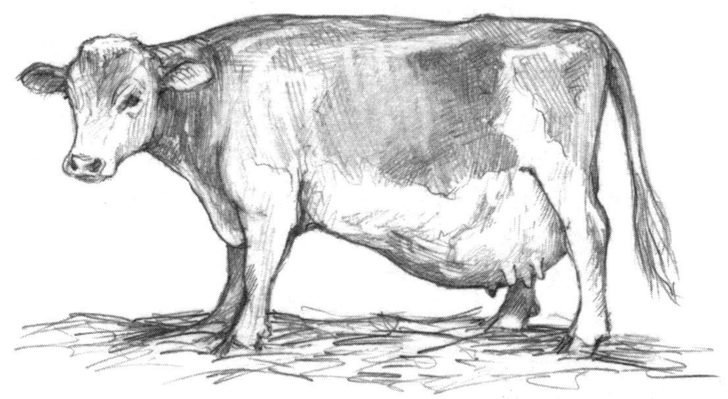

When a cow has an abdominal hernia, she suffers muscle separation due to a weakness or trauma, which allows the heavy uterus to drop through the abdominal wall.

Grass tetany (a condition caused by mineral deficiency) sometimes occurs when pregnant cows are on lush pastures, especially cereal crops such as wheat pastures in fall or early spring, that are deficient in some minerals because they're so fast growing. In these cases the cow usually recovers if she's given calcium or magnesium.

Milk fever, in which a high-producing dairy cow develops a sudden drop in blood calcium and cannot get up, usually occurs soon after calving (see chapter 6) but may also occur just before calving.

Ketosis (pregnancy toxemia) is an occasional problem in fat beef cows that suffer lower levels of nutrition during the last two months of pregnancy and results from changes in the liver due to the metabolic demands the cow faces at this time or, as in the case of dairy cows, in early lactation. Heavy demands for energy in a dairy cow right after calving or in a pregnant beef cow carrying twins cause an increased rate of fat metabolization from body reserves. Overly fat cows and cows carrying twins are more at risk.

If a beef cow is affected by ketosis shortly before calving, she may become restless and aggressive or excited, uncoordinated (with a stumbling gait), and have difficulty getting up and down. She won't pass much manure, and what she does pass is very firm. She may develop muscle tremors and fall down as a result. If this occurs as much as a month or two before calving, she stops eating, is dull, and eventually gets to the point when she can't rise again. The breath of some afflicted cows smells like acetone.

Treatment for ketosis usually consists of giving glucose and electrolyte solutions intravenously and propylene glycol orally. The cow should be encouraged to eat as much good-quality hay as possible. A cow with a severe case of ketosis may die, even with treatment, but mild cases usually recover with treatment, especially if a cow continues to eat even small amounts of good hay.

Ketosis can be prevented by properly feeding the cow during late pregnancy. Adequate nutrition supports cows but doesn't allow them to become too fat. Remember: If any cow is down and unable to get up, consult your vet immediately for diagnosis and treatment.

Ingestion of Hardware

Cows that ingest a sharp object such as a nail or piece of baling wire are at risk for *hardware disease.* Action of the digestive tract may push the sharp object into or through the gut wall, causing peritonitis. When a cow is thought to have swallowed a metal object, a cylindrical cattle magnet is put down the cow's throat with a special "balling gun" for administering pills or boluses orally. After the cow swallows the magnet, it goes into the stomach, where it stays for the life of the animal and collects any metal objects she may have inadvertently eaten with her feed.

Cows are more at risk with this during late pregnancy because the increased size of the uterus puts more pressure on the digestive tract. A foreign object that was sitting harmlessly in the stomach or was partially embedded in the lining before pregnancy may get pushed clear through the stomach wall when the gut is short on space.

Cows in late gestation have a higher incidence of the problem. If a heavily pregnant cow becomes dull, goes off feed, or shows other signs of illness, hardware disease may be a cause, which your veterinarian can determine through an examination. If the cow was not given a magnet earlier in life, it is worthwhile to use one if hardware disease is suspected. If the sharp object has not already gone clear through the stomach wall, a magnet may pull it back.

Premature Birth

Sometimes a calf is born too early. *Premature* birth is caused by some of the same factors that can cause an abortion, with the difference that the premature calf is closer to term and has more chance for survival.

One way to know if a calf is full term is to check his mouth. A full-term calf has one or two pairs of *incisors* erupted, whereas a premature calf has no teeth yet, and his gums may be dark pink.

If a premature calf is a victim of late-term abortion, isolate the cow in case she has a disease and have the vet examine her and the calf. The placenta should also be sent to a diagnostic lab if there's any suspicion of disease.

If the premature calf seems healthy, you may be able to save him with intensive care (see chapter 9).

Chapter 3

Normal Calving and Difficult Deliveries

THE RISKIEST TIME IN A CALF'S LIFE MAY BE his entrance — the birth process. It's estimated that each year more than 3.5 million calves in the United States alone are lost during or shortly after birth and that 45 percent of these deaths are due to *dystocia* (delayed or difficult birth).

Factors that affect birth size, weight, and calving ease include the sex of the calf, the age of the dam, breed and birth weight of the sire, breed and birth weight of the dam, gestation length, environment, and nutrition of the dam. Birth weight and size, like gestation length, are often inherited; therefore, calving problems can be minimized if you select cows and bulls that were small- to medium-sized at birth. Birth weight is also lower in hot seasons and higher in cold weather because in cold weather the blood circulation of the dam is concentrated internally, leading to a bigger fetus. Feeding cows high levels of protein the last 90 days of gestation can increase size of calves at birth: Pregnant cows need adequate energy and protein for fetal growth and for their own body condition, but overfeeding protein may result in big calves and more calving problems.

The main cause for dystocia is a big calf and a small pelvic area in the dam, who is sometimes a small heifer. It's important for heifers to be well grown by calving time and to be bred to bulls that sire small calves. Generally, the larger the dam, the bigger her calf. In addition, male calves tend to be larger than females, and they may be born after the due date, whereas heifer calves often come before their due date: Because the fetus grows fastest in the final stage of gestation, several more days of growth create a larger calf. One study suggests that each extra day of gestation amounts to about a pound's increase in the size of the calf.

Most cows give birth without problems, especially if they're bred to bulls that sire small or average-sized calves. Even then, however, challenges sometimes occur. This chapter looks at the birth process — both in the best scenarios and when difficulties arise.

Minimizing Calving Problems

When cattle were wild, they gave birth quickly and easily, much like bison, and calves were small. Further, those calves with problems did not survive to have offspring themselves. Mother Nature ruthlessly culled and selected for easy calving.

With domestication, however, we've created animals that are bigger, meatier, and faster growing. In selecting for "improved" beef traits, we have also inadvertently selected for animals that are larger at birth. Hence, the domestic cow has more calving problems than did her wild ancestors.

After experiencing some horrible difficulties with large calves, especially in the 1970s and 1980s, when stockmen in this country were experimenting with larger continental breeds such as Charolais and Simmental and crossing them with smaller British cattle, many cattle breeders realized they needed

Calving Necessities

Before the start of our calving season, we try to have everything we might need on hand and the calving barns ready, with machinery out and straw in. Since we tend to park tractors and store odds and ends in the barns, under shelter, during the 10 months we're not calving, it can be a mad rush if we're not quite prepared when the first calf arrives. If a cow or heifer surprises us by calving early and needs assistance, we don't want to be caught scrambling to find the OB chains or searching for that new box of OB gloves we bought nine months ago.

We were caught off guard one season when we'd only used the calf puller once the year before and couldn't remember where we had left it. When you're lying on your face in the pen with your arm in a cow, you may have to ask your child to run and get the chains or the OB lubricant. We learned that it pays to have a specific place for certain things and to have everyone in the family know where they are so they can always be located in an emergency. And make sure you order a new jug of iodine before the start of the calving season if the old one is nearly empty.

Here's a calving-season list of things to have on hand:

- Halter and rope, in case you need to tie a cow to assist her
- Disposable obstetrical gloves or sleeves
- Plastic bucket for wash water and rag(s) for washing the cow
- Obstetrical lubricant and disinfectant in a squeeze bottle
- Clean obstetrical (OB) chains and handles for pulling a calf. *Note:* OB chains and handles are preferable to nylon straps, which are more difficult to keep clean. Chains and handles can be boiled, they don't cut off blood circulation to the calf's lower leg when constant tension is applied, and handles can be attached anywhere along them for easier pulling.
- Mechanical calf puller, kept in a handy location
- Flashlights for checking cows at night
- Strong (7 percent tincture) iodine for dipping the calf's navel stump
- Nolvasan (chlorhexidine) disinfectant solution
- Uterine boluses (large, oblong pills) if recommended by your vet
- Injectable antibiotics for the cow or calf, prescribed by your vet
- Syringes and needles in various sizes for cows and calves
- Bottle and lamb nipple for feeding a calf
- Stomach tube or esophageal feeder for a calf unable to nurse
- Suction bulb to suck fluid out of a newborn calf's nostrils
- Tool box to hold any needed items in one handy place
- Your veterinarian's phone number
- Alarm clock

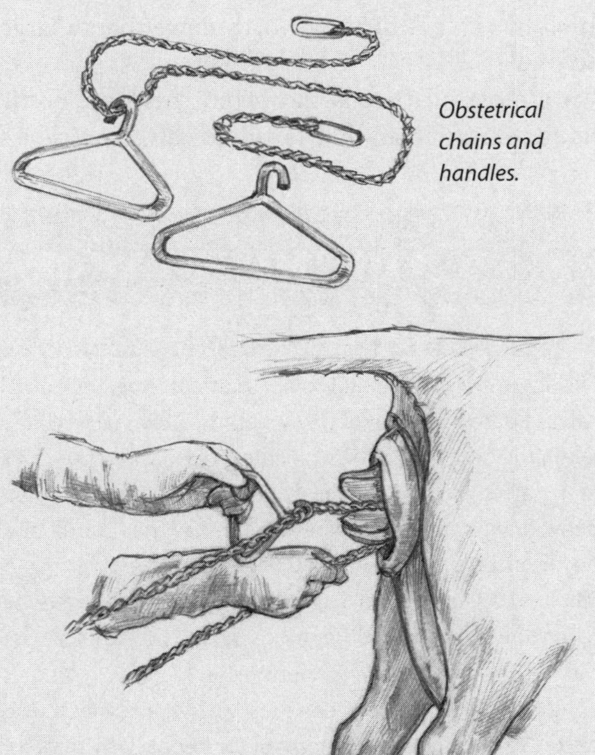

Obstetrical chains and handles.

One advantage to using a chain is that pulling handles can be attached anywhere you need them along the chain.

to select for smaller birth weights and calving ease. Breeds with large muscle mass (called *double muscling*) such as Charolais, Belgian Blue, and Piedmontese have more calving problems. Some British breeds such as Angus and Hereford also have some calving problems. Herefords were originally draft animals selected for large size and large bone structure. Consequently, Hereford heifers often needed help with calving. Angus were originally known for small calves and easy calving (they ranged semiwild in the Scottish Highlands), but in recent years Angus breeders have worked to increase the size, frame, and growth of these cattle and in doing so have created larger calves and more calving problems.

There are advantages to using some of the minor breeds that haven't been "improved" for increased beef production. If you select a breed known for small calves and easy calving, you'll probably have a decreased loss rate at birth when you are unable to be there for the birth process. Calves from some of these breeds may not be as big at weaning time, but a small live calf at birth is worth more than a large dead one!

In almost all breeds, however, there are some bulls that sire larger-than-average calves or calves with wide hips and shoulders that don't pass through the birth canal easily. Finally, some cows always have big calves and hard births, regardless of the size of the bull that sires their offspring.

No matter what breed or crosses you use, the key to calving ease is selecting breeding stock to combine ease of calving with other traits you desire. The goal of most cattle raisers is a herd of easy-calving cows whose calves grow fast.

The Role of Hormones in Calving

Hormones influence ease of birth. Cows carrying bull calves have more difficulty calving, not only because of the larger size of males but also because cows carrying males have higher testosterone levels than do cows carrying females.

Cows experiencing dystocia also have different estrogen and progesterone levels than cows that give birth easily. These hormones influence the degree of relaxation and expansion of the birth canal and the force of labor contractions.

THE IMPORTANCE OF CALVING RECORDS

WE KEEP DETAILED CALVING RECORDS on every cow, including due date, the sire, the actual calving date, the time of day when the cow started early labor, the time when she broke her water, when the calf's feet started to show or the amnion sac appeared, when delivery was complete, whether the cow had a bull or a heifer, and anything abnormal (if we have to assist her and why). In calving season, I always carry a pocket notebook to jot down the exact time things occur and later transfer this information to a permanent record.

With these notes, we can look back at a cow's calving history and know what's "normal" for her at each stage of labor and delivery. The record reminds us that a cow may require more frequent checking or assistance, or that she is a fast and easy calver and that something may be wrong if she's taking too long. Some cows have such consistent histories that we always remember whether they calve fast (such as between checks) or not, or that an old pet always waits for assistance even when she doesn't need it. But often I refer back to the calving records to have more clues about what to expect, since most cows have consistent delivery times.

Our records-check saved Ginger's calf in 1987. Her first five calves were born quickly and easily but she was taking just a little longer with number six. Recognizing that extra time was not normal for her, we put her in the barn, tied her up and checked her, and discovered that the calf was crooked and not coming readily into the birth canal. The placenta was also starting to detach; part of it was coming ahead of the calf. We pulled him and delivered a live calf, Gingivitis. The record book saved the day.

Stages of Labor in the Normal Birth

As the cow or heifer nears the end of gestation, her body makes changes to aid the birth process. One of the first signs that she's near calving is development of her udder. It may begin enlarging six weeks before she calves, especially in heifers, or may fill just in the last few days of gestation. Some cows and heifers have so much udder development that you think calving is imminent, yet many more days of gestation pass before the actual event. Others will "bag up" almost overnight right before the calf is born and fool you into thinking that they aren't yet ready to calve.

Impending Calving

Signs of impending calving:

- Mucus is discharged from the vulva as the cervical plug softens and is expelled.
- The vulva relaxes. This doorway becomes enlarged, soft, and flabby as the birth canal prepares for birth. *Note:* Some cows will get a loose and floppy vulva a few weeks before they actually calve, keeping you guessing.
- The *pelvic ligaments* relax. These are located at the back end of the cow or heifer, in the area between the tailhead and the point of buttock (pin bone) on each side of the tail, and are about 1 inch (2.5 cm) in diameter. They attach the pin bones to the spine. While they're easier to see in most diary cows than in beef cows, you can feel them easily in beef cattle. When they appear loose and sunken and completely relaxed, calving will usually begin in about 12 hours.

  To assess these ligaments, if cows are gentle, walk slowly among them a couple of times a day while they're eating and approach from behind those you think are close to calving. Rub your hand alongside a tailhead to feel the pelvic ligaments (most cows enjoy this scratching; it's a place that's hard for them to reach). The ligaments are very difficult and tight except during the few hours just before labor begins, when they loosen up to enable the birth canal to expand.

Early (First-Stage) Labor

Though labor is categorized into three stages, none of them starts or ends abruptly; each stage flows gradually into the next.

Changes that take place in the cow during the first stage of labor are not visible but are preparing both the birth canal and the calf.

Physical Changes in the First Stage

- Cervix structure changes so it can relax and dilate.
- Uterine contractions begin, stimulating the calf to move into position for birth and extend his front legs. Contractions also start to soften placental attachments so that the placenta can more readily separate from the uterine lining. First contractions, and brief signs of uneasiness, last a few seconds and occur every 10 minutes or so, gradually coming at shorter intervals and increasing from 12 to 24 per hour during the last two hours of early labor. They occur at about one per minute as the calf starts into the birth canal.

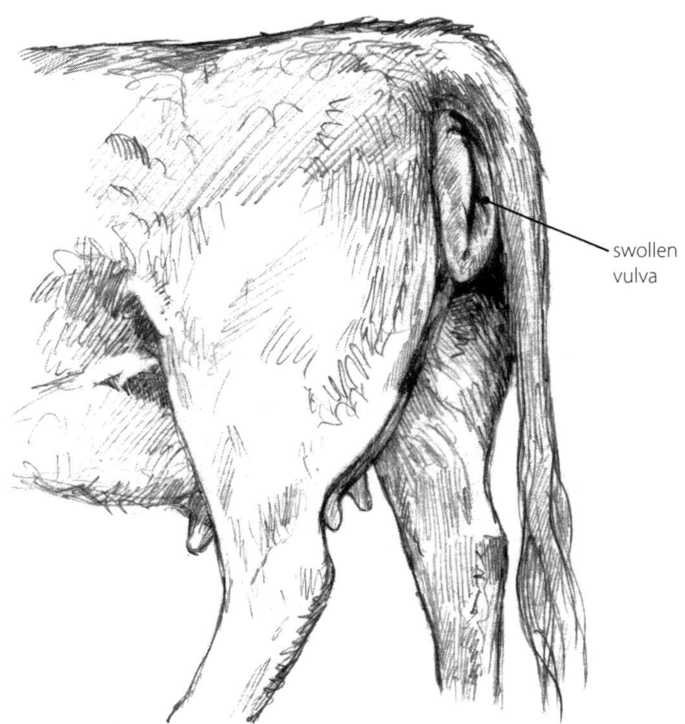

The vulva becomes swollen and floppy as the tissues relax in preparation for calving.

Behavioral Changes in the First Stage

- The cow is very alert and may become restless as uterine contractions begin: Even if the cow is lying down chewing her cud, she's more alert than usual. It's her instinct to watch and to be aware of any prowling predators that could be a danger to the calf she's about to have.
- The cow may leave the herd and find a secluded spot. A confined cow may pace the fence.
- She shows discomfort as uterine contractions occur. She may swish her tail, kick her belly, look at her flank, and get up and down, but she seems largely unconcerned between contractions. She may continue to graze or eat or chew her cud between spasms.
- Some cows, especially easy calvers, show few external signs of early labor except a more rapid respiration rate or some muscle twitches. Unless you're very observant, you might not realize that they're calving.

First-Stage Labor Specifics

Rather than take a quick look when checking the herd, watch the pregnant cows for 10 to 20 minutes. It's easy to miss some early labor signs because cows behave normally between contractions. Every time a contraction occurs (that is, the muscular wall of the uterus contracts), the cow feels a sharp pain. The wave of contraction starts at the bottom of the uterus (the tip that's low and forward in the abdomen) and moves along the entire organ like a swallowing motion, putting pressure on the fetus. *Note:* The unborn calf is called a fetus until delivery is complete, but for simplicity, we'll often refer to it as a calf while we're talking about the birth process.

These periodic waves of contraction are uncomfortable both to the calf and to the cow, and the calf becomes more active. He squirms, which helps him move into position for birth. The pressure generally makes him straighten his front legs, aiming for the birth canal. A large calf has probably already run out of wiggle room in the uterus and has been lying in proper birthing position for a while. He may simply need to straighten his legs. Conversely, a large calf may be in an abnormal position and not have

Teats Can Indicate When Calving Will Occur

A clue that calving may take place within 24 hours is the filling of the cow's teats. Even if the udder is large, the teats don't generally become full and distended until the cow is nearly ready to calve. Occasionally the plug in the end of a teat will start to come out, and a bit of secretion will appear at the end of the teat. Some cows will actually drip milk.

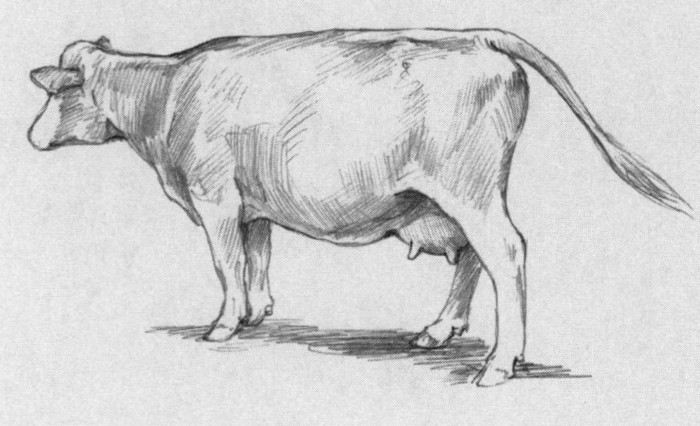

Teats are empty.

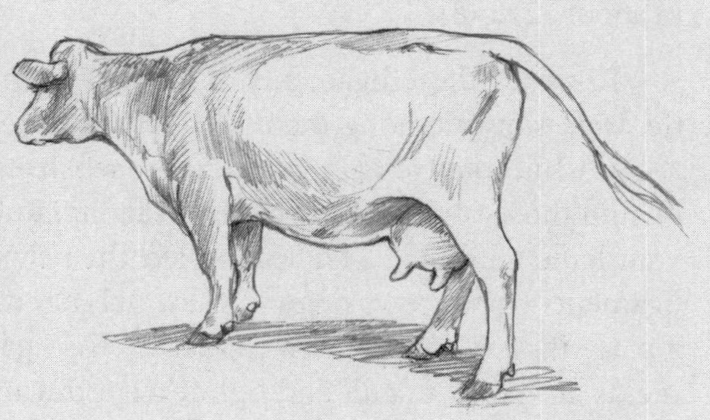

Teats are full and distended.

enough room to move. This improper positioning is one reason some calves need assistance at birth.

The length of early labor is unpredictable. Sometimes cows take longer in early labor because it takes more time for the calf to position himself for starting through the birth canal. In such cases, the cow may repeatedly get up and lie down, which helps rearrange the calf as he works toward proper direction.

As the calf and the fluid-filled membranes that surround him are pushed toward the cervix, the water bag around the calf is often pushed against the cervix first. As a result, the cone-shaped cervix shortens and dilates even more, making the uterus and vagina one continuous canal. When the water bag is the first thing to come through the cervix into the birth canal, it pushes ahead of the calf and helps to open the cervix more fully.

The cow may strain for only a moment but keep her back arched and tail slightly out because of her discomfort. This is one of the most obvious clues that the cow is actually calving: Even if she's not visibly straining, she holds her tail out a bit so that it remains away from her body.

As early labor progresses, contractions become stronger. Once the water bag enters the birth canal, the pressure it creates against the pelvis may stimulate the cow or heifer to arch her back and strain. Contractions now begin to involve her abdominal muscles —a voluntary straining — as well as the uterine muscles. The cow may strain for only a moment but keep her back arched and tail slightly out because of her discomfort. This is one of the most obvious clues that the cow is actually calving: Even if she's not visibly straining, she holds her tail out a bit so that it remains away from her body, as she normally does when she urinates and defecates. This is particularly evident when she walks around. On our ranch we often remark about a cow beginning labor that her tail is "out two degrees."

When Will She Calve?

If you have a breeding date on each cow, you have an idea when each will calve, though the sex of the calf, the season of the year, and the gestation length determine whether calves come ahead of or after their due date. Weather also makes a difference. A falling barometer (meaning a storm is approaching) seems to trigger labor in cows and heifers that are near to term. Most cows begin labor in a low-pressure period rather than when the barometer is rising.

Some stockmen try to time a cow's calving for the daylight hours instead of in the evening by feeding most of the cow's hay ration late at night. Some claim this works because the cow spends much of the night eating rather than calving. Nevertheless, it never worked well in our herd; two-thirds of our calves always came at night. Then again, calving in January at our latitude means that two-thirds of the 24-hour period *is* night!

Contractions become more frequent and occur at regular intervals, and the cervix dilates more fully. Near the end of first-stage labor, the cow may strain a little more, which causes her to empty her bladder and move her bowels. If the cow is restless, she passes manure frequently as she paces around. This helps to make more room for the calf to come through the birth canal without additional pressure from a full bladder or colon.

Active (Second-Stage) Labor

An average, active labor, from the time straining begins or the water bag appears or breaks, takes about 70 minutes, but it may take from 15 minutes to four hours. This stage usually takes longer in heifers than it does in cows that have calved before.

Physical Changes in the Second Stage

- Some part of the calf comes through the cervix to enter the birth canal. Once the calf starts to enter the pelvic cavity, the pressure on certain nerves stimulates the cow to start straining with her abdominal muscles, which will look similar

Weak Contractions Affect Presentation

Until the start of labor, the calf's legs are flexed in the uterus so they take up less room. His knees are often the first part of his body to push against the dilating cervix, but soon his legs straighten and his feet start through it. If for some reason the cow does not have strong uterine contractions (*uterine inertia*; see page 86), the calf may fail to straighten his legs or extend his head and neck. Thus, inadequate uterine contractions are one reason for the malpresentation of head or legs turned back at birth.

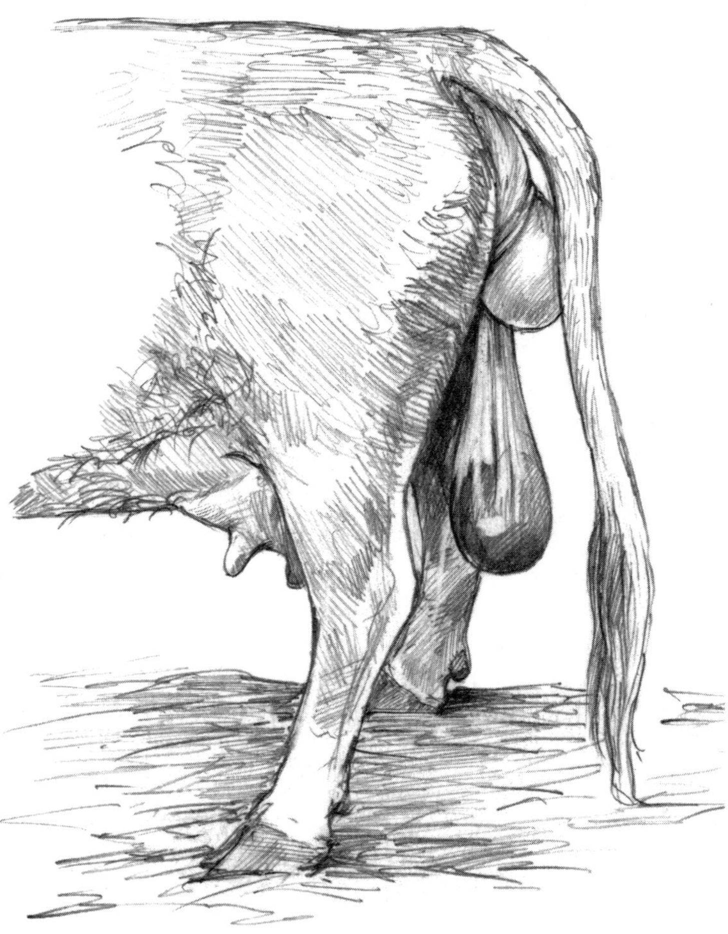

If the "water bag" has not already broken in a flush of amber fluid, it emerges first and may hang down toward the cow's hocks. The amnion sac, which is full of clear fluid and encases the calf, is next to come out, and the calf's feet should soon appear within it.

to the response to the stimulus that causes her to pass manure.

- The cow's straining forces the calf against the dilating cervix, stimulating release of *oxytocin* in the cow, which causes stronger uterine contractions at shorter intervals.
- The water bag, a thin membrane filled with dark, amber fluid, often breaks at the beginning of second-stage labor as it is pushed ahead of the calf through the birth canal. It may protrude from the vulva as a big membrane balloon, about the size of a basketball and somewhat maroon in color, or break before it gets to the vaginal opening. To an observer, it will look like a flood of amber fluid gushing from the cow.
- The calf's feet push through the dilating cervix, then his head presses against it each time the cow strains, opening it up more fully. By the time the calf's head comes through the cervix, the front feet are well into the birth canal. The amnion sac is often still intact when it protrudes from the vulva. The calf's feet should be visible within it, though sometimes you can't see them immediately.
- After the head emerges, the rest of the calf soon follows, as a result of increased uterine contractions.

Behavioral Changes in the Second Stage

- The cow becomes more focused on her internal pains and more oblivious to you.
- Most cows lie down and start straining hard in intermittent series.
- If the cow is standing up, her back is arched and her tail is extended.

Second-Stage Labor Specifics

Some textbooks claim that the breaking of the water bag or the appearance of the water bag at the vulva signals the start of active labor, but judging the arrival of second-stage labor by this appearance alone can be deceptive and unreliable: Sometimes the water bag comes alongside the calf as he is born or even

PROGRESSING THROUGH ACTIVE LABOR

The cow may get up and down a few times after the calf's feet and nose appear, or she may just lie there and continue to strain until she calves. Once the calf's forehead starts out through the vulva, however, she will generally not get up again unless you disturb her, finishing the delivery with a series of hard contractions.

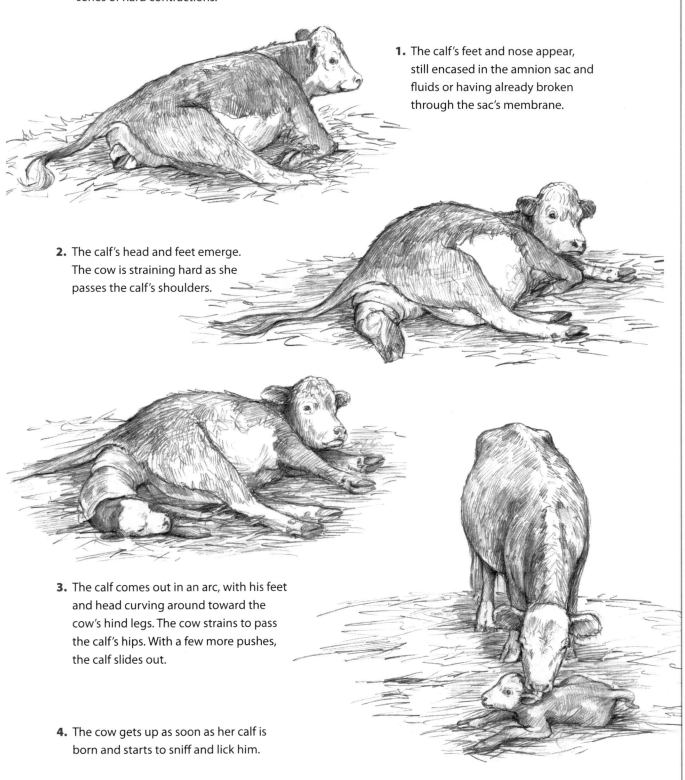

1. The calf's feet and nose appear, still encased in the amnion sac and fluids or having already broken through the sac's membrane.

2. The calf's head and feet emerge. The cow is straining hard as she passes the calf's shoulders.

3. The calf comes out in an arc, with his feet and head curving around toward the cow's hind legs. The cow strains to pass the calf's hips. With a few more pushes, the calf slides out.

4. The cow gets up as soon as her calf is born and starts to sniff and lick him.

after the calf emerges. If you wait for the water to break in order to time the length of second-stage labor, you may not judge it correctly.

Don't confuse the water bag with the clear, white amnion sac that encases the calf. The amnion sac is filled with a lighter-colored, thicker fluid and often appears intact at the vulva with the calf's feet clearly visible within. If the calf is big and is birthing slowly, the amnion sac may appear first and is about the size of a large grapefruit.

If all is normal, the cow makes steady progress once the amnion sac or the feet appear. Sometimes the sac has broken — there may be a dribble of thick clear or whitish fluid from the vulva — and the feet appear with the membrane draped over them instead of with the sac surrounding them. Usually one foot is ahead of the other because the tight space makes it necessary for one shoulder to come through the cow's pelvis ahead of the other.

It may take several moments of hard straining to pass the calf's head. His nose may appear, and progress will slow for a time until the vulva is stretched enough to pass his forehead. Once the forehead passes through the vulva, the rest of the calf usually emerges swiftly. The cow may rest for a moment once the calf's head is out, then give a series of intense contractions without any rest between them while she passes his shoulders and rib cage.

The bulky mass of the calf's shoulders stretches the birth canal even more than the head does, which stimulates more release of oxytocin from the cow's pituitary gland. This, in turn, accentuates her uterine contractions, which work with abdominal contractions to expel the calf. Another wave of strong contractions is similarly triggered when the calf's hips come through the birth canal.

As the calf's rib cage comes through, fluid emerges from his mouth and nose as a result of pressure on his chest. This helps clear the calf's airways for his first breath.

The calf curls around toward the cow's hind legs as he slides out. His hind legs may remain in the birth canal a few moments until the cow gets up or until the calf struggles free.

If the umbilical cord has not broken, the calf may lie there a moment before breathing. If the cord breaks as the calf emerges, he will try to breathe very soon, once the sac and fluids are away from his face, because he has no oxygen. Generally, the calf will raise his head and shake it to help clear his nostrils before he takes his first breath.

The cow often gets up immediately after the calf is born and turns around to sniff and lick him, unless she's a first-time mother. If both mother and calf lie there a few moments, the cord may not break until one or the other moves. In breaking, the umbilical blood vessels and the *urachus,* the tube that runs from the calf's bladder to the navel and through the

A Calf's First Breath

The calf is stimulated to breathe when his nostrils are uncovered and he feels air on his face. About 20 percent of calves are born with the amnion sac intact, often with fluid still in it. If the amnion sac does not break and this membrane and its fluid remain over the calf's head, the animal will not take a breath. This *immersion reflex* keeps the calf from drawing fluid into its lungs — but it also means that some calves die soon after birth. It's important that the sac break. The cow should start licking it off and nudging the calf with her nose and head to get him moving and breathing. If the calf goes too long without oxygen, he will suffocate.

When Is It Time to Jump In?

During the birth, it's time to help if the process is slow — for instance, when the amnion sac is visible for 30 to 40 minutes with no feet inside it. It's a definite sign that the birth is taking too long if fluid in the amnion sac is a dirty yellow-brown: This means that the calf is stressed and may be in trouble; he has defecated into the amniotic fluid because of uterine pressure on his abdomen or because he is short on oxygen. Act quickly to help complete the birth.

umbilical cord, are ruptured. Because they're somewhat elastic, they retract toward or up into the calf's abdomen. The torn ends of the arteries then shrink to prevent hemorrhage.

The calf should get up within 10 to 13 minutes of being born and look for the udder.

Third-Stage Labor

The final stage of labor and birth, shedding the placenta, takes one to three hours but can sometimes last longer.

Third-Stage Labor Specifics

Continued uterine contractions open the cups on the uterine lining so they'll let go of the corresponding attachments on the placenta. The cow has more contractions as the uterus shrinks and pushes out the detaching placenta. The placental mass starts through the birth canal and enters the cow's pelvis, stimulating the cow to add abdominal straining to uterine contractions, which helps expel the membranes.

The calf should get up within 10 to 30 minutes of being born, though a big calf that had a slow birth may take longer, and should begin looking for the udder. Usually the cow licks the calf and encourages him to get up, aiming him toward her udder with licking and nudging once the calf rises. Sometimes the contractions as the cow works at shedding the afterbirth will make her lie down again for a while. At this time, her calf may blunder about until she finishes expelling the placenta ("cleaning") or becomes so worried about the calf that she gets up again so he can nurse.

The calf's sucking stimulates the release of oxytocin in the cow, which triggers milk letdown and stimulates more uterine contractions to get rid of the placenta and hasten shrinking of the uterus to normal size.

Once the cow passes the placenta, she usually eats it — instinctive behavior that protects the calf from predators. After he nurses, the calf lies near the birth area and sleeps, hidden while the cow leaves to graze or go to the feeding area. If allowed to remain there, the placenta's odor, especially on a warm day, would attract scavenging birds and animals that might endanger the calf. Sometimes a cow can choke on her afterbirth. Because of this, it's advisable to remove it from the stall or area after she cleans.

Occasionally, a cow is slow to clean and retains the placenta for several days or even a week or longer. In some of these instances, antibiotic treatment becomes necessary (see chapter 6).

Helping in the Birth Process

Recognizing the normal stages and progress in birth as outlined in the previous sections enables you to judge whether a cow or heifer needs your help. It's important to decide how long and in what circumstances to leave her laboring on her own and when to help her yourself or seek help from your vet.

The Dangers of Calf Death during Labor

A calf may die from lack of oxygen any time during labor if the placenta detaches — and it always detaches after a long labor.

If the cow is not assisted and the calf can't be born, he will die after 3 to 12 hours of active labor. By that time, the cow or heifer is exhausted and is not straining anymore. The open cervix allows pathogens into the uterus, which multiply in the tissues of the dead calf. Gas production and swelling of the calf begin 24 to 36 hours after the beginning of labor, and there may be a putrid discharge from the cow's vulva.

Trying to pull a dead calf from a cow that's been in labor too long can be risky and difficult because the cervix is closing and the calf is swollen. This is a life-threatening situation for the cow or heifer and requires veterinary help. If you observe your cows closely as calving approaches, you won't have this difficulty. You'll know when labor begins and can assist in a timely fashion.

Remember: Don't intervene too soon — that is, before the cervix is well dilated. Doing so could injure the cow as you attempt to pull the calf through a narrow cervical opening. Forceful pulling before the birth canal is ready can rupture the cervix or tear the vagina and vulva. The cervix is programmed to relax and open fully as the top of the calf's head presses intermittently against it with each contraction. Your hard, steady pull on the calf can actually delay this process.

When to Intervene

Once the calf is in proper position and the cervix is fully dilated, there's no point in waiting for the calf's birth if the animal is taking too long to come through the birth canal.

There are a number of reasons to intervene at this point. The calf is subjected to a great deal of pressure, both from uterine contractions and from the constricted area in the birth canal, and each time the cow strains, her abdominal contractions constrict blood vessels to the uterus, resulting in a diminished oxygen supply to the calf. If all of this goes on too long, the calf may be born weak, unconscious, or dead from oxygen shortage. In addition, if the calf is short on oxygen and is also born in cold weather, he won't be able to shiver to keep himself warm and is more at risk for severe chilling or freezing.

Outside of the threats to the calf, waiting too long to intervene in a prolonged birth means the heifer or cow is exhausted and thus unable to strain productively. Much of the lubricating fluid around the calf may be gone because the sacs have ruptured and lost fluid.

If a cow spends too long in labor before you jump in to help, the vaginal wall becomes swollen, making it harder to put your hand and arm into the birth canal and providing less room to manipulate the calf if he's in the wrong position.

Finally, if the cervix and uterus of the cow have already started to shrink, correcting a *malpresentation* by pushing the calf back into the uterus is difficult or impossible.

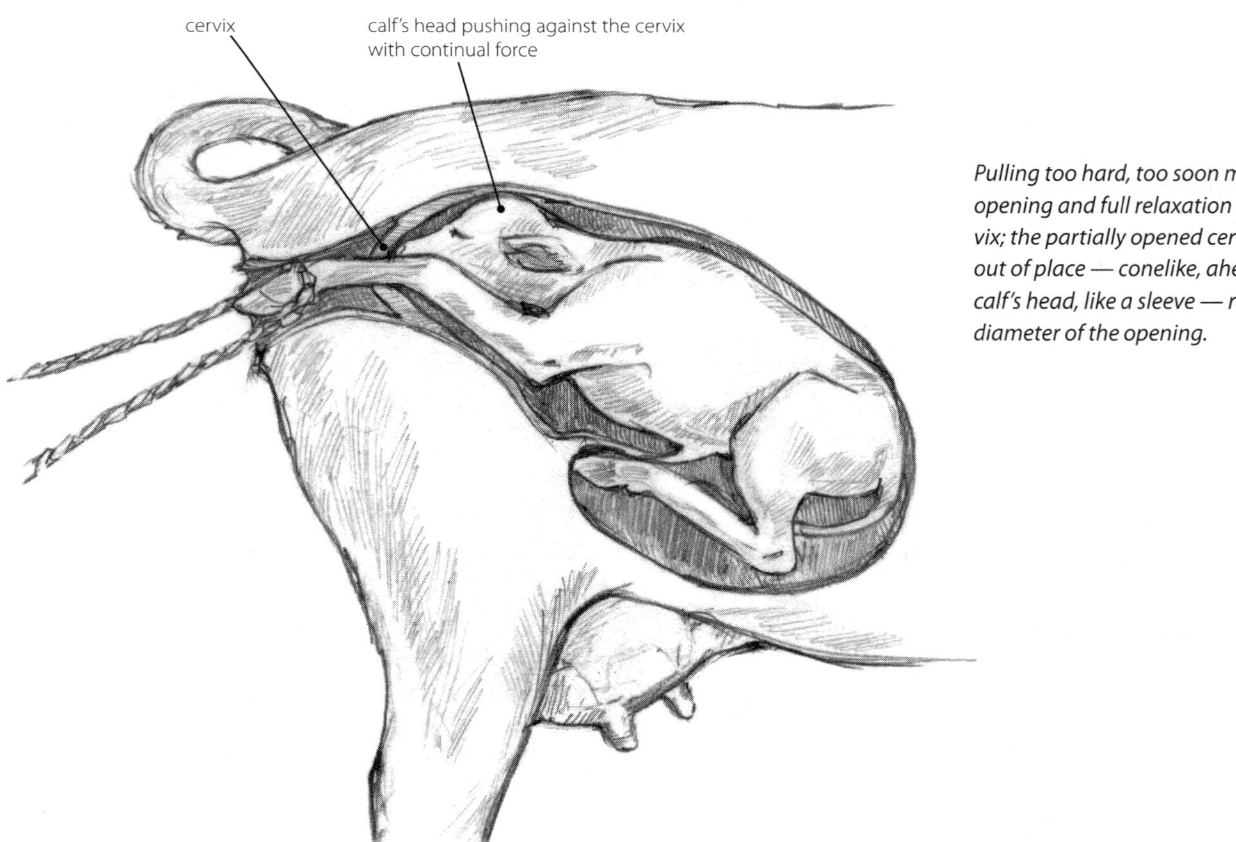

Pulling too hard, too soon may delay the opening and full relaxation of the cervix; the partially opened cervix is pulled out of place — conelike, ahead of the calf's head, like a sleeve — restricting the diameter of the opening.

Remember that a calf that spends minimal time in the birth canal (that is, experiences an easy or properly assisted birth) is more lively and strong and is able to get up and find the udder more quickly.

Check the Cow

If nothing of the calf shows after the cow has been straining intensely, check her to see if the calf is not presented normally or if he is too large to be easily born. It's more beneficial to both cow and calf if you begin assisting before the cow is fatigued and the calf is compromised — or dead.

There are a number of factors that can signal it's time to check the cow during labor:

- The cow is off by herself and is restless for more than six to eight hours.
- The cow has been straining hard for more than one hour and either no calf is showing or the calf's feet are showing when she strains but go back in when she rests.
- Yellow-brown fluid is present in the amnion sac or in the vaginal discharge.
- The feet of the calf are upside down (bottoms of the feet are up instead of down) or only one foot is showing.
- The calf's birthing progress has halted altogether.

How to Check a Cow in Labor

Restrain the cow. In order to check most cows, they must be restrained, especially if there are no calf feet showing yet and a calf doesn't appear to be entering the birth canal. Once the calf is in the birth canal, the cow or heifer is usually less mobile and more apt to continue lying down even if you check her. If the cow is standing, to make sure you can check her properly, tie her or put her in a stanchion or head catcher.

Approach the cow calmly and quietly. If you're taking a heifer to a chute or head catcher, take a gentle cow with her to keep her calm. If she's in a barn stall and you need to tie her, quietly corner her to put a halter on. (Never tie a cow with only a rope around her neck.) Attached to the halter there should be a long rope that you can hold on to while you put it around a corral post or solid barn support. Gradually take up the slack in the rope until the cow is close to the tie spot. If she's flighty, stand on the other side of the fence or panel while tying her, or just loop the rope around the post and take it to the next post to tie it. This way she can't smash into you while you are securing it. Be sure to tie short; don't have so much slack in the rope that the cow can fling herself around while you're checking her. Also, tie close to ground level; if you tie the rope too high, the cow will pull downward as she hangs back on the rope and will be more apt to end up on the ground while you're still trying to check her, when you want her standing. If she goes down, you want the rope tied low to keep her from hanging by her head.

Be prepared. Bring warm water containing mild disinfectant, a rag for scrubbing, a squeeze bottle of lubricant disinfectant, and OB chains and handles. If you don't have a helper to hold the cow's tail, tie it to a string around her neck so she won't swat you in the face with it or flip manure. Wear a short-sleeved or sleeveless shirt because you may have to insert your whole arm into the cow to determine what's wrong. Take time to scrub your hand and arm, and wash

What Part of the Calf Am I Feeling?

You can recognize the calf's head easily by feeling the mouth, tongue, eyes, and ears. It's a bit harder to determine if you're feeling a front leg or a hind one. If the bottom of the foot is facing downward, it's usually a front foot. To make sure, feel farther up the leg to the knee or hock. If that joint is round and bends in the same direction as the *fetlock joint* (the big joint at the end of the lower leg, at the *dewclaws*), it's a knee. If it bends in the opposite direction, it's a hock (you'll be able to feel the point of the hock).

If you have trouble feeling through the amnion sac surrounding the calf and are certain you won't be calling the vet for the birth, carefully break the sac or find the already torn edges and insert your hand so you can feel the calf's body parts directly.

the cow's vulva and anus thoroughly by scrubbing them with a clean rag or towel and OB scrub solution (such as Betadine, which is a "tamed" iodine, a compound used as a disinfectant that is not as harsh as iodine). Merely putting disinfectant over the top of manure will not kill bacteria!

Because the cow may defecate several times during your exam, have extra wash water on hand to rinse her again. Note that putting your hand into the vagina will make her strain and pass more manure and will mean you'll have to wash her vulva and your arm again. It's handy to have extra water in squeeze bottles; they are not spilled as easily as a bucket, and they're easy to manipulate with one hand.

It's wise to use a clean, disposable OB glove or sleeve to cover your hand and arm after you wash them. This keeps your arm cleaner and minimizes the introduction of contamination into the cow. Coating the glove or sleeve with obstetrical lubricant reduces irritation to membranes of the birth canal. A protective sleeve also helps guard against animal-to-human infections such as brucellosis and salmonellosis.

Start the check. Insert your hand slowly and gently into the vulva, making sure to cause the least discomfort possible. If the water bag is in the birth canal, don't rupture it; in case you find a problem you can't deal with and must call the vet for help, it's best not to allow all the fluids to escape the cow. If the fluids are gone, the uterus, like an empty balloon, will be shrinking by the time the vet gets there, and important lubrication will be lost.

If, however, you determine that you can give the cow assistance yourself, then rupture the membranes so that you can manipulate the calf or put chains on his legs.

Next, put your hand into the birth canal as far as necessary to find the calf. If the feet are right there, reach a little farther to make sure the head is coming; you should feel the nose a few inches beyond the feet. If the head isn't there or there's nothing yet in the birth canal, reach farther into the canal until you come to the cervix.

Make an assessment. If the cervix is fully dilated and you can easily put your hand through it, there's probably a reason that the calf is being prevented from starting into the birth canal. Reach into the uterus to feel the calf and determine which way he's lying and perhaps why he can't proceed. If the cervix is not fully dilated, it will feel like a small opening in the end of the baglike birth canal and may still have sticky mucus in it. If you can put only one or two fingers through it, the cow needs more laboring time. If the cervix is partly open, you may be able to put your hand through it to reach the calf and determine why his feet are not starting to enter the birth canal. If the vagina abruptly ends at the pelvic brim and is pulled into tight, spiral folds, you may be encountering a uterine torsion (see page 57). If all you feel

Birth Losses

All too often a cow loses a calf at birth because of a simple problem that could have been corrected by giving help at the right time.

A 1993–1994 survey of 2,000 Alberta cattle ranchers by researchers at Western College of Veterinary Medicine in Saskatoon, Saskatchewan, sought to identify primary causes of death in calves. Survey records were completed by 426 ranchers, giving information on a total of 63,500 calves, including 6,751 calves that sickened in those herds and 3,292 calves that died. Surprisingly, and by a wide margin, stillbirths topped the 10 causes of death, followed by calving problems, pneumonia, and, in fourth place, scours (diarrhea), which is usually considered the number one killer.

The term "stillbirth" is deceptive, however. Very few calves are actually dead at the time they are being born. Most calves classified by ranchers as *stillborn* were found dead by someone who wasn't there at birth to know what happened. I would guess that almost all calves classified as stillborn were actually alive during birth but died because birth was too slow (perhaps the calf was too big); the placenta detached (because the birth was too slow); the amnion sac surrounding the calf did not come off after birth and he suffocated (oddly enough, a problem that often happens after a swift birth); or some other complication occurred. Almost all these calves would have been alive with a little assistance from the stockman.

upon checking is the spongy mass of placenta coming ahead of the calf into the birth canal, the placenta is detaching too soon and the calf will soon run out of oxygen. You must deliver the calf quickly.

Your assessment of the situation will help you determine whether to give the cow more time, call the vet to correct a malpresentation or a uterine torsion, or go ahead and pull a calf that has started into the birth canal in proper position but is simply coming slowly because he's large. To determine if the calf is too large to be pulled and must be surgically delivered, see Checking a Heifer, page 79.

If the calf responds with a reflex action when you touch his eye or grab his tongue (he will move his head), stick a finger in his mouth (he will suck) or into his anus, if he's backward or breech (he will contract the anal sphincter), or pinch the skin between his toes (he will jerk his foot), then he's still alive.

When to Call the Vet

If you can't ascertain what is abnormal in the calf's position or you've worked for 20 to 30 minutes on a problem and have not been able to correct it or extract the calf, call your vet. In order to save the calf, don't spend too long in futile efforts.

Call the vet immediately if you determine that the calf's head is too large to fit through the pelvis, you note abnormal discharge or a foul odor coming from the cow, or you feel any abnormality in the cow, such as a tear in the vagina or uterus, a torsion shutting off the birth canal, or a prolapsed bladder. Also call the vet immediately if you see or feel any

EVERY CALF BORN ALIVE

IN THE YEARS WHEN WE CALVED OUR COWS at pasture in March and April and observed them only sporadically, we averaged a 4 percent birth loss due to a variety of factors, including slow births (of large calves), malpresentations, coyotes, lack of mothering from first-time mothers, or something as simple as the amnion sac not breaking, which resulted in the suffocation of the calf. In contrast, in the 35 years we calved in winter and diligently observed the cows, checking them every hour or less, we've averaged a 0.3 percent birth loss. In most years, in fact, we lose no calves.

In our own herd, which for many years was made up of more than 170 cows, we've found that almost all calves can be saved if we are present at the proper time. During the years we closely observed cows, we had only one stillbirth in which the calf was obviously dead before delivery. All the other calves were alive at the start of active labor and we've been able to save almost all of them.

For many years we calved in January so that cows could be bred in April before going to summer range on mountain pastures. Because it was often subzero at that time of year, we put almost every cow in the barn when she went into labor, and we were there for every birth so that no calves would freeze to death. Because we were there, aside from saving almost every calf, we also learned a great deal about normal and abnormal births. We've learned that if you're there to give assistance, you can cut birth losses to virtually nil.

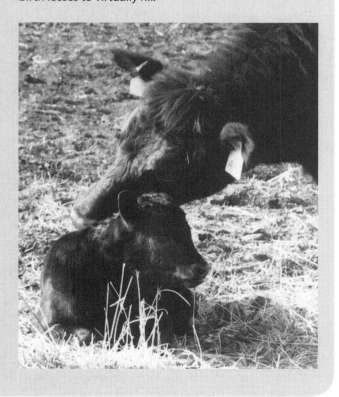

abnormality in the calf, such as leg joints "fixed" at an odd angle or an oversized forehead. The calf may need to be delivered by cesarean section or, if he's dead or dying, by *fetotomy* (cutting the fetus apart to bring it out in pieces).

Call the vet immediately if you determine that the calf's head is too large to fit through the pelvis, you note abnormal discharge or a foul odor coming from the cow, or you feel any abnormality in the cow.

If the calf is dead upon delivery, you can usually tell if he died during birth or was already dead before you gave assistance. If the calf's body tissues have started to swell and the hair coat is coming off (slipping), the calf has been dead at least 24 hours. If there is no tissue swelling but the corneas of the eyes are cloudy and gray, the calf has probably been dead at least six hours.

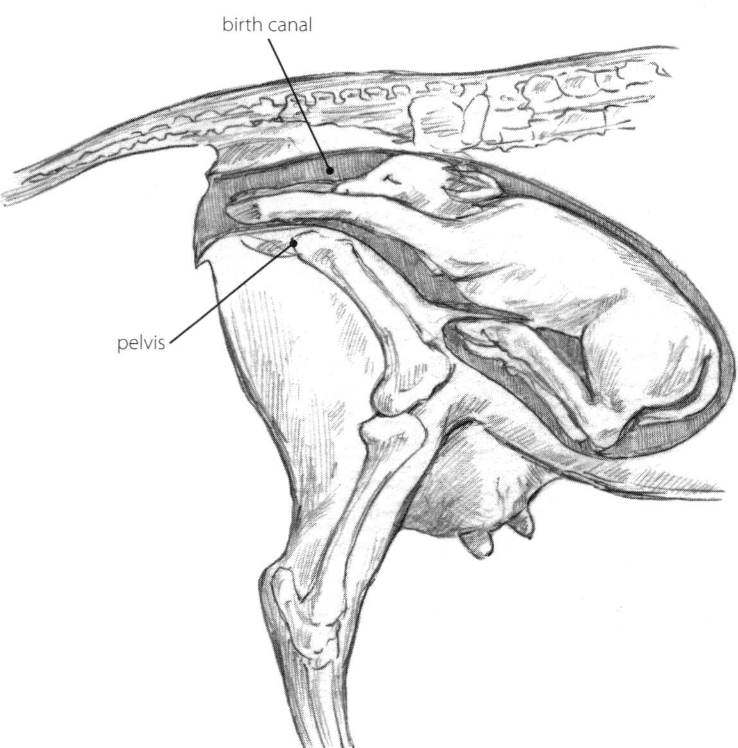

As he is entering the birth canal, the calf must come up and over the pelvis in this normal, frontward-facing calving position.

Pulling the Normal Calf That's Just a Little Too Big

Pulling a calf should be attempted only when the calf is in proper position — that is, normal *anterior position* (frontward, with front feet and head coming into the birth canal) or *posterior position* (hind feet coming into the birth canal). See chapter 4 for more on these positions.

In a normal anterior position, the head should be resting on the legs, with the eyes at about knee position. If the head is turned back and only the legs are there, feel up the legs to make sure they are front legs (see page 71, What Part of the Calf Am I Feeling?). Any deviation from front feet and head first or hind feet first must be corrected before you can pull the calf.

First Pull without Chains

If the head has not yet entered the birth canal and goes off to the side when you start pulling on the legs, the calf may be too big and needs help to be born. Keep one hand on his head to keep it straight as you pull on his legs. You may have to insert both arms into the birth canal to get the calf entering properly before you attach chains to his legs. You can grasp the lower jaw of the calf to keep the head coming straight. Once the head enters the pelvis, it should keep coming as you pull on the legs. Don't use excessive force when handling the jaw or you could break it. Also, if you move the head by hanging on to the jaw, take care that the calf's incisors don't cut the cow's uterus; keep your hand between the calf's teeth and the cow's tissues.

Attaching Chains to the Legs

Once the head enters the birth canal, you can attach chains to the calf's legs, to pull the calf (see page 75). If it's not already broken, break the water bag to allow more room to work. You'll also need to break the amnion sac to get chains on the calf's legs. Use plenty of lubricant — as one vet said to me, "An ounce of lubrication is worth a ton of traction pres-

Attaching Chains

Obstetrical chains work better than a strap or rope because chains don't totally restrict circulation and are easier to clean between calves. They're also handier because you can attach a handle to them anywhere for a proper grip.

When attaching chains to a calf, first encircle them around the calf's legs (one chain end to each leg) above the fetlock joints so they won't pull on the joints and feet. Never put a chain just above the calf's foot or it might injure the joint or pull off the hoof shell. Make a double loop (especially if you'll be exerting a strong pull, as with a calf puller) and place the first loop above the fetlock joint and the second around the *pastern*, above the hoof. A single loop may pull the leg at an awkward angle, and if you exert a lot of pressure (as with a calf puller), you can cause joint injury or even a broken bone. The double loop ensures a straighter pull on the leg and spreads the stress over a greater area with less risk of injury to the calf. The pull should come from under the leg; pulling from the side may break a leg.

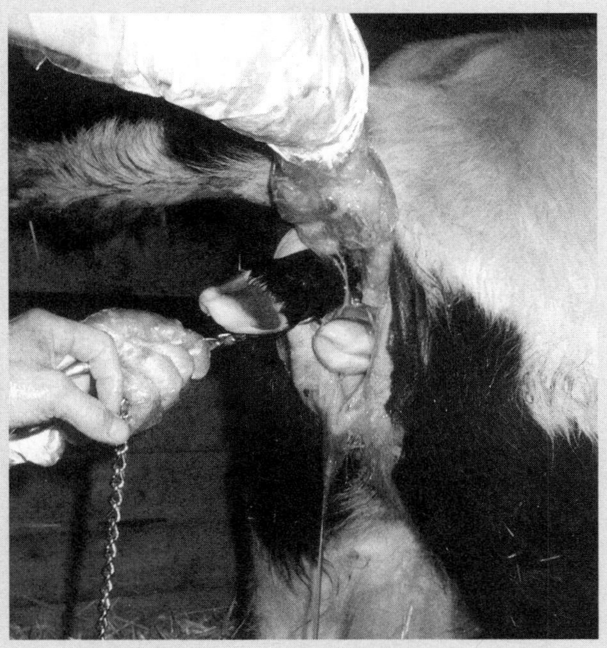

Attach the chains far enough above the fetlock joint, and make sure that the pull will be from the underneath part of the leg.

sure." The calf will be relatively dry, and there will be more friction without the fluid from the water sac around the calf making him more slippery. Apply the lubricant to your hand from a squeeze bottle and force it in around the calf and birth canal. Commercial obstetrical lubricants can be obtained from your vet or a livestock supply catalog, but if you don't have any, a generous amount of liquid soap and water, or soap flakes and water, will work if it's a very mild type of soap.

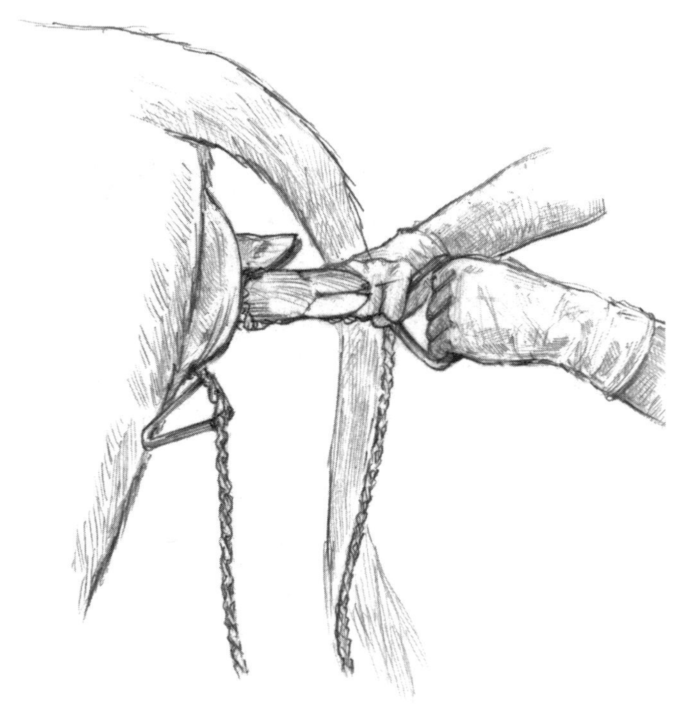

You'll have to break the amnion sac and let out the fluid, in order to attach chains to the calf's legs.

Pulling with Two People Is Best

If we assist a birth, my husband and I work as a team, pulling the calf by hand (with chains on his legs) rather than using a calf puller. We rarely use a calf puller except for backward calves. In almost all other situations, the strength of two people is adequate even for a very difficult birth, and you are less apt to injure the cow or calf. Also, when you pull the calf by hand, you can pull at the best angle without the calf puller getting in your way.

Direction of Pull

Many calf pullers limit your options and pull at the wrong angle part of the time. It's important to remember that the calf has to come in an arc: He starts from down in the uterus and must come up over the cow's pelvic brim. When his feet are coming through the birth canal and starting to protrude from the vulva, you should pull straight back and a little upward. After you get his head and shoulders out, however, you should change the angle of your pull and begin pulling slightly downward, toward the cow's legs.

> PULLING POSITION
>
> On a hard pull, it helps if the cow is down; she strains more effectively, and you can get more leverage sitting behind her bracing your feet against her hind end. Some people brace themselves on a bale of straw placed behind the cow, out of the way of the emerging calf.

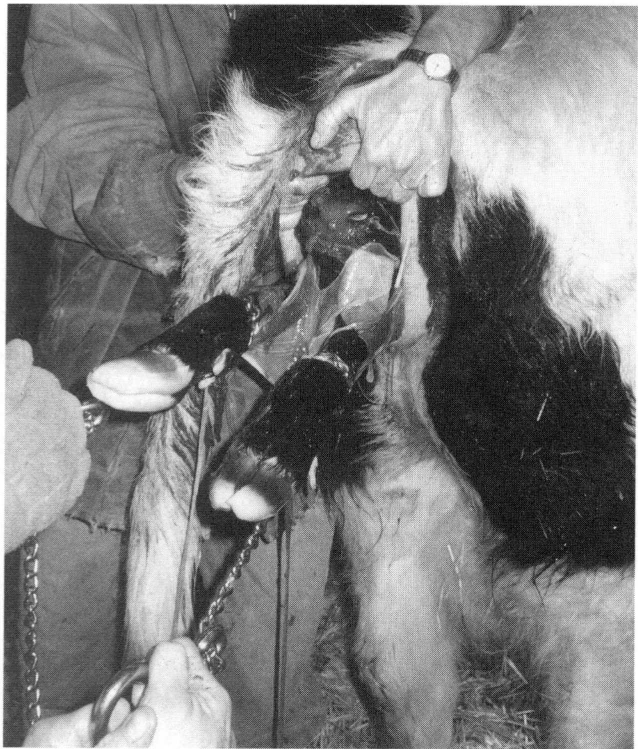

One person stretches the cow's vulva so the calf's head can come through more easily, while the other person pulls on the calf's legs with obstetrical chains.

Once the calf's rib cage is free and clear of the vulva, you can pull straight down toward the cow's hocks; the calf's body must arc up and over the pelvis and then come down. In a normal birth, with the cow lying on the ground in labor, the calf curves around toward the cow's hocks and feet as he slides out. This is the arc you must duplicate when pulling a calf for easiest delivery and for minimal trauma to the calf.

Stretching the Vulva

On a difficult pull, it helps if one person pulls on the calf's legs while the other person stretches the cow's vulva. When we work as a team, my husband pulls on the calf while I stand or sit beside the cow or heifer (depending on whether she's up or down), facing the rear, and put my fingers between the calf's head and the vulva so I can pull and stretch the tissue of the vulva.

Together my husband, Lynn, and I pull and stretch the vulva each time the cow strains to give birth to the calf and rest when she rests. Stretching the vulva as the calf's head comes through allows it to come more easily and more quickly with less wear and tear and fatigue for the cow. Once the calf's head is out, the rest of his body comes out more easily. If it's a big calf or a hard birth, after we get the head out, I help Lynn finish pulling the calf with the chain handles.

Special Considerations for First-Calf Heifers

Most times, situations in which labor takes too long involve first-calf heifers. They are often not yet fully grown and typically have a smaller pelvic area than that of a cow.

Signs of Early and Active Labor

If you're watching a heifer, you'll know when she begins early labor. A heifer in labor is often easier to recognize than an older cow that's starting labor:

- She's restless and uncomfortable and may become quite upset. She hasn't experienced uterine contractions before and may pace. The restless stage, when uterine contractions start moving the calf toward the birth canal, can take two to six hours and sometimes longer.

- A heifer will progress through early labor, her water may break, and the calf may start to enter the birth canal — then progress may slow or stop. The tips of the calf's feet may show at the vulva and come no farther, or the heifer may strain and have nothing to show for it. The calf may be too big or it could have a malpresentation.

Does the Heifer Need Me?

If a heifer is not working hard to calve within two to four hours of breaking water, you must check her. Keep in mind, however, that breaking water is not a reliable guide to length of labor (see page 66): A heifer's water may not break at the start of active labor, and if you wait for this sign, you may wait too long to help her.

Remember, too, that heifers are tricky in that they often take longer than cows to go through early labor, meaning it's hard to judge how much time to give them. A nervous, confined heifer may pace the stall or pen and not settle down to serious labor. She may put off straining, but if she puts it off too long, the placenta will detach and the calf will die.

You don't want to intervene too soon, especially if the heifer is nervous or wild, thereby upsetting her and risking that she'll not mother the calf after it's born. Yet it's better to assist the delivery than to run the risk of losing the calf because you didn't help the birth in time.

One Shoulder at a Time

A big calf with wide shoulders may stop as the shoulders try to come through the pelvis; the shoulders must come through on a slant, one at a time. If both feet are out at equal distance, pull one leg until it advances several inches, meaning the shoulder attached to that leg has eased into the pelvis. Keep easy tension on that leg while pulling more strongly on the other one, to bring that shoulder through also. After the shoulders are through, apply traction equally on both legs to complete the birth.

BETTER SAFE THAN SORRY

It's always smart to detect and correct problems early in labor while you still have a live calf. On our ranch we feel it's best to check the heifer and pull her calf if there's any question about whether she needs help. We've found that it's better to assist a heifer that might not need us than it is to neglect one that does need help.

Even if he survives the prolonged birth, a calf that spends a long time in the birth canal with continuous pressure on his head will be compromised. His circulation will be impaired, his tongue may be swollen, and he'll be short on oxygen if the umbilical cord was pinched or the placenta started to detach.

If you know when a heifer started second-stage labor, you'll have more information by which to judge how long you can safely wait before intervening. If the heifer is straining hard but making little progress, don't leave her in hard labor more than an hour. If left to her own devices, the heifer will labor and eventually have the calf (unless it is too big to come through the pelvis) but will wear herself out in the process, and the calf may be dead by the time she delivers him.

Even if he survives the prolonged birth, a calf that spends a long time in the birth canal with continuous pressure on his head will be compromised. His circulation will be impaired, his tongue may be swollen (making it difficult or impossible for him to nurse until the swelling goes down), and he'll be short on oxygen if the umbilical cord was pinched or the placenta started to detach. In addition, the exhausted heifer and her stressed calf may both be slow to get up. If the weather is cold, this slow rising will mean the calf may chill and the tired heifer may be slow to mother him. This is not the way to get off to a good start in life!

Assisting Early

When it's done properly, assisting early is not as damaging or potentially fatal as giving assistance too late.

If you pull only when the heifer is straining, you'll give the cervix and birth canal time to dilate. Apply traction only when the heifer strains; never pull steadily. Intermittent straining and pulling allows blood flow to the calf to resume when the heifer rests. Constant pressure constricts blood vessels and the umbilical cord (which is squeezed between the cow's pelvis and the calf) and is hard on both the heifer and the calf.

When you do pull, never jerk. Go slowly, to avoid tearing the soft tissues of the birth canal and to allow time for it to expand as the calf comes through. If you're pulling on the legs and the head has not yet appeared and the calf can't make any more progress (as if there's a sudden obstruction), stop and check inside the heifer again to see what's wrong and to make sure the head is still coming.

Timely Assistance = Healthy Heifers

In earlier times, textbooks and veterinarians warned stockmen to be patient and never try to pull a calf too soon. They stressed the risk of injuring the cow, heifer, or calf by pulling before the birth canal was dilated. But not much was said about drawbacks of waiting too long. Many heifers were allowed to labor fruitlessly for two or three hours before they finally delivered a calf or assistance was given. By the time the calf was born, both Mama and baby were exhausted, slow to get up, and slow to nurse.

A number of more recent studies have shown that it's best to assist heifers no more than one hour after active labor begins. Timely help results in a healthier, more vigorous calf and dam. In addition, assisted heifers breed back faster: The reproductive tract returns to normal sooner because it's been less stressed. In fact, proper intervention in birth shortens the interval between birth and the first subsequent heat cycle for the heifer. Generally, each 10 minutes the delivery is delayed adds two days to this interval, and some heifers that didn't have help when they needed it do not become pregnant again that season.

When to Help a Heifer

A heifer that is giving birth for the first time can run into a number of difficulties. Here are some guidelines on when to take action if the heifer seems to be struggling without making progress or if she is growing exhausted.

- Allow no more than an hour to pass once the calf's feet show at the vulva. This gives enough time for the cervix and birth canal to dilate so that the calf can be pulled without injuring the heifer. Even if the feet and nose are showing after an hour of hard labor, it's best to pull the calf unless visible progress is starting again.
- If the calf's tongue is sticking out, it may be due to swelling. It usually means the heifer has been in labor too long and needs help.
- If you can see that the whole head is coming out, the calf has probably stretched the tight membranes just inside the vulva and the heifer may be able to complete the birth without assistance.
- Many heifers need only a little help because they have a constricting ring of tissue (called a *persistent hymen*) in the birth canal. The stretching and tearing of this band as the calf comes through is painful, so painful that some heifers quit straining. This is one reason to pull a calf even if the heifer and calf do not appear to be in trouble.
- Any time a heifer takes more than a four- to five-minute break between straining episodes, she's getting tired. If she becomes too tired, she can't strain effectively, even if you help her, and the calf will be stressed and weak from being in the birth canal too long. If a heifer takes more than a 10-minute break, it's definitely time to help.

How to Check a Heifer

Restrain her. If the heifer is not wild and continues to lie there and strain as you quietly approach, you may be able to check her right where she is, wit out getting her up. If the heifer jumps up when you approach, you'll have to put her into a head catch or chute or tie her up to restrain her while she's being checked.

Start the check. Kneel down behind her, and with a clean hand and arm (as described on page 71, preferably using a sterile obstetrical glove and sleeve), gently reach into the vulva and check to see if both of the calf's front feet are coming.

When you reach into the birth canal, both front feet and the calf's head should be aimed toward the birth canal or should be starting through it. If feet and head are in proper position, check to see if the head will fit through the pelvis. If the feet are starting to come through but you don't feel the calf's nose, the head may be turned back with the nose pointing toward the front of the heifer. In an adult cow, if the calf's head is turned back, it may indicate insufficient uterine contractions, but in a heifer, it often means lack of room for the head to enter the pelvic cavity.

If the heifer jumps up when you approach, you'll have to put her into a head catch or chute or tie her up to restrain her while she's being checked.

Make an assessment. If the calf's head is aimed properly, his nose and/or his tongue should be starting through the birth canal a little behind the feet. If the pelvic opening is small and the calf's forehead is hitting the top of the pelvis, however, there may not be enough room for the calf to fit through. By reaching in with your hand, you can tell if the head is too big: You should be able to push at least one or two of your fingers over the top of his head (pushing your fingers between the cow's bony pelvis and the calf's forehead). If the pelvis is hitting the calf's head at eye level, you won't be able to pull the calf; he won't fit. Call your vet so that the calf can be delivered by cesarean section (see chapter 5).

Checking a Flighty Heifer

If the heifer is not yet in hard labor and you need to check her to determine why she's taking so long, she'll likely still be very mobile, getting up and down and pacing around. At this stage she is quite capable of running off and probably won't let you approach. You'll have to restrain her by tying her up or putting her in a stanchion or head catcher so you can reach inside the birth canal.

Be aware that a heifer is also liable to kick when you start to check her — unless the calf is already in the birth canal. Once the calf has started through or once the heifer starts straining again, she is less likely (or able) to kick.

Pulling a Big Calf from a Heifer

We prefer to quietly help a heifer without having to tie her up or put her in a head catch; she's more likely to mother the calf if you don't upset her. If she's been down for a time, straining, and is tired, the heifer may be cooperative when you sneak up behind her to start pulling the calf. She may also be unable to jump up due to the pressure on her pelvis from the calf in the birth canal.

Usually, once you start pulling, even if it's just on one leg at first, it stimulates the heifer to start hard straining again, and she won't jump up. If you approach quietly and are quick about getting the chain around one foot and starting to pull, this often buys you time to get the chain on the other leg, and later you can reposition the chain on the first leg when the heifer settles into straining. It's safest to do this in a barn stall or small pen in case the heifer does try to jump up and run away.

While the heifer is straining, keep tension on the calf's leg with one hand and reach in with your other hand to make sure the head is coming if it's not yet visible and to determine if there's room for the head to fit through the pelvis.

Once you get chains on the calf's legs, it's easiest to help the heifer if she's lying down, preferably on her right side with all four legs sticking out to the side (which is the natural position for hard labor). The largest stomach (the *rumen*), on her left, takes up a great deal of room. Lying on her right, she can strain more effectively than on her left side or

HELPING A HEIFER GIVE BIRTH

Most heifers don't need the extra traction of a mechanical calf puller. Chains on the calf's legs and pulling one leg at a time to ease his shoulders through the pelvis is generally adequate.

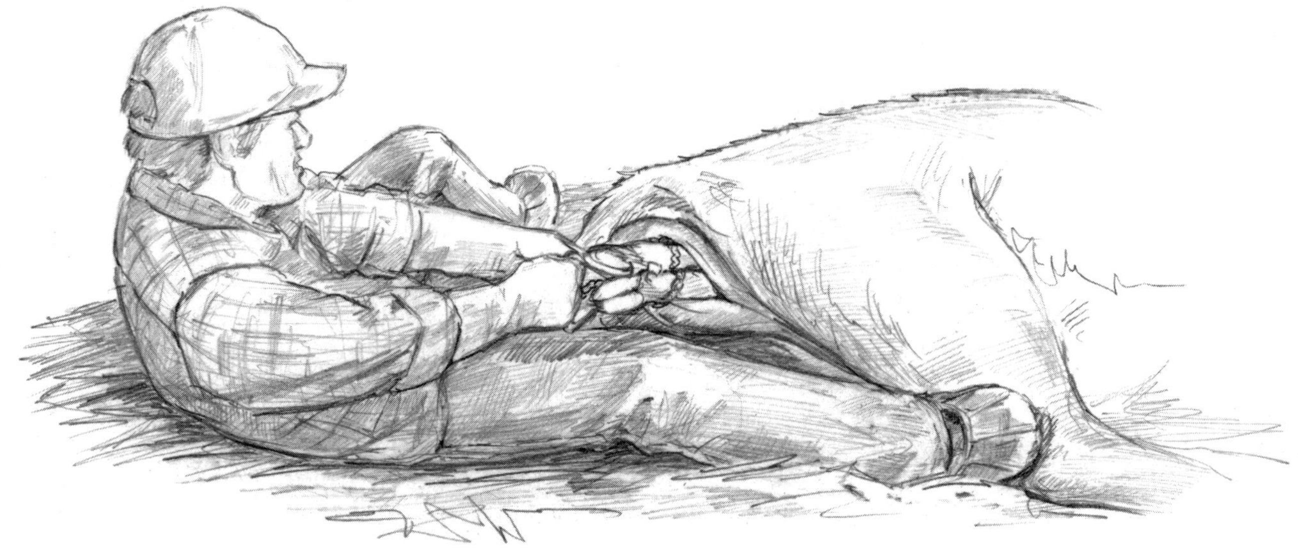

Leaning into the pull may be all the extra tension that's needed if she's making progress.

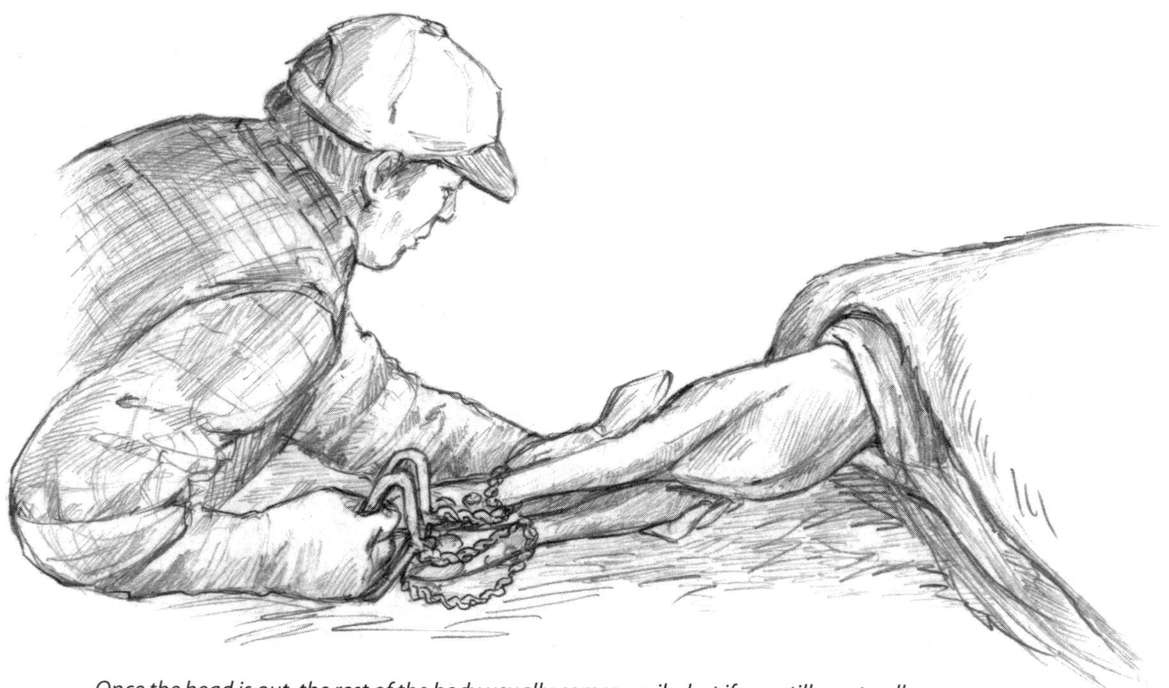

Once the head is out, the rest of the body usually comes easily, but if you still must pull, ease off for a moment as the rib cage comes out, so the chest can expand and enable the calf to take a breath. Constant tension on his legs hinders chest expansion.

standing up, and also presents a better angle for the calf to come through her pelvis. Note, however, that an easy-calving cow may not lie flat.

Most heifers need only minimal assistance and don't need the help of a calf puller. Pull one leg at a time, to ease the shoulders through the pelvic opening one at a time. You can "walk" the shoulders through the pelvis, starting with the lower leg near the ground; you should be able to feel the shoulder move as you pull. The fetlock joint will be about 4 inches (10 cm) outside the vulva when that shoulder comes through. Then that leg can be held in place with steady tension on its chain while you apply traction to the other leg. At this point, the direction of pull should be straight back from the heifer, which is difficult unless she's lying down. With a helper stretching the vulva as you pull, the head will come through much easier, with less strain on you, the heifer, and the calf.

If the calf is trying unsuccessfully to breathe, it's a sign that the umbilical cord is restricted and the calf is running out of oxygen.

After the calf's head emerges, the heifer may take a short rest before she resumes straining. She may also stop straining for a moment after passing the calf's rib cage. This is usually not a problem (and allows you to rest, too), as long as the calf can start breathing. Even though the umbilical cord may be pinched off at the time (because the calf's abdomen and navel area have entered the pelvis), when his rib cage emerges fully so that it can expand, the calf can start breathing. If the calf is trying unsuccessfully to breathe, it's a sign that the umbilical cord is restricted and the calf is running out of oxygen. Make sure his ribs are out, then ease off on your pulling; constant tension on the calf's legs can hinder expansion of his chest and the calf may suffocate. Once you get him breathing, you can finish the delivery.

Persistent Hymen

In some heifers, labor progresses nicely until the feet and possibly the nose show, then progress suddenly stops. If you reach into the vulva and birth canal, you'll find the hymen, a strong band of connective tissue a few inches inside the vulva that makes a narrow opening and a tight fit for the calf. As you pull the calf, the ring will stretch or break and the calf can come through the canal.

Hiplock

Sometimes you have made good progress and you get a calf partway out of the birth canal only to have him hang up at the hips. It's a bad combination if the big baby calf is wide in the hips and the cow or young heifer has a narrow pelvis.

To solve the problem, you must take advantage of every bit of room the cow has. Remember that the calf must come up and over the pelvic brim in an arc. As his body comes out, start pulling more toward the cow's hocks. Get the calf out far enough that his rib cage is free of the birth canal before you pull sharply downward or you'll hurt his ribs. Once his ribs are free of the birth canal, the rib cage can expand, and even if the calf is hiplocked and therefore stuck there for a few minutes with his hind end inside the cow, at least he can take his first breaths.

Next, put lubricant around the calf as far in between him and the birth canal as you can reach. Then pull straight down toward the cow's feet and pull the calf underneath her, between her hind legs if she's standing while laboring. This raises the calf's hips higher in the pelvis to the space where the pelvic opening is widest, making it more likely that the calf will come through than if you try to pull him straight out with his hips jammed against the cow's pelvic bones. If the cow is lying down during the birth, pull the calf between her hind legs, toward her belly. It also helps to rotate the calf 45 to 90 degrees; with the calf half turned on his side, his hips will come through the up-and-down axis of the cow's pelvis, which has a little bit more room than her side-to-side width.

RESOLVING A HIPLOCK

When the calf's hips are jammed against the dam's pelvis, try pulling him straight down toward her feet and then under her belly. This can be tricky if the cow is standing and able to walk around. On several occasions my husband and I have waltzed around a barn stall with the cow, trying to keep her standing still (and not kicking us!) as we pulled the calf between her hind legs.

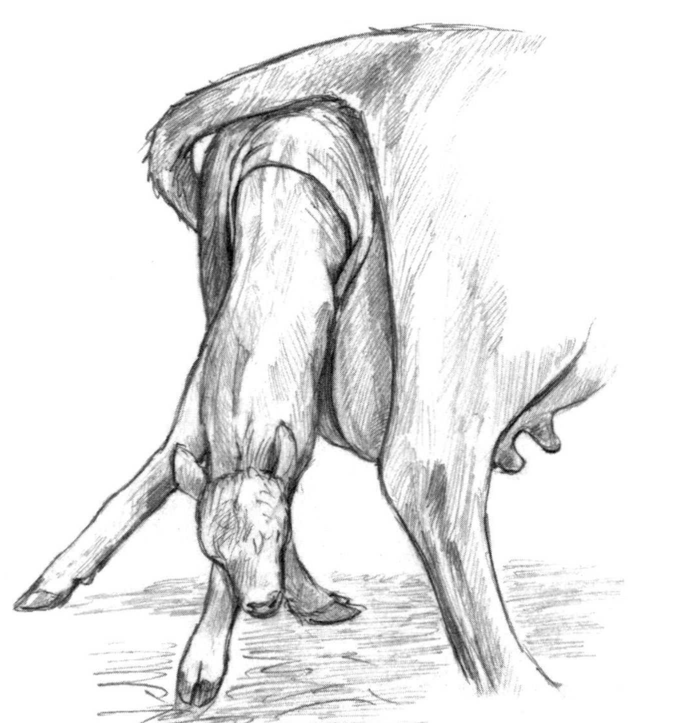

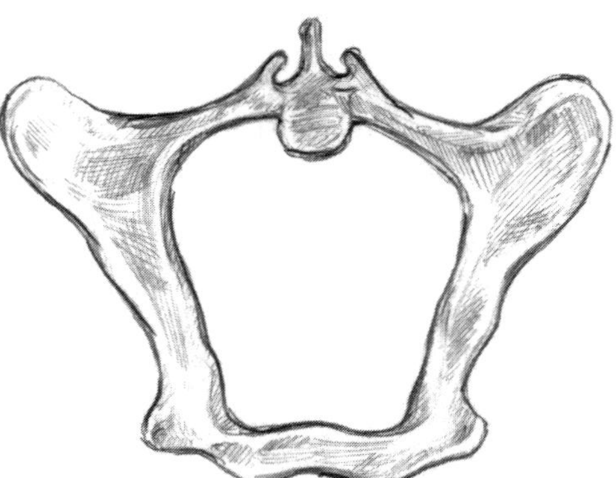

When trying to correct hiplock, keep in mind that the pelvic opening is widest at the top, more narrow at the bottom.

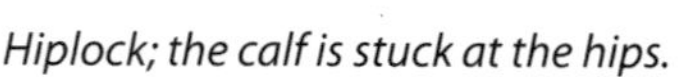

Hiplock; the calf is stuck at the hips.

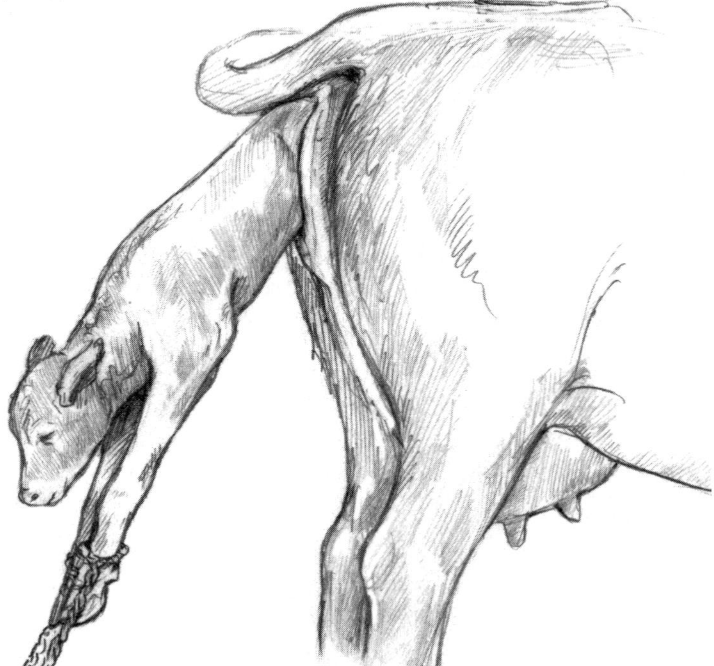

After getting the calf to breathe, put more lubricant around the calf's hips and pull him straight down toward the cow's feet. This raises his hips higher in the pelvis, where the opening is widest.

It's easiest to rotate the calf before he gets stuck in his mama's pelvis. Thus, if a calf is big and you fear he might hiplock, rotate him as soon as his head emerges. Two strong people can usually do this sucessfully: One pulls the calf's legs in a twisting motion while the other puts a half-nelson wrestling hold on head and legs and twists until the front of the calf is basically sideways. By rotating his front to this degree, the calf's hips start to rotate before they hit the pelvis. They'll then come through at a slant, which gives the calf more room.

If the hiplock is severe, roll the cow temporarily onto her back: With two strong people, each person can grab one of the cow's legs and roll her over, though if she's a heavy cow, it might take several people to do it. The idea is that as she rolls over, the hind legs of the calf will flop one way or the other in her uterus, thereby rotating the calf's hips so they're on a diagonal and can pass more easily through the pelvis. In addition, while she's on her back, the extra weight of the cow's abdomen pushing down on her uterus helps expel the calf. To finish the birth, use plenty of lubrication around the calf and give alternating side-to-side pulls to create a rotating motion that can free one hip and then the other. Pull the calf directly between the cow's hind legs, arching him toward her belly.

ALLERGIC TO COWS

During the 1980s I suddenly developed a troublesome sensitivity to amniotic fluid. After more than 25 years of handling birth problems and newborns without even a hint of an allergic reaction, my hands and arms suddenly began to swell, itch, and turn red after I had had them inside a cow to check or correct the position of the calf or after handling a wet newborn calf. I didn't want the inconvenience of using plastic gloves, so I endured the pain and itching, which were not too intense if I was able to wash my hands very soon after having the fluid on them.

As is often the case with allergies, I had this problem for several years during calving season and then it subsided. I am no longer bothered with this nuisance.

How to Use a Calf Puller

The less you use a calf puller, the better. If you do use one, do it very carefully or it may put so much pressure on the calf that it will seriously injure or kill him or the laboring cow. In our herd we've used a calf puller only for backward calves, except for a handful of situations in which the strength of two people was not enough to pull a large calf. In most instances, heifer's calves or any other too-large calves can be pulled by hand. In addition, when you pull by hand, you are more likely to stop in time and make that vital call to the veterinarian if a calf needs to be delivered by cesarean section.

The less you use a calf puller, the better. If you do use one, do it carefully, or it may put so much pressure on the calf that it will seriously injure or kill him or the cow.

In situations when a calf is coming out backward, however, usually the only way you are going to get him out alive is by using a calf puller, unless you have three or four strong people to help.

According to our veterinarian, a common misconception regarding the calf puller is that it's just a winch that allows more and more pressure to be applied to a calf. Many people don't understand that the calf puller is designed to be used as a lever, with the added advantage of allowing you to keep and hold whatever progress the cow has made so the calf doesn't slip back each time she quits straining.

Warning about the Calf Puller

Remember that two strong people can exert a force of more than 400 pounds and can't pull hard enough to hurt a cow or calf, while a calf puller may apply more than 2,000 pounds of pressure. Traction with a puller should be applied only when the cow is actively straining, so that it adds to her laboring efforts. Never exert pressure when the cow is at rest, except in the final delivery of a backward calf.

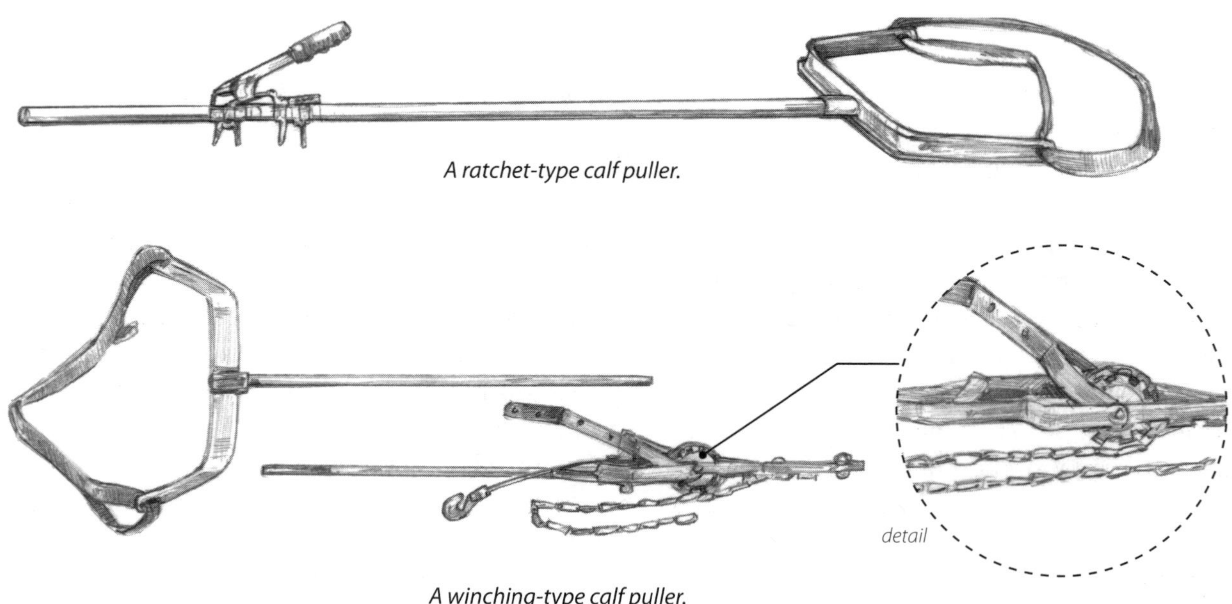

A ratchet-type calf puller.

A winching-type calf puller.

Attaching the Chains

A rancher's improper use of a calf puller can result in the calf's bones and joints being seriously fractured. However, if the puller's chains are applied carefully and properly to the legs, there is less stress on the calf's bones and joints.

When you attach the chains to the calf during delivery, make sure the first loop is completely above the fetlock joint. Then make a half hitch below it, around the calf's pastern. Before hooking the chains, properly adjust the rump strap of the puller on the cow. Many people leave it too loose or don't use it at all, but its purpose is to hold the puller in the correct position. It should be adjusted so the calf almost rubs over the metal plate of the puller as he emerges. This position — with the plate pressing against the cow's rear end and pelvic bone — helps push her pelvis into the angle that allows the most room for the calf to come through.

Next, hook the calf's leg chains to the puller, and apply traction only when the cow strains. Whatever you do, don't be in a hurry. *And remember to pull on both legs at the same time!* Pulling on the legs one at a time with a calf puller, as you might do when pulling by hand, exerts so much force that you can easily kill the calf or paralyze the cow in the birthing process. If the calf won't come through readily when you pull both legs together, it's a sure sign that the calf should be delivered by cesarean section.

Working the Puller

The most important aspect of the calf puller comes from its up-and-down motion. After the chains are properly applied to the calf's legs, shorten the puller or extend its cable to obtain as much leeway as possible for pulling. This is especially important if the calf is backward because you're apt to run out of room to winch (on a cable-type puller) before his shoulders and head come out of the cow (see chapter 4).

When pulling a normally presented calf (front-feet first), position the puller straight out behind the cow at the level of her back. After taking up all available slack on a cable-type puller (that is, the cable is tight and is hooked to the chains on the calf's legs) or ratcheting all slack out of the chains with the newer ratchet puller, slowly bring the end of the puller as close as possible toward the level of the cow's feet while she's straining. This puts more pressure on the calf's legs.

Then lift the puller back up to its original position, taking up the slack you gained, and repeat the process when the cow strains until the calf's head (or hips, if the calf is backward) emerge.

Repeat this cycle several times as you bring the calf's head, shoulders, and rib cage through the vulva. Once the rib cage is fully out, release the puller tension and pause for a moment to let fluid come out of the calf's nostrils and to start the calf's breathing. His chest cannot expand while his front legs are

HOW TO USE A CALF PULLER

Most calves can be pulled by two strong people. Every once in a great while, however, as in when a calf is coming backward, use of a calf puller is necessary. One should have a complete understanding of the mechanism and the risks of injury related to it before using the puller.

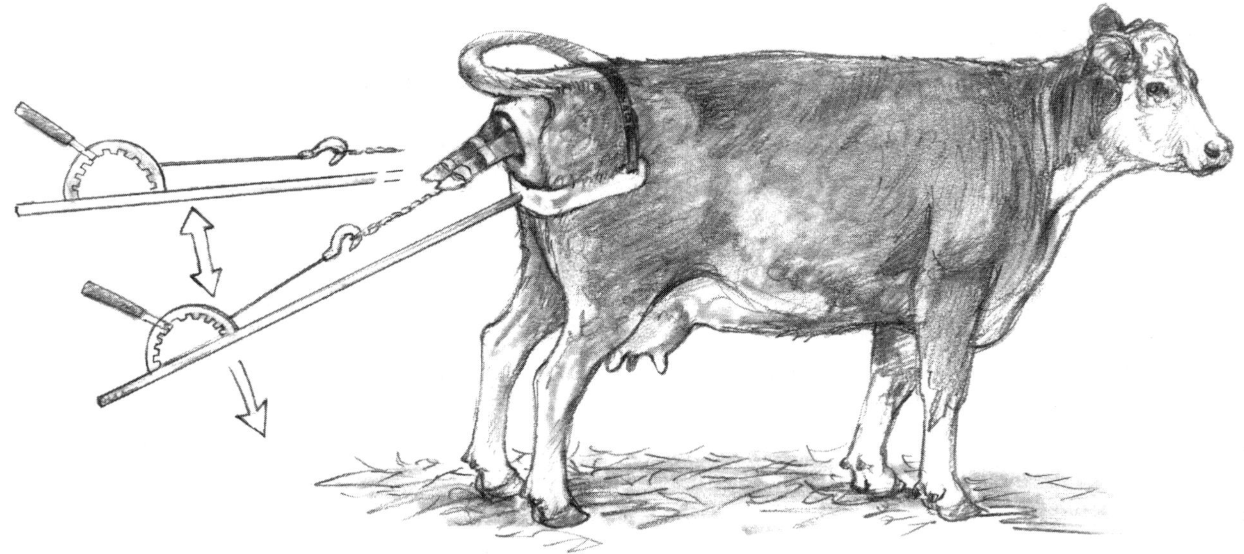

Start by holding the puller straight out, parallel with the cow's back, and take up all the slack in the chain with the winch or ratchet. Then slowly bring down the puller toward the level of the cow's feet as much as possible. Lift it back up, taking up the slack you gained. Repeat this process until the calf's head comes out. Then use the winch or ratchet to bring him on out.

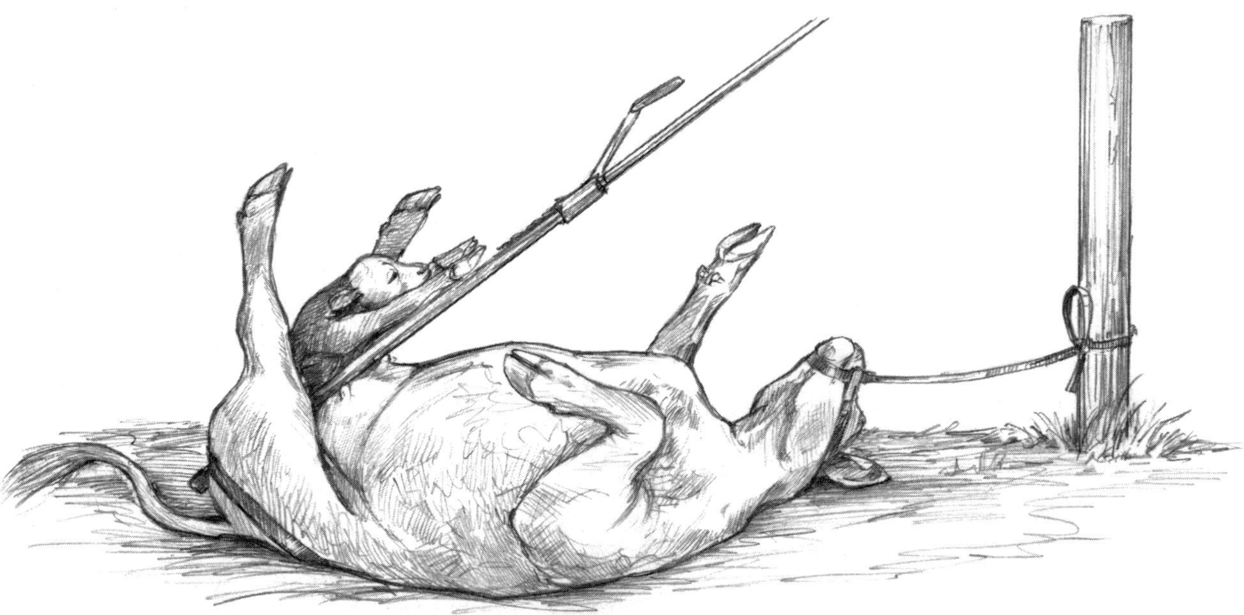

If a calf hiplocks when you are using a calf puller, release the tension on the puller, roll the cow onto her back, bring the puller upright, and retighten the tension, pulling the calf between the cow's hind legs. Bring the end of the puller down toward the cow's belly and head.

being pulled. Poke a finger in his ear to make him shake his head to clear the mucus and fluid from his nose and mouth. Tickle the inside of the calf's nostrils with a piece of hay or straw to make him sneeze and cough, which will draw air into his lungs and get him started breathing. If it's been a hard pull, let the calf lie there a few moments to breathe. Once he's breathing normally, hook the leg chains to the puller again, then use the winching or ratcheting aspect of the puller to bring the calf out fully. Keep the handle down toward the cow's hocks as you ease the calf's hips through the pelvis and continue to put gentle pressure on the chains, thus helping to lift the calf's hips up into the widest part of the pelvis.

If you're using a puller and the calf hiplocks, loosen the tension on the puller, get the calf breathing, and roll the cow onto her back with all four legs straight up. With the cow on her back, bring the puller to an upright position and regain the tension on the chains so that you're pulling the calf between her hind legs. With the tension tight, bring the end of the puller down toward the cow's belly and head. This leverage will rotate the calf's hips a bit more so the widest part of his hips is brought forward into the widest part of the cow's pelvis.

Prevent Uterine Infection

After any difficult birth, whether you pulled the calf by hand or with a puller and especially if you had to reach into the uterus to manipulate the calf into proper position, your vet may advise you to insert antibiotic *boluses* (large oblong pills) into the uterus soon after delivery, while the cow is still down or is still restrained.

To do this, use a sterile OB glove and, reaching in past the open cervix, deposit two or three boluses far enough into the uterus that they won't be expelled by the cow when she is straining to shed her placenta. Alternatively, your vet may tell you that giving the cow an injection of broad-spectrum antibiotic is more beneficial than inserting boluses into the uterus.

When the puller rod passes center and starts down toward the cow's head, the breech spanner plate that was originally positioned just beneath her buttocks and vulva will slide off the cow and push into the calf's abdomen. This won't hurt the calf; it will only help push him out of the cow.

Uterine Inertia

Primary *uterine inertia* can be a cause of a difficult birth and results in the cow's being unable to expel the calf.

Sometimes if a cow or heifer has had no exercise during pregnancy (perhaps if she's been confined in a stall or small pen), she has poor muscle tone. This may result in the inability of the uterus to contract strongly when she goes into labor, but more often it results in poor condition of the abdominal muscles, and the cow may simply wear out during active labor.

A genuine lack of strong uterine contractions, however, is generally due to a problem beyond insufficient exercise, such as low levels of calcium or magnesium, though this is more common in dairy cows than beef cows; an improper ratio of estrogen to progesterone; or not enough oxytocin or prostaglandins produced during labor. Anything that interferes with proper hormone balance in the cow may lead to uterine inertia.

Because the uterus is not contracting as it should, the calf is not pushed up into the birth canal. The cow is in labor, but she doesn't seem to progress to second-stage, active labor.

Uterine inertia is fairly common in older cows that have a large belly and a sagging uterus so that the calf sits very low in the abdomen. The cow starts labor, but she doesn't strain much and no calf appears. When you reach into the birth canal to check, the cervix is wide open and the cow is definitely in second-stage labor but the calf is still down in the uterus and hasn't yet started up over the pelvis, and the cow is having very few contractions or none at all.

If the calf is in normal position, you can reach in and find the front feet, attach OB chains, and pull him out. Nevertheless, there are two potential dangers that can arise from uterine inertia: First, you may not check the cow in time because you think

A Dutch Method for Pulling a Calf

An effective method for pulling calves was developed at the University of Utrecht by using specific positioning of the cow. The main idea is to work with the cow instead of against her.

While she is restrained and still standing, wash her hind end and check her to determine size and position of the calf and to correct any malpresentation (see chapter 4). Next, the cow should be lying on the ground rather than standing when you pull the calf; she can't strain as effectively when standing. Make sure the cow is lying on her right side. You can accomplish this by securing a rope around her flank and one around her chest, behind the elbows, in half hitches, and by tying a rope to her right hind leg at the pastern. In this squeeze method, the cow usually goes down when the right hind leg is pulled forward and under the cow at the same time that the other body ropes are pulled.

When the cow is lying down, her pelvis is more straight up and down, which makes a straighter opening for the calf to come through, especially as the cow strains. Pull when she strains, using the force of only one person per leg. Pull first on the calf's leg that is lower in relation to the vulva (that is, nearer the ground) in order to pull through that leg's shoulder, then pull on the other leg. The direction of traction is straight out, which is difficult unless the cow is down.

When the cow is lying down, her pelvis is more straight up and down, which makes a straighter opening for the calf to come through, especially as the cow strains.

Once the shoulders are out, two people pull on the calf at the same time, one on each leg, rotating the calf 45 to 90 degrees as he emerges so that the widest area of the calf's hips pass through the roomiest part of the cow's pelvis. You can often accomplish this simply by crossing the chains and rotating the calf as you pull. In this method, pull straight out or slightly up relative to the backbone of the cow as you rotate the calf out.

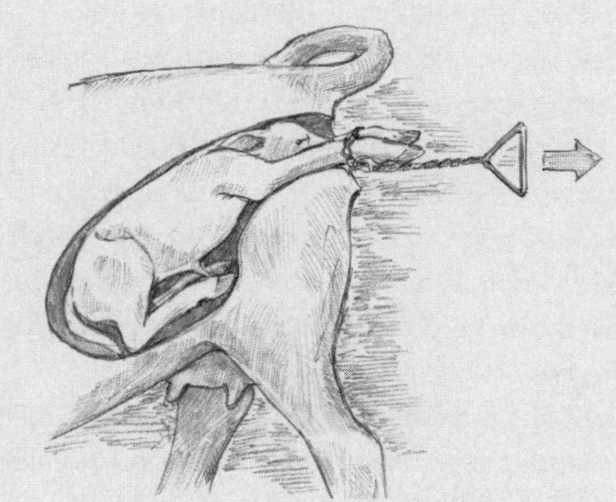

1. The cow is lying down on her right side. Traction is applied to one leg at a time, to walk the calf through the pelvis one shoulder at a time.

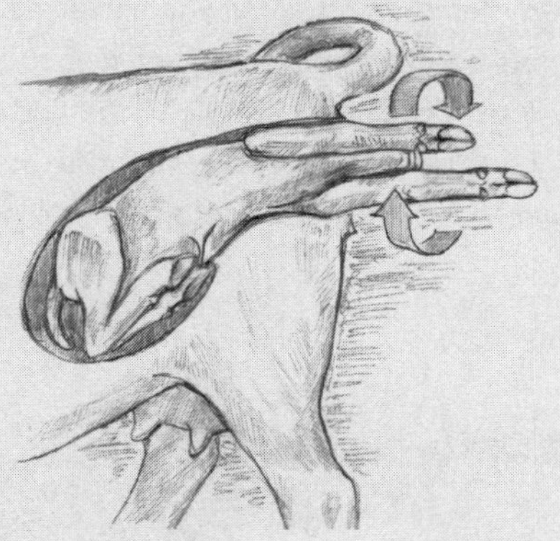

2. After his shoulders are through the pelvis, a large calf can be rotated to bring him through the widest part of the cow's pelvis.

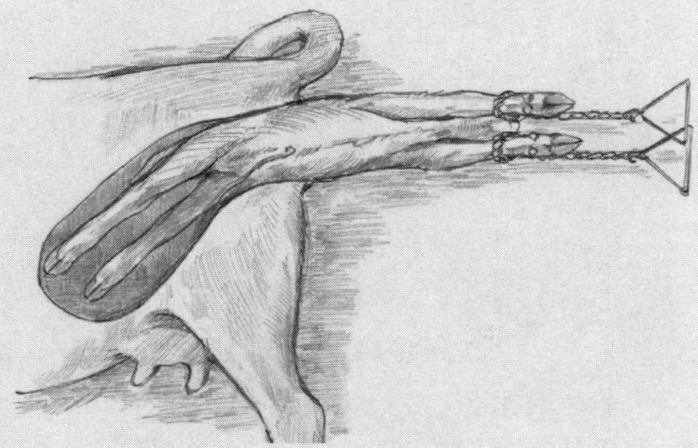

3. Pull out the calf by applying traction on both legs at once, pulling straight out or slightly upward relative to the cow's backbone.

SAVING GOLIATH

THE MOST SPECTACULAR SAVE we ever performed was on a bull calf we pulled from a heifer in 1974. Beauty Spot was a medium-sized Hereford heifer bred to a Hereford bull. In those days, our bulls sired large calves, and we often had to pull heifers' calves. On that spring day, Beauty Spot took a long time in labor, but after she'd been straining awhile, we helped her. She was a gentle heifer and didn't protest when we hooked chains onto her calf's legs while she was lying down.

We knew her calf was alive when we started pulling; his feet jerked in protest. When we finally got out his head, his nose was blue, but he still had a blink reflex. He was a huge calf, and pulling by hand was hard for both of us, and by the time he was born, he seemed dead: His mouth and gums were blue and he was limp, with no reflexes. Yet I felt a heartbeat, so we immediately began giving him artificial respiration. Lynn massaged the calf and moved the legs vigorously, which helps stimulate heart and lungs, and he checked the calf's heartbeat as I blew air into his lungs with my mouth over one nostril and holding the other one shut.

After 30 minutes of our unceasing efforts, the calf began to lose his blue color and started to breathe on his own. He was still unconscious, though, so we kept rubbing and stimulating him. After another 15 minutes, he woke up and was able to hold up his head and look around. His mama was still lying down, tired from her labors, so we fed Goliath via stomach tube because he was not strong enough or capable of sucking. It took a few hours for his swollen tongue and nose to return to normal.

His mother was interested in what we were doing with him, but she was tired and wobbly from the hard birth. We helped Goliath accomplish his first nursing with both mother and calf lying down. We moved him closer to her udder and stuck a teat in his mouth, and he eagerly nursed. Soon after, he was able to stand. Mama and baby quickly recovered from the hard birth.

Since those early days of big calves, we've selected for smaller-birth-weight genetics in our cow herd and have reduced the incidence of hard births, but we'll always remember saving Goliath.

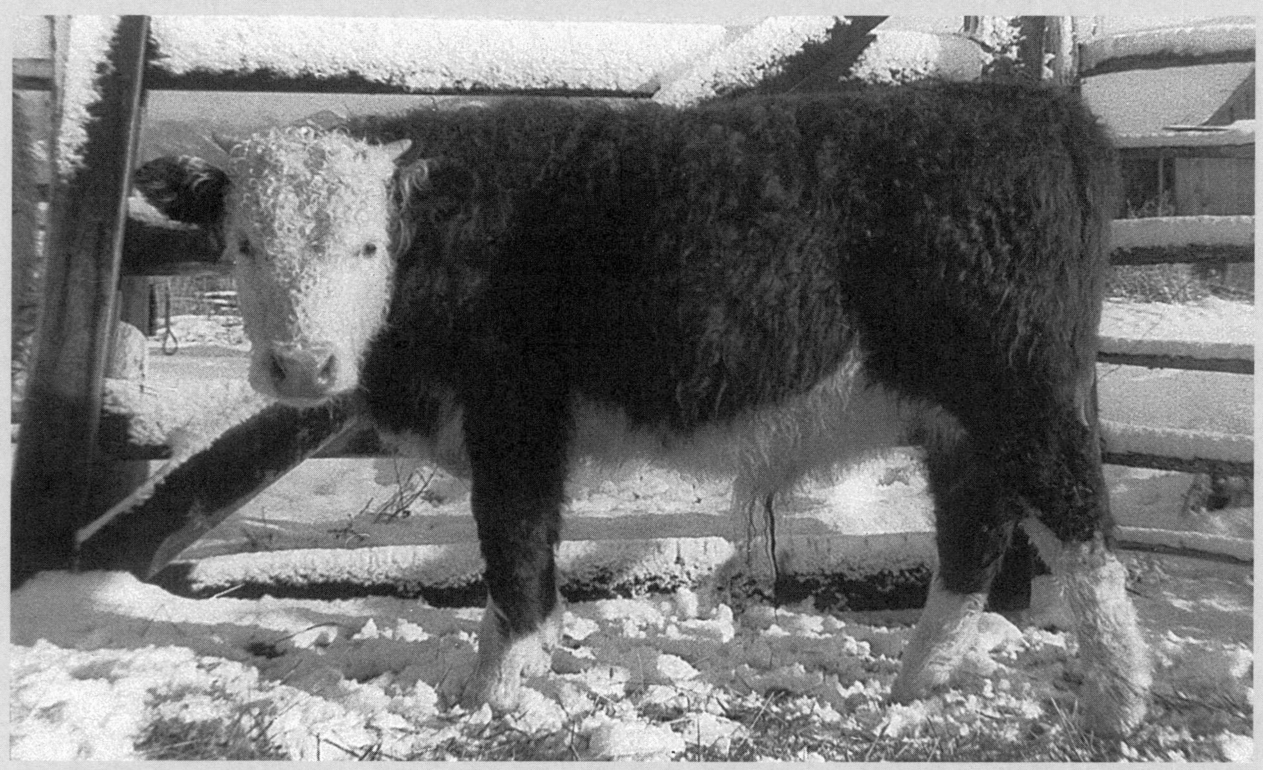

Goliath at six months of age.

she's still in early labor, and if you fail to check her, the placenta will eventually detach, and the calf will be dead by the time you realize there's a problem.

Second, the lack of uterine contractions may result in a malpresentation of the calf. During early labor, uterine contractions put pressure on the calf, stimulating him to move and aiming him toward the birth canal and into proper position for birth. If the uterus is not putting pressure on him, the calf may be in any position, unable to be born without help. This situation must be discovered early, while the calf is still alive, so that the malpresentation can be corrected.

Secondary uterine inertia is the result of, rather than the cause of, difficult birth. If a cow or heifer has a malpresentation, a large calf, or some other problem that hinders delivery, she may strain in vain and become exhausted so that uterine and abdominal contractions become weaker and cease. The best way to prevent this problem is to keep a close eye on the calving cow or heifer and be ready to give assistance early on.

When to Give a Calf CPR

Sometimes a calf doesn't start to breathe immediately after birth, and if you don't get him breathing, he will die. If he's been out of oxygen for a while during a hard birth, you have only a couple of minutes or less to get the calf breathing. There are several causes for breathing failure in a newborn calf.

The Sac Doesn't Break

Some calves are still encased in the amnion sac and fluids after sliding out of the birth canal. This happens fairly often with a fast, easy birth; the sac is more apt to break during a long labor. In many instances the sac simply doesn't break. Unless the calf struggles and breaks it or the cow jumps up directly after birth and starts licking the calf's head or nudging him around with her head, the sac remains intact and suffocates the calf.

Sometimes the membranes are thin and easily broken; the calf must only lift or shake his head and they separate. Other times, the membranes are thick, and the calf can't break them by himself; if the cow doesn't get up and help the calf immediately, he dies. Even if the calf is running out of oxygen, he instinctively holds off breathing if his head is still surrounded by fluid or his nose is covered. This immersion reflex (see A Calf's First Breath, page 68) keeps the calf from drawing fluid into his lungs and drowning.

The cow's instinct, however, is to get up and start licking her calf as soon as he's born, but if she's a little tired from labor or if she's a heifer, she may not rise in time. In fact, most of the losses from failure of the sac to break are in first calvers and from an easy birth in which the calf slides out very quickly. In these instances, the heifer may not realize she has a new baby and doesn't get up immediately.

If you are present at the birth and the sac does not come off the calf's head, break the membrane and quickly remove the fluid from the calf's nose and mouth so he can breathe.

It's a Hard Birth

Another common cause of failure of the calf to breathe is a hard or long birth. The calf may be exhausted or unconscious. In addition, if he was in the birth canal a long time, his nose and tongue may be swollen and his air passages restricted. The umbilical cord also may be pinched during final stages of slow birth (for instance, if the calf is delivered backward), meaning the calf is short on oxygen and unconscious.

Special Concerns for the Backward Calf

In a backward birth, the calf's head is inside the cow until the last stage, and his air passages stay full of fluid. In addition, the umbilical cord is pinched as the calf's hindquarters pass through the cow's pelvis, so he's out of oxygen and must start breathing as soon as you pull him out.

Traditionally, vets advised holding up a calf by the hind legs, with his head hanging down so that fluid could drain from the airways, but they've found this doesn't help. In fact, this position puts more pressure on the calf's lungs from the weight of his abdomen. It's better to suction out what fluid you can, then get the calf to cough.

GETTING A NEWBORN CALF TO BREATHE

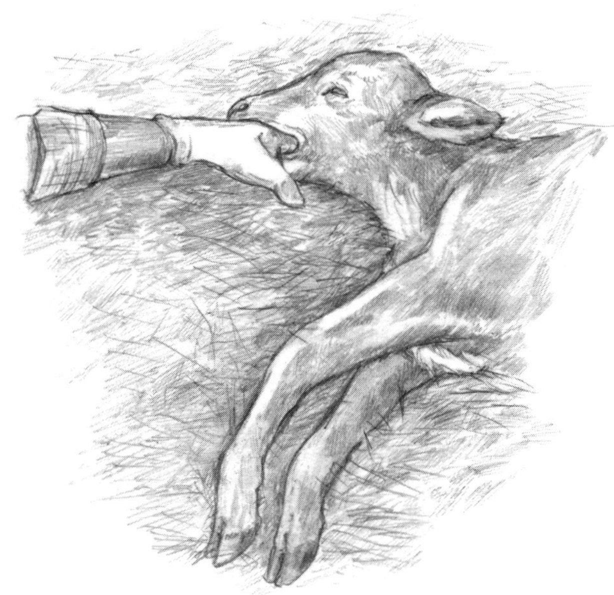

Clear some of the mucus and fluid from the calf's airways so he can start breathing.

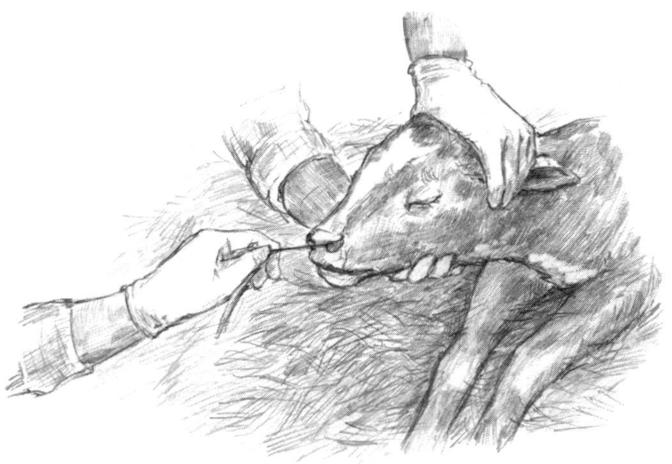

If the calf still isn't breathing, you can often get him started by tickling the inside of a nostril with a clean piece of hay or straw to stimulate him to cough or sneeze and draw air into his lungs.

The Placenta Detaches

Sometimes the placenta detaches from the uterus before the calf is fully born. Because the placenta feeds the calf and provides the calf with oxygen via the umbilical cord, once the cord detaches, both supplies are removed.

The placenta starts to detach after the cow has been in labor for a time whether or not the calf comes through the birth canal. Thus a breech calf, for example, may be dead by the time you discover there's a problem. If you're pulling a big calf or it's a slow birth in which the cow finally has the calf without help, the placenta may be detached by the time the calf is born. You'll see some of the thick membrane and its red buttons coming out with the calf or emerging right after him. If the calf has been short on oxygen for a while, he may be limp and unconscious. In almost all such cases, the calf is normal; he simply needs to begin breathing immediately. To start this, you can give him CPR.

Administering CPR to a Newborn Calf

Knowing what to do and taking immediate action are crucial in saving a calf that fails to breathe. If the heart is still beating, there's hope. In a limp, unconscious calf, the heart may be hammering hard and loud as the body struggles desperately to survive without oxygen. If the calf doesn't start breathing soon, however, the heartbeat becomes weaker, slower, and very faint. Heart rate is one way to tell if a calf is in respiratory distress. It drops as body tissues are deprived of oxygen. Normal heart rate in a newborn calf is 100 to 120 beats per minute. If the calf fails to start breathing within about 30 seconds of being born, however, and has a heart rate that's lower than normal, the calf is in trouble.

Checking a Calf's Heart Rate

Place your hand on the lower left side of the rib cage, just behind and above the elbow of his front leg. A newborn calf's heartbeat is easy to feel because the heart is beating strongly and there's little tissue between it and the chest wall. If the heart rate has dropped to as low as 30 to 40 beats per minute, the calf's condition is critical.

Checking a Calf's Mucous Membranes

The color of the calf's *mucous membranes* will give you important information about his oxygen status. Normally the newborn calf's gums are pink. Even in a black calf with a black tongue there are some nonpigmented areas inside the mouth or under the tongue, and these should be healthy, bubblegum pink. If the gums and other nonpigmented tissues are gray, blue, or colorless, the calf is in trouble and must start breathing immediately.

How to Give Artificial Respiration to a Calf

First, clear the airways. Roll the calf onto his breastbone in an upright position (rather than flat on the ground), with his head and chin resting on the ground and his nose as low as possible. This position allows fluid to drain from the nostrils. If the calf's airways are still full of fluid, use your fingers to strip fluid from his nose and mouth in a suctionlike action, much like squeezing a tube of toothpaste. The best method is to use a rubber suction bulb to clear the nostrils; you should carry one in your pocket.

If the airways are full of fluid, the calf's first breath may draw fluid into the windpipe, and it may take him awhile to cough it out. He will have rattly breathing for several hours. If the calf is weak and tired from a hard birth and doesn't immediately start breathing, this fluid makes it more difficult for him to breathe properly, so it helps if you can suction some out.

Next, massage the calf. Brisk massage of the calf's body and legs helps increase his circulation and stimulates breathing. Flexing the legs also prompts lung action. If the calf doesn't take a breath within one minute of birth, even after you've tickled his nose with a piece of straw, blow air into his lungs. It is better if there are two people: One person can rub and massage the calf, check his heart rate, and gently work his legs for heart and lung stimulation while the other person periodically blows into one nostril.

Administer artificial respiration. Lay the calf on his side with his head and neck extended. Cover one nostril tightly with your hand, holding the mouth shut; this will prevent air from escaping out of the mouth or nose when you blow air into the other nostril, forcing air into the calf's windpipe and lungs. Gently blow a full breath into the nostril. Don't blow rapidly or forcefully; doing so could rupture a lung.

STARTING THE HEART AGAIN

OCCASIONALLY you can restart a calf's heart if it stops during a hard birth. A few years ago our son and his wife pulled one of their heifer's calves, a big bull calf they knew was alive when they started pulling. When he was delivered, however, the calf was limp and his eyes were glazed; he was technically dead, with no heartbeat.

Desperate and frustrated, because he knew the calf had been alive just moments before, our son slammed the calf's rib cage very hard with his fist, directly over the heart — and it started beating again! His wife immediately began blowing into the calf's nostril, and our son rhythmically pushed on the rib cage to stimulate the heart, which soon started beating strongly on its own.

After many minutes of artificial respiration, the calf regained consciousness. It took about 12 hours for that calf to recover enough to nurse its mother (it was fed colostrum by tube in the interim), but the recovery was complete and the calf showed no ill effects.

Keep blowing into the nostril until you see the chest move and rise. Then let the air come back out on its own. Blow in another breath until the chest wall rises again, showing that the lungs are filling.

Continue filling the lungs and letting them empty until the calf starts breathing on his own. It may take just a few breaths or quite a while, depending on the calf's condition. Usually, once the body tissues become less oxygen starved, the heart rate will rise and the calf will regain consciousness and start breathing. Respiration may be erratic at first, but if everything else is normal (there are no birth defects or other difficulties that are compromising his health), he will develop a more regular breathing pattern in a few minutes.

Artificial respiration can save calves that would otherwise die following birth complications, a hard birth, or a backward birth. Remember: If there's a heartbeat, the calf is still alive. With a little effort, you can give a second chance to a calf compromised in this way.

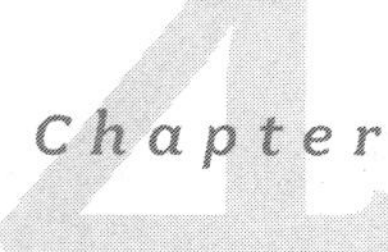

Chapter 4

Handling Malpresentations

Sometimes a calf can't be born because he is in a position that won't allow him to come through the birth canal. Often malpresentations are simple problems that hinder forward progress: The calf's fetlock joint may be turned back, or both of his front legs are presenting on the same side of the head, or his elbow is hung up on the brim of the cow's pelvis. Other positions are more difficult to correct — a turned-back head or a breech presentation in which the calf's rump is all that's aimed toward the birth canal.

Knowing what can go wrong and how to correct it may make the difference between life and death for the calf. In some instances, correcting malpresentations requires a lot of experience, and you must call your vet. However, if the slowdown is something simple, you can probably correct it yourself. This chapter will help you decide if a vet's help is needed and, if not, how you can get the calf and cow out of a tricky birth situation.

Consider the Possibility of a Malpresentation

Before labor begins, the large, full-term calf is cramped for space in the distended uterus, since there isn't much room. His extremities are tucked close to his body. His neck is bent (his head is tucked around by his side) and his legs are flexed; his knees and hocks are bent, with his feet drawn up next to the body. At the beginning of labor, the first parts of the calf to press against the dilating cervix are usually his knees. Thirty minutes later, with uterine contractions putting pressure on the calf and stimulating his movement, the calf's head and neck have extended, his forelegs have straightened, and his feet enter the cervix. This head-and-front-feet-first position is the most streamlined way to be born and the only way calves fit through the limited space of the pelvis — for a live birth — without help.

Problems arise when the calf does not or cannot extend his head, neck, and legs to start through the birth canal. Malpresentations are common if a calf is too big to fully extend his legs in the limited uterine space, or if the calf is already dead and therefore can't respond to uterine contractions.

Watching the Birthing Clock

The calf's deadliest enemy during birth is time. As a general rule, you can assume that he has roughly three to four hours of oxygen after the cow's water breaks, or whenever she starts second-stage labor. After that length of time, the placenta will often start to detach from the uterine lining. If the time limit is approaching and the cow is not straining hard or is straining and no visible progress is being made, she needs help. We always check a cow within two hours of breaking her water if she has not shown obvious progress.

Any number of things can happen to slow down a cow giving birth to a calf. The cow may be in early labor too long or may break her water, signaling the end of early labor and the beginning of active labor, and then do nothing. She may or may not start straining. Strong abdominal straining is stimulated only when part of the calf starts through the cow's pelvis. If a calf is premature, the cow's contractions may not be as strong (uterine inertia), and the calf may not be stimulated enough to extend the limbs.

In many types of malpresentations, the cow will strain. The calf's head or one leg or both may come into the birth canal, but he comes no farther because one leg or the head is turned back, for example. The cow may continue to strain, putting pressure on the calf. If she's been straining for a while and nothing appears, you need to reach into the birth canal to see what the problem is.

The calf's deadliest enemy during birth is time. He has roughly three to four hours of oxygen after the cow's water breaks, or whenever she starts second-stage labor.

Sometimes it's okay to give a cow a little more time, but in other instances you may lose the calf if you wait to check the cow. It's easy to know the cow is in active labor when the calf's foot starts to protrude from the vulva. Then you have something to judge the time frame by and can check her and help her if birth does not progress. If nothing shows, you must try to judge how long she's been in early labor, or active labor, and look at your records to find out what might be typical or abnormal for that particular cow.

Keep Records of Each Birth

If the cow does not begin hard labor after a reasonable time in early labor, it may be because the calf can't start through the birth canal because of how he is positioned in the uterus. If you suspect a cow has been in early labor more than six hours and has not begun straining, she should be checked. It helps to know your cows individually and to keep records on their calving history. If a cow that's typically a "fast calver" takes too long in early labor, you know there's a problem. In our calving records we note the time the cow's early labor begins, the time the water breaks, when a part of the calf becomes visible, and when the calf is born, among other things, including any problems we encounter and how we dealt with them.

The Older Cow

An old cow with a saggy belly and large uterus — with a calf positioned low in her abdomen — may take a long time to calve if her uterine muscle tone is poor. She can't push the calf up over the pelvic brim. If she takes too long, the placenta detaches and the calf dies. Or she may have a malpresentation due to lack of uterine contractions. Even if the calf presents normally, she may need help to calve.

Recognizing and Correcting Abnormal Birth Positions

Because time is crucial, it pays to check the cow and see if it's something you can correct. If it's a breech calf whose legs you can't reach or a torsion of the uterus, don't spend time trying in vain before you call the vet. He or she will probably be able to correct it but in some cases the vet must remove the calf surgically. If you recognize a problem early, you can get help before a cow is in serious trouble or a calf has died.

Pushing the Calf Back In

In most instances when you need to correct the position of the calf or his leg, you must push him back into the uterus where there's more room to manipulate his body parts. To do this, put pressure with your hand on the portion of the calf already in the birth canal. If you push hardest when the cow is not straining and try to hold ground as she strains, this will be easier. The simplest way to push a calf back is to lean your weight against him continuously, rather than pushing with brute strength and wearing yourself out. Each time the cow quits straining for a moment, your leaning will push

CALVING RECORDS
AT THE SKY RANGE RANCH

COW #249

Crystal, ***daughter of Christy and Little John, born Jan. 17, 1978***

1980 (her first calf) Due Jan. 6 (bred to Joe)

Calving Jan. 7. Started obvious labor by 5 p.m. Put her in the barn at 6:40 p.m. Straining hard at 8:50 p.m., but nothing showing yet. Calf's feet appeared at 9:05 p.m., then calved swiftly at 9:15 p.m. Small white-faced red heifer calf. Calf a little slow to get up. Uncoordinated at first, and we had to help her nurse, then she seemed ok. Cow didn't clean 'til January 11 (a possible sign that something was a little wrong with the birth).

COW #14

Camero, ***daughter of Liza and Sigfried, born Jan. 18, 1986***

1989 (her 2nd calf) Due Jan. 30 (bred to Danny Boy)

Calving Jan. 27. Started labor 10 a.m. Put her in barn at 11 a.m. Amnion sac showing at 1:30 p.m but no feet in it. No progress. Finally tied her up and checked her at 3:15 p.m. Head entering birth canal but no feet. Had to push calf back and bring both legs into birth canal, then pull the calf. HARD pull with chains but did not have to use calf puller. Delivered calf at 3:30 p.m. Red bull calf.

COW #282

Camilla, ***daughter of Cammie and Waffles, born Jan. 12, 1994***

2000 (her 6th calf) Due Jan. 8 (bred to Polar Bear)

Calving Jan. 13. Noticed her in labor at 5 a.m. Broke her water at 5:45 a.m. Put her in the barn at 6 a.m. Calf's feet showing at 6:50. Calved swiftly at 7:05. Black brockle-faced bull.

COW #504

Bluebird, ***daughter of Syringa and Samson, born Jan. 24, 2001***

2003 (her first calf) Due March 28 (bred to an Angus/Gelbvieh bull)

Calving March 31. Restless all morning. Broke water at 11:40 a.m. Put in barn at 11:50 a.m. Did nothing. A little bloody mucous discharge at 3:30. Put her in the head catcher to check her. Calf upside down and not entering birth canal. Rotated the calf and pulled him (just chains, didn't need calf puller). BIG black bull calf, delivered at 3:45 p.m. Cow confused and bunted him with her head when he tried to stand up. Had to separate them. Put her in head catcher and helped the calf nurse. Left a halter on her, dragging a rope, and kept them in separate stalls. Had to tie her each time we helped him nurse for the first 36 hours, then she mothered him ok.

HOW TO MAKE ROOM FOR MANIPULATING BIRTH POSITIONS

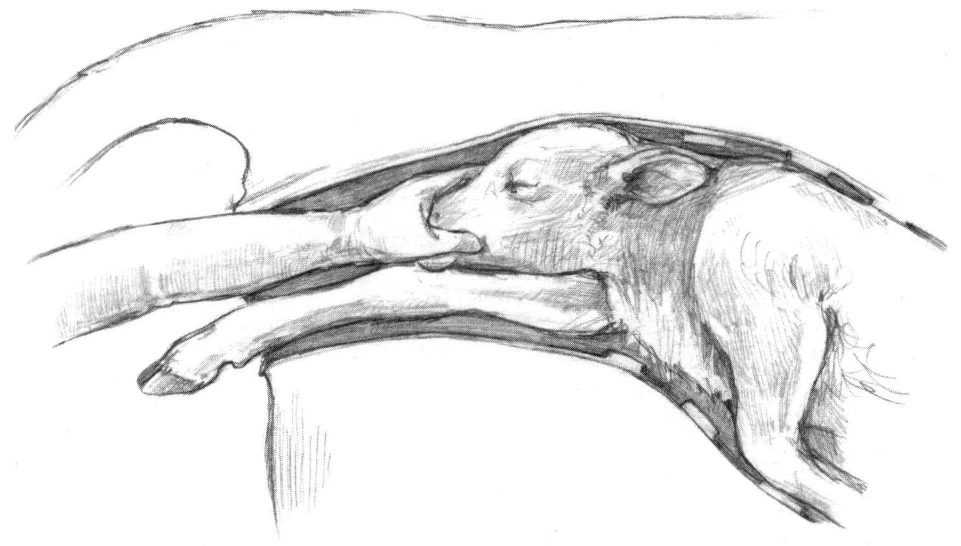

Push the calf back into the uterus, where there will be more room to manipulate the turned-back leg and bring it into the birth canal.

the calf back. Put your hand on his head, breastbone, or rump (whatever is presented) and lean steadily. You'll gain a few inches between each contraction.

Use of Epidurals When Pushing Calf Back

Sometimes when a veterinarian is trying to manipulate a difficult calf, he or she may give the cow an *epidural* injection of anesthetic into the spinal column near the base of the tail to keep her from straining while the calf is pushed back and the malpresentation is corrected. This can help if a cow is lying down and straining hard, and won't get up on her feet. She may stand up after the injection, as she no longer feels pelvic pain, which makes it easier to manipulate the calf because it takes the abdominal pressure off the cow's uterus.

A big disadvantage to giving an epidural, however, is that she won't be able to strain after the calf is repositioned; she'll be no help in expelling him. All effort must come from the person(s) helping to deliver the calf by pulling. The most beneficial use of an epidural is when your vet is trying to replace a prolapsed uterus and needs the cow to quit straining (see chapter 6).

Cautions When Repositioning a Calf

Always be careful when correcting any malpresentation, and use lots of lubricant. Disinfectant obstetrical soaps provide lubrication as well as being antiseptic. Keep a bottle on hand for calving season. Other water-soluble soaps will work in a pinch to provide slippery liquid; use a mild soap that contains no artificial scents or coloring agents that might be irritating.

When trying to straighten a leg or turn the calf's head around, always keep your hand protectively between the calf's head or foot and the uterine wall. If you tear a hole in the wall by pushing or scraping part of the calf against it, this is a life-threatening situation for the cow.

On occasion the cow's own contractions will push a hoof or a nose through the uterine wall, especially if a calf is situated in the wrong position, but tears in the uterus occur much more frequently with human intervention and delivery manipulations. More than half the cows with this type of injury will die, even if a veterinarian can surgically repair the tear immediately after the birth.

Push the Calf while Straddling the Cow

One of the easiest ways to straighten a malpresented calf if the cow or heifer goes down and won't get up (without resorting to an epidural injection to keep her from straining) is to pull her hind legs straight out behind her. This forces her to lie on her belly, *stifles* (the large joint high on the hind leg), and *brisket* (the area between the front legs). You need a helper to straddle her back and sit facing her tail, lean back, and forcefully hold her tail straight up over her back. Sitting on the cow provides the weight to help keep her in this position, while holding the tail straight up reduces her ability to strain and puts her hindquarters higher than her front, which makes it easier to push the calf back into the uterus and correct its position.

After you have pushed and leaned on the calf enough to get him back into the uterus with room to reposition him, grab and move his leg (or head) in one quick motion just after one of the cow's contractions, bringing it around before the cow can strain again. Once you have the legs and head coming properly through her pelvis, reposition the cow onto her right side, with all four legs out to the side (a natural position for calving), so she can now strain more effectively.

A Stuck Toe or Elbow

Sometimes the toe of one foot is bent backward or the foot has knuckled under, catching on the vulva and impeding progress. Once you straighten that out, the calf should come easily.

Especially with a large calf, one or both elbows may catch on the cow's pelvis and the foot or feet will be advanced only as far as the calf's nose. When a front leg is too far back at the elbow and the shoulder blade is thrust forward, sometimes all you need to do is pull the leg that is not advanced and it will unstick.

If the leg won't advance easily, however, you must push the calf back a little in order to get the elbow unstuck. His head will be well along in the birth canal, and you must push on it to back him up. To do this, push on the head when the cow is not straining. This is not always easy, because your hand in the birth canal stimulates the cow to strain against you. If you can push the calf back a bit, however, this gives room to reposition the leg that was hindered by the elbow catching on the pelvis. Then you can pull the stuck leg upward in a rotating manner, to lift the elbow joint over the pelvic brim. Once you get the leg coming, the calf should come more easily, and you can pull him out.

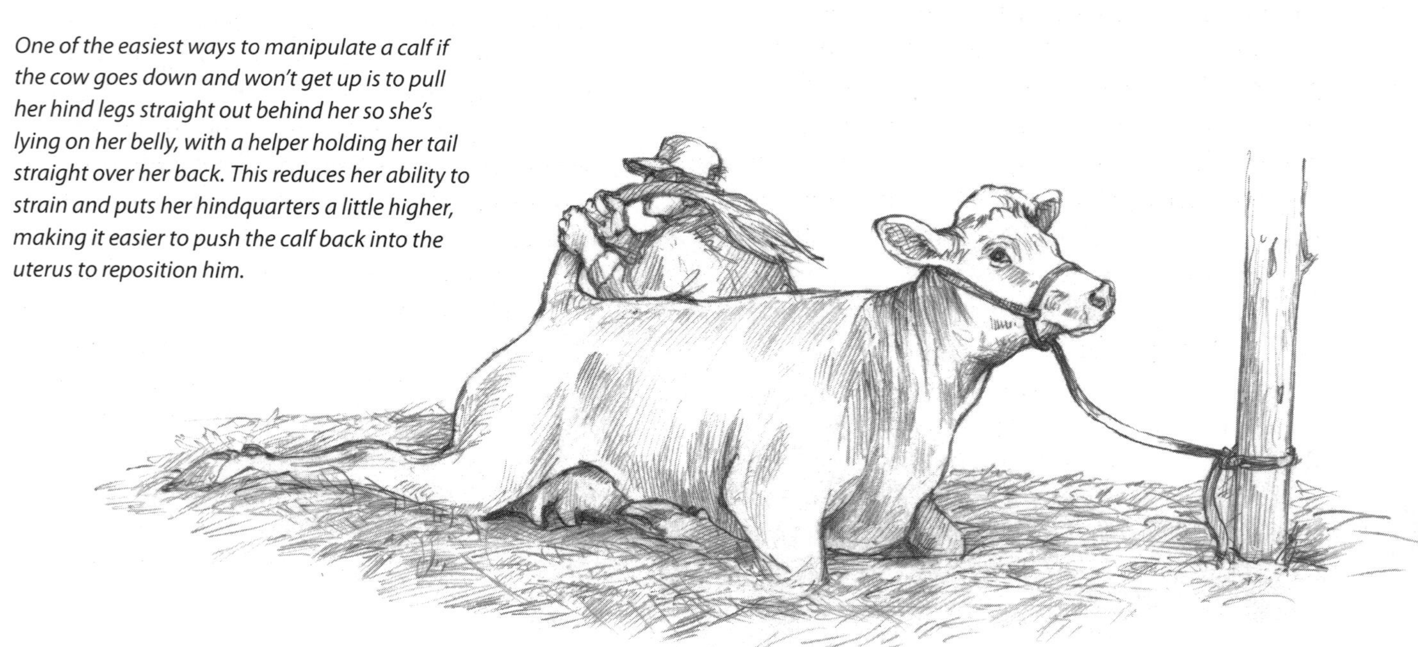

One of the easiest ways to manipulate a calf if the cow goes down and won't get up is to pull her hind legs straight out behind her so she's lying on her belly, with a helper holding her tail straight over her back. This reduces her ability to strain and puts her hindquarters a little higher, making it easier to push the calf back into the uterus to reposition him.

CALVES WITH HUNG-UP TOES OR ELBOWS

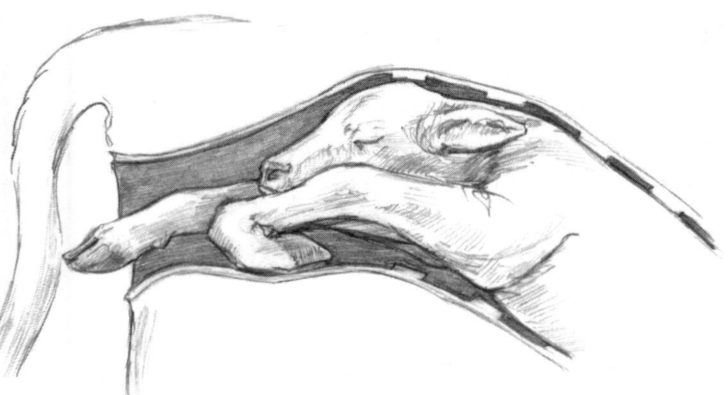

Bent Toe

Toe bent back (one front foot knuckled under), hindering the calf's progress through the birth canal.

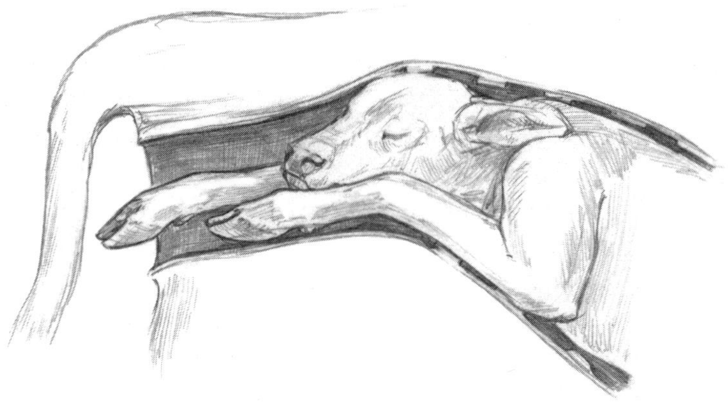

Caught Elbow

One elbow caught on the cow's pelvis.

Sideways or Upside Down

A sideways calf has feet and head pointing to the side instead of coming straight out. The sideways or upside-down position is easily mistaken for backward, since the upside-down feet look like hind feet until you reach in and find the head is there. You can usually correct either position enough to deliver him.

To do this, you can push him out of the rigid pelvis back into the uterus, where he floats more freely and there's room to rotate him. It's easier if the cow is standing up, with her uterus hanging freely in the abdomen, rather than lying down, when there is more pressure on the uterus and calf from abdominal contents. Don't start pulling a calf through the birth canal until you have pushed him back into the uterus and rotated him into the proper position or you may hurt him and the cow, especially if he is completely upside down.

It's rare to find a calf upside down, but this can usually be corrected by twisting the legs to rotate him — if you get him far enough back into the uterus to do so. Have the calf provide part of the necessary movement by using one hand to provoke him into moving as you put a rotational twist on his leg with your other hand. To stimulate him to move, press on his eyeballs (which are protected by his eyelids) with your thumb and middle finger. This triggers a convulsive reflex movement, which can aid your effort to turn him.

Don't start pulling a calf through the birth canal until you have pushed him back into the uterus and rotated him into the proper position or you may hurt him and the cow.

Another method for rotating the calf requires crossing his legs before applying traction via leg chains. This tends to turn the calf as you pull. If he's lying with his back to your right, with his legs aimed toward your left as you're facing the back of the cow, cross his legs with his left leg uppermost, since that's the shoulder that's down too far, and pull on that leg the hardest. This raises that shoulder as you pull, twisting the calf into a more upright position as his legs uncross, helping straighten the calf. It also helps if you can hold on to his jaw and twist (rotate) his head at the same time, to help turn him. If you have a helper, one person can pull on the leg chains while the other twists the head. Push him as far back in the uterus as you can, apply the chains, and cross the legs in the appropriate direction to turn him as you pull. The crossed legs and chains should become parallel as the calf twists into proper position. If this doesn't turn him enough, push him back into the uterus again and repeat the process until he is in proper position to be pulled out.

If the calf is completely upside down and you can't rotate him, it helps to have the cow lying down so you can roll her onto her back temporarily while you attempt the rotation. It also helps if her hindquarters are higher than her front end. If this doesn't work or you don't have enough helpers to roll the cow, call your vet. Then if the vet can't rotate the calf either, there's the option of surgical delivery. This is especially important if the calf is backward. An upside-down, backward calf may be impossible to rotate and must be delivered by cesarean section.

Foot or Leg Turned Back

If one or both front legs are turned back, one front foot may appear and not the other, or just the nose and no feet, and the cow makes no more progress. If you are not watching the cow very closely and she continues to strain, she may start to push the head through the vulva even though one or both legs are turned back. Most calves cannot be born in this position, unless they are very small and the cow has an extra-large pelvis; the calf won't fit through the birth canal with a leg turned back, and definitely not with both legs turned back. She will just keep jamming the calf's shoulder against the pelvis, and he is stuck.

It's best if you discover this problem before the head is completely out, so you can push the calf back into the uterus, where there is more room to maneuver the leg. If the head has come through the vulva, this becomes much more difficult. Get the cow up, if she will get up, since it's easier to push the calf back in if she's standing. She won't strain quite as hard, you have more room to work, and you're not in such an awkward position as when lying behind her, struggling to manipulate a leg.

Push the calf back into the uterus by pushing against his head or the point of his shoulder and reach farther to find that leg. A leg turned back at knee or fetlock joint is fairly easy. You just need to straighten it and bring it into the birth canal if turned back at the fetlock joint, or push the knee up if turned back at the knee, moving the foot outward in an arc over the pelvic brim and being careful the hoof does not scrape the sides of the uterus or birth canal. Cover it with your hand as you raise it up.

A leg turned back at the shoulder is harder to reach and bring forward properly. You may need both arms in the cow to accomplish this, holding the calf back in the uterus as far as you can with one hand while you lift the leg up and straighten it so it can come into the birth canal. If both front legs are turned back, you must push the calf back and get the legs straightened out one at a time.

Once you get the leg straightened or any other abnormality corrected, so the calf is now aimed into the birth canal, it's easier to deliver the calf if the cow is lying down. She can strain more effectively, and you can also get more leverage to pull by sitting behind her, bracing your feet on her hindquarters. If she wants to lie down after you've corrected the malpresentation, give her a chance to do so, then continue with the delivery.

A LEG AHEAD

WE'VE HAD OCCASIONS in which a calf had to be pushed way back into the uterus so we could bring a turned-back leg into the birth canal. One such situation occurred during the labor of Brazen Britches, daughter of Fancy Pants. She was typically a fast calver and on this occasion nearly had the calf's head out by the time we noticed there was only one leg. We quickly caught her and repositioned the calf.

More recently our son had to deliver a calf without retrieving the leg. One of his cows had pushed the calf's head clear out by the time the problem was discovered. There was no way it could be pushed back in, but luckily the cow was roomy enough that Michael was able to pull the calf out with a little traction on the one leg. It's much easier on the cow and calf, however, if the problem can be corrected early.

REPOSITIONING A TURNED-BACK FOOT OR LEG

If you discover that a calf's leg or foot is turned back, take the following steps to reposition the calf for normal delivery. If the calf's head has already emerged from the vulva before you notice the malpresentation, you'll need to stand the cow up and try to push the calf back in before manipulating the leg and foot.

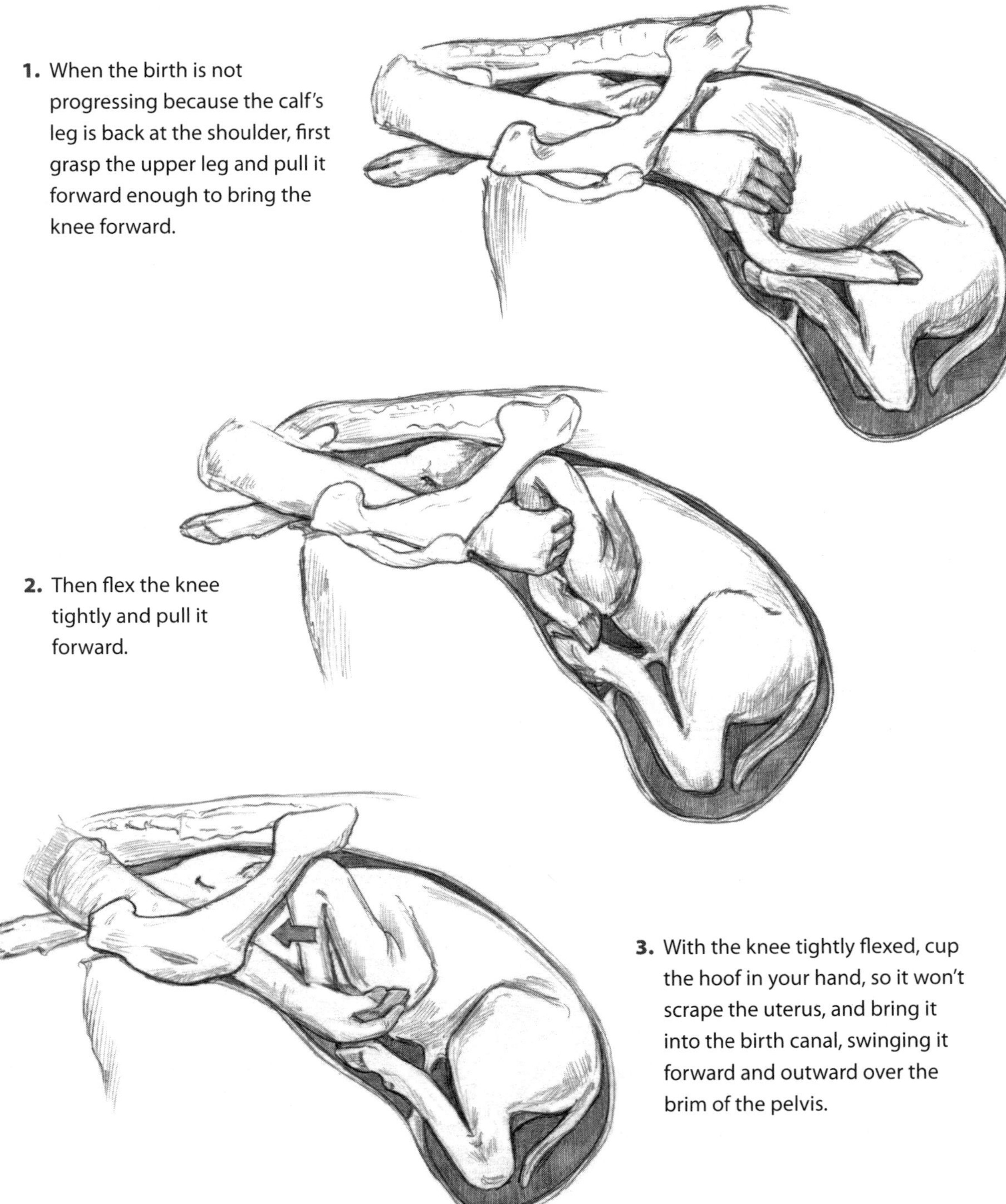

1. When the birth is not progressing because the calf's leg is back at the shoulder, first grasp the upper leg and pull it forward enough to bring the knee forward.
2. Then flex the knee tightly and pull it forward.
3. With the knee tightly flexed, cup the hoof in your hand, so it won't scrape the uterus, and bring it into the birth canal, swinging it forward and outward over the brim of the pelvis.

Head Turned Back

Sometimes the calf's head fails to enter the birth canal. Due to lack of space in the uterus during late gestation, the head is bent around to one side and sometimes can't extend during early labor. One or both front feet may show at the vulva, but the cow makes no more progress; or nothing shows. If the front feet appear and the legs protrude as far as the mid–*cannon bone* (the bone between knee and fetlock joint) and there is no sign of the calf's nose, you should suspect the head is turned back.

The sooner this problem is corrected, the better. Reach inside the birth canal to feel for the head. It should be coming 6 to 12 inches (15.2 to 30.5 cm) behind the feet, depending on the size of the calf and the length of his legs; the head should be positioned above the legs, the calf's eyes at about knee level. If the head is turned back, try to stand the cow up if she's down, as there's more room inside the uterus to manipulate the calf if she is standing, and it's easier for you to get both arms into the birth canal.

Put a halter on before you make her get up, so you can tie her to restrain her. If she won't get up, have her lie on the side that makes accessible the part of the calf you need to work with, even if you have to roll the cow over. If the calf's head is turned back toward her left flank, position the cow on her right side so the calf's head is uppermost rather than down under everything.

A head turned back can be a difficult challenge. Some people try to use a *head snare* (a loop of stiff cable) or chain or rope around the calf's head to help guide it into the birth canal. This is risky; you are more likely to damage the uterus if the calf's nose or jaw rubs or pushes against the uterine lining as you pull the head around. The calf's teeth may cut the uterus, since his mouth gapes open as you pull his head with a loop. It's much better just to use both hands. Hold the calf as far back as you can with one hand while grasping his lower jaw with the other to bring the head up into the birth canal, keeping your hand between the jaw and the uterine wall. If you can't quite reach his jaw, get hold of the corner of his mouth to bring the head around to where you can.

If you have trouble getting both arms into the cow, try pushing the calf as far as you can with one hand, then quickly transfer that hand to the calf's jaw and pull the jaw around in an arc until the nose is pointed into the birth canal. It's much easier, however, if you can keep pushing on the calf as you reach for the jaw; you won't lose ground if the cow is straining. Once you get the head started into the birth canal, put chains on the legs to pull the calf.

PERSEVERANCE PAYS WHEN REPOSITIONING A CALF

A TURNED-BACK HEAD can be one of the most difficult malpresentations to correct. Often it takes a very long arm and brute strength to reach it and get the head and neck maneuvered into corrrect position without it flopping back out of line again. If the cow is lying down and won't get up, it may require time lying on the ground behind her, struggling to reach the head after pushing the calf's feet back (the head and neck can't be brought around if the front legs are already jammed into the birth canal). It takes strength, endurance, determination, and sheer willpower to keep working at it.

Some vets give the cow an epidural block in this instance to keep her from straining against them while they try to manipulate the calf. But it's better if the cow's hind end is not anesthetized. You want her to be able to call on all her power to deliver the calf after you get the head and neck straightened out.

There's been only one occasion during which my husband was not able to reach and bring a turned-back head into the birth canal and we had to call our vet. But the vet couldn't get the calf straightened out either, and finally had to do a C-section to deliver the calf.

REPOSITIONING A TURNED-BACK HEAD

Although repositioning a turned-back head is challenging, you'll need to correct it as soon as possible. Rather than reaching for a head snare, which can lead to damage to the uterus, try the techniques on page 100, and refer to the illustrations below.

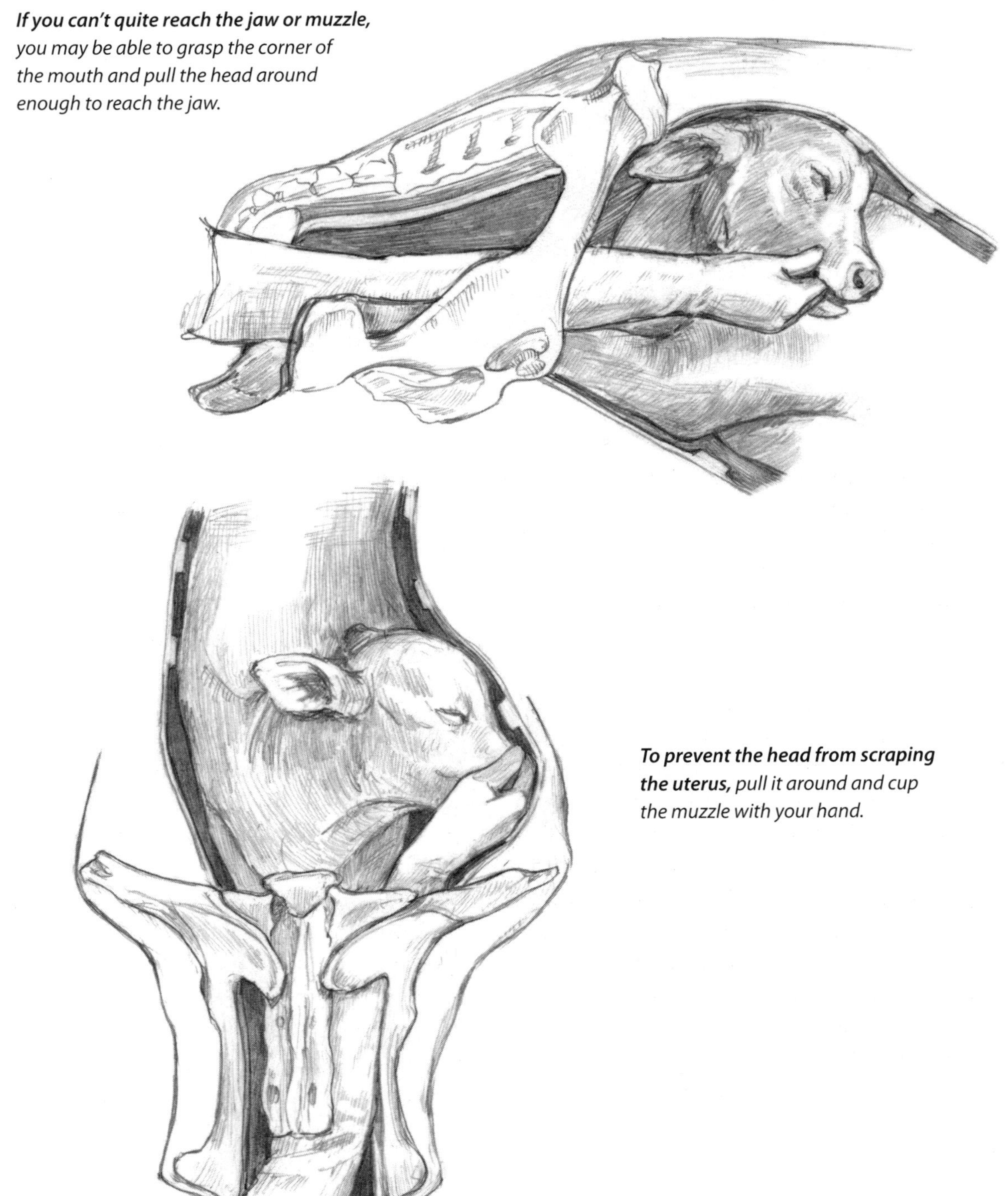

If you can't quite reach the jaw or muzzle, *you may be able to grasp the corner of the mouth and pull the head around enough to reach the jaw.*

To prevent the head from scraping the uterus, *pull it around and cup the muzzle with your hand.*

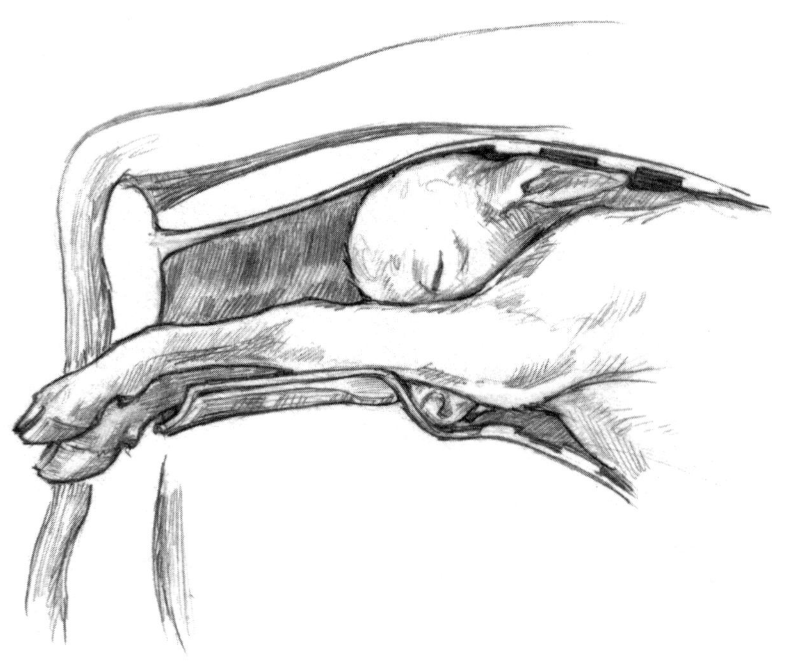

REPOSITIONING THE CALF WITH FOREHEAD UP, NOSE DOWN

When the forehead is up and the nose is down, the calf must be pushed back far enough to lift his nose and jaw up into the birth canal. If the calf's head has dropped down between his front legs, you must push the calf back far enough to get one of the front legs back into the uterus and out of the way. This will give you room to pull the head to that side and then up over the pelvic brim. Once the head is in place, you can bring the leg back into the birth canal and attach chains to pull the newly positioned calf.

Keep checking, though, to make sure the head is still coming before you pull much. Sometimes it will flop to the side again until you get it well started. On occasion you may need to use a head snare to keep it coming into the birth canal. If you have to pull the head through the pelvis with traction, however, this often means the calf is too big; it would be safer to deliver via cesarean section.

Forehead Up, Nose Down

The forehead up–nose down malpresentation may be easy or hard to correct, depending on how quickly you discover it. If the head is just approaching the pelvis, you can grab the calf's mouth or nostrils and pull the head up into normal position above the front legs, guiding it into the birth canal. But if the cow is already shoving him hard against the pelvis or if you've been pulling the legs without first checking to be sure the head was advancing and his nose is down and rammed against the brim of the pelvis, he can't come through. His head may drop down between his front legs, with his neck jammed against the cow's pelvis.

Push the calf back far enough to bring the head up into proper position. Then make sure it continues to come into the pelvis when you pull on his legs. To bring the calf's head into the birth canal when his face is jammed, push on the forehead with one hand (back away from the pelvic brim) while lifting the jaw up over the brim with your other hand.

If the calf's head is clear down between his front legs (the top of the neck hitting the cow's pelvis), it's harder to get. The calf must be pushed back enough to get one of the front legs clear back into the uterus and out of the way to give you room to pull the head to that side and then up over the pelvic brim. Then you can bring that leg back into the birth canal, attach chains to the legs, and pull the calf.

In a really difficult case, it may be necessary to push both legs back into the uterus in order to get the head up into proper position. An alternative is to rotate the calf by twisting his legs, putting him temporarily upside down (which makes it easier to extend his head). Some vets recommend rolling the cow onto her back, which may help you maneuver the calf's head into the pelvis.

Back or Belly Presentation

The back or belly presentation is rare in cattle, and if it occurs, you need your vet to help. Instead of having the feet aimed toward the birth canal, the calf's back or belly is jammed against the pelvis. In the latter situation, all four feet may be trying to enter the birth canal (and can be mistaken for twins). The vet may try to push the calf back and reposition him so the closest end of the body (front or rear) can be moved into position to come through. This is often difficult or impossible, however, and the best solution is to remove the calf by having your vet perform a cesarean section (see chapter 5).

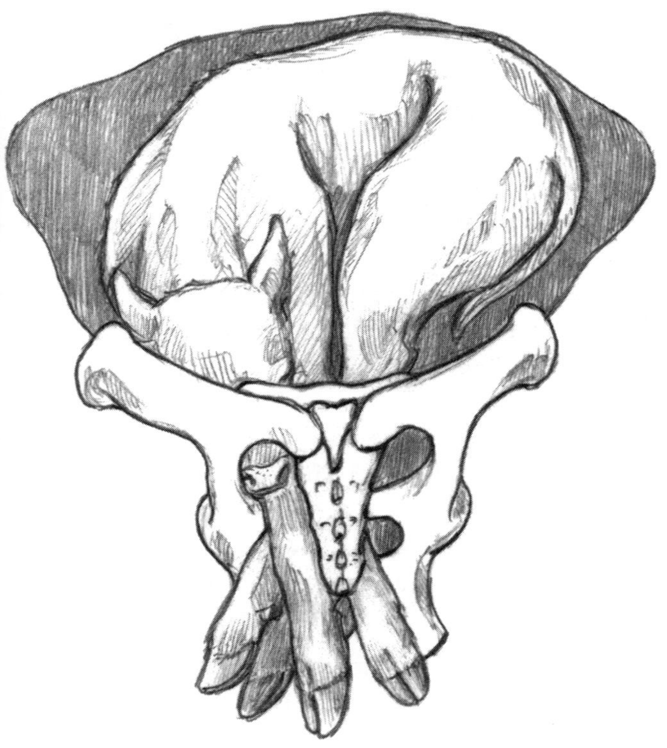

You'll need to call the vet if a calf presents all four legs during labor. Belly presentation is very rare in cattle. This position is hard to correct; the calf is usually delivered by c-section.

Why Do Calves Come Backward?

Several factors can influence whether a calf ends up backward at birth, but the biggest may be heredity. English vet G. H. Arthur found, during the 1960's, that many fetuses are carried backward and upside down during the first 6 to 6½ months of gestation and then rotate to a frontward, right-side-up position. By the end of the sixth month, there are equal numbers of fetuses in both positions, but by the middle of the seventh month most are facing forward, with 5 percent still posterior.

The numbers of fetuses in posterior position may increase because calves sired by certain bulls have grown too large (with length exceeding the width of the uterus) to rotate into the correct position by 6 to 6½ months — the turning stage of gestation. Final birth weight doesn't mean a calf will be backward, since many huge calves are properly positioned, making more of their growth spurt after they shift position, but there may be a correlation between fetal growth stages (which may be influenced by heredity) and whether or not the fetus shifts its position by the time it is 6 to 6½ months along in gestation. Some bulls' offspring may grow faster than others during early gestation, becoming too large by that stage to rotate. If a herd suddenly has more backward calves than usual, it could be due to a new bull.

Other factors that may influence the number of backward births in any given year include the sex of the calf, the age of the dam, nutrition — anything that has a bearing on the rate of fetal growth during the stage of gestation when the calf shifts position. Another factor is body condition of the dam. Increased numbers of backward calves in pregnant feedlot heifers have been noted and may be due to large amounts of fat deposited in the pelvic or abdominal area of the cow that prevent the repositioning of the fetus.

Backward Presentation

A calf coming backward will be a slow birth unless he is very small, because he is not streamlined in this position. Nature has things programmed for a normal frontward delivery. Usually, the calf stretches the cervix and vulva gradually as the front legs, head, and then larger shoulders pass through. But with hind legs coming first, the big hindquarters of the calf must come through early on. This takes a lot of stretching. The hips are often difficult to pass through the cow's pelvis, and the rib cage tends to catch on the way through. Even the lay of the hair is wrong for smooth delivery on a backward calf. When pulling a backward calf, use lots of lubricant and put it as far into the birth canal — alongside the calf — as you can.

It may take the cow longer in early labor to get the calf's hind feet aimed in the right direction. When his feet do start to show through the vulva, you can tell they are hind feet instead of front feet because heels will be up, with bottoms of the feet showing. If you see the bottoms of the feet, however, don't just assume the calf is backward and start pulling. Reach inside to get a feel of the whole leg to determine if there are knees (which are front-leg features) or hocks (hind legs). If you feel knees, the calf is sideways or upside down instead of backward and must be rotated. If they are front feet (the legs just twisted because the calf is a little sideways), make sure the head is there and not turned back. Remember always to be sure which part of the calf is presented before you put on chains and start pulling.

You also need to check the cow if she's taking too long before she presents feet. By reaching in, you can tell if the calf is started into the birth canal and, if so, whether you are finding front feet or hind feet. If you think they are hind feet, make sure by reaching along the legs until you find the tail.

Assisting in a Posterior Delivery

Once you determine that the calf is presenting backward, take the following steps to assist the cow and deliver the calf safely. (See drawings on page 106.)

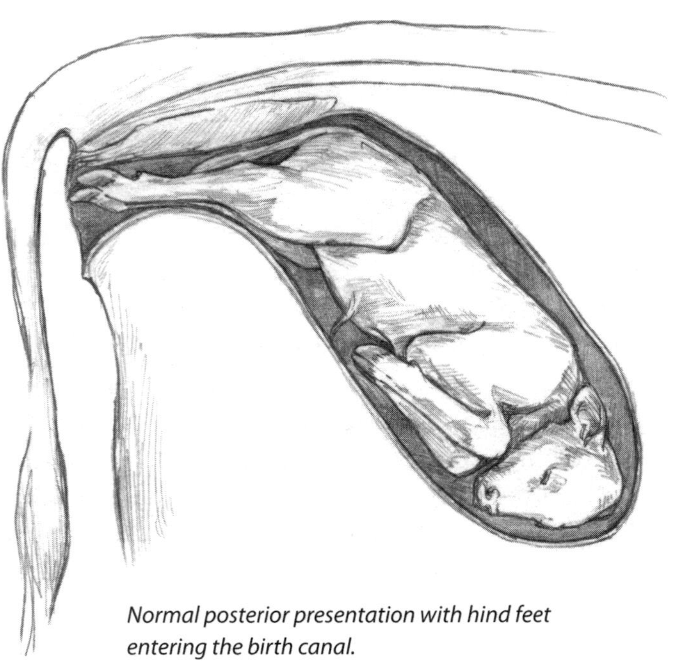

Normal posterior presentation with hind feet entering the birth canal.

A Backward Birth Is an Emergency

It's important to recognize the signs of a backward (posterior) birth so you can assist in the delivery. In a normal posterior presentation, the calf is right-side up and both hind feet are first to enter the birth canal. The legs are stretched out behind the calf, which puts the bottoms of the feet facing upward when they emerge from the cow's vulva.

The head and front legs will be the last part of the calf to emerge, so there is danger of suffocation. Never try to turn around a backward calf; there is not room and not enough time. This feat is nearly impossible, and to attempt it would seriously injure the cow. The backward calf can be safely delivered just by helping him through the birth canal in the position he's in.

After delivering a backward calf, your most urgent task if he is still alive is to get him breathing. Quickly get the fluid out of his air passages, then tickle his nostril to stimulate a cough. If he is limp and unconscious but his heart is beating, you still have a chance to save him if you give him artificial respiration (see chapter 3).

1. ***Restrain the cow*** in a place with plenty of room behind her to use a calf puller and to maneuver it easily. You don't want her in the corner of a small barn stall, with her back end too close to the wall. This is one instance where you definitely need to use a calf puller unless the calf is very small. Only a few backward calves are small enough to be pulled by hand. A rare few will survive an unassisted birth if the cow calves fast and jumps up immediately as the calf's front end comes out, pulling the membranes and fluids away from his face so he can start breathing. But most calves will not survive unless you use a calf puller to get them out quickly, since pulling by hand is usually extremely difficult and slow unless you have three very strong people delivering the calf. The calf's umbilical cord will be pinched off or broken during the birth, making it urgent that he's born immediately.

Reposition Chains Ahead of Time

We learned to place chains above a calf's hocks the hard way, while delivering one of the first backward calves we lost. We winched him out swiftly, until we ran out of cable. His shoulders and head were still inside the cow, but there was no time to undo everything and put the chains above the hocks. Instead, Lynn and I grabbed his legs and pulled with all our strength, but we could not get the calf out of the cow quickly enough, and he died.

After that loss we always took time, on every backward calf, to reposition the chains before the crucial moments when delivery must be swiftly completed.

2. ***Complete a more thorough check*** to know what's happening. Sometimes the umbilical cord has caught over a hind leg if the leg passed under the cord while straightening to enter the birth canal. If this happens, the cord will stretch and break before you've pulled the calf halfway out. If the cord is caught, you can correct the situation. Push the calf back into the uterus if you can, far enough to manipulate the entangled leg (by flexing the hock tightly) and release it from the cord. Also make sure that the calf's tail is not stuck straight up and over his back, or his tailhead will jam into the pelvis and impede the birth process.

3. ***Attach chains to the calf's legs*** in a double loop above the fetlock joints and start pulling him. Go slow and easy, giving the cervix plenty of time to dilate fully as the calf's buttocks start through it. Traction should be applied on just one hind leg at a time until its stifle joint has been drawn up over the pelvic brim. Bringing legs into the bony pelvis one at a time enables the wide hindquarters to come through more easily.

4. ***If hindquarters are still stuck, cross one leg*** over the other and pull harder on the lower one to rotate him to one side and ease the stifles through the pelvis more readily. Another way to rotate him a little is to bend the hind legs a bit and use them as levers in a circular motion to twist the calf's hindquarters. If he is rotated 45 to 90 degrees, so he is nearly lying on his side, this takes advantage of the widest diameter of the cow's pelvis.

5. ***Make sure the calf's tail is not protruding upward*** as the hindquarters start through the pelvis. If the tail is up over the calf's back, it may damage the birth canal as you pull him through or the pull may break his tailhead. Put your hand over his rump and make sure the tail is down between his hind legs as he is entering the pelvis. You'll have to pull fast and forcefully at the end, so you don't want to damage the cow. Make sure everything is coming properly — tail down, stifles coming through the pelvis one at a time. The calf's umbilical cord won't pinch off and make him vulnerable for suffocation until his hindquarters are going through the cow's pelvis, so you have time to go slowly, until the hind legs are far enough out to get past the hocks. Using a calf puller or three strong men, pull equally on legs in an angle that is straight out and slightly upward from the back of the cow.

PULLING A BACKWARD (POSTERIOR) CALF WITH A CALF PULLER

When a calf is coming through the birth canal backward, a mechanical puller is necessary for adequate traction.

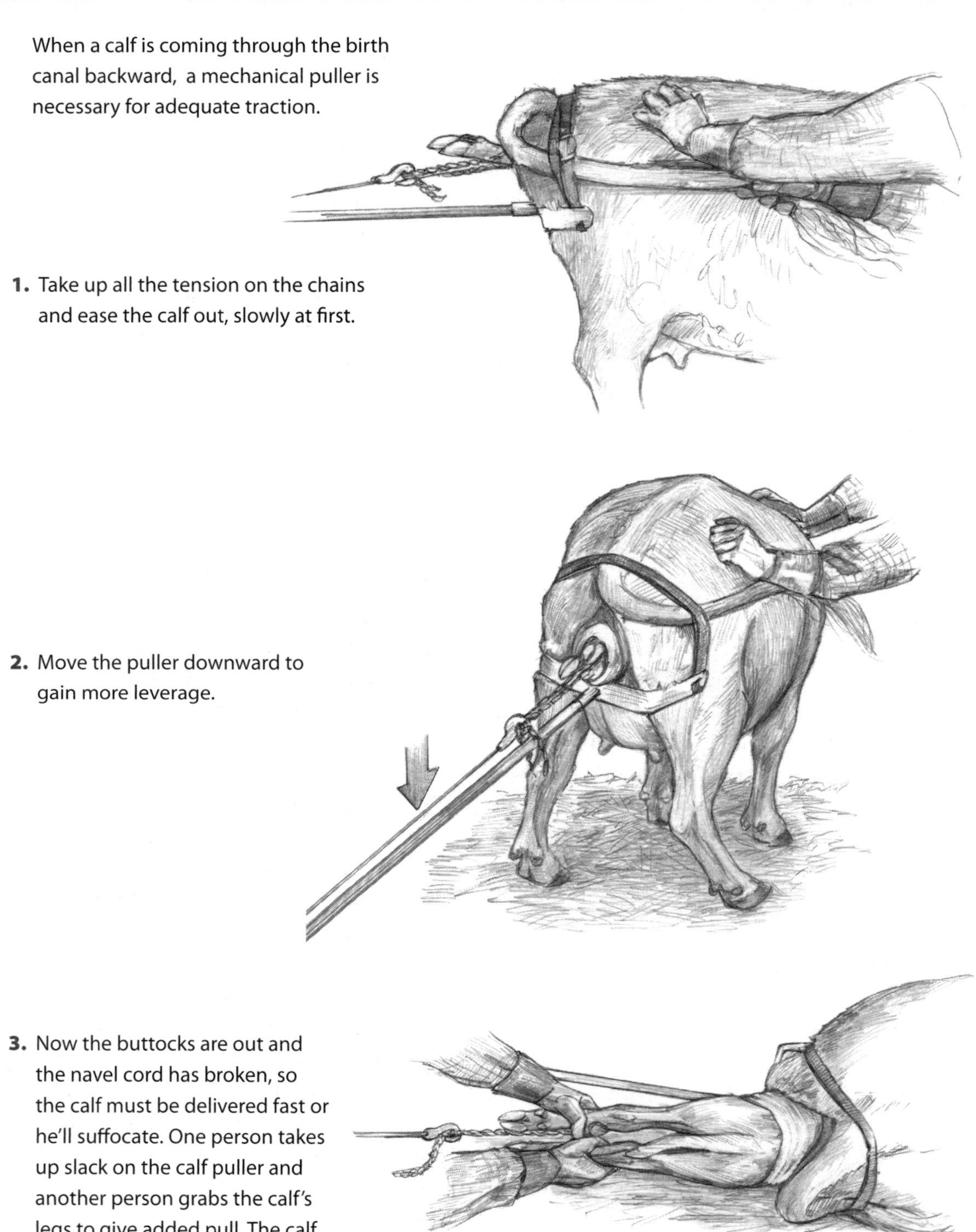

1. Take up all the tension on the chains and ease the calf out, slowly at first.

2. Move the puller downward to gain more leverage.

3. Now the buttocks are out and the navel cord has broken, so the calf must be delivered fast or he'll suffocate. One person takes up slack on the calf puller and another person grabs the calf's legs to give added pull. The calf is pulled swiftly out of the cow before he suffocates.

6. ***Reposition the leg chains above the hocks,*** once you've pulled the legs out past the hocks, especially if you're using a winch puller with cable. This gives you more room to winch. Otherwise you may get a big calf more than halfway out and run out of cable room. At that point you don't have time to reposition the chains; the calf will be short on oxygen and suffocating because the umbilical cord has already been pinched or broken. You usually don't run out of pulling room with the extra-long, ratchet-type pullers, however.

7. ***Before pulling out the calf, rotate him back*** into the normal position if you had to rotate his hindquarters to get his hips through the pelvis. Go slowly and carefully until the calf's tailhead and anus emerge, to be sure the back of his rib cage has started through the pelvis. You don't want the calf's rib cage to catch on the pelvis and be crushed because you are swiftly jerking him through. Once his rib cage has entered the pelvis, as his hindquarters are emerging from the vulva, hurry him on out as fast as you can before he suffocates. As before, the direction of the pull should be straight back out of the vulva.

The Backward Odds

Most calves are born with front feet extended, head resting on the knees. But a few come out backward and may not survive unless you are there to help. Many years ago one of our vets told us that a person is lucky to save one out of ten backward calves. This is probably true when cows calve at pasture and aren't checked frequently. But with close observation, and assistance given at the proper time, you can beat those odds.

During 40 years of calving we've had more than 80 backward and breech (rump first) presentations — an average of two per year — and we've lost only four of those 80 calves. One died because we didn't check the cow soon enough. The calf was breech (no legs in the birth canal; see page 108) so the cow was not straining yet, even though she'd been in labor too long and the placenta had detached. Another was fatally injured during delivery; he had a crushed rib cage — from catching on the cow's pelvis — and a punctured lung from broken ribs. Two other losses were big calves that suffocated because we couldn't pull fast enough, but most posterior and breech presentations can be safely delivered.

On average, 5 percent of all calves are positioned backward at birth, although the number of posterior presentations in any herd in any given calving season will vary. . . . The position of a fetus when a cow is checked for pregnancy is not necessarily the way it will face at birth.

On average, 5 percent of all calves are positioned backward at birth, although the number of posterior presentations in any herd in any given calving season will vary. When a fetus is growing, it's quite active and can readily change position, especially when it's small. During the first three months of gestation, there are equal numbers of fetuses facing backward and frontward. From the fourth through the middle of the seventh month of gestation, the majority of fetuses are positioned backward but then rotate.

The position of a fetus when a cow is checked for pregnancy is not necessarily the way it will face at birth. Out of curiosity one fall, after a calving season in which we had five backward-facing calves in our herd of 170 cows, we asked our vet to see which way each calf was lying when he checked the cows. He said that at that particular stage of pregnancy (about five months), many calves are backward but shift to proper position before they reach full term. Of the calves he could reach, we took note of the dozen that were facing backward at that time. Surprisingly, none of the original dozen was backward at birth, but three that were not backward when the vet checked at five months presented backward at birth.

Breech Presentation

A calf in a breech position is one of the most common reasons a cow does not progress to hard labor after the cervix dilates. The only part of the calf's anatomy that can enter the birth canal is his tail or maybe his hocks.

Due to long hind legs and limited space in the uterus, a number of calves that are backward in late gestation fail to extend their hind legs during labor. The calf can come no farther as the feet cannot enter the birth canal and the rump is jammed against the cervix. His legs are forward or down instead of extended behind him. He's usually in a "sitting" position with hind feet toward his head. The legs may put pressure on his abdomen, and this may cause him to have a bowel movement. If this happens, the fluids surrounding the calf, or discharging from the cow's vulva if the sac has broken, are yellow-brown. On occasion the hind legs are flexed, not forward, with the hocks trying to come through the cervix.

Due to limited space in the uterus, backward calves may fail to extend their hind legs during labor.

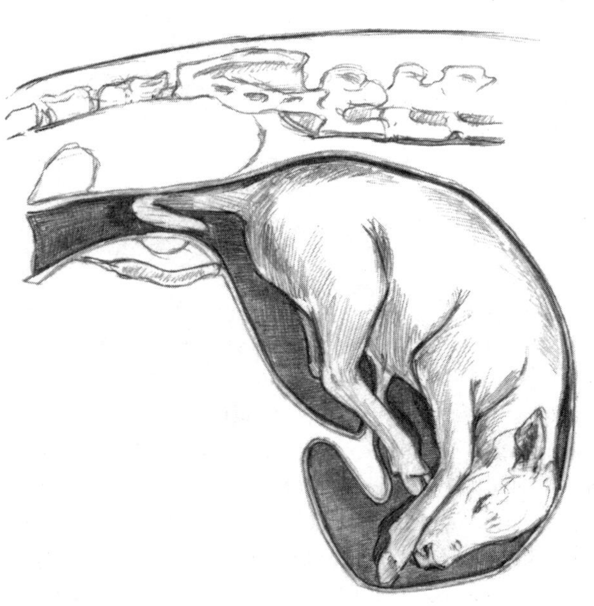

In a breech presentation with his hind legs up toward the calf's head, sometimes the only thing entering the birth canal is the tail.

"NATURAL" BACKWARD BIRTHS

OF ALL THE BACKWARD BIRTHS we've experienced, only two calves were born without help. One was a tiny calf that emerged swiftly. The other was a streamlined calf sired by an Angus bull that threw small calves. Lynn and I arrived on the scene just as the cow was in labor, with the calf halfway out. Seeing he was backward, we ran up behind the cow to try to grab on to the calf and pull him out.

We startled the cow when we ran up behind her, and she jumped to her feet. The calf fell out as she sprang up. He had been moving readily through the birth canal as she labored and had not yet suffocated; the cord was probably just starting to pinch off when we approached, as the calf's hips and rib cage were passing through the birth canal.

The cow's jumping up was fortunate. If she had continued to lie there a few more moments with the calf not yet out of the birth canal, he would have suffocated.

To Check or Not to Check?

A breech presentation can't be detected without reaching into the birth canal to check what's happening. The cow may or may not break her water. She appears to be still in early labor. Since no feet enter the birth canal, there is nothing to stimulate her to begin hard straining. If no water bag is observed, there may be no visible sign that second-stage labor has begun. If she does start to strain, it is usually because she is jamming the calf's hocks or hips through the cervix, but he cannot be born.

The cow may not start straining at all if the hind legs are forward because nothing enters the birth canal. But if you wait too long to check her, the calf will die. This can be a difficult decision to make. Should you restrain and check a cow that is obviously calving but not yet in hard labor? Ultimately, it's better to check her on a "false alarm" (finding that the feet and head are indeed coming and the cow just needs more time) than to wait too long and have a dead calf.

BREECH CALF WITH HOCKS FEXED

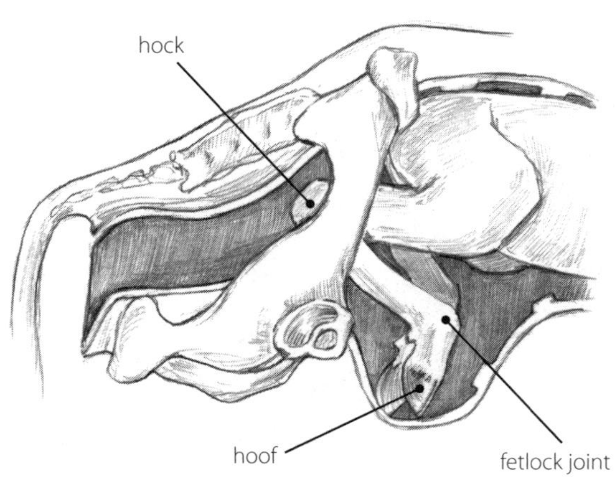

The calf's hocks are pressing against the cervix in this breech position, and the cow may start to strain.

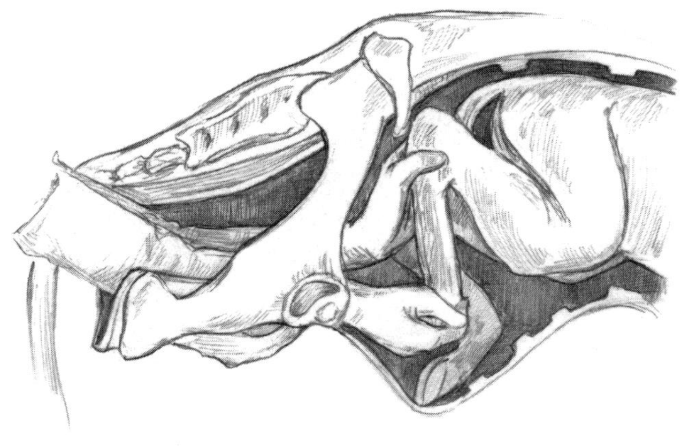

Using both hands in the birth canal, the calf can be pushed forward and manipulated. The hock is flexed and lifted with one hand while the other hand is cupped around the flexed fetlock joint and hoof to bring it safely over the pelvic brim without scraping the uterine lining.

Repositioning a Breech

If the calf is breech, you'll find only the tail or rump or hocks after reaching way in through the cervix to touch him. To reposition the calf, his rump must be pushed forward (so it's not jammed against the cervix or pelvis) to make room to maneuver each hind leg and bring it into the birth canal. It's easier to get both arms into the birth canal and to push the calf if the cow is standing and not lying down where she can push the hardest. If you are a small person, you'll probably need someone with a longer arm to do this maneuvering for you.

With one hand, push the calf's rump forward into the uterus as far as possible. Then, with the other hand, grasp one of his legs, bend the hock joint, and lift this joint upward. Reach farther forward along that leg until you find the foot. Draw the calf's foot backward in an arc, with your hand cupped protectively around his toes so they won't scrape or tear the wall of the uterus as you bring that foot around to the rear. (See drawings on next page.)

Keep the hock joint flexed tightly and the calf pushed as far forward with your other hand as you can. Lift the calf's foot up over the cow's pelvis, keeping your hand cupped around the hoof since this narrow passage is most likely where it will scrape. Do the same with the other hind leg after you have the first one straightened out behind the calf and in the birth canal. Make sure the umbilical cord does not get caught over one of the legs as you lift it up. Once both hind legs are extended behind the calf and in the birth canal, attach chains and pull the calf.

If you try the above techniques and still find it is impossible to bring the legs into the birth canal, the calf must be delivered by C-section.

> **IT TAKES TWO HANDS**
>
> It's a tight fit to get both arms in the cow's birth canal, especially if you have big arms, but it's the best way to get a breech calf repositioned. There is always enough stretch in the vulva and vagina to get both arms in; remember that a calf coming through this narrow space is wider than your two arms.

REPOSITIONING A BREECH PRESENTATION

1. Push the calf forward into the uterus so there is room to pull one of the legs into a flexed position.

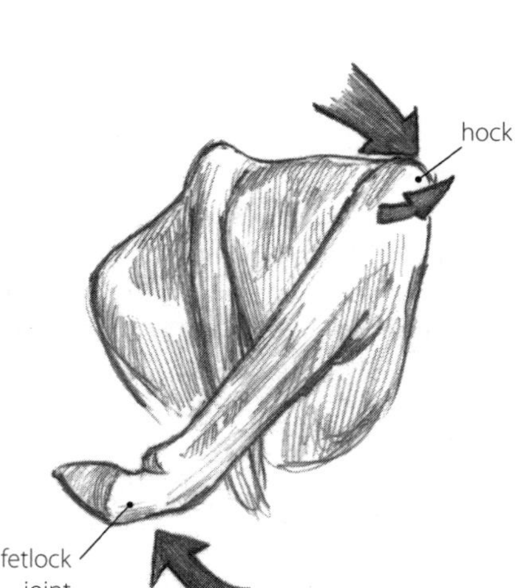

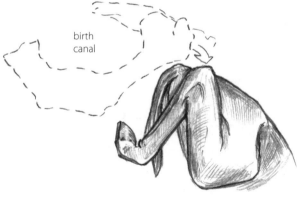

2. Push the flexed hock outward and swing the flexed fetlock joint back.

birth canal

3. Keep hock and fetlock joints tightly flexed and bring the fetlock joint and foot over the pelvic brim . . .

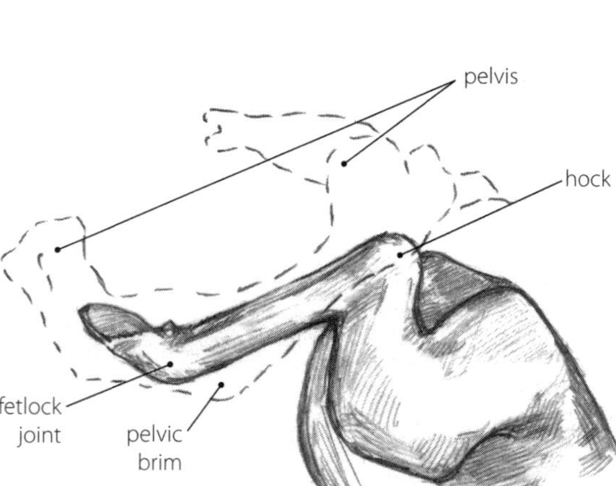

4. . . . and into the birth canal. Repeat the process with the other leg.

BREECH BIRTH LESSONS

PIGGY, A YOUNG ANGUS COW, gave us our first experience with a breech calf in 1969. She took a long time in early labor, and we kept waiting for something to show. We finally ran her into the corral, tied her, and checked her, only to discover that the calf was breech, with nothing entering the birth canal.

When Lynn felt inside the cow, he could feel part of the placenta alongside the calf, detached. The calf was already dead. We did not know how to correct this type of malpresentation and called our vet. He came out to the ranch and delivered the dead calf, first bringing the hind legs into the birth canal so the calf could be pulled.

From that sad loss we learned that waiting too long before checking a cow can be fatal for the calf. We resolved to be aware of when each cow starts early labor and to check any that we feel are taking too long. Since then, we've delivered a number of breech calves and have not lost any. In fact, we had to call our vet only once, to come with his long arms and help us reach a calf whose hind legs were too long for us to reach for repositioning.

Torsion of the Uterus

If a cow is suffering from *torsion of the uterus* (the uterus has flipped over), there will be a corkscrew twist in the cervix. The torsion is more often twisted counterclockwise, when viewed from behind the cow. This sometimes happens during gestation and may cause problems then (see chapter 2), but it more frequently occurs during early labor when violent movements of the calf in response to uterine contractions cause the uterus to swing and rotate, especially when the cow is getting up or lying down. When she gets up, she first raises her hindquarters as she lurches forward, kneeling on her forelegs, and may pause for a moment before making the final effort to stand. In this position, the uterus hangs almost vertically, enabling it to rotate quite easily if the calf makes a sudden movement.

If the torsion is mild (45 to 90 degrees), it may correct itself during labor as the calf heads into the birth canal and the cow gets up and down (cows often get up and down a lot if a calf is not coming right, which helps the calf reposition). Many mild torsions are not recognized as such by the cow's human assistants. Rather, they are seen as just abnormal positions for the calf: The calf seems to be positioned sideways or upside down and can be rotated into proper position before you pull him.

In a more serious torsion (180 degrees or more), however, the twist shuts off the birth canal and the calf cannot come through. The cow is obviously in labor but may not progress to active labor; there is no stimulus to strain if the calf cannot enter the birth canal. The cow may be in pain, very upset, and difficult to handle. In a severe torsion, the vulva may appear pulled forward at the top and tilted to one side or the other (usually to the right).

CROOKED CALF

Often a calf will be aimed a little crooked when entering the birth canal, perhaps due to slight torsion of the uterus. Most of these calves will straighten as the birth progresses, and the situation corrects itself. But sometimes you must help. A rotated calf can't come through the canal readily; he's not streamlined in this position.

Methods for Returning the Uterus to a Normal Position

When you put your hand in to determine why the cow is taking so long, instead of finding a closed or partially open cervix, you come to some folds and twists of tissue that block the birth canal. In this situation, call the vet. If it's only a partial torsion, the vet may be able to rotate the calf and uterus back into the proper position by twisting the calf's legs, but if it's a complete torsion, it may be necessary to roll the cow (see pages 113 and 114). If there is not enough help available to roll the cow, the vet may cut an incision in the cow's flank, reach through, and turn the uterus back over. This works only if the cow is standing.

The most common sign of uterine torsion is a cow in early labor (restless, signs of abdominal pain) but not progressing to active labor or straining hard. If assistance is not given, the placenta detaches and the calf dies. If you or your vet can reach through the twisted constriction and grasp the calf by elbow, shoulder, or leg and he is still alive, there's a chance he can be turned over by first getting him swinging back and forth to get some momentum, then making a major push to roll him over completely. This works better if the cow's hindquarters are higher than her front end, allowing the uterus to swing more freely. Be sure you're turning it in the proper direction or you'll make the twist worse. It also helps if the calf is still alive. The vet may press on the calf's eyeballs (which are protected by the eyelids) while starting to swing the uterus over; this causes a violent movement of the calf, which helps to turn the uterus.

Flipping over the womb by hand. The vet will try to determine, by vaginal and/or rectal palpation, the direction of the torsion. After cutting a slit in the flank, the vet will reach in and confirm the direction of the twist, then try to turn the uterus back over. If the twist is to the left, the hand is passed down between the uterus and the cow's left flank and some portion of the calf is grasped, with the uterine wall between the calf and the hand. An effort is made to rock the calf and uterus back and forth, creating an arc with 10 to 12 inches (25.4 to 30.5 cm) of swing, and then to rotate it by lifting and pushing strongly to the right. For a twist to the right, the hand is

PANDORA'S BOX

ON A COLD DAY IN JANUARY 1972, one of our high-strung, cranky Angus cows, Pandora, was taking too long in early labor. She became more upset as the day wore on and kept trying to get out of the pen.

Day faded into evening, and after several hours of waiting and watching, we resigned ourselves to manually checking Pandora and took on the challenge of tying her up. She was the nervous kind of cow that can pivot and jump around so fast — even with her head anchored to a post — that she's a danger to the person trying to check her. She could create a "crack-the-whip" effect on your arm, banging you into the fence first on one side and then the other, if you could keep up with her that long.

Needless to say, the manual check didn't work very well, so we ran her into the lane to our barn and caught her in a head catcher, where she couldn't sling herself around so much. Lynn checked inside her. The calf was still alive, but the feet hadn't come through the cervix, and the legs seemed twisted around. Things weren't right.

We called our vet, who arrived at midnight in very good spirits after just returning from a country barn dance. It was a cold, dark night (8°F/–13.3°C) with a nasty wind blowing. Jeep lights and a flashlight provided illumination. I held the light in one hand and Pandora's protesting tail in the other as the vet examined her and diagnosed the problem: torsion of the uterus. She had a corkscrew twist near the cervix — and in her case it was more than 360 degrees.

We'd never heard of this problem, and our vet said he usually dealt with about six a year, out of 35,000 cows in our county. He told us a rotation can happen with an overactive calf or if the cow has been fighting, which we knew could be a factor in Pandora's case: She was *always* fighting some other cow. Trouble was her personal theme. We named her after the mythical character who opened the box and let out all the troubles into the world.

When we told the vet her name, he chuckled and said she just needed to have her vagina straightened out. He cut a slit in her left side, reached his arm in, and began heaving, turning the uterus and undoing the twist.

It took a lot of effort. The calf, uterus, placenta, and fluids together weighed well over 100 pounds, but his strong arm and good-humored determination eventually got the job done. Then we pulled the calf. Pandora needed help; with the slit in her side she couldn't push. Each time she strained, air rushed through the hole in her side and she couldn't put any pressure on the calf. Thus we pulled him, sewed up the hole, and put the pair in the barn, out of the wind.

We named the calf Torque. He was one of our biggest steers that fall, so we were glad we got Pandora's vagina straightened out.

CORRECTING UTERINE TORSION WITH A PLANK

One method for correcting uterine torsion is to have someone stand on a plank or ladder resting on the cow's abdomen while others roll the cow using leg ropes.

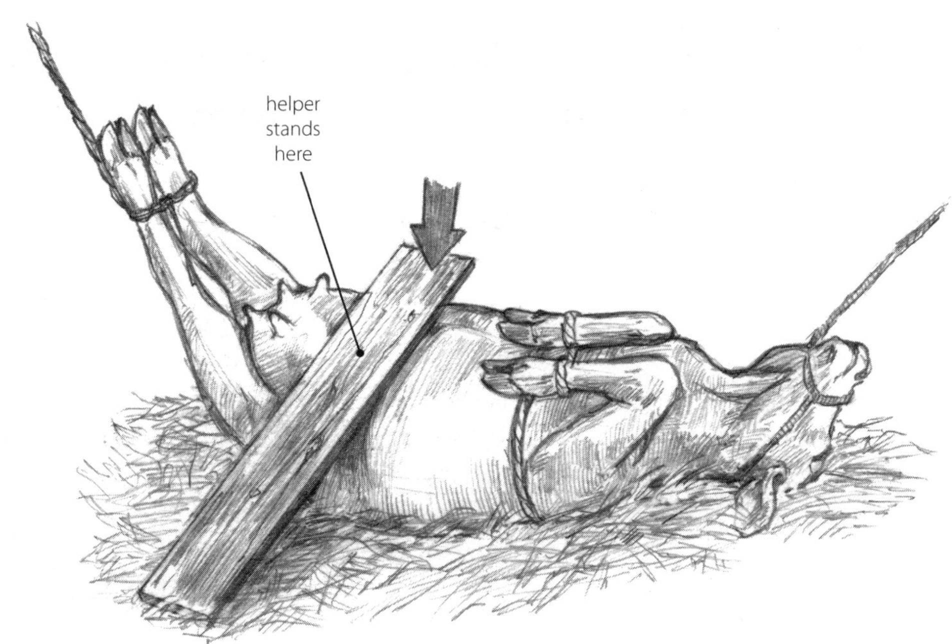

passed over and down between the uterus and the cow's right flank, and the same technique is used to swing and then rotate the uterus. This method is easier if the vet is tall and strong, with long arms, and the calf is not huge.

Rolling the cow. Another method requires using ropes to put the cow on the ground if she's standing and rolling her over with three or four strong people. The goal is to roll her body so quickly in the direction of the twist that it rotates faster than the heavy uterus, correcting the twist. To accomplish this, the cow is held down by one person holding her head while her front feet are tied together with one rope and her hind feet tied together with another. With two people holding each rope, at a given signal they all give a hard pull so the cow is rapidly turned from one side to the other, rolling over on her back from right to left or left to right — whichever direction is needed to resolve the torsion.

She is then examined again, by a hand in the birth canal, to see if the twist has been resolved. If so, there will be access into the cervix and uterus to reach the calf. If the torsion was not resolved, the cow can be slowly returned to her original position and another attempt made to pull her over quickly. One person might keep a hand in the vagina during the procedure to make sure the rolling is in the proper direction. If the folds in the vagina are tightening instead of loosening, this is a clue that the cow is being rolled in the wrong direction.

The weighted-plank method. When there are not enough people to roll the cow quickly, you can put a wide wooden plank or a ladder (9 to 12 feet [2.7 to 3.7 m] long) on the cow's flank while she is lying down, with one end of it on the ground. The cow must be lying on the same side as the direction of the torsion. One person stands on the plank where it rests on the cow's abdomen while the cow is very slowly pulled over by use of leg ropes. The object of this method is to hold the uterus stationary by means of the weighted plank as the cow's body is rotated around the uterus. The weight of the person and plank creates pressure first on the upper abdominal wall, then the belly, and finally the opposite side of the abdomen as the cow is rolled, and this holds the uterus in place, correcting the twist.

As soon as the torsion is corrected, the calf should be pulled, since the cervix is usually fully dilated and may start closing up again soon. There is also more chance to get the calf out alive if you don't delay. If the torsion can't be corrected by any of these means, or the cervix is not dilated or will not dilate after the calf and uterus have been rotated, he must be delivered by c-section. One problem with delivering the calf by c-section before the torsion is corrected is that the incision into the uterus may be inaccessible for suturing after the calf is removed and the uterus put into proper position. It's always best to try to get the torsion resolved before resorting to a c-section (see chapter 5).

ROLLING THE COW TO CORRECT A UTERINE TORSION

If there are enough people available to help, your veterinarian may decide not to cut open the cow to correct the uterine torsion, but to use ropes to roll the cow instead.

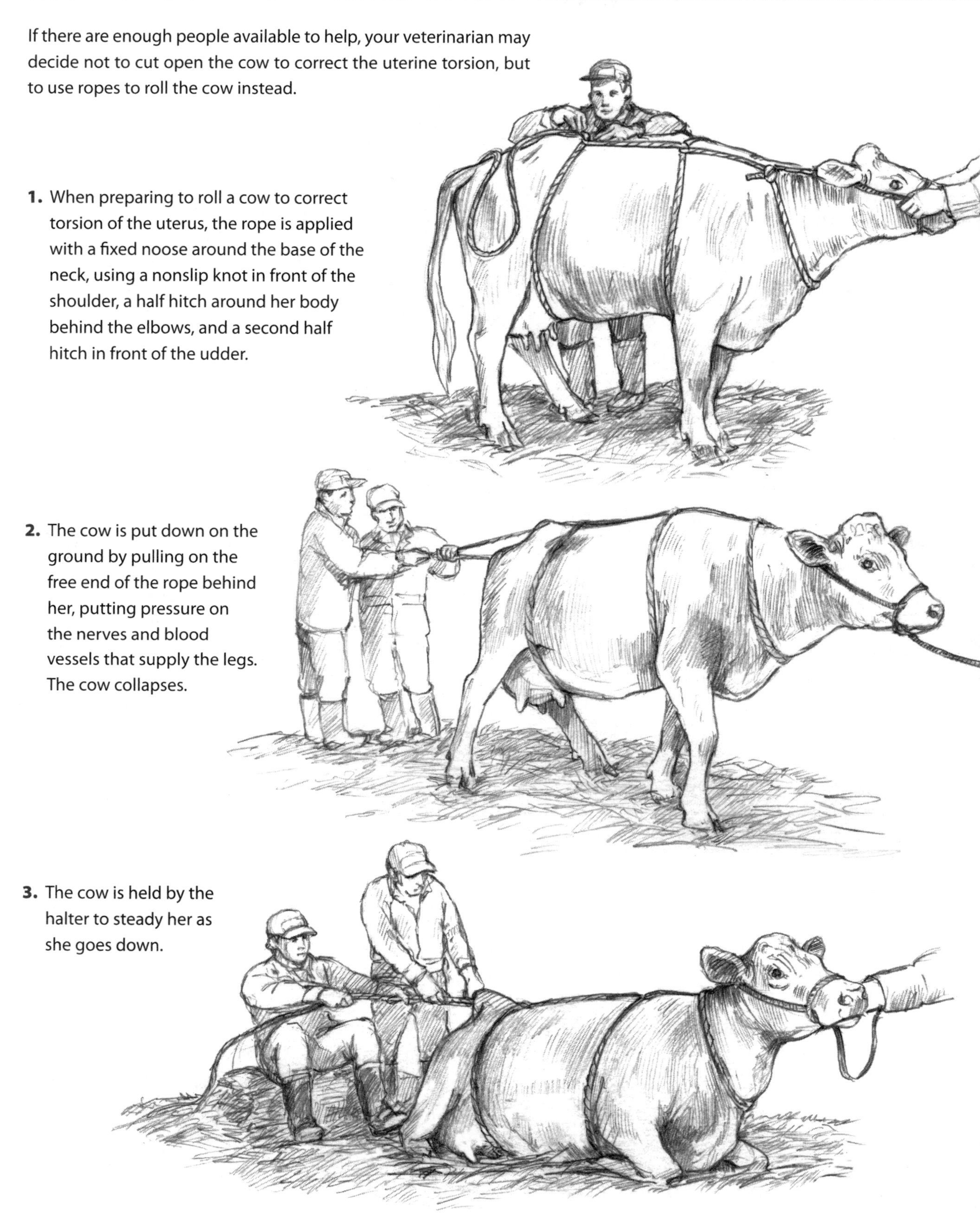

1. When preparing to roll a cow to correct torsion of the uterus, the rope is applied with a fixed noose around the base of the neck, using a nonslip knot in front of the shoulder, a half hitch around her body behind the elbows, and a second half hitch in front of the udder.

2. The cow is put down on the ground by pulling on the free end of the rope behind her, putting pressure on the nerves and blood vessels that supply the legs. The cow collapses.

3. The cow is held by the halter to steady her as she goes down.

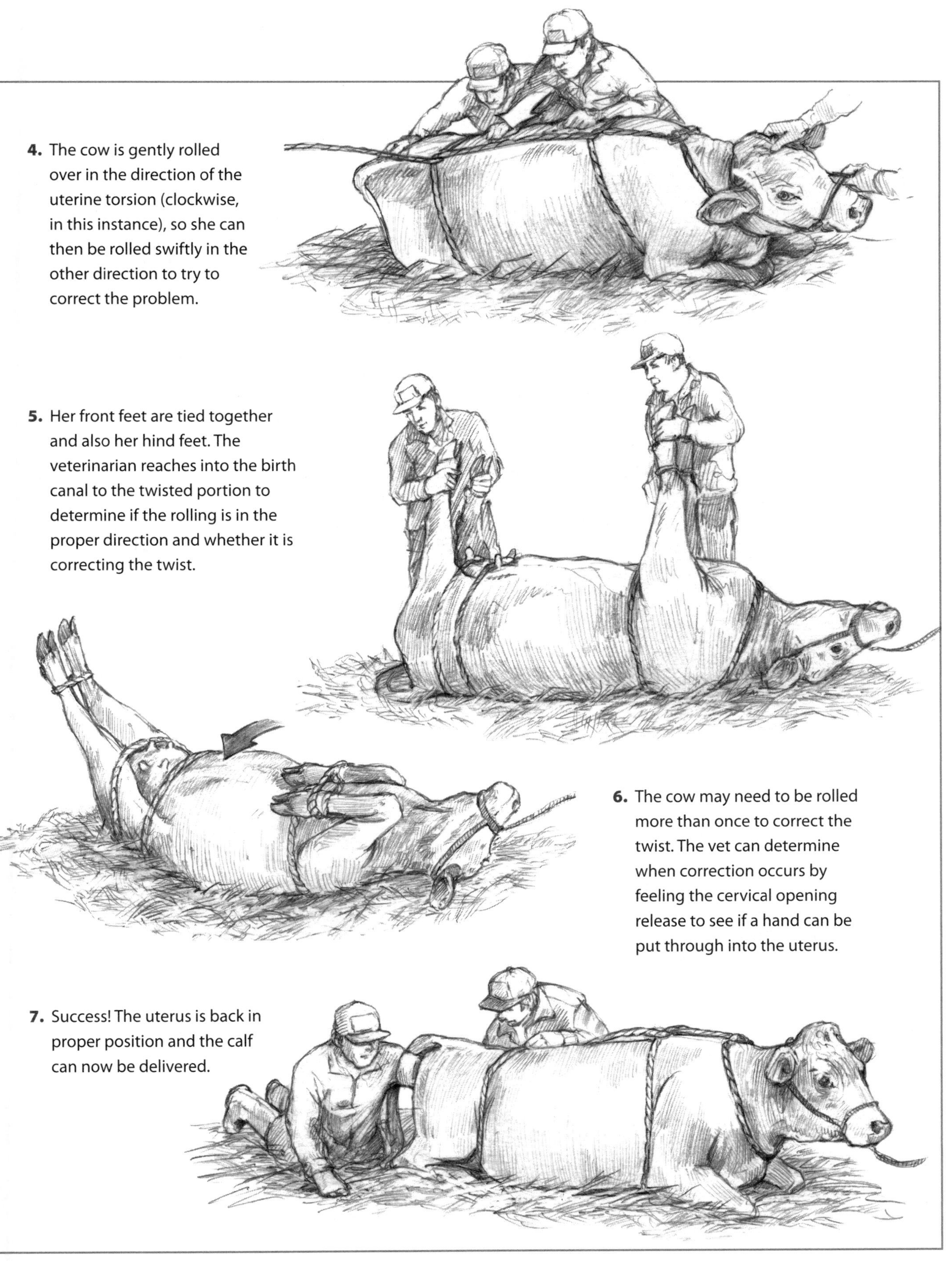

4. The cow is gently rolled over in the direction of the uterine torsion (clockwise, in this instance), so she can then be rolled swiftly in the other direction to try to correct the problem.

5. Her front feet are tied together and also her hind feet. The veterinarian reaches into the birth canal to the twisted portion to determine if the rolling is in the proper direction and whether it is correcting the twist.

6. The cow may need to be rolled more than once to correct the twist. The vet can determine when correction occurs by feeling the cervical opening release to see if a hand can be put through into the uterus.

7. Success! The uterus is back in proper position and the calf can now be delivered.

Twins

Twins are created when a cow has two eggs develop at the same time (often one from each ovary, with a fetus developing in each horn of the uterus) or when a fertilized egg splits. If the two fetuses are in the same horn, their amniotic sacs are adjacent; if there's one twin in each horn, only their allantoic sacs are adjacent. In most cases the tissues between bovine twins' adjacent allantoic sacs break down, and they share the fluid in which the amniotic sacs float. This usually occurs about the 40th day of gestation. Each fetus may still have its own water bag, which precedes it through the birth canal, or there may be only one water bag for both.

Many sets of twins are born without assistance. They may come one at a time, anywhere from a few minutes to a few hours apart. Even if both twins are in the same horn, one may be closer to the pelvic opening than the other and is born first — if it can get into proper position to start into the birth canal. Unless they are in abnormal position, twins are often born easily because they tend to be a little smaller than singles.

The cow may give birth quickly and be up licking her new calf, then have more contractions and lie down again to deliver the next one. In many cases she'll start intense straining again about 10 minutes after the birth of the first calf. Or she may have taken care of the first calf (it's been up and nursing) and a few hours later lie down and give birth to the second. On occasion she will lie there and deliver one right after the other, with risk of one or both of them suffocating if the water bags or amnion sacs don't break. The twins may be piled on top of one another. Even if they do not come this closely together, the second calf usually has the better chance of survival. Although he is in the uterus longer, in most cases he's not compromised because no part of him is yet in the birth canal, and while in the uterus he has his own "lifeline." After the first calf is delivered, the second calf also has more room to straighten and get

TWINS IN A SINGLE UTERINE HORN

If twins are in the same horn of the uterus, their amniotic sacs are adjacent and usually grow together; they share the amniotic fluid.

TWINS IN SEPARATE UTERINE HORNS

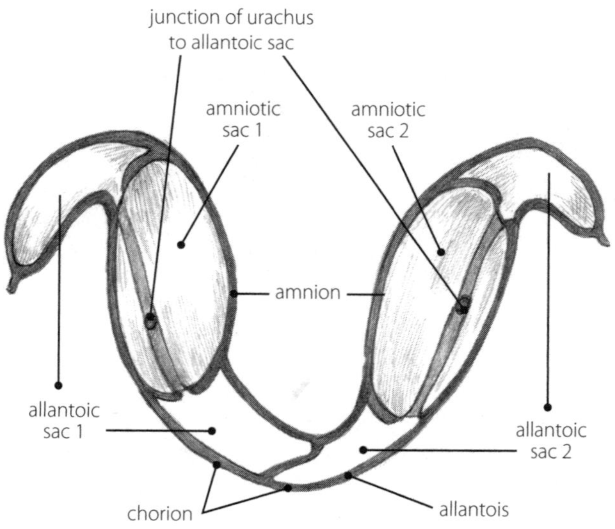

If twins are in separate horns of the uterus, they each have their own amniotic sac and fluid.

into a proper position for birth. Sometimes the first calf's health is compromised because it took too long to get into this birth position.

Sometimes twins need assistance, especially if they both try to come at the same time, blocking the entrance to the birth canal. Sometimes one twin delivers headfirst and the other is backward, or the first one may be in the wrong position for birth (head or legs turned back), due to lack of space or uterine inertia. The cow may have uterine inertia because of excessive stretching of the uterine tissues or the extra weight and mass of two calves. Without strong uterine contractions, the calves may not position properly for birth, and the cow will not progress to active labor although the cervix is fully dilated. Unless you suspect a problem and check her, the placentas will eventually detach and the calves will die.

If the cow is taking too long in labor and you check her and find the cervix open, you can reach into the uterus and find a calf, and then pull it if it's in the proper position. Sometimes the second twin is not discovered until after you've pulled the first one. If a calf seems smaller than it should be, or the cow gives you any reason for suspicion, such as uterine inertia or anything else not quite right, or if she has been known to have twins before or comes from a family line that often has twins, it's a good idea to reach back in after delivering the calf to check if there's another one there. If so, it may need to be pulled out as well.

Always Consider the Possibility of Twins

When you check a cow that's taking too long in labor and there are two legs in the birth canal, don't assume they belong to the same calf. You may be feeling a front and a hind leg of different calves. Follow each leg up to where it joins a body, especially if there is no head in the birth canal, and determine whether you are dealing with one or two calves. If one or both twins are presented abnormally, push everything back into the uterus far enough to straighten things out. Always be careful in any manipulations and in pushing twins back, since there's more risk of injuring or rupturing the uterus than with just one calf. Sometimes when both twins are located in the same horn the uterus will rupture just from the cow's own efforts at labor.

Untangling Twins

When you know you have two calves to be delivered instead of just one, you must determine where the calves are in relation to the birth canal, untangle and reposition them if necessary, and then determine which calf should be pulled first.

- If you can carefully push the calves back to where you can correct the posture of the first one or to allow room to deliver it, try to pull the closer calf.
- If you are unsure which calf to pull first and one calf is backward, pull the backward one first, after reaching in through the cow's birth canal and pushing the other as far back into the uterus as possible.
- Never pull on a calf until you are sure both legs belong to the same calf.
- If you can't get the twins straightened out, call the vet before you spend much time trying and while you still have a chance to deliver them both alive.

TWICE AS NICE

WE'VE HAD ONLY SIX SETS OF TWINS in our beef cows in 41 years, in contrast to the numerous twins in our Holstein dairy cows and our son's beef herd, which has four to seven sets each year. Our first beef twins surprised us in 1977 when Jokasta had a small heifer calf and then gave birth to an identical little heifer 3 hours later. We named them Melva and Marla and gave them to our kids, age seven and nine. Since then, we've had five more sets and were lucky on most of them, losing only one premature twin and saving his brother, in 2005.

Chamelean put forth a head and one leg while calving in 1997. We corrected the problem and delivered the calf, and 15 minutes later she lay down and pushed out a huge water bag. Our daughter realized it looked too big and dashed back into the stall to break it, and discovered the second calf right under the water bag. It would have suffocated if she hadn't been there.

OUR EXPERIENCE WITH LUPINE CALVES

A FEW YEARS BACK, one of our son's cows took too long in early labor, and he became suspicious. This was her fifth calf, and she'd always calved quickly. He put the cow in our head catcher and checked her. The calf had not yet entered the birth canal; it was breech (buttocks pressing against the open cervix) and upside down. Feeling farther in to try to reach a hind leg, our son suspected the calf was dead, and discovered that the leg joints would not flex. He struggled briefly with the legs, then realized it was a "lupine calf" and called the vet.

The vet arrived an hour later and confirmed that the calf's hindquarters were too large to come through. Hoping to avoid surgery, he used a wire saw to take a hind leg off the dead calf in the uterus to reduce the total size of the haunches and then tried to pull the remainder of the calf. This didn't work. He finally had to do a c-section, making the incision in the cow's flank and uterus twice as long as usual to extract the deformed calf without tearing the uterine wall. Not only were the leg joints fused in abnormal positions, but the head and buttocks of the calf were too broad and the neck was fixed in bent-around position. There was no way it could have come through the birth canal. This grotesque monster was created because the cow ate lupine in early pregnancy.

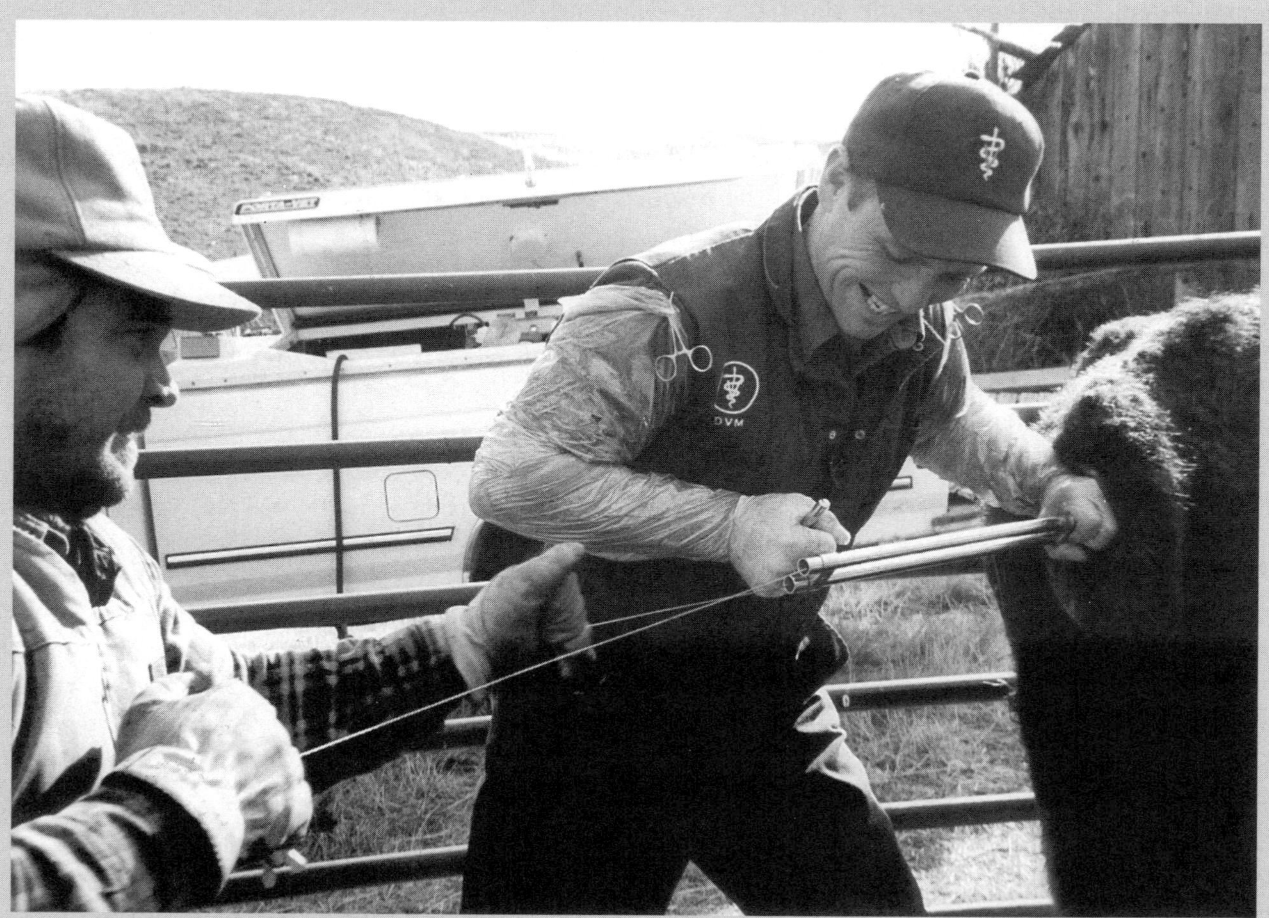

Our son and the vet are using a wire saw to remove one leg of the fetus.

Abnormal Calves

Any time you check a cow, keep in the back of your mind the possibility of an abnormal calf inside. This may be what's hindering progress or making it impossible for the legs to straighten enough to enter the birth canal.

On occasion, due to some accident of gestation or toxic influence at a certain stage (such as toxic alkaloids in lupine ingested by the cow) or a genetic defect, the calf is malformed. In certain instances a calf may be a "monster" with acute angulation of the backbone (with the tail close to the head) or the chest and abdominal wall incomplete, with internal organs and intestines exposed. Leg joints may be fused and unable to bend, as in the case of "lupine" calves (see page 118 and chapter 15), or the calf may have extra body parts (extra legs or two heads). A full-term hydrocephalic calf (with a large head) or any calf with unusually large or swollen parts may be impossible to deliver normally and require emergency surgery.

In many cases an abnormal calf is aborted or born prematurely, which makes for smaller size and easier delivery, but if carried to term, some can't be born. Your vet may choose to cut the calf in pieces (fetotomy) that can be brought out through the birth canal or deliver him by c-section if cutting him up poses risk to the cow.

Sometimes the monstrosity is not obvious at first, and you may attempt to pull the calf but find you can't continue at a certain point. This sometimes happens if the part of the calf first entering the birth canal seems normal, as in the case of a hydrocephalic calf coming backward (he comes through until the large head reaches the dam's pelvis), or a backward calf with extra front legs or two heads, or a frontward calf with hind leg joints that are fused at an angle and unable to bend.

In instances of abnormal calves, being able to detect a problem that would make normal birth difficult can give you the opportunity to call your veterinarian before the situation becomes life-threatening for the cow. The calf may or may not be normal enough to survive, but delaying delivery too long can put your cow at risk. It's always wise to check the cow and be able to make a judgment call on whether or not to call the vet. In certain instances, the calf will have to be delivered by c-section.

WIRE SAW USED FOR FETOTOMY

This wire saw is used by vets to cut the calf in pieces (fetotomy) so that he can be brought out through the birth canal. The vet gets the wire "saw" into proper position, making sure the wire is over the limb that needs to be removed. The steel tubing protects the cow as the wire — pulled back and forth — creates friction and a cutting action to saw through the portion of the calf that must be removed.

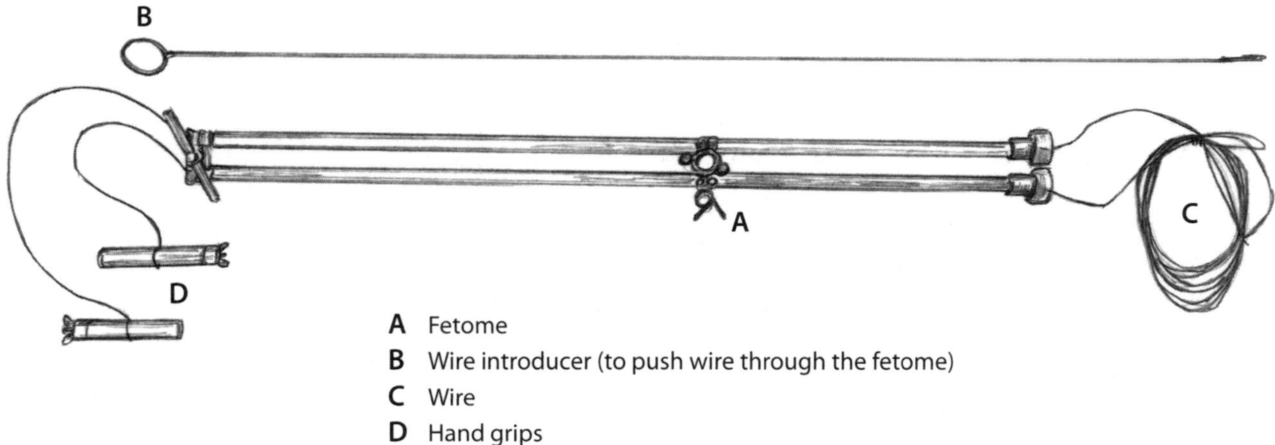

A Fetome
B Wire introducer (to push wire through the fetome)
C Wire
D Hand grips

Chapter 5

Cesarean-Section Delivery

A CESAREAN SECTION, often called a c-section, is the surgical delivery of a fetus when it cannot be born by natural means. An incision is made through the cow's abdominal wall, the *peritoneum* (the inner lining of the abdominal cavity) and then through the uterine wall so that the fetus can be retrieved.

Human babies have been delivered this way since the time of the Roman Empire. Roman law stated that every woman dying in advanced pregnancy or labor should have the fetus removed in this fashion, to save the child or provide for separate burial if it did not survive. Legend has it that Julius Caesar was born this way, hence the term, though some historians say the term is derived from the Latin word *caesaro,* which means "I cut." It is doubtful that Julius Caesar was born in this way, as his mother survived the birth; medical procedures were too crude then to keep the mother alive while cutting the baby out of her uterus.

By the 1830s, c-sections were performed successfully on cows and ewes, though these surgeries were performed without benefit of anesthesia and before the use of antiseptics and antibiotics. Cattle c-sections were done only sporadically before World War II but were commonplace by the 1950s.

No matter how persevering and innovative you are as a midwife, there are times when you and the cow or heifer simply cannot deliver the fetus through the birth canal, even with the help of your vet. Then the only option for saving the life of the calf is a c-section birth.

Reasons for C-Sections

There are many situations in which a fetus can't be delivered by ordinary means, including incidents of large calves and/or small pelvises, incomplete dilation of the cervix, the development of fetal "monsters," malpresentations or uterine torsion that can't be corrected, and the death and swelling of a fetus inside the uterus. Sometimes it's easy to determine that surgery is the only option. You'll know it's time for a surgical delivery when you assess the size of the calf in the birth canal and realize the head won't possibly fit through the pelvis (see chapter 3) or after you have struggled to correct a malpresentation and then called your vet, only to watch the professional be just as unsuccessful as you were at making it work.

CALF SIZE IS IN THE GENES

Genetics is a major factor in determining calf size, and this trait comes from both parents. Even when bred to a low-birth-weight bull, a large-frame heifer may produce a calf too large to be born if she herself was a large-birth-weight calf. Selection for moderate-frame cattle with average or less-than-average birth weight is the best way to reduce calving problems that require a c-section because of mismatch between the calf size and the cow's pelvic area.

Young Heifers and Big Bulls

Births commonly cannot proceed when the dam is physically immature. This may happen when heifer calves are bred too young (when bulls or bull calves are allowed to remain with the herd) or when a bull gets through a fence and breeds young heifers. Well-fed heifers may reach puberty and have fertile heat cycles at a young age. They may become pregnant if bred, even though they're not mature enough or their pelvic area is not large enough to deliver the calf when it reaches full term.

Heifers bred to bulls that sire large calves present the most common cause for c-sections; the calf is too large to pass through the heifer's small pelvis. There are bulls in many breeds that should be used only on mature cows. Most stockmen try to select a low-birth-weight bull for breeding heifers. Since most heifers are bred as yearlings to calve at age two, they are not yet full size and don't have as much pelvic area as a mature cow.

Heifers bred to bulls that sire large calves present the most common cause for c-sections; the calf is too large to pass through the heifer's small pelvis.

YOUNG HEIFERS AND C-SECTIONS

IN OUR HERD we've had two instances in which young heifers were accidentally bred. The first, a Hereford heifer named Portia, bred several months too early, calved before she was two years old. We asked our vet if she'd need a c-section, since she was small and bred to a bull that sired large calves, but he said not to worry, just to wait and see. Indeed, she had a small calf, calving without assistance.

The second case was more worrisome; Prunella was only seven months old when she was bred — and still nursing. We didn't realize she'd been bred and the next spring we put her on the range with the other yearlings. We soon noticed that she was getting an udder and was very round in the belly, so we brought her home and watched her closely. She was unable to give birth, and the calf had to be delivered by c-section. Prunella was immature and not very motherly; she did not want anything to do with the calf, so we raised her calf, Prune, on a bottle.

Double-Muscled Calves

Cesarean section may be needed for calves with excessively large body mass due to double muscling. This occurs frequently in breeds such as Charolais, Belgian Blue, Piedmontese, and South Devon. Even though the skeletal frame of the calf may be no larger for a double-muscled 140-pound calf than it is for an 80- or 90-pound calf, the muscular *hypertrophy* (double muscling) of the heavier calf makes normal birth impossible.

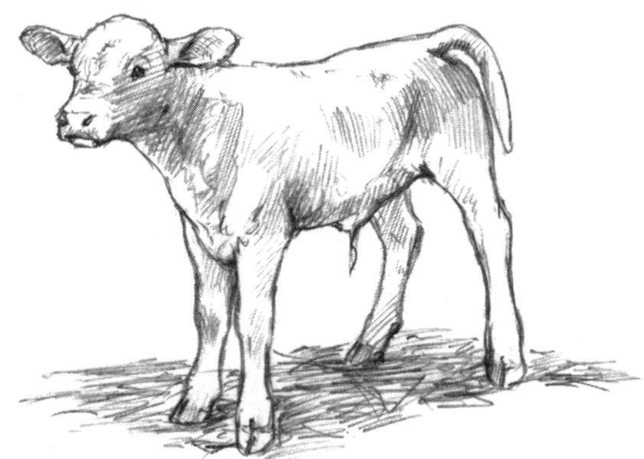

Day-old calf with normal muscling.

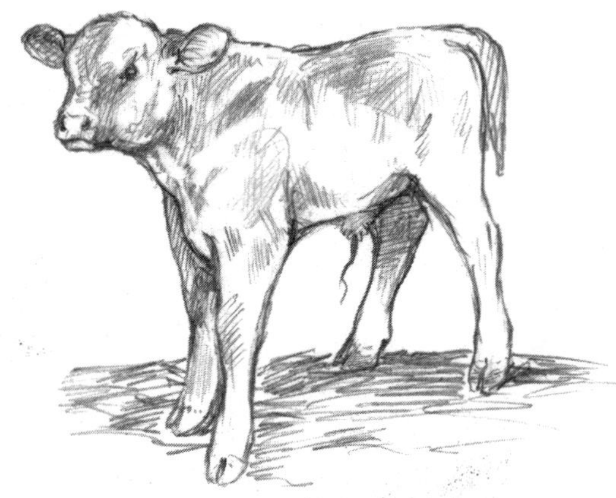

Day-old "double-muscled" calf with thicker shoulders and extra muscling on the hindquarters.

Dead Fetus

Sometimes a dead fetus must be delivered by c-section, if it is not pulled soon after it dies. Massive swelling of *subcutaneous* (under the skin) tissues may make its body mass too large to come through the birth canal. If a fetus dies due to an undiscovered malpresentation or because the placenta detached during long labor and the situation was not soon resolved, the dead calf may be too swollen to be pulled. In cases where the fetus has been dead for some time or in instances when the calf has a deformity or *contracture* of limbs (cannot straighten limbs enough to come through the birth canal), the veterinarian may decide to do a c-section. He or she may also choose to dissect the dead calf, using a saw wire to carefully sever the limbs from the body, in the uterus, and bring it out through the birth canal in pieces.

CERVIX CLOSED BEFORE CALVING

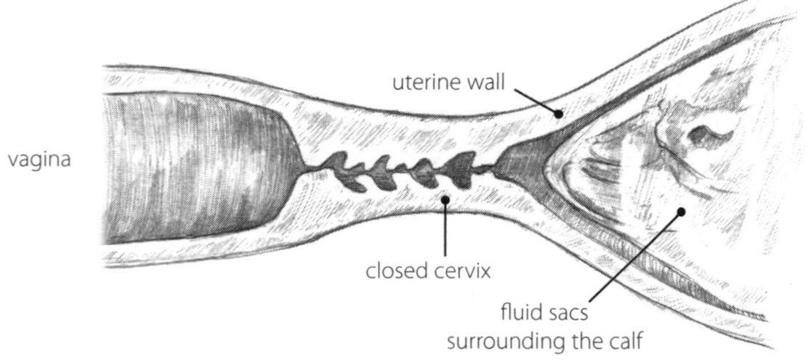

CERVIX OPENING DURING LABOR

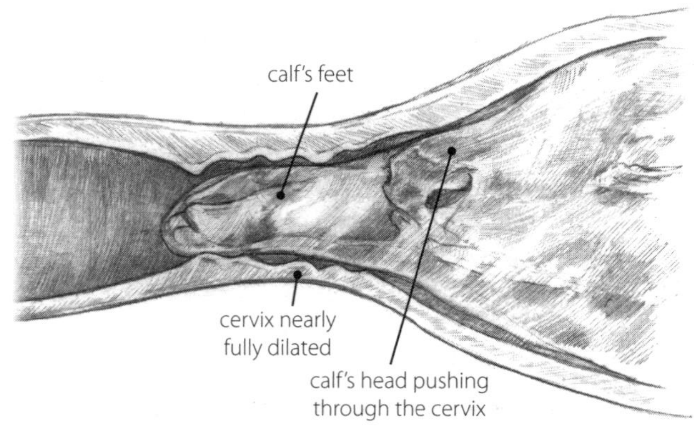

Failure of Cervix to Dilate

On occasion the cow's cervix remains narrow and constricted. The mucus plug has come out, which indicates the cow has been in labor and should be delivering the calf, and the calf's feet may start through the partially opened cervix but cannot proceed. The constricted opening that has failed to dilate allows you to insert only one to four fingers, not your whole hand, when you check the cow.

The cervix may be constricted by fibrous scar tissue resulting from injury during a previous calving, but this is not common. More often the problem is hormonal dysfunction; the cervix fails to "ripen" in the final days of gestation so it can begin to dilate during early labor. If it fails to dilate, the cow shows typical signs of early labor but won't progress to active labor if no portion of the calf can make it through the cervix. It may be difficult to tell how long she's been in labor. If you wait too long for the cervix to dilate more fully, the calf will die.

If the cow's cervix is not dilating normally, your vet may recommend an injection of oxytocin. This hormone stimulates uterine contraction and labor; usually the cow shows an effect within an hour or two. If this does not cause the cervix to relax enough for normal delivery, the calf must be removed by c-section. Sometimes incomplete cervical dilation accompanies uterine torsion (see chapter 4). The cervix may continue to be constricted even after the torsion is corrected by the vet.

If the cervix fails to dilate, the cow shows typical signs of early labor but won't progress to active labor if no portion of the calf can make it through the cervix.

On occasion the cervix opening is not large enough because it is actually closing up again after prolonged labor, even though one of the calf's legs has come through. Or the cervix may close after birth of one twin before you can get the other twin delivered, such as in a breech delivery that had to be corrected. The cervix often starts constricting soon after being fully dilated.

A UTERINE TEAR AND THE MISSING CALF

IN APRIL 1971, one of our Hereford heifers, Rapscallion, was taking a long time calving, so we checked her and discovered that her calf's feet were huge. We tried unsuccessfully to pull the calf, and then called our vet for help.

When he arrived, he felt inside Rapscallion and was surprised to discover that there was no calf in the uterus. He then got an incredible look on his face as he reached in her abdomen through a tear in her uterus, felt for the calf among her intestines, and said, "It's still alive!"

He surgically removed the calf from her abdomen and sewed up the tear in her uterus as well as the abdominal incision. He said that with such a huge rupture and repair, the cow had one chance in a hundred to survive, but if she made it through the night, she might have a fair shot.

Rapscallion lay there, subdued and dull in the calving pen, and that night it started to snow. We feared moving her but were even more worried that the shock of being wet and cold would kill her, so we got her up and gently herded her across the lane and into our calving barn.

It snowed three feet that night, and then we were afraid the barn roof would collapse! But it didn't, and we shoveled off the snow. Even though she was unable to become pregnant again, probably due to adhesions and scar tissue, Rapscallion recovered. Needless to say, she was in no shape to tend to her bouncing baby that spring. We raised her calf Rascal on a bottle.

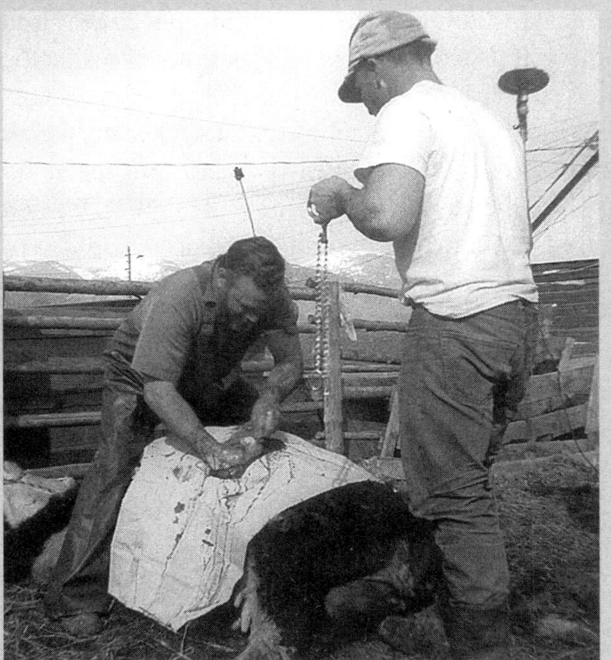

Rapscallion's calf dropped out of her uterus through a tear in the uterine wall and slipped down into her abdominal cavity. Dr. Pete South made an incision into Rapscallion's abdomen and reached inside to search for the calf. Here, he pulls out the amnion sac encasing the calf and a hind foot through the incision. Moments later, Lynn pulled the calf out by his hind legs.

Tear in the Uterine Wall

The uterine wall may be torn by the calf's putting a foot through it during the cow's contractions or in a case of uterine torsion; failure of the cervix to dilate; excessive pressure from an enlarged uterus, with twins or excess fluid around the calf; or during attempts to correct a malpresentation. In rare cases the uterus ruptures due to external injury, such as a kick or being hit in the belly by a horned cow. On occasion a calf's rump in a breech presentation completely blocks the pelvic opening so that no fetal fluids escape, and the pressure of continued uterine contractions against the full uterus causes it to rupture.

If the tear is discovered before the calf is delivered, the vet may choose to do a c-section to reduce chances of enlarging the tear, which would put the cow at risk for contamination of the abdominal cavity and resultant *peritonitis.* If the calf can be taken by c-section, sometimes the tear can be successfully sutured via the incision to remove the calf, and the cow will recover.

Too Much Fluid

Occasionally during late gestation, excessive fluid accumulates in the amniotic or allantoic membranes around the fetus. The cow's belly becomes progressively larger (see chapter 2), and she has trouble getting up and down. In these instances, or in situations where the fetus itself is swollen with fluid, it must be removed by c-section before it is full term, to save the cow. For this to be successful, the vet will usually first drain the fluid through a tube inserted into the uterus — slowly, so the cow doesn't go into shock.

Torsion of the Uterus

If uterine torsion (see chapter 4) cannot be resolved or if the cervix does not dilate after the torsion is corrected, the only way to deliver the calf is by c-section surgery. If the condition is recognized early, while the calf is still alive, he can be successfully delivered surgically. But the cow risks complications, since the uterus may be swollen because the twist is blocking the blood supply to the uterus. The uterine wall may be damaged or even perforated by the calf's head or foot.

The surgery is also made difficult if the uterus is still twisted and therefore in the wrong place. Portions of small intestine may be displaced and thus hinder the veterinarian's access to the uterus. After the calf is removed and the uterus is turned back to proper position, the incision into the uterus may not be on the same side as the incision through the abdominal wall, and it may be hard to pull the uterus up out of the abdomen for suturing because it is still rather full of fluids, since those were unable to escape via the vagina.

Miscellaneous Reasons for C-Section

Other situations in which a c-section may be employed are when the birth canal or cervix is constricting after a prolonged labor (when the optimum time for pulling the calf through the birth canal is past), the birth canal is constricted from tumors or extensive scar tissue from injuries in earlier pregnancies or deliveries, or there is a fracture of the pelvis or a mummified six- to eight-month fetus that's too large to be expelled through the undilated birth canal. Recognizing the imminent death of the cow from hardware disease, cancer, or severe injury, for example, is another reason to call the veterinarian for a c-section surgery. If the fetus is near term, the vet can remove the calf to save him and then humanely euthanize the cow.

We're Not Always Successful

Our one instance of uterine torsion in which the vet could not correct it and chose to do a c-section resulted in the birth of a live calf but the loss of the cow. Melia was laboring too long, so we checked her and discovered a torsion. We called the only vet available that night. After unsuccessful attempts to turn the uterus, the vet performed a c-section but was unable to control the bleeding and found it very difficult to suture the uterine incision.

OUR FIRST EXPERIENCE WITH C-SECTION

OUR FIRST C-SECTION DELIVERY was performed when one of the pregnant heifers we bought at the start of our ranching venture did not progress to active labor. She had a hormonal problem that kept the cervix from dilating. We checked her several times, but there was no progress. We called our vet, who told us to bring her to his clinic for surgery, and we hauled her to town in our horse trailer. We named her Cearie, and though she did not want to mother her calf, and we had to give him to another cow to raise, we kept her. She had only normal pregnancies and deliveries from that point on.

When to Perform a C-Section

There are times when, despite your best efforts, you must allow the calf to be delivered by c-section. Below are two surefire signs that the calf will not progress normally. It is not wise to continue pulling on the calf; you will only injure or kill him or the dam if:

1. *The calf does not make adequate progress* through the birth canal with two or three people pulling, or with the use of a calf puller, after a few minutes of applied traction.
2. *The calf is simply too large to fit* into the pelvic canal. The head and both elbows of the calf (or both stifles, if backward) cannot be pulled into the pelvic canal by the efforts of one strong person.

Surgical success often depends on the time spent and degree of traction applied before you realize a calf can be delivered only surgically. It's always best to make the decision while the calf is still alive and the cow is not yet injured by futile attempts to pull the calf. The worst situation is to pull a calf partway out and then find that he cannot be delivered. At that point he's too far out to push back into the uterus for a successful surgical delivery and must be cut apart instead. It's best to err on the side of caution and call your vet when you have serious doubts.

If the fetus is dead, the vet may opt to cut it up in the uterus in order to bring it out, but if it's still alive, the choice is a c-section. If cow and calf are not yet compromised, surgery is generally successful and both survive. A c-section should not be considered a last resort but rather an alternative way to deal with a difficult situation and have a successful outcome.

The Surgery

After you've determined you can't pull the calf or correct a malpresentation, or that there's some other problem you can't handle, your vet will assess the situation and correct it or decide that surgery is the best option for saving the cow and/or the calf. The cow should be sheltered in a clean, well-lit area where she can be restrained — tied or in a head catcher. A barn with clean bedding and good light is ideal. Outdoors works fine if the weather is nice and it's close to an electricity source for the vet's equipment or a light.

Before the operation, the vet typically clips the surgical site and scrubs it with disinfectant. The operation can be performed with the cow standing or lying down (see pages 126–127 for depiction of surgery on a standing cow).

C-Section on a Cow Lying Down

If the cow is lying down and can't get up, there is no choice about how to position her when operating. Some veterinarians prefer the cow to be lying down on her side and making the incision lower in the flank. Rather than the vertical cut in the standing cow, the incision is an oblique line, below the fold of skin in the flank and above the udder attachment, following an imaginary line between stifle and navel. There is less risk of the intestines coming through the incision if the cow is on her left side. If she's lying on her right side, the vet may want two or three people to roll her onto her left side.

Other vets prefer to make the incision along the midline under the belly, with the cow rolled onto her back. This incision starts near the udder and extends forward 12 to 14 inches (30.5 to 35.6 cm). The uterus can then be pulled to the incision and partway out of the cow's belly, preventing contamination of the abdominal cavity if the uterine contents are infected.

Most veterinarians use a drape of cloth around the surgical site to help keep foreign matter or fluids from seeping or dropping into the abdomen. With the cow on her back, the intestines tend to stay where they belong, since the uterus, which has been pulled up through the incision, keeps them from coming out. The abdominal wall at this site is not as thick as in the flank, and there is also less muscle tissue and fewer blood vessels to cut through. However, the abdominal wall at the bottom of the belly is largely fibrous tissue and does not stretch as much as muscle, making a longer incision necessary.

LOCAL ANTIBIOTICS A MUST

ON RARE OCCASION a cow will develop a fatal infection due to clostridial infections (such as blackleg and malignant edema). This is a good reason to use adequate local antibiotic in the surgical site. The first c-section done at our place by a new vet who'd just come to our community ended tragically, even though we got the calf safely out of the heifer (he had a ridge on top of his skull that made it impossible for him to fit through her pelvis) and she was mothering him nicely. The vet did not put any antibiotic into the incision, nor give her injected antibiotics.

By the next day she was ill with high fever. Though we started her on massive doses of antibiotics, it was after the fact, and it was too late. When she died two days later, we cut her open, and all the tissue around the incision was black. The vet looked at it and said that she had malignant edema.

CESAREAN SECTION DELIVERY ON A STANDING COW

Most veterinarians prefer to operate on a standing cow, making an incision in the upper left flank. Sometimes the upper right flank is used when torsion of the uterus is the reason for the c-section.

Disadvantages of a right-flank incision in most situations include more difficulty in bringing the uterus up to the incision (unless there is a torsion) and more risk of contaminating the abdominal cavity with uterine contents. This is not so serious if the calf is alive and there is no infection present, unless the uterine contents have been contaminated by attempts to manipulate a malpresentation. It can be very serious, however, if the calf has been dead awhile and the uterus contain pathogens.

If the incision is in the right flank and is a little too long, it can be difficult to keep the cow's intestines where they belong. If she coughs, strains, or moves around, a mass of small intestine may be pushed through the incision. The left flank is usually a safer site, since the intestines are not directly under the incision and the rumen helps keep the intestines in place.

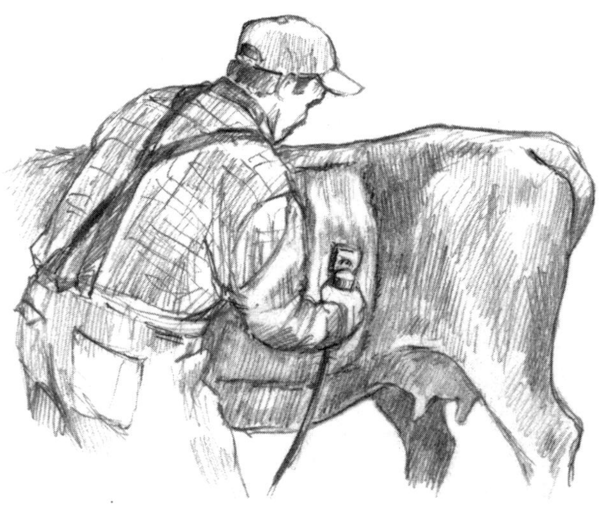

1. The cow's left flank, just behind the last rib, is shaved.

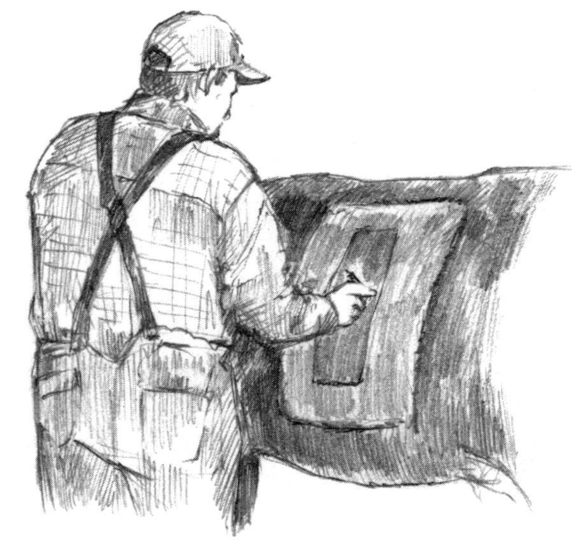

2. Local anesthetic is injected to deaden the area.

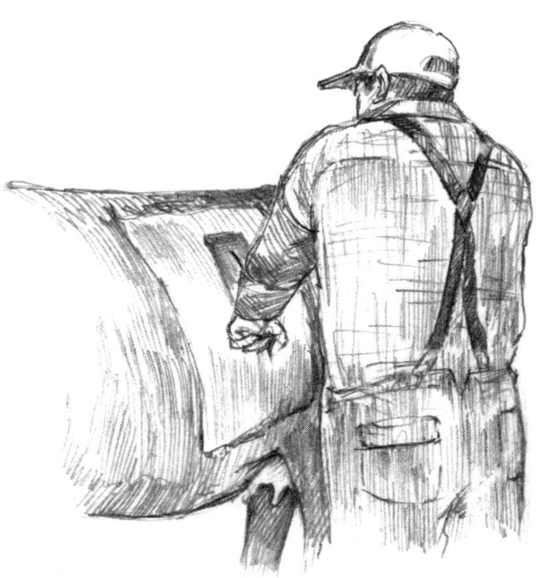

3. An incision is made through the skin and into the abdominal cavity.

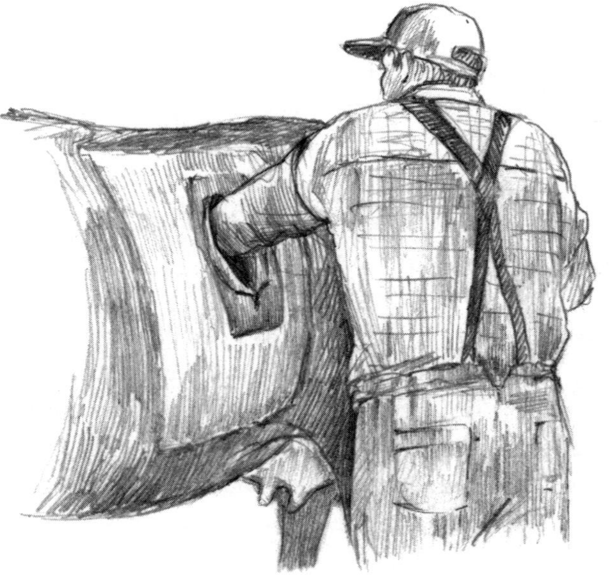

4. The vet reaches in to find the uterus.

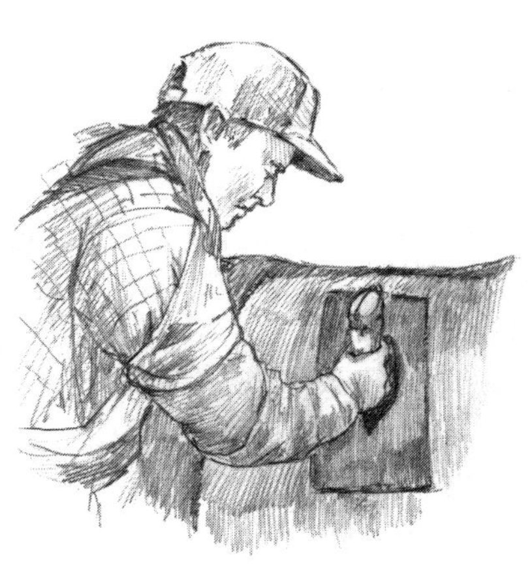

5. After pulling the uterus to the outer incision, a cut is made through the uterine wall, and one of the calf's hind feet, still within the amnion sac, is pulled through the incision.

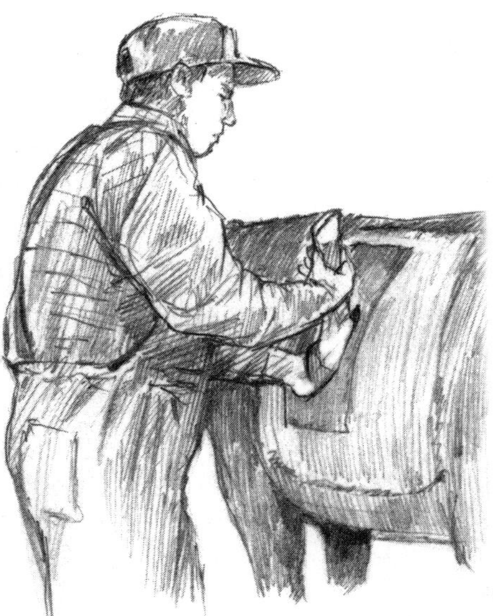

6. The amnion sac is ruptured and the leg is grasped as the vet holds the uterus in position against the outer incision.

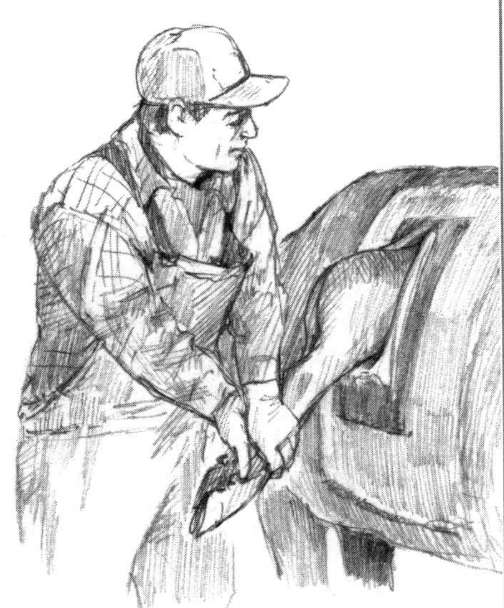

7. He reaches in to find the other hind leg and starts pulling on both hind legs to bring the calf out of the uterus.

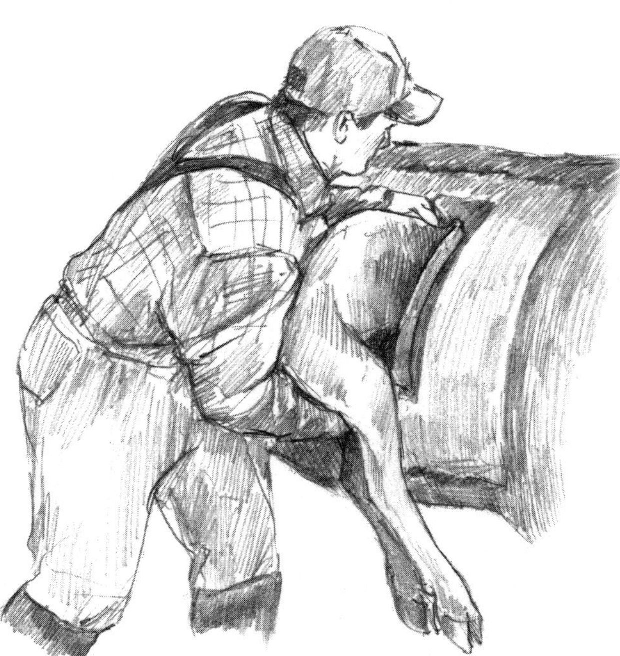

8. The calf is quickly brought out of the cow, as the umbilical cord is now ruptured and the calf must soon start breathing.

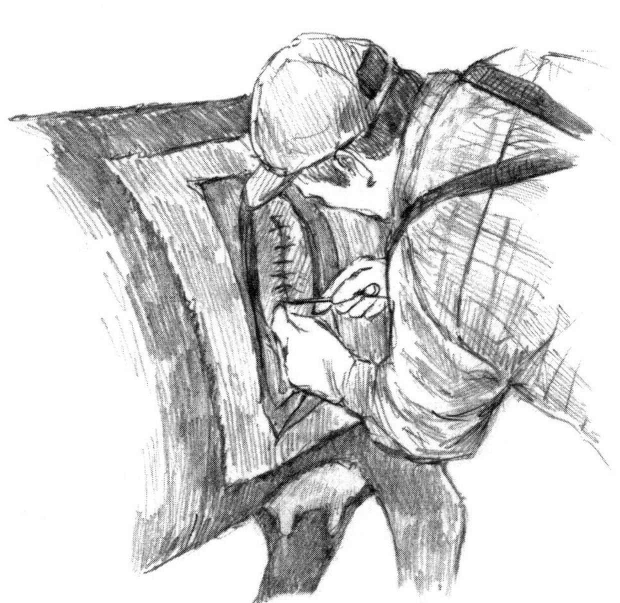

9. The uterine incision has been sutured, and the uterus is now ready to be pushed back into place so the abdominal wall and then the skin incision can be sutured.

Proper suture material and technique must be used to ensure that the incision does not break open with the weight and pressure of the abdominal contents once the cow gets up.

The Procedure

The cow is usually tranquilized and local anesthetic is given before the incision is made through the abdominal wall. After the skin and the abdominal wall beneath it are slit, the vet reaches in, finds, and pulls the uterus to the surface by grasping one of the calf's legs within, and then makes an incision into it. The incision is usually directly over the calf's leg and is made from toe to hock. The vet then reaches in to grab the hind legs of the calf, which are usually closer.

The incision must be long enough that the calf can be pulled through it without tearing the uterine wall. He is pulled out through the incision by his hind legs if he's lying in a normal position, with front legs and head pointed toward the birth canal. If he's lying backward, with hind feet aimed toward the birth canal, he is pulled out by his front legs and head.

The uterus has an extensive blood supply; after the calf is removed, hemorrhage from the incision must be controlled by clamping off major blood vessels. Resorbable sutures are used when closing the incision in the uterus and the abdominal wall. Stronger sutures, which later must be removed, or staples are used to close the skin.

LIFE-AND-DEATH DELIVERY

We've had several situations in which a cow was dying but the calf was close enough to term that we had our vet deliver him by c-section. Two were older cows with tumors in their abdomen, but Oh Susannah was a young cow. She was due to calve March 16, but in the middle of February we noticed she was only picking at the hay we fed. We brought her down to the corral and tried to entice her to eat and drink. But she refused, so we gave her fluids via stomach tube.

We had our vet examine her, and he suspected a blocked digestive tract. He gave her mineral oil by stomach tube, antibiotics, and a magnet in case she had ingested some kind of hardware. She was not passing manure, and her rectum was raw and infected. She was weak, and we realized she could not recover.

The vet came again the next morning to do a c-section and remove the calf — still alive and four weeks premature. We brought the calf, Suzette, into the house for a few days of intensive care and raised her on a bottle. After euthanizing the cow, our vet performed a postmortem exam and discovered she had an impacted *omasum* (third stomach); it was huge and hard and full of dried-out material. She had a hairball in her intestine, a bruise on her rumen, and some adhesions, but no hardware. Her gut was completely blocked by the impacted omasum; there was no way she could have survived. We felt fortunate we were able to save her calf.

After the Surgery

If the calf is alive, the vet will hand him to you to take care of while he or she attends to the cow, checking to make sure there's not a second calf (that is, a twin) and no other tears or injuries to the uterus. Then the vet disinfects and closes up all incisions.

Your immediate task is to get the calf breathing. Fluid must be drained from his air passages (a suction bulb works well for drawing fluid from his nostrils), and the calf must be stimulated to take a breath. If he doesn't start breathing immediately, stick a clean piece of hay or straw up his nose to make him cough and begin to breathe. After he's breathing, disinfect his navel stump and put him in a clean place where he can safely attempt to get to his feet.

The cow is given an injection of antibiotics and powder or boluses directly into her uterus before suturing. One of the greatest risks to her life — besides possibly bleeding to death if major uterine arteries have been cut and not properly sealed off afterward — is infection resulting from surgery, so she needs adequate antibiotic coverage to prevent serious infection.

If the calf is alive, the placental membranes are usually left within the uterus, to be shed naturally. Trying to remove them often results in excessive bleeding. If the calf is dead and the uterus is already infected, the placenta may come away more readily, and the veterinarian may try to remove it before suturing the cow. In either case, the vet may give her oxytocin to help stimulate the uterus to contract back to normal size.

The cow should be monitored closely for 24 hours to make sure that she doesn't suffer hemorrhage or shock and should be watched for several days for signs of infection. She should be kept on antibiotics for three to seven days, depending on her risk for infection as assessed by the vet. Keep her apart from other cattle so they won't pester her and possibly injure the surgical site. The vet may give her anti-inflammatory medication. If there's evidence of shock, she may need intravenous fluids. A mature dairy cow may also need an intravenous administration of calcium solution to prevent "milk fever" and to help the uterus shrink up.

The cow may have to be checked again by your vet 24 to 48 hours after the surgery, just to make sure she's doing okay. If she has any fever at all, is dull and not eating normally, or has diarrhea, this is cause for alarm and may be an indication of peritonitis. The skin sutures or staples can be removed once the skin is adequately healing and growing back together — in about 14 days.

TRAUMA AND THE MOTHERING INSTINCT

CEARIE WAS NOT INTERESTED in her calf; perhaps the same hormonal problem that caused her cervix not to dilate during labor also made her less motherly. We raised her abandoned calf on another cow. Prunella was an immature heifer, not ready to be a mama. She was more concerned about her own pain than mothering a calf. Like Prunella, many heifers are "turned off" to motherhood by the stress and trauma of surgery.

In contrast, a cow that's had calves before will generally go ahead and care for her calf. Cammie, for example, was a second calver when our vet had to surgically remove her calf; the head was turned back, and neither we nor our vet could get it into the birth canal. After the c-section, we kept Cammie on antibiotics and anti-inflammatories for several days because she was so dull and not eating. In spite of her extreme pain and a tough recovery, Cammie very much wanted to mother her calf and would get up and stand patiently for him to nurse.

Caring for the Calf Post-op

If the calf survives, he should be given adequate colostrum in the first hour. If the cow is not too traumatized to mother him, he can be left with her. If she's dull and uninterested, you may have to help him accomplish his first nursing. Most cows will mother the calf in spite of their pain, but a heifer, being a first-time mama, may be less inclined to mother the calf. Trying to make her mother him by tying her up, putting her in a head catch so she won't bunt or avoid the calf, or hobbling her hind legs so she can't kick him adds more stress to her already stressed condition, and it's often better not to traumatize her further with efforts to make her mother a calf she doesn't want. In these instances, it's usually better to let her recover in peace and raise the calf on another cow or on a bottle.

Stress and trauma from surgery may inhibit the cow's appetite for a few days. It's often beneficial to give painkillers (such as Banamine) to help reduce inflammation as well as pain for the first day or two so she'll feel well enough to eat. She must eat and drink to produce milk. Most cows will rebreed again after a c-section, if the vet did a good job of surgery and there is no serious infection afterward. The conception rate after a c-section in mature cows may be only slightly lower than herd average but can be quite a bit lower for first calvers if they are raising their calves. It takes them longer to recover and cycle again after the surgery, and they may not breed before the end of the breeding season.

Scar tissue from the incision may interfere with fertility or cause the cow to abort her next pregnancy. Adhesions sometimes develop between the uterine incision, the abdominal wall, and the peritoneum (the lining around the abdominal contents). Your vet can examine the cow rectally 5 to 10 days after the surgery to detect any adhesions that might be forming. These can often be resolved by gently separating them via rectal palpation.

Chapter 6

Complications Following Pregnancy and Birth

THERE ARE SEVERAL PROBLEMS that can arise for the cow after the calf is born. Problems range from mild to serious. Some can be temporary and readily resolved — naturally, with time. Others require assistance from you. Still other complications are life-threatening to the cow and will require your immediate action. This chapter will help you prepare for all the possible postnatal developments in the health of the cow.

Paralysis after Calving

Sometimes after a long birth, in which a cow tries to have the calf without help and he is in the birth canal too long, or after a hard pull, the pressure of the large calf coming through the pelvis affects the main nerves that go to her hind legs.

Nerve Damage

Pressure on the *gluteal nerve* (which serves the large muscle of the buttocks) during birth may make it hard for the cow to get up. If she can get up, she may wobble when she walks. Damage to that nerve may cause the muscle on that side to atrophy or shrink up, but in most cases it will eventually recover.

The *obturator nerve* also runs along each side of the pelvic cavity to serve the thigh muscles and is more commonly damaged than the gluteal nerve. If there's been too much pressure on this nerve or it's stretched during birth as the calf is forced through the pelvic circle, the cow may not be able to get up. She can't pull her hind legs inward to stand. Often one leg is affected more than the other, depending on which side the cow was lying on. If both legs are affected, she can't get up without help; her legs slide outward when she tries to stand. If just one leg is affected, she can get up and stand, with help, if the weak leg can be kept from sliding out to the side.

This paralysis may last a few hours or a few days. In some instances, as when a cow calved unattended and lay too long with the calf in her pelvis, or if a pulled calf should have been taken by c-section, the cow may never stand up again. You may find her lying there with the dead calf stuck in the birth canal or unable to get up after a hard pull with calf pullers (which may have killed the calf).

Paralysis can occur from a hard pull by hand, too, but it is usually not as serious or long lasting. Most commonly, the cow is unsteady and has trouble getting up. But if she can stand for a while with her pelvis and hind legs in the proper position, she quickly improves. Risk for paralysis is minimized if you can get her to stand up very soon after the birth. Often the longer she lies there, the worse it will be, especially if she's lying in an awkward position.

Getting the Cow to Stand Up

It may seem cruel to force the cow to get up, but this may minimize or prevent what might otherwise be a very serious problem. She will be tired after a difficult delivery and may just lie there. If she won't try to get up, encourage her by twisting her tail or startling her. A flighty cow will try to rise if you startle her with a sudden movement or noise, but a gentle one may not try.

If startling her doesn't work, one trick that often helps is to put your hands firmly over her nostrils, tight enough that she can't breathe. When she starts to worry about being short of air, she will usually try to get up. If that doesn't work, touching the hairless area under her tail with a hot shot/cattle prod (giving an electric shock) will startle almost any cow into trying to get up. The suddenness of this unexpected shock will take her mind off her tiredness, and she'll usually lurch to her feet. Before you try to get her up, move her calf safely away from her, so that if she wobbles and staggers, she won't step on or fall on him.

If she's unsteady on her feet, grab her tail and keep her from falling. You don't want to risk a leg fracture or dislocation of the hip joint. If you can keep her on her feet a few minutes, she will generally be less helpless the next time she tries to get up. The longer she stands, the better. It may take two people to steady her and keep her from falling over on her numb side, and she may try to swing or kick that hind leg a little because it feels funny (like when you hit your funny bone or when your arm or leg has "pins and needles" resulting from abnormal pressure).

If she goes down again right away, let her rest a few minutes, and then get her up again. Make sure she can stand and walk on her own before you leave her and her calf unattended; you don't want her to fall on him. If she tries to turn around, the leg that's wobbly may collapse under her and down she'll go. Monitor her until you are sure she has figured out how to manage on her own. Usually, once she's up and around, the leg will soon be back to normal; she can mother the calf without further problems.

Extended Care for Paralysis

If she absolutely can't get up, make her comfortable. Move her hind legs into a more normal position if she tried to get up and failed, leaving her hind legs askew. Milk colostrum from her while she is lying there if she has a live calf, and feed him with a bottle, or bring him to the udder and keep him lying down so he's at a level where he can nurse if you guide his mouth to a teat.

If you think there's a chance that she'll try to get up when you're not there to assist and monitor her, partition the calf away from her if she's in a barn stall,

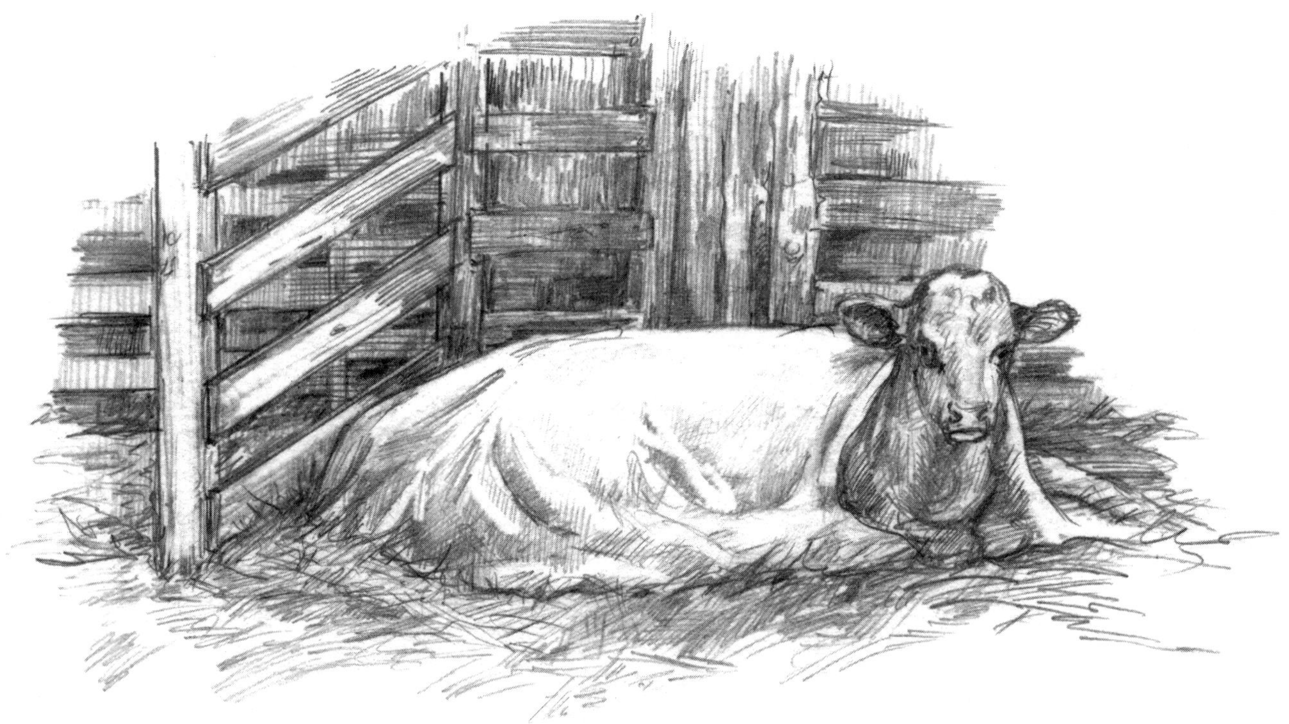

Occasionally a cow will calve and then be unable to get up. Simply placing a tarp over her can protect her from windy or wet weather and keep her warm between efforts to help her stand.

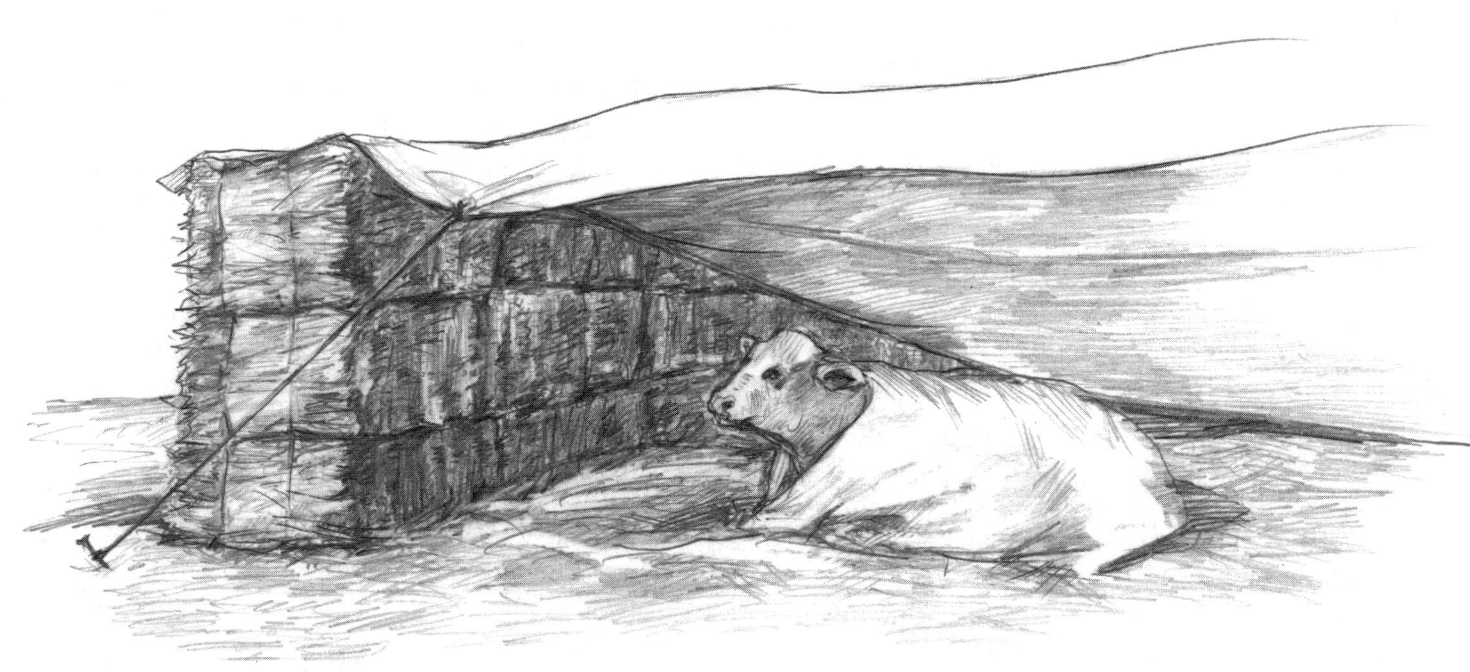

If weather is cold and wet, a windbreak of bales and a tent will keep off the rain and snow.

or make a temporary pen for him nearby if she's in a larger area, so that she can see and smell him but there's no danger of her falling on him if she struggles to get up. Hobble her hind legs so they won't do the splits if she tries and fails (see chapter 8). Tying the legs together reduces the chances of tearing leg muscles or fracturing an upper leg bone. Position the legs 16 inches (40.6 cm) apart, and tie a strap or baling twine above the fetlock joints in nonslip knots so it can't tighten and cut off circulation.

Keep her well bedded and change it often, so her rear end and udder will stay clean. Your vet may prescribe vitamin E and selenium for the cow and steroids to help reduce swelling and assist nerve healing. Check the cow often and try to get her up. If she cannot stand, find a way to hoist her up, using an overhead beam in the barn or a tractor loader if she's outside, so that twice a day she's standing with support for 15 to 20 minutes. Wide belting of some kind can be used as a sling, going around her front end behind the elbows and her rear end at the flanks. There are devices to clamp onto hipbones to hold up a cow's hind end, and you may be able to borrow something like this from your vet. It also helps to turn her over a couple of times a day, so she isn't always lying on the same side. Otherwise she will get "bedsores" from constant pressure, and the muscles on which she is lying will become fatigued.

If you think there's a chance she'll try to get up when you're not there to assist and monitor her, partition the calf away from her if she's in a barn stall, or make a temporary pen for him nearby if she's in a larger area, so that she can see and smell him but there's no danger of her falling on him if she struggles to get up.

Most cows get up in a few hours or a few days, especially if you keep helping them. Periodically stand her up if she'll try. Several people can "tail her up" and hold her steady a few minutes or longer, until she collapses again. The more you get her up, the quicker she will recover. If she's been down awhile when you find her, however, the outcome may not be as good.

COWS WHO COULDN'T GET UP

THE WORST CASE OF PARALYSIS we ever had was a heifer whose calf hiplocked when the vet pulled it. We'd hoped for a c-section delivery, but he thought he could be pulled. He couldn't get the calf out using a calf puller, so we rolled her onto her back. The vet pulled the calf directly across the cow's udder and belly with a calf puller to get him out. The calf was stuck in the heifer's pelvis too long, however, putting pressure on her nerves, and she could not get up following the birth.

We had to leave the paralyzed cow in the barn, where she occupied a stall for two weeks during the peak of calving season, leaving us short on barn space. We got her up several times a day, rolled her from side to side, and eventually she was able to stay on her feet.

We had to leave the paralyzed cow in the barn, where she occupied a stall for two weeks during the peak of calving season, leaving us short on barn space. We got her up several times a day and rolled her from side to side, and eventually she was able to stay on her feet. She soon wobbled out of the barn under her own power to a nearby pen where she could continue her recovery.

Another serious case occurred more recently, when our son had to pull a calf from one of his cows that had excess fluid in the uterus. The calf was abnormal — large and swollen — and difficult to pull. The cow was able to get up briefly, but then she went down and couldn't get up for many days. We finally carried her with a tractor loader into a barn where we could use a hoist to suspend her and get her standing up.

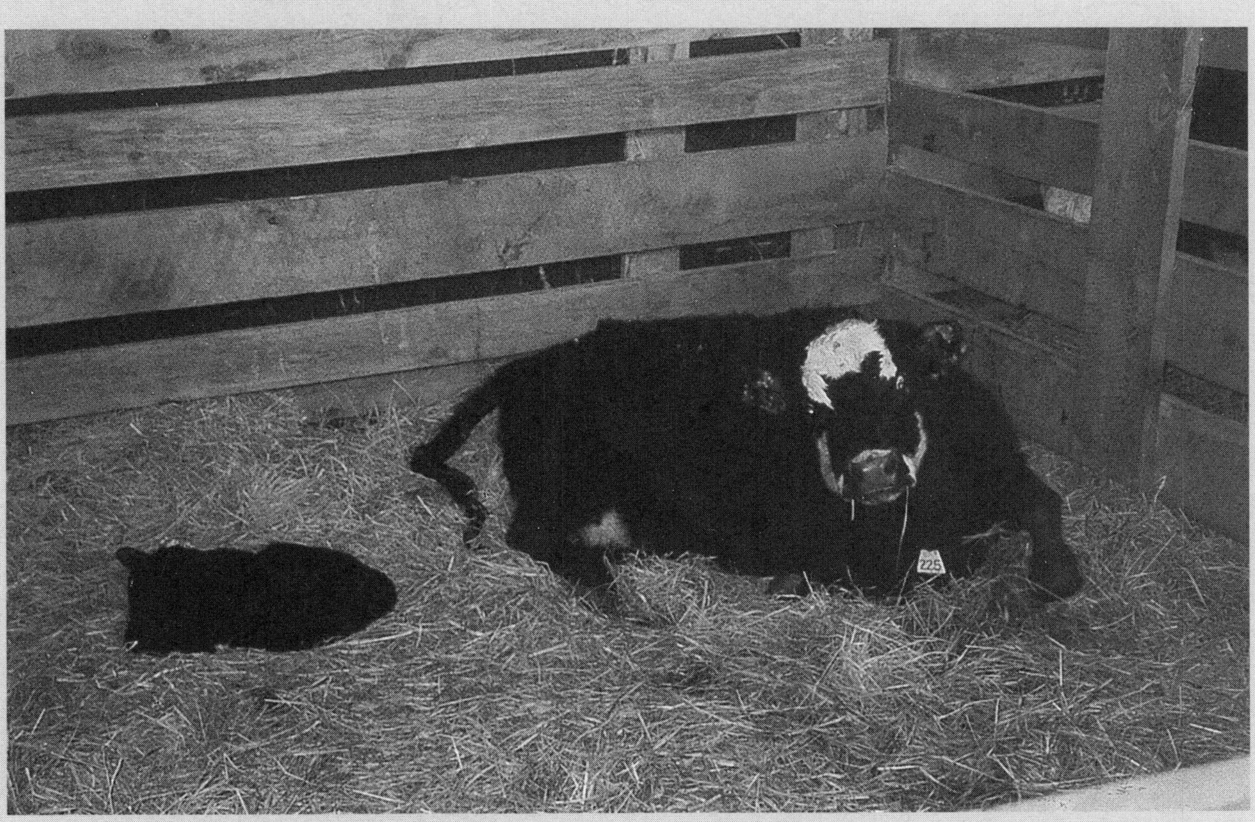

HELPING A PARALYZED COW TO STAND

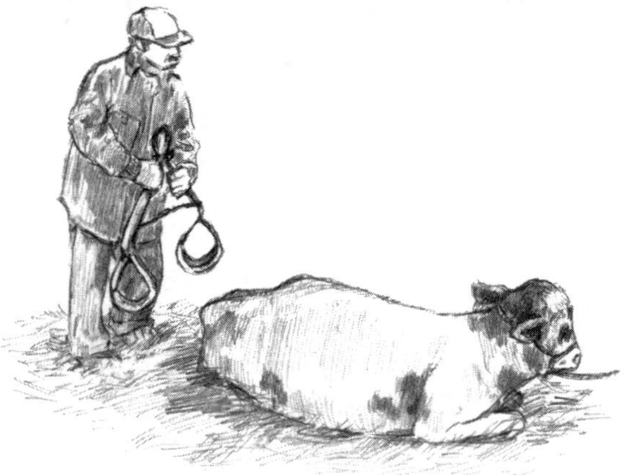

1. Use a hip hoist to lift a cow that can't get up. Pad metal rings with old socks held in place with duct tape to make it easier on her hip bones.

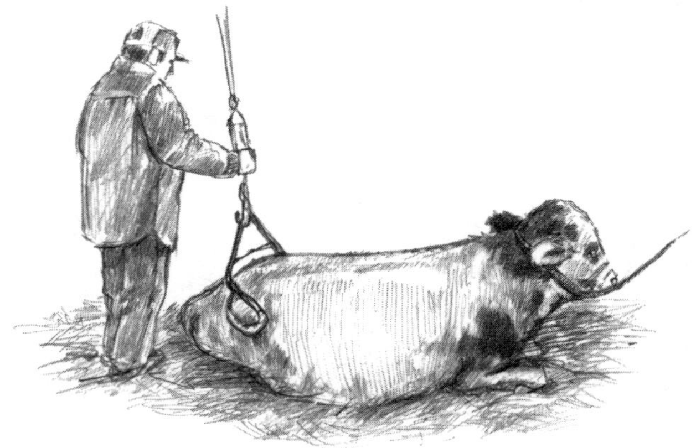

2. The metal rings should fit around and under the hip bones. Tighten the bar/span between them to hold the hoist in place while lifting the cow with a come-along winch.

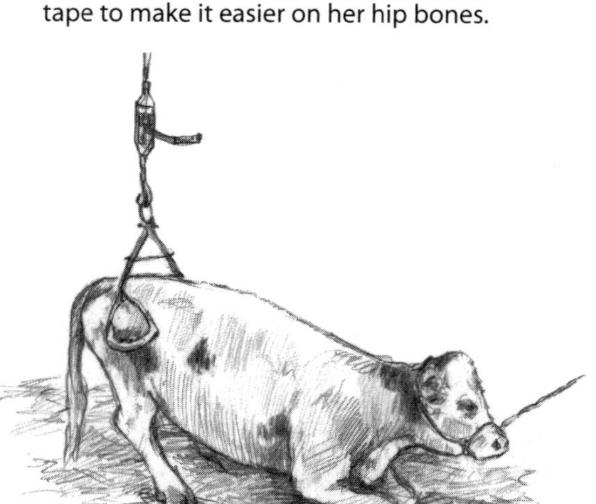

3. With the pulley winch attached to a chain between two of the support posts of the barn, the cow can be winched up off the ground.

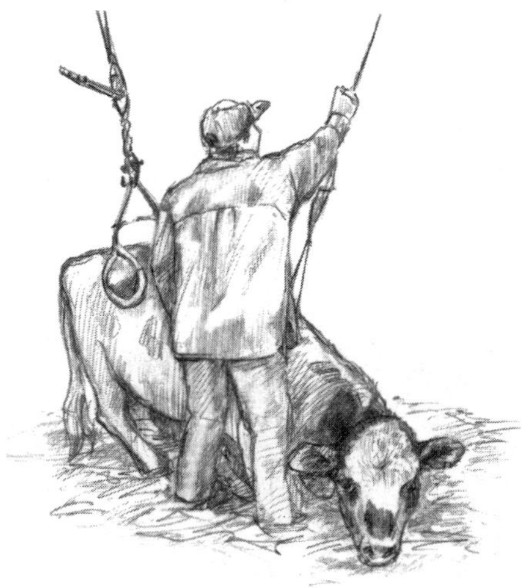

4. If a cow has been down awhile, she'll be weak and will need support for her front end as well as her rear. Use a wide belt, such as a lash cinch from a pack saddle, as a sling for her front.

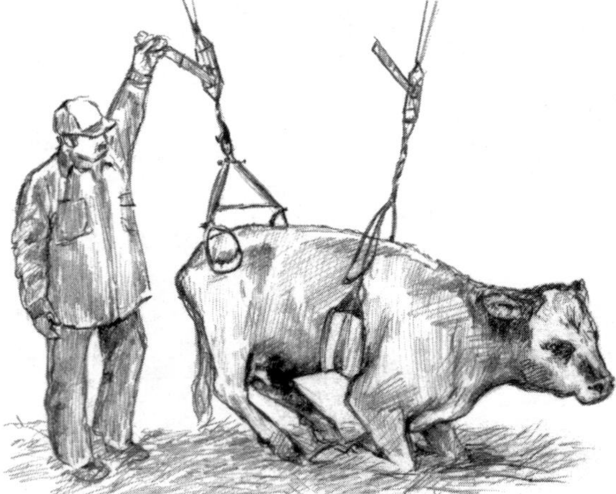

5. Winch her up.

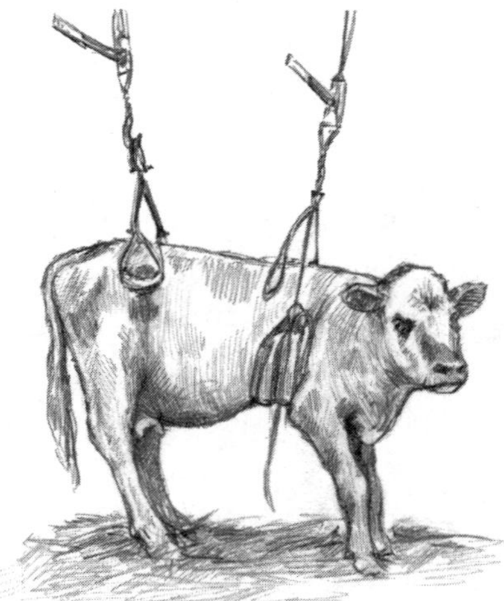

6. The cow is on her feet and on her way to recovery.

Injury to the Cow or Heifer

Damage to vaginal or uterine tissues after a hard birth can lead to bleeding or infection. Other injuries include bruising and tears in the uterine or vaginal wall. Injuries are most likely to occur when cows have been in labor for a long time and when the vagina is dry and not lubricated. Damage to the tissues makes them vulnerable to infection, so it's wise to give the cow antibiotics.

Simple swelling after an injury will eventually subside, but if swelling is large (due to accumulation of blood inside damaged tissues), it may need to be opened and a clot removed. Have your vet examine and treat any cow that suffers a tear or swelling of the vulva or vagina after calving. A tear in the vulva (due to excessive stretching) should be repaired so that it will heal properly. Otherwise the vulva may not close completely, allowing for the possibility of fecal contamination.

Postpartum Hemorrhage

Bleeding after calving may occur if the reproductive tract is damaged and a major blood vessel is torn. This can happen if the uterine or vaginal wall is punctured by the calf's foot, a person's hand, or an obstetrical instrument while the calf is being pulled or manipulated. After the calf is pulled, blood from the torn vessel may accumulate in the uterus and seep out through the vulva later, or it may leak into the abdomen if the uterus was torn.

If You Suspect a Tear

Have your vet examine the cow if you think there may be a tear. If the bleeding is from a uterine laceration, it may halt if the uterus shrinks up quickly; an injection of oxytocin stimulates uterine contractions and helps it to shrink swiftly. If the uterus is completely torn (ruptured), your vet will repair it by stitching the rip. If bleeding is from a vaginal laceration or broken blood vessel, the vet may try to clamp off the bleeding vessel or pack the vagina with something like a large clean towel to put pressure on the vessel and halt the bleeding until it clots and seals off.

If blood streams from the vulva immediately after the birth, it's more likely that the umbilical cord was pulled apart before most of the blood from the placenta was pumped into the calf by the contractions of the uterus. The blood is coming from broken vessel ends in the umbilical cord, which has drawn back up into the vagina.

This is most likely to happen if a cow had uterine inertia (see chapter 3) and poor uterine contractions that failed to pump the placental blood into the calf via the umbilical cord during final stages of birth. This type of bleeding won't continue and is not life-threatening for the cow. It may mean the calf was deprived of part of his blood supply and will be weak for a while.

Injuries are most likely to occur when cows have been in labor for a long time and when the vagina is dry and not lubricated.

Bleeding may also occur if the placenta is forcefully or too quickly removed, especially following delivery of the calf by c-section. Severe and sometimes fatal hemorrhage may result after removal of a placenta during a c-section. It's always best with a live calf and a healthy placenta to leave the placental tissues alone and allow them to come loose on their own (see chapter 5).

Prolapse of the Uterus

This serious emergency occasionally occurs after calving. It may happen following a hard birth (a calf being pulled or the cow having a slow, difficult birth), but prolapse is more common after a normal, easy birth. The cow continues to strain as she lies there because of continued contractions and after-pains, and out pops her uterus. Or you check on a calf that was born normally and unassisted and find the cow standing there licking him, with her uterus hanging down behind her.

A prolapsed uterus can occur right after birth or up to two hours later, while the cervix is still dilated. The wide-open cervix allows the uterus to turn inside out and come through the birth canal after the calf. In some instances, gravity is a contributing factor; a prolapse may be more likely if the cow is lying on a downhill slope, with hindquarters low, or if the weight of the partially shed afterbirth is pulling on the uterus as she lies there. When the far end of one or both uterine horns begins to turn inside itself, the cow keeps straining because it feels like there's something still in there that she must push out.

To reduce risk for uterine prolapse, try to get the cow up and moving around as soon as possible after pulling a calf. The cow's activity helps the uterus to drop back down into the abdominal cavity rather than remaining up at the level of the pelvis, poised to invert itself through the birth canal. If the uterus drops back down, this also straightens the uterine horns. Without a partially inverted horn to push against, the cow is less likely to prolapse.

PROLAPSED UTERUS

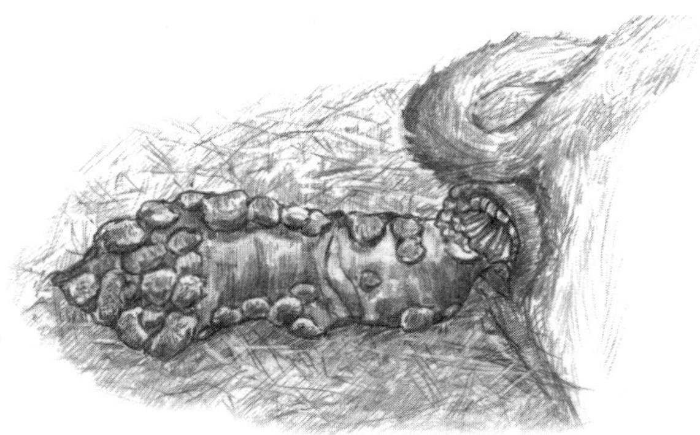

A prolapsed uterus is a mass of fragile tissue weighing more than 40 pounds. Call your vet the minute you discover a prolapse and try to keep it as clean as possible until she arrives.

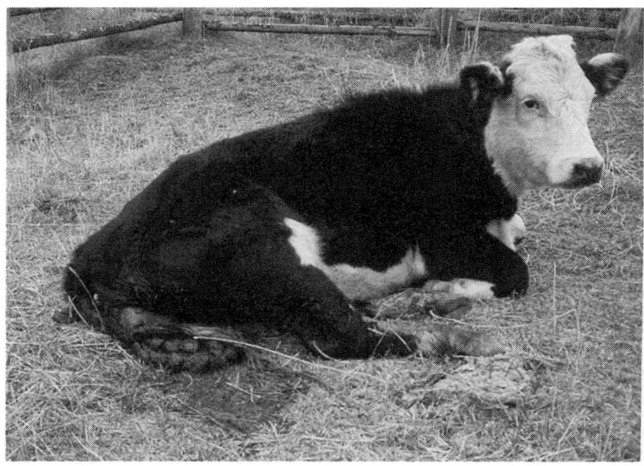

When a uterine prolapse occurs, even if the exposed uterus does not suffer major damage, it is easily bruised and will become infected if the cow is lying on the ground or if it gets covered with manure, which will happen soon if it hangs out for long.

Get Help Quickly

A prolapse is a serious emergency; call your vet as soon as you discover it. The uterus is a 40-plus-pound mass of fragile tissue hanging out and can be very difficult to push back in. If the uterus falls out, it must be replaced quickly or it may hemorrhage or become damaged and you may lose the cow. If the weather is cold, the cow will swiftly lose body heat through the exposed tissue. The cow may chill or go into shock and die. If she steps on, lies on, or kicks this mass of tissue hanging down past her hocks, she may rupture a major artery and bleed to death.

> *If the uterus falls out, it must be replaced quickly or it may hemorrhage or become damaged and you may lose the cow.*

During pregnancy, the uterus develops a large blood supply to take care of the growing fetus. These large arteries by late pregnancy are nearly the size of a garden hose. When the uterus turns inside out, the arteries are just inside the exposed surface. If one of them ruptures, the cow can bleed to death in 5 to 10 minutes. By the time you realize what's happening, it's too late to do anything.

Even if the exposed uterus does not suffer major damage, it is easily bruised and will become infected if the cow is lying on the ground or if it gets covered with manure, which will happen soon if it hangs out for long. The sooner it's replaced, the less damage it will suffer and the less chance there is for serious complications. While you wait for the vet to arrive, keep the inverted uterus as clean and undamaged as possible. If the cow is lying down, wrap a large clean towel around the prolapsed organ. If she's standing, keep her from walking around (tie her if necessary), and support the uterus with a large towel or sheet held by two people.

Replacing the Uterus

The vet will probably give the cow an epidural injection (spinal block) to keep her from straining and from passing manure; this makes the job of replacing the uterus less difficult. Without a spinal block

OUR EXPERIENCE WITH PROLAPSES

IN 40 YEARS OF CALVING, we've had only five prolapses. The first was a Hereford heifer in 1969; she prolapsed right after we pulled her calf. We called our vet, who created a tripod using poles that enabled us to hoist her hind end higher, to facilitate easier replacement of the uterus without the heifer straining so much. She recovered, had many more calves, and never prolapsed again.

The next case was Brighty, in 1984. She was a fat crossbred cow who prolapsed 30 minutes after delivering her fifth calf.

Chub prolapsed two hours after giving birth to her third calf. She was the daughter of a cow that in later life had a vaginal prolapse, so we wondered if it was an inherited weakness.

The only instance of a vaginal and uterine prolapse in the same animal was in a heifer that prolapsed her vagina before calving and immediately prolapsed her uterus when she calved. We sold her after she raised the calf.

The fifth case was a heifer that aborted at seven months and then prolapsed her uterus. We didn't find her right away, since it was late fall and the cows were still on our mountain pasture. Her uterus had probably been hanging out at least a day. I herded her slowly down out of the mountains with my horse. Her uterus was bruised, dry, and very cold. We were afraid she'd suffered too much trauma and shock to have a chance for survival, so we chose not to treat her and butchered her instead.

to keep her from straining, about the only way to get the organ back in is to raise the cow's hindquarters and try to drop and push it into place — but as one vet noted, this is like trying to push a watermelon into a pop bottle.

The inverted organ must first be thoroughly cleaned. Some vets replace the uterus a little at a time while the cow is standing there, starting with the part closest to the vulva, using gentle pressure. Others use some method to raise her hindquarters, which puts the weight of the abdominal contents farther forward, leaving more room. This can be done with a rope tied to a barn beam or tripod or by standing her hind legs on a bale of straw. If she's down, she can be put on her belly with her hind legs out behind her temporarily, with her weight resting on her stifles and an assistant straddling her, facing to the rear and hanging on to her tail. If she was not given an epidural, pulling the tail up vertically helps keep her from straining and also tilts her vulva upward, making it easier to replace the uterus. The person replacing the uterus can kneel behind the cow, between her hocks, supporting the organ on his or her thighs while replacing it little by little. Or two people can hold a board or tray to support the uterus as it is being pushed back in.

If placental membranes are already partially detached, the vet may carefully remove the rest from their buttons before the uterus is replaced. But if the placenta is still well attached, it's better to avoid the risk of bleeding and leave the membranes intact, to come out later on their own. As the last portion is replaced, the person doing it should continue to press forward with closed hand into the vagina, to make sure that the whole organ is pushed past the cervix so it will drop down through the pelvis into proper position. Both horns must be fully pushed into their positions; if any portion is still inverted, it will give the cow something to strain against.

Without a spinal block to keep her from straining, about the only way to get the organ back in is to raise the cow's hindquarters and try to drop and push it into place — but as one vet noted, this is like trying to push a watermelon into a pop bottle.

The next step is to keep her from pushing it right back out again. The cow may need another epidural injection to keep her from straining for a bit longer. Or you or the vet can put several sutures across the vulva opening to keep the uterus from being pushed out again until the cervix has closed and there's no longer any danger. These stitches can be removed in a few days. Stitch as you would to keep a vaginal prolapse in place (see chapter 2).

Prolapsed Uterus Aftercare

The cow needs antibiotics and close monitoring to make sure she doesn't develop infection. Shock and stress, even if she doesn't develop infection, may decrease her appetite, and she may have poor milk production for a few days. You can supplement her milk for the calf, if necessary, until her milk flow increases.

If the uterus was not out for long and was kept clean and undamaged until replaced, the cow or heifer generally recovers. In most cases, even when there is swelling, bruising, and contamination, it will heal and the cow will survive and recover; the recuperative ability of this organ is quite amazing. Sometimes, however, the prolapse is followed in an hour or so by the cow's death, due to internal bleeding. The weight of the heavy uterus hanging down can tear some of the tissues, rupturing major arteries.

Most cows that prolapse don't have lasting ill effects; the uterus shrinks back to normal size, and the cow rebreeds on schedule. Exceptions are cases of severe damage to uterine tissues (from freezing, drying, laceration, etc.) that might cause infertility.

Prolapse of the uterus is generally a one-time occurrence. Repetition of this condition is the exception rather than the rule, so if the cow raises a good calf, it's usually worth the gamble to keep her. If, however, she tends to prolapse the *vagina* before calving and then prolapses her uterus after calving, this is a bad combination and a good reason to sell the cow; you know she will have problems again with vaginal prolapses (see chapter 2), and this may increase the risk of another uterine prolapse.

KNOW WHAT'S GOT THE BUTTONS

Prolapse of the uterus should not be confused with prolapse of the vagina, a condition that usually occurs before calving in a heavily pregnant cow. The vaginal prolapse is a pink mass of tissue the size of a large grapefruit or volleyball, whereas uterine prolapse is a much larger, longer mass; deeper red in color; and covered with darker red "buttons" by which the placenta is attached.

Retained Placenta

Most cows clean soon after calving, shedding placental membranes within 2 to 12 hours. The uterus is shrinking up, having stretched greatly to accommodate the growing fetus, and contractions continue for several days, though in decreasing frequency and intensity. These contractions aid the shrinking process and help flush fluids and tissue debris from the uterus. The cervix constricts again, often very rapidly. Ten to 12 hours after normal calving, when placental membranes have usually been shed, it becomes difficult to insert a hand through.

A retained placenta is a common complication after calving. It generally has no long-term ill effects but in some instances will lead to serious infection within the uterus (see page 139), which can have detrimental effects on the future fertility or health of the cow. Factors leading to a retained placenta include anything that interferes with the "unbuttoning" of the cotyledons that attach the placenta or anything that limits uterine contractions. The contractions help cause physical separation of these buttons by distorting the shape of the *placentomes* (attachment spots where the cotyledon of the placenta hooks into the maternal caruncle).

Primary or secondary uterine inertia (insufficient labor contractions; see chapter 3) often leads to a retained placenta. Contractions are weak or lacking before and after calving; the uterus is slow to shrink and therefore slow to shed placental membranes. The action of suckling triggers uterine contractions, so a cow that loses her calf or doesn't have a calf nursing immediately after birth may be slow to clean.

For proper detachment to occur, the placentome protuberances must be mature and ready to loosen. This maturation process occurs during final stages of pregnancy and depends on rising levels of estrogen; it is usually complete two to five days before calving. If anything interferes with proper maturation, such as premature birth or an abortion, the placenta may be retained. Abortion almost always results in

UTERINE INFECTION LOSS

WE'VE LOST ONE HEIFER TO UTERINE infection. Slippers, a daughter of Bootsie, had a huge calf we had to pull. We got him out alive and the young cow seemed fine for a week, but then she quit eating. She had a high fever. We gave her antibiotics and fluid, but she had developed peritonitis, and we couldn't save her. Our vet suspected that a tiny uterine tear was caused by the traumatic birth and that uterine fluids may have seeped into the abdominal cavity.

the cow retaining the placenta. Twins are often a little premature, so birth of twins may also result in a retained placenta. Anything that causes the calf to come early (heat stress, inflammation of the placenta from infectious disease) can lead to a retained placenta. Other factors include nutritional deficiencies (lack of vitamin A or selenium) and lack of exercise before calving. In some instances, overly fat cows are slow to clean.

If a cow does not shed her placenta within 36 hours following the birth, there's a good chance she won't shed it for a week to 10 days, since uterine contractions have ceased. Retained membranes then depend on shrinking of the uterus and disintegration of the attachments to come loose. The shedding is often hastened, however, by an increase in exercise. If the cow is out at pasture moving around, she sheds the membranes more quickly than if confined.

Placental retention generally requires no treatment unless the cow suddenly gets sick, which is rare, or develops endometritis — in both cases she needs antibiotics. Injections of oxytocin can help the uterus shrink up and shed the placental membranes, but this is helpful only during the first 48 hours. The membranes should be left to slough away on their own. Even careful removal by a vet causes some damage to the uterus, and small pieces of membrane are invariably left inside to cause problems later.

If the cow does not develop serious infection following a retained placenta (and most do not), she will eventually clear the temporary inflammation and infection and have normal fertility, especially if she is not bred again until at least 60 days after calving. In our herd, for example, we've had numerous instances of retained placenta, but those cows rebred on schedule.

Uterine Infection

Sometimes a cow or heifer develops infection after calving, even if calving was normal and she shed the placenta normally. It's more common, however, for infection to follow a difficult birth. Uterine infections most often follow births in which the calf scraped the uterine wall, births that are prolonged and stressful, births that require manipulation of the calf, and cases in which the cow did not shed the placenta for several days following the birth.

Use of Antibiotics

As a precaution against infection, some vets recommend inserting antibiotic boluses into the uterus (and there are boluses marketed for this purpose) if you give prolonged assistance to pull a calf or put your hands into the uterus to manipulate the calf. Boluses can be put carefully into the uterus soon after the calf is born with a clean, disposable OB sleeve covering your hand and arm. Other vets feel boluses aren't very effective and recommend systemic antibiotics instead, if there's a chance the cow is at risk for uterine infection. Intrauterine antibiotics may do more harm than good, by reducing the rate of disintegration of placental attachments and reducing the level of white blood cells that "clean up" debris and contamination within the uterus.

A mild and temporary infection is common after calving, since the vulva and cervix were relaxed during birth, enabling bacteria to gain entrance. Blood and sloughed button tissue (the caruncular attachments between uterus and placenta) provide an ideal environment for bacterial growth. But in most cases, bacteria do not persist because continued debris-flushing uterine contractions and migrating, bacteria-devouring white blood cells get rid of them.

Bacterial Infection

In some cases, bacteria multiply rapidly and take up residence in the uterus. *Metritis* (infection of the uterus) may occur after an abnormal birth, especially a difficult delivery with prolonged traction on a calf or manipulation of a calf. Infection may also develop after uterine inertia, twins, or retained placenta.

If bacteria become well established in the compromised and still stretched uterus after calving, some may produce toxins that are absorbed into the bloodstream and cause serious illness (*septicemia*). On rare occasions, infection is due to clostridial bacteria, which can be rapidly fatal. If a cow becomes dull and goes off feed after calving, she needs immediate treatment.

Her temperature may be high (fever) or subnormal. Heart rate will be elevated. Respiration will be too fast, and you may think she has pneumonia. She usually won't eat or drink much, is dehydrated, and has diarrhea because of *toxemia*. The infection may spread to the abdomen, to cause *peritonitis*. The cow may go into shock. There may be putrid discharge from the vulva, and she may stand with her back humped up and her tail out or may strain, especially if she has not yet shed the placenta.

To save her life, she needs antibiotics and good supportive care. Get help from your vet. A broad-spectrum antibiotic will usually be prescribed, along with anti-inflammatory drugs (like Banamine) and fluid. If the cow is not drinking, she needs fluid by stomach tube or IV. The vet may flush her uterus with warm saline solution to get rid of infected material. The flushing intervention also has a soothing effect and stimulates the uterus to contract and flush itself. Saline flushings may be followed with an antiseptic solution. If the cow survives, she may or may not be fertile again, depending on how much uterine damage was done.

FOOLED BY ENDOMETRITIS

A DAIRY COW gave us our only experience with persistent endometritis. Lynn and I had a dairy for a short time after we were married, before we came back to the ranch to raise beef cattle. When we sold our dairy cows at a farm sale, the vet checked them ahead of time.

One cow, judged to be pregnant and sold as such, began to discharge pus a few days later. The man who bought her had her checked by another vet, who diagnosed *pyometra* (a pus-filled uterus). We returned the farmer's money and took back the cow. Because we knew she would probably never be fertile, we sold her for butchering.

Endometritis

Mild infection after calving resulting in *endometritis* (inflammation of the uterine lining) is fairly common. This is not life-threatening, as the infection remains confined to the uterus, but unless resolved it may become chronic and render the cow infertile. Causes of endometritis include retained placenta, twins, abortion, difficult birth (with damage to tissues and more risk of bacteria entering on the hands of a person assisting delivery), and a dirty environment at calving. Symptoms include white or yellow-white discharge from the vulva in the days or weeks after calving, increasing in volume during the cow's first heat period, when her cervix is dilated and there is more vaginal mucus to help flush pus from the uterus. Endometritis may eventually clear up after she starts having heat cycles again, as the uterus naturally flushes itself.

In some instances, however, infection does not clear up and leads to accumulation of pus in the uterus. The uterus ceases to produce or release the hormones that trigger degeneration of the corpus luteum (CL) in the ovary. The CL persists, so the cow does not come into heat (see chapter 1). The uterus is under continual influence of progesterone, which makes more ideal conditions for bacterial growth, and the infection is never eliminated. The cervix remains tightly closed, so pus continues to accumulate within the uterus, though occasionally there will be discharge of pus from the vulva. Since the cow never comes into heat, and the uterus is slightly enlarged, the owner and veterinarian may mistakenly think the cow is pregnant when checking her later in the season.

Because most cows with endometritis eventually clear up on their own, many stockmen don't bother to treat them. This always leaves some risk, however, that the problem will progress to pyometra (pus accumulation in the uterus) or long-term damage and changes within the uterus that might interfere with conception. Consult your vet for advice on treatment. Some vets recommend a broad-spectrum antibiotic infused directly into the uterus.

Milk Fever

A cow that produces a lot of milk may develop an acute lack of calcium at calving or soon after, because so much of her body's store of calcium is being shunted into sudden production of milk. She can't remove calcium from where it's stored in her bones quickly enough. This happens most commonly in dairy cows but may also happen in beef cows. Most cases of *hypocalcemia* (low calcium) occur within 48 hours after calving, and most often in mature cows during their peak years of milk production (their third through seventh calves). Cows on legume forages are more at risk.

As calcium levels drop, the cow may become excited or quit eating, with muscle tremors in head and legs. The muscles are unable to function properly. She may not want to move, and if she does, she walks stiffly, is uncoordinated, and may fall. Soon she lies down and is no longer able to get up, seeming weak and dull or sleepy, with her head turned back toward her flank. Temperature and heart rate are low. If not treated soon, the cow drifts into unconsciousness, goes into shock, and dies.

Treating Milk Fever

Give the cow who is ill with hypocalcemia at least 14 to 28 ounces (400 to 800 mL) of calcium solution, administered slowly (over 20 to 30 minutes) intravenously or injected under the skin. Sometimes the vet will give half the dose via IV and the rest subcutaneously for slower absorption, to prevent side effects from rapid absorption. Reducing the rate of milk removal, by not milking the cow or giving her calf a supplemental feeding so it won't nurse her as much, can help. Treatment usually results in dramatic improvement, and the cow soon recovers. In some instances, however, the condition is complicated by *grass tetany* (low levels of magnesium), and she needs supplemental magnesium as well.

> **MILK THERE FOR THE CALF WHEN HE NEEDS IT**
>
> Some cows have more milk than the calf can handle for a while; a large unsucked quarter stops producing milk due to the constant pressure. It dries up and becomes smaller. At that point the calf may start nursing it; he can now get his mouth on the teat that was too large and awkward before. Once he starts nursing it, that quarter will start producing milk again.

Grass Tetany

Similarly to milk fever, a cow may lose large amounts of magnesium if she milks heavily after calving. If feed is low in magnesium (such as pasture grasses growing in cool, cloudy weather) or cows are exposed to cold-weather stress after calving, blood levels of magnesium may drop enough to cause grass tetany. Affected cows are restless, stop eating, and have an unusual high-stepping gait. Some become aggressive. As the problem progresses, they fall down and have convulsions. Treatment is intravenous administration of magnesium, but some cows do not respond and die. This problem can usually be prevented by feeding hay, which is high in magnesium, to lactating cows grazing lush grass pasture during cool, wet weather.

Mastitis

A cow may develop inflammation and infection in the udder following calving. This is primarily a problem in dairy cows, due to the complexity and quantity of *mammary tissue* in these high-producing cows. But *mastitis* can also occur in beef cows and can be quite serious. Depending on the pathogen involved, a bad case may be fatal. Mastitis may develop if one or more *quarters of the udder* become infected due to contamination, as when a cow lies in mud and manure. Infectious organisms may enter the teat canal.

Mastitis may also be a sequel to bruising and trauma if the udder is bumped; the damaged tissue creates ideal conditions for infection. If a cow has a large, distended udder at calving or shortly after, before her calf nurses or if he cannot consume all the colostrum and one or two quarters are very full, she may bruise it. If she has to travel fast — being chased into a calving pen or if you are trying to get her to the corral for some purpose, she may bang the full udder with a hind leg and bruise it.

If a cow has a large udder and more colostrum than her calf can consume at first nursing, it often helps to milk some of the extra, so the full quarters won't be so distended and easily bruised. Save and freeze the extra colostrum for emergencies (see chapter 7). By milking the full quarters, you increase the chances that the calf can suck them the next time he nurses; they won't be as huge, nor the teats so distended, and hard to get onto. Often, by milking out the big quarters, you reduce the risk for mastitis.

On the flip side, if a cow is in a dirty environment, there may be more chance of mastitis in the unsucked quarters if you milk them, forcing the plug out of the teats and opening the way for infection. This can happen if a cow has more milk than her calf can handle for a while, and the unsucked teats stay huge until he has a bigger appetite. Of course, if the seal comes out of the teat readily, a cow may leak streams of colostrum from all four teats when her calf starts to nurse, stimulating milk letdown. In that case, the teat duct is already open.

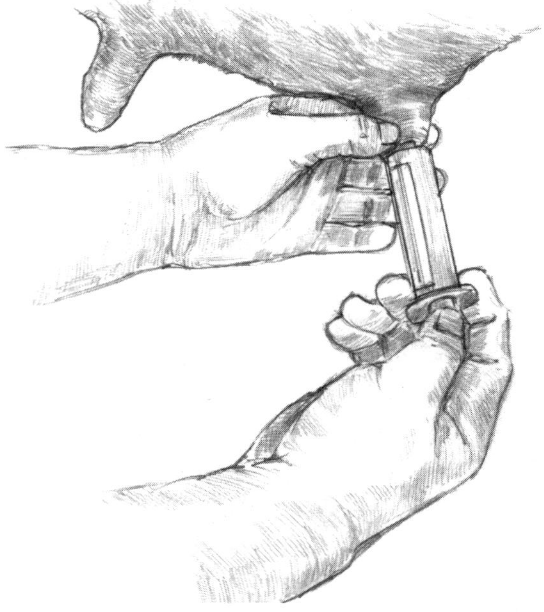

To treat mastitis, milk out the infected quarter and inject a mastitis antibiotic up into the teat.

Treating Mastitis

If a cow gets mastitis at any time during lactation, it should be treated as soon as possible. If infection stays localized in the udder (usually just one quarter), the mammary tissue may be damaged, but the infection is not life-threatening. That quarter may be permanently damaged, however, without prompt treatment. It will be small — and dry — the next time she calves or may produce a little fluid right after calving and then dry up.

If the infection does not stay localized and gets into the bloodstream, as some pathogens do, the cow is sick. She'll go off feed and develop a fever. Unless treatment is swift and diligent, part of the udder may slough away, and she may die. In a serious case of mastitis in which the cow is ill, she needs injections of *systemic* antibiotics as well as local treatment. Otherwise, antibiotic squirted into the infected quarter may be adequate.

Mammary infusion products for dairy cows also work for a beef cow. Once or twice a day the medication is squirted from a small syringe into the teat opening after that quarter has been milked out. Consult your veterinarian for advice on products to use and how to use them. The main thing is to keep that quarter milked out twice daily, if the calf is not nursing it. Milk out as much as you can. It may be lumpy, clotted milk or watery fluid. Continue milking and treating until the infection clears and the quarter is producing normal milk again.

Most types of mastitis infection will not hurt the calf. If he nurses that quarter, it saves you the task of milking it out, but often the cow won't let him nurse because it's sore, or the calf may not like the taste of the milk and refuse to nurse. If the cow is sick or quits eating, consult your vet, and use an appropriate systemic antibiotic until the cow has fully recovered. Mastitis can be very serious; diligent and proper treatment can make a difference in whether you lose that quarter — or even the cow.

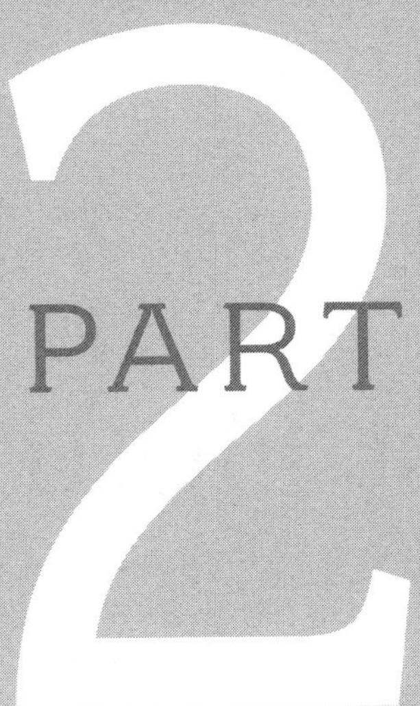

PART 2

Care of the Newborn Calf

Chapter 7

The First Hours of Life

The calf is safely born. Now you need to make sure he's breathing and gets up soon and finds the udder. The cow usually stands up immediately after delivery and starts licking the calf, pushing him around vigorously with her nose, nudging him to get up. He falls down a few times and then wobbles toward the udder, helped by Mama's licking and pushing at his rear end to guide him in the right direction. That's the way we like to see it happen, but sometimes a calf needs more help getting his life started.

The abrupt move from the safe environment of the uterus to the risky outside world requires great adaptability. Most newborns can manage this drastic change — unless they've been stressed by a difficult delivery or have complications immediately following their birth. In these instances, they need help from you to survive.

Make Sure He's Breathing

In most normal, uncomplicated births, the calf begins breathing within 30 to 60 seconds after he's born. If he's not breathing, clear the fluid away from his nose with your fingers and tickle the inside of one nostril with a clean piece of hay or straw. If that doesn't work, you may have to give him artificial respiration (see chapter 3).

Traditionally, compromised calves (with fluid in their airways, not breathing) were held up by their hind legs to allow fluid to drain from the airways, but now most vets do not advise this. They say that most of the fluids that drain are stomach fluids that are important to the health of the calf. Holding him up by the hind legs puts pressure on his diaphragm from abdominal organs, interfering with normal respira-

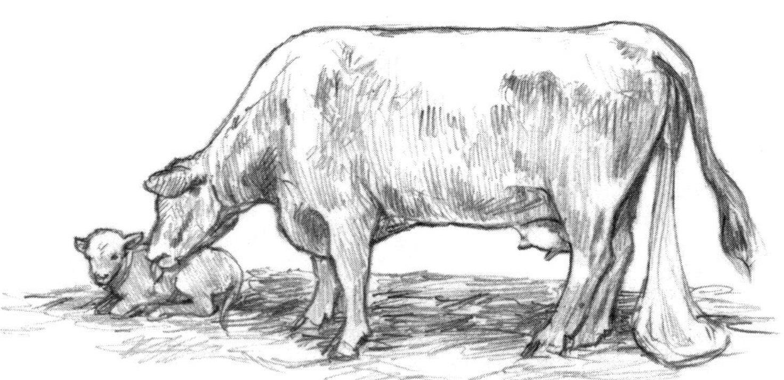

The cow usually gets up immediately after delivering the calf and starts licking him.

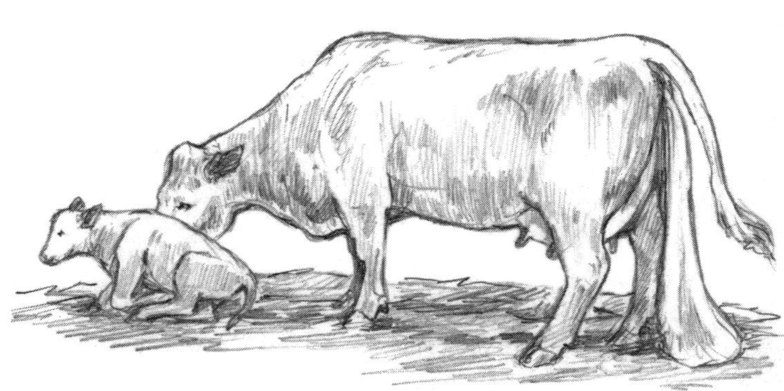

She pushes him around vigorously with her nose, urging him to get up.

tory movements and inhibiting breathing. It's better to use a suction bulb to clear the airways.

If a calf was stressed during birth and doesn't start breathing immediately, it may be a sign that he's suffering from *acidosis* (a pH imbalance caused by stress and a shortage of oxygen that can have adverse effects on proper functioning of heart and lungs). It may take several hours or even days for his body to correct this. One way to tell whether the calf is normal or metabolically compromised is to observe how soon he assumes a more upright position — lying on his breastbone with his head up, rather than out flat.

After a normal birth, the calf is usually raising his head and looking around or trying to get up within 2 to 5 minutes. After a hard birth, it may take a calf 6 to 12 minutes. If he just lies there and has not tried to raise his head after 3 to 5 minutes, rub him briskly with a towel or a handful of straw to stimulate circulation, and prop him up a little. Respiration is aided when the calf is more upright; lung function and rib cage movement are impeded when he's lying flat.

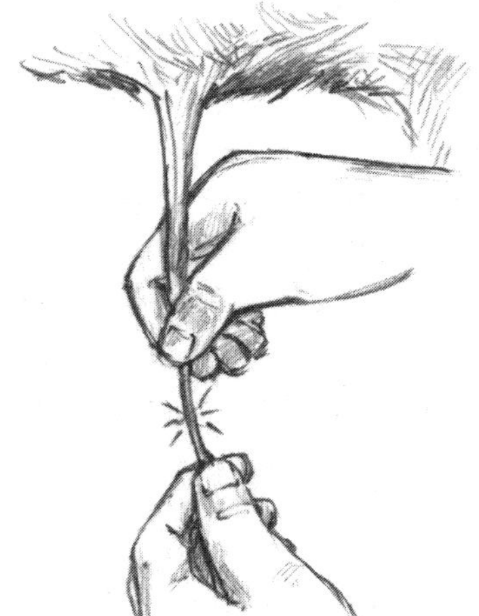

When the navel stump (the umbilical cord) is too long, carefully pull it apart about three inches (7.5 cm) from the abdomen with very clean hands, being careful not to pull or jerk on the calf's abdomen.

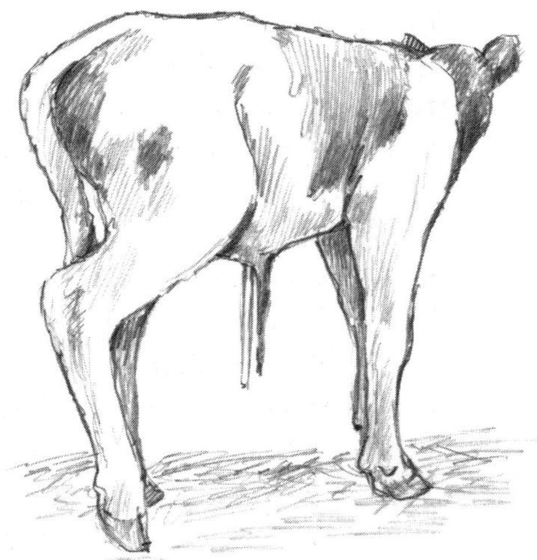

On rare occasions a calf has an "extra" white tubular cord at birth. This should be cut with a very clean, sharp knife.

Care of the Navel Stump

Once the calf is breathing, disinfect his *navel* stump. If a cow calves on clean grassy pasture rather than dirt or mud, there is less chance of bacteria entering the calf's navel stump. If she calves in a pen or barn stall, there is risk for infection. Head it off by using a good disinfectant right after birth, before the wet, bloody navel stump is dragged in the dirt, mud, or manure as the calf struggles to get to his feet.

Most stockmen use strong iodine (7 percent tincture of iodine) to disinfect the navel. It acts not only as a disinfectant but also as an astringent to help the stump dry more quickly and seal off, preventing entrance of pathogens. The best way to disinfect it is to dip the entire stump in a small widemouthed jar containing about a half inch (1.25 cm) of iodine. If the cord broke off long and drags on or near the ground, break it — don't cut it — to about 3 inches (7.5 cm) long. Do it with very clean hands, and break it between your hands; never create a pull or jerk on the calf's belly. Once the stump is a reasonable length, immerse it in disinfectant. Make sure the entire stump is dipped and saturated; swish it around, holding the jar up to the belly.

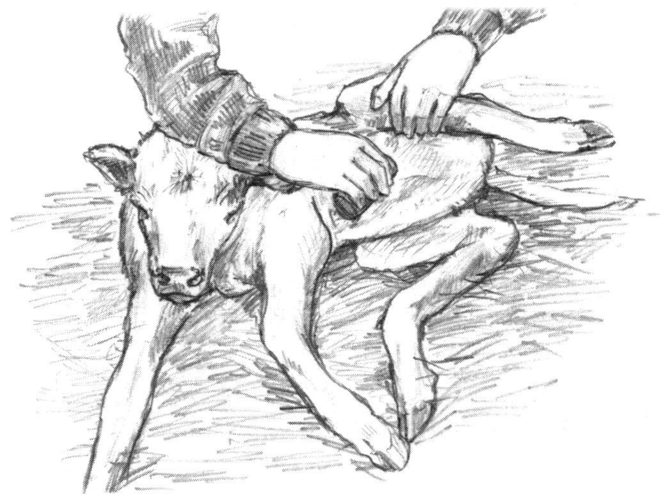

After you make sure the calf is breathing, disinfect the navel stump, immersing it in a small jar of iodine. You may have to lift the calf's hind leg to be sure that you immerse the entire navel cord stump. Repeat the iodine application a few hours later and as many times as needed, until the navel stump is completely dried up.

One application of iodine may not be enough to dry the stump quickly. You may have to repeat it a couple of times in the first 24 hours or until the stump dries, to prevent *navel ill* (see chapter 14). Bull calves take longer for the cord to dry than do heifers, since urine may keep a bull calf's navel area wet if he urinates while lying down. Many cows will lick and chew at the calf's navel and may try to lick all the iodine off as soon as you apply it. You may need to reapply it and monitor the calf to make sure the cow leaves the navel stump alone for a bit, or distract her with hay.

On occasion you'll see a calf with an unusual cord. Sometimes tubular tissue that was part of the *umbilicus* inside the calf has a portion remaining outside the calf. A firm white tube may extend several inches from the navel with the umbilical membranes. This firm tube won't dry up and fall off as readily as the other tissues. It is a solid structure without blood vessels and can be cut. If it hangs down very far, carefully cut it off near the navel with a clean knife, then disinfect the navel stump.

On rare occasions you may see a newborn calf with a hernia (see chapter 14). If it's a fairly large hole at the navel, allowing abdominal tissue or intestines to bulge through, call your veterinarian and have it checked. If the hole is very large, and there's risk that loops of intestine might come through, your vet can stitch it right up.

Keep Iodine away from Eyes

Take care not to spill iodine on the calf. It burns the tissues and can make the skin raw and sore. Avoid splashing any into his eye (or yours!), since it's very caustic. Once when I was applying iodine to a newborn calf outdoors on a dark night, using a flashlight for illumination, I had trouble immersing the stump while he struggled on the ground trying to get up, and he kicked the iodine jar with a hind foot. It spilled, and some of it splashed into one of his eyes. The eye turned blue and cloudy, and it was several months before he could see again in that eye.

A Bleeding Cord

Once in a while a cord bleeds when broken. Usually when it breaks naturally, as the cow gets up or the calf tries to get up, the torn vessels draw back into the calf's abdomen and seal off, and there's not much bleeding. Never cut the cord with a knife or scissors; a cut cord bleeds more readily than a torn one.

Sometimes a cord bleeds profusely, even if everything is normal. You can halt the bleeding by tying or clamping the stump for a few hours so blood can clot and the vessels can seal off. For instance, after a normal delivery, one of our calves began bleeding and we didn't notice because we didn't have to assist with the birth. Our daughter, who was in the barn attending other calves, looked into that stall to make sure the calf was up and nursing and saw spots of blood on the straw. She saw blood streaming from the calf's navel and used one of her hair clips to clamp it off. Whatever you use to tie or clamp the cord to halt bleeding, make sure the cow doesn't try to chew it off. Don't leave it there, because there's usually some drainage from the navel cord and you don't want to inhibit this. Carefully remove the tie or clamp after one or two hours and reapply iodine to the stump.

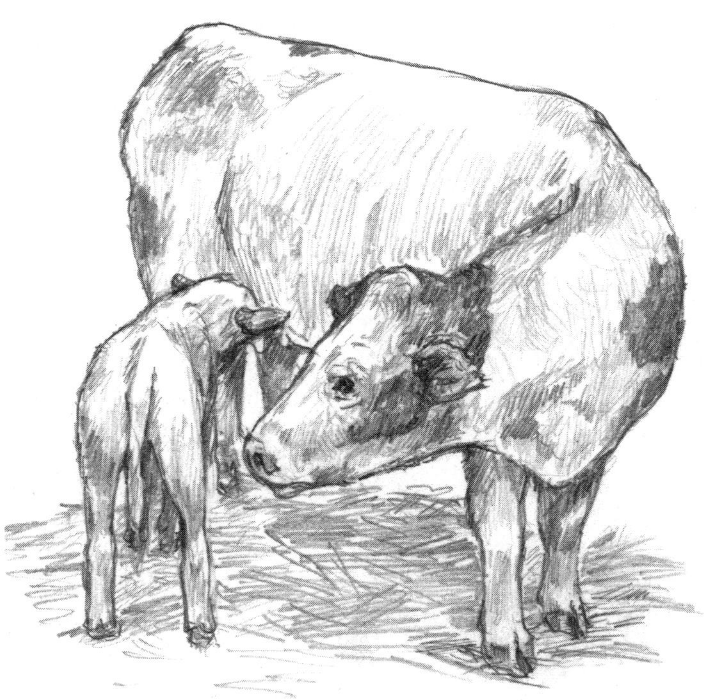

The cow licks and nuzzles her new calf and guides him to her udder because it is very important that he nurse colostrum soon after he's born.

Make Sure He Nurses Right Away

It is crucial that the calf get up and nurse soon after birth. If he can't accomplish this on his own, you must help him by guiding him to the udder and putting a teat into his mouth or feeding him by bottle or stomach tube if he's unable to nurse.

The Importance of Colostrum

The cow's first milk, *colostrum,* is vital to the health and survival of the calf. It contains special ingredients that give him a good start. It gives him a burst of energy for body warmth and strength, and important *antibodies* to help him fight disease. The antibodies he absorbs directly into his bloodstream can help him fight blood-borne infections such as salmonella, pasteurella, and *streptococcus,* any of which could cause septicemia. The antibodies that stay in the gut can attack any scours-causing pathogens the calf ingests. Colostrum also serves as a gut stimulant to help him pass his first bowel movements.

Laxative Effects

A calf that gets adequate colostrum passes bowel movements within the first several hours after birth, and the dark green-brown sticky *meconium* soon gives way to bright yellow *feces* as the colostrum passes through. A calf fed regular milk or milk replacer may take a long time to pass his first bowel movements.

During late gestation, the fetus continually swallows some of the fluid in which it floats. It does not pass bowel movements, however, until after it's born, unless the calf is severely stressed during birth — then he'll pass meconium into the amniotic fluid, turning it yellow-brown. The swallowed fluid condenses into

The Role of Antibodies

When viruses or bacteria enter the body, they cause damage by multiplying and creating toxic products, stimulating the body to create antibody proteins *(immunoglobulins)* to react with the invading agent and neutralize it. Some types of antibodies are carried through the body via the bloodstream.

The main role of one kind of white blood cell is to produce antibodies. If an animal has antibodies against a specific disease organism, any time that pathogen invades the body again, an army of white blood cells with their antibodies converge on the site to kill the invader. Exposure to one strain of pathogen may result in immunity to that strain but may not protect against other strains of the same organism. Immunity depends on level of exposure, stress on the animal, and current health. A severe disease outbreak in a herd may eventually break down a healthy animal's immunity and will overwhelm a stressed animal's defenses even sooner.

Vaccination can stimulate production of antibodies, serving as the *antigen* (any foreign substance entering the body that causes the body to create antibodies). The body makes protective antibodies to fight the invader. Later when the animal comes in contact with the actual infection, antibodies in the bloodstream can inactivate the pathogen. If enough antibodies are present to inactivate all the agents that invade, the animal won't get sick, and the invasion stimulates rapid production of more antibodies for future protection. With vaccination and natural exposure to various pathogens, a cow develops many antibodies and strong immunity. During late pregnancy she puts these in her colostrum so that her newborn calf has some instant immunity after he nurses.

The fetus begins to produce antibodies against some pathogens at various stages of development, since some invaders pass through the placental barrier from the dam if she becomes infected. A fetus can be infected with BVD, *leptospirosis*, or other diseases, and may be aborted (see chapter 2), be born diseased, or start making antibodies of its own, depending on its stage of development. But fetal immunity doesn't do the calf much good when he's born. For a few weeks before calving and a short while after, the calf's immune system is hindered by the high levels of *cortisol* (one of the hormones that stimulates birth) present in both cow and calf. Young calves are very vulnerable to disease and must absorb antibodies from the dam's colostrum.

dark, soft-to-firm material in the intestines and must be passed after the calf is born. Colostrum triggers intestinal contractions to move this material out.

High-Energy Food

Colostrum contains creamy fat, is high in energy (twice the calories of regular milk), and is easily digested. A calf that gets right up and nurses is more vigorous and better able to stay warm even if he's born on a cold night. A newborn calf that has nursed will generally buck around afterward, feeling good. A calf that hasn't nursed may be sluggish and easily chilled.

When it's cold, one way to determine if the calf has nursed is to feel inside his mouth. If his mouth is cold, he hasn't nursed; if it's warm, he probably has. If the weather is cold, it's very important to get colostrum into the calf within the first hour of birth, not only for energy to keep warm but to make sure he absorbs antibodies from his dam's colostrum. Stress, which includes being chilled, quickly reduces his ability to absorb these large molecules.

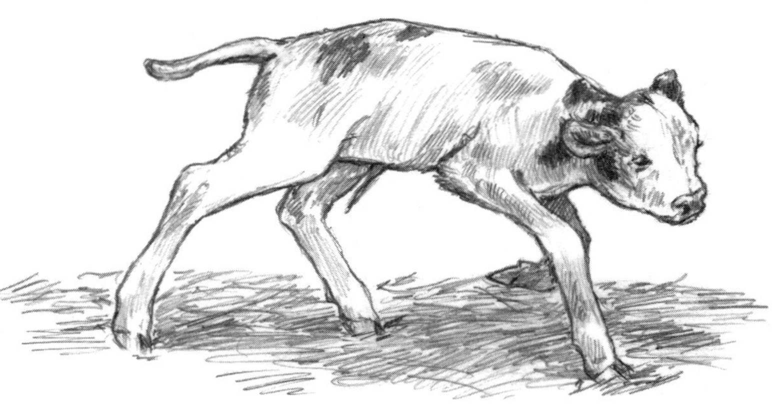

A newborn calf that has nursed is vigorous and feeling good. He often runs and bucks around after he finishes nursing.

Antibodies

The calf is born with no immunity to disease. If he fails to obtain colostrum soon after birth, he must rely on his own immature immune system to develop protection, and this process isn't quick enough to avoid disease. For most infections, it takes the immune system 6 to 10 days to respond adequately and fight pathogens, and in many instances, as when challenged by gut or respiratory infections at an early age, the immunological response is not timely enough to keep a calf from becoming seriously ill or dying.

But Mother Nature has this loophole covered. The calf has a good chance of staying healthy if he acquires temporary protection *(passive transfer)* from his dam's colostrum. The antibodies in a cow's bloodstream can't cross the placenta because these molecules are too large, but the calf can receive them right after birth by drinking her colostrum. During the last three weeks of gestation, she accumulates antibodies from her blood into her mammary glands. Her colostrum contains a high level of the various antibodies circulating in her bloodstream. Thus, it is important to keep cows healthy and on a good vaccination program against the diseases in your region or on your farm. A well-fed healthy cow produces an abundant amount of colostrum and a large volume of antibodies — most concentrated at the time of birth.

If a cow's vaccinations against viral diseases (IBR, BVD) and clostridial diseases (blackleg, malignant edema, enterotoxemia, etc.) are up to date, this helps protect the calf. The cow also has antibodies against common disease organisms in her environment, including pathogens that cause some types of diarrhea or pneumonia in calves. On some farms it helps to vaccinate cows ahead of calving with a "scours" vaccine to create antibodies against the deadly pathogens that cause intestinal infection early in a calf's life. Common culprits are certain types of *Escherichia coli* (the infamous *E. coli*) bacteria, *rotavirus,* and *coronavirus.* Most of these vaccines must be given at least three weeks ahead of calving; some must be repeated later if the cow does not calve for a couple of months after vaccination, while others are still protective for several months. Your vet can advise you on precalving vaccines that might be helpful for your calves.

It does no good to vaccinate cows for these diseases, however, unless calves are able to absorb antibodies from colostrum. The best insurance you can give a newborn calf is to make sure he nurses his dam within an hour or two of coming into the world. If he doesn't get that protection, he is at risk for life-threatening disease. In these instances, give him substitute colostrum from another cow. If that isn't possible, give the calf a commercial preparation of concentrated antibodies or an oral *E. coli* vaccine soon after birth, if this type of scours infects your calves (see chapter 11).

Substitution

A calf that does not get colostrum at birth is at risk for life-threatening disease unless he gets an adequate substitute. If he doesn't nurse soon enough, he doesn't get the protection. Even if he eventually gets a full belly of colostrum some hours later, his gut lining is thickened, and he can't absorb antibodies through it, into the bloodstream and lymph system.

It's good to have frozen colostrum for emergencies, in case a calf can't nurse the cow and it's difficult to milk the cow to obtain some. Colostrum substitutes are handy in an emergency and better than nothing but not as good as the real thing. Frozen colostrum from one of your own beef cows is better. Dairy-cow colostrum may not contain as many antibodies per quart, due to the immense volume produced, and may be risky: You might get salmonella or some other pathogen from a dairy farm.

A calf that does not get colostrum at birth is at risk for life-threatening disease unless he gets an adequate substitute.

A partial feeding of a commercial product or frozen colostrum can be used to jump-start a slow calf and possibly stimulate him soon to nurse his dam. A partial feeding also can be counterproductive, however, if the calf doesn't get more colostrum right away. The little bit you fed him more quickly closes the antibody absorption window of opportunity in his gut. If he might not nurse his dam very soon, give him a full dose of substitute colostrum.

Absorbing Antibodies

There are several types of antibodies in colostrum, including *IgG* and *IgA*. Their absorption rate and role in disease prevention varies. IgG antibodies are absorbed immediately and directly through the

Passive Transfer

Temporary protection gained by a calf from his mother's colostrum gives him immunity against certain diseases until his own immune system starts producing antibodies. This temporary protection lasts three to six weeks or longer, depending on the quality of his dam's colostrum and how much he absorbed — how soon after birth he nursed and how much he nursed.

But calves' antibody levels begin to drop at three to four weeks of age, or sooner for some heifers' calves that don't get strong colostrum. Colostrum from a first-calver does not contain as many antibodies as the colostrum from an older cow. Protection from the experienced cow may last longer. The time it takes for the calf's own immune system to kick in and ward off invaders varies, depending on the strength of the passive transfer. If he received a high level of antibodies from colostrum, which would effectively neutralize invading pathogens, his own defenses are not stimulated to develop until the temporary protection wears off. Since no antigen is being transferred with passive immunity, the calf's immune system is not stimulated until the transferred antibodies are gone and he encounters antigens from his environment or from vaccination.

Antibodies gained via colostrum can interfere with the effectiveness of vaccinations. If the calf is vaccinated against a disease while he still has high levels of maternal antibodies, his immune system won't bother to respond to antigens in the vaccine; they're being neutralized by the maternal antibodies still circulating in his bloodstream. Some vaccinations given to calves at an early age (two to three weeks) will not give him much protection since they cannot stimulate immunity. Most calf vaccines should be given at six to eight weeks or older and repeated with a booster two to six weeks later, to make sure the calf's immune system responds. Consult your vet, and follow label directions on vaccines for calves.

intestinal wall to enter the lymph system and bloodstream ready to fight disease organisms, while IgA antibodies stay in the gut and attack any pathogens found there, such as *E. coli* bacteria. A calf must nurse soon to absorb IgG antibodies through the intestinal wall before it thickens and must continue to have colostrum in his next several nursings to keep IgA antibodies in his gut to protect against scours pathogens he may ingest from dirty teats or a dirty environment. The IgA antibodies in his mother's dwindling supply of colostrum (as it is diluted with regular milk) continue to be of benefit even though he can no longer absorb any antibodies through the gut lining.

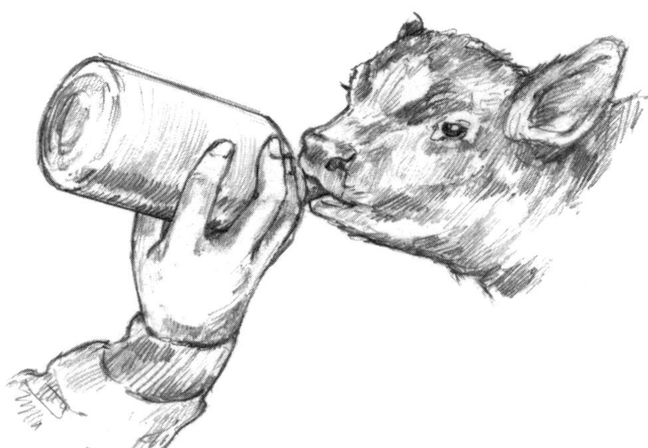

If the calf won't be nursing his dam very soon, feed him a full ration of colostrum.

Factors that Affect Colostrum Absorption

Things that can interfere with a calf's timely absorption of colostrum include

- ***Hard birth.*** A calf may be slow to get up or be unable to suck because of a swollen tongue.
- ***Adverse weather.*** A calf may be chilled or overheated before he can nurse.
- ***Birth space.*** Calves born in a crowded pen may not bond with the cow or may try to nurse the wrong cow and get kicked off.
- ***Cow's temperament.*** A cow may refuse to mother the calf.
- ***Human interference.*** If you are too quick to tag, give selenium injections, band bull calves, etc., you may upset a first-time, timid, or wild mama, so she doesn't mother the calf.

When first born, a calf can absorb large antibody molecules directly through the thin gut lining of the intestinal wall in a process called *pinocytosis,* which involves creation of a fluid pocket that aids movement of antibodies through the wall of the intestine and into the lymph system.

Years ago people thought a calf had 24 hours to absorb maternal antibodies, but studies showed that as soon as calves are born, the gut lining begins to thicken and the rate of pinocytosis decreases as the calf's age increases. He has maximum antibody absorption if he nurses within the first 15 to 30 minutes of life. By 4 hours of age, a calf has lost 75 percent of his ability to absorb them. Soon the antibodies destined to go through the gut lining can no longer get into the bloodstream to give protection against systemic illness.

The Antibody/Pathogen Race

A newborn calf's "open gut" allows not only antibodies to slip through, but pathogens as well. It is a race between pathogens and antibodies. Once he starts to nurse, gut closure is hastened. This is nature's way of insuring that nothing else slips through, such as bacteria or viruses, after he is up and sampling his new world. It helps if the cow is clean, rather than with teats covered in mud and manure. If cows must be in a corral to calve, use straw for bedding if conditions are wet, and keep udders and flanks clean. Otherwise the new calf will ingest a lot of pathogens in his attempt to find the teats and nurse.

Because of the newborn calf's open gut, make sure antibodies get there first. Colostrum stimulates systemic immunity when antibodies slip through into the circulatory and lymph system and go to all parts of the body. Other ingredients coat the gut. If the good guys in colostrum get to the gut first, they close the door to pathogenic organisms that the calf ingests in his first days, preventing penetration of the intestinal lining by bacteria and toxins. Absorption of antibodies hastens the thickening of the gut lining, further halting passage of bacteria through the intestinal wall.

There are also some immune-stimulating cells in colostrum (nonantibody immune cells) that help the calf's immune system mature and develop. Research has shown that without these cells to help stimulate his immune system, a calf is more susceptible to disease throughout his life than are calves that received adequate levels of these immune-stimulating cells via colostrum during the first minutes of their life.

Cow's and Calf's Health and Breed Make a Difference

Many factors can influence the quantity and quality of colostrum. These include age of dam, breed (beef cows usually have more concentrated colostrum than high-producing dairy cows), precalving nutrition, and precalving vaccinations. Undernourished cows have lower colostrum quality; an adequate protein level in the diet is necessary to create antibodies. Thin cows may give birth to weaker calves that don't get up as quickly or nurse as vigorously as they should, and the dams may have lower levels of antibodies.

Heifers tend to have fewer antibodies in colostrum than mature cows. Heifers are still young and growing, their bodies are still responding to new antigens, and even if they are vaccinated, they don't always respond to vaccine as well as an adult cow. A heifer's calf's immunity from her colostrum may start to wane after three weeks, whereas an older cow's calf may have good protection for a couple of months. Heifers have less colostrum, due to less udder development, and their calves may not absorb as many antibodies as necessary, if they are slow to nurse their mamas.

HOME COWS = HEALTHY CALVES

A cow raised on your own place has more immunity against the pathogens her calf will face than a pregnant cow you purchase and bring home from somewhere else. Precalving vaccinations can help, but home-raised cows give their calves the best protection against the pathogens on your place.

Cow/Calf Stress Affects Calf Health

Studies at Colorado State University showed that antibody levels obtained by calves at first nursing were much lower in calves that experienced a difficult birth, even when the cow was milked right after calving and the calf was force-fed colostrum. If a calf is short on oxygen during birth he may suffer temporary acidosis, which hinders the gut's efficient absorption of antibodies from colostrum. Thus, calves with prolonged or difficult delivery are more at risk for disease in the first weeks of life.

They are also more prone to digestive disorders and stomach ulcers. University of Nebraska studies showed that stress from a hard birth raises cortisol and other hormone levels in cows and heifers and in their calves too, because until a calf is born, his blood is affected by whatever is in the bloodstream of the dam. They found that higher blood levels of cortisol, *epinephrine,* and other hormones evident in calves born of stressed dams resulted in higher incidence of stomach ulcers and other digestive-tract disorders than in calves born to dams that were not stressed.

The Nursing Schedule

If a calf has not suckled within one hour of birth, help him nurse the cow or feed him fresh colostrum or a substitute, or milk the cow and tube the calf with her colostrum if he can't nurse. In the first nursing, a calf needs to consume about 5 percent of his body weight (1.5 quarts [1.4 L] for a 60-pound [27.2 kg] calf, 2 quarts [1.9 L] for an 80-pound [36.3 kg] calf, 2.5 quarts [2.4 L] for a 100-pound [45.4 kg] calf) and the same amount again six to eight hours later. Also keep in mind that stress can greatly shorten the window of time in which a calf can absorb antibodies. Cold weather, hot weather, a hard birth, and so on, make it even more imperative that you get colostrum into the calf immediately.

Make sure the calf is able to nurse again on his own, especially if you had to help him the first time. Calves usually load up on colostrum at their first nursing, instinctively gaining a high level of antibodies and sufficient nutrients and energy to get them off to a good start. They will nurse until they have completely drained the udder or are too full to consume any more. After that they usually buck around a little, then lie down to nap, getting up to nurse again six to eight hours later. A calf that wants to nurse sooner than that probably didn't get quite enough the first time. If a strong, healthy calf is not interested in nursing again until eight or nine hours later, he probably got an adequate amount.

Calves usually want to nurse about every 8 hours, and if you are feeding a newborn calf by bottle, or supervising the nursing if a heifer doesn't want him to nurse, make sure that he has his meals that often. Don't wait 12 hours; that's too long between meals for a newborn calf. Feedings during the first 24 to 48 hours should be from his own mother or should contain some colostrum even if you feed him yourself. One good feeding of colostrum is imperative, but continuing to get colostrum after the first feeding and through the first 24 to 48 hours is best, even if he must then go to regular milk or milk replacer because something happened to his mother or because she's a dairy cow.

MAKE SURE A CALF GETS HIS FILL OF COLOSTRUM IN HIS FIRST DAYS

Time Nursed	Size of Calf	Amount to Be Consumed
*Within first two hours**	60-pound calf (27.2 kg)	1.5 quarts (1.4 L)
	80-pound calf (36.3 kg)	2 quarts (1.9 L)
	100-pound calf (45.4 kg)	2.5 quarts (2.4 L)

**A newborn calf needs to nurse the same amount of colostrum as shown above 6 to 8 hours later. He will nurse three to four times in 24 hours, with the stretch in between nursings depending on the volume of colostrum consumed each time he nurses his mama.*

Don't wait 12 hours; that's too long between meals for a newborn calf.

Collect Colostrum for Emergencies

A cow with extra colostrum can be milked and the colostrum frozen for future use. Store it in small plastic containers (empty pint or quart tubs from margarine, whipped topping, or other grocery items). Or you can use ziplock freezer bags that store flat in your freezer (thereby taking up less space) and can be thawed more quickly in warm water. Label each container or bag with the date collected and the name of the cow it was collected from. Colostrum should be frozen quickly and kept frozen at low temperature.

The potency of frozen colostrum will be high for several years. When kept in a freezer a long time, it loses some of its antibody quality, but faced with a choice of using five-year old colostrum or none, use the old colostrum. It won't keep as well in a self-defrosting freezer as in an old-style freezer. The automatic-defrosting system may damage some of its protective antibodies and almost all the immune-stimulating cells during storage. In spite of this, most frozen colostrum collected from a beef cow with high-quality colostrum is more protective, even after freezing and thawing, than commercial colostrum substitutes.

Collect colostrum from a cow that has not already been nursed, or from an udder quarter the newborn calf has not sampled. Antibody levels are highest at calving and decrease rapidly after the calf nurses; any remaining colostrum is diluted with production of regular milk. Antibody concentration in the first milking or nursing is more than twice the level present in the second milking and more than five times higher than that in the third milking. The best and easiest time to obtain colostrum from a cow for freezing is when her calf is nursing for the first time. If she has an abundant supply, the calf won't be able to consume it all during his first nursing, and you can steal a quarter or two of her udder that he doesn't need.

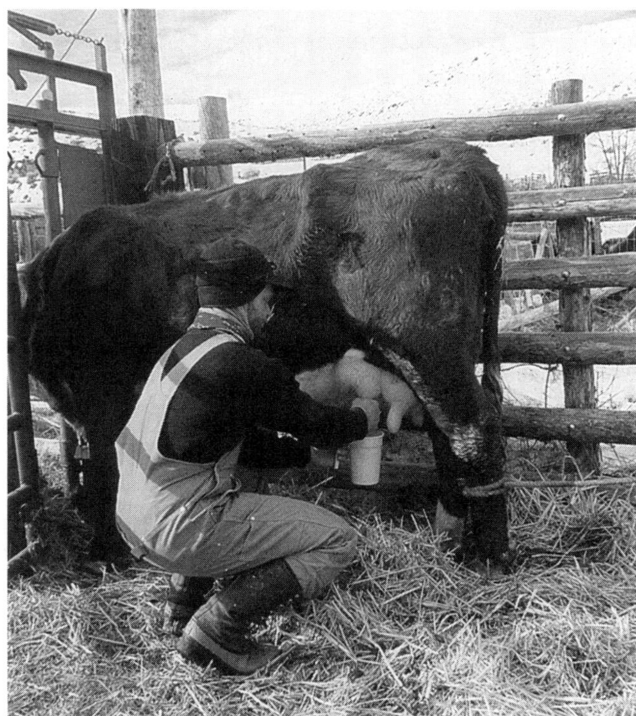

Milk extra colostrum from a cow that has more than her new calf can drink to freeze and save for emergencies.

Is It Good Colostrum?

You can tell if colostrum is high quality — containing lots of antibodies — just by the look and feel of it. Good colostrum is thick and yellow, with a slippery, waxy feel, and dries on your hands in thick flakes like wax. Poor colostrum has a thinner consistency, more like milk, and is not as bright yellow. It isn't as creamy; it does not contain as much protein, fat, and vitamins. If you put some in the refrigerator, because you know you'll need some soon and don't want to freeze and thaw it, good colostrum is almost all thick yellow cream, whereas poor colostrum or diluted colostrum will have only an inch or two (2.5 to 5 cm) of yellow cream that rises to the top.

MINE THAT LIQUID GOLD

Every year during calving season we milk colostrum from a few gentle cows or a cow whose quarter her calf didn't nurse. If you have to restrain a cow that's just calved and has extra colostrum, use this to your advantage and milk out some to freeze.

Colostrum Collection Made Easy

The easiest, quickest way to steal colostrum with the least stress to the cow or risk of spilling is with the Udderly EZ pump for mares, sheep, and goats. The trigger-operated pump has a flange that fits over the teat and a collection bottle beneath it, so the milk can't spill or get dirty. A few pulls on the trigger handle create a vacuum, and the milk flows into the collection bottle.

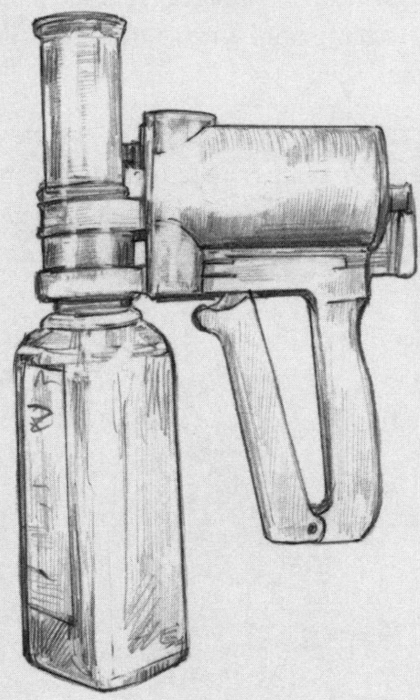

This hand-held pump is an excellent tool for easy colostrum collection from a nervous cow since it's much faster to use than collecting colostrum by hand. The cow does not have to stand still as long and there's no spilling if she moves around or kicks. It's also safer — you can stand or squat alongside the cow and reach to the udder with one hand, leaving the other hand free for fending off kicks or a quick escape. If the flow stops, squeeze the trigger a few times to create a vacuum. The bottle fills quickly, and when it's full you just unsnap it from the pump, and put a nipple on it to feed the calf, pour it into another container to freeze, or label and freeeze the collection bottle itself. You can order extra plastic bottles for this purpose.

Methods for Collection and Use

- If a cow is gentle and a good mama, she won't mind if you sneak up next to the calf and gently milk while he's nursing. Squat quietly right beside the calf, with him between you and her head so that when the cow reaches around to see what's going on she smells him, and she will be less apt to kick. She wants her calf to nurse and won't disrupt his nursing.
- Clean the udder with a warm damp cloth before you start milking, if the cow will tolerate it.
- Milk into a clean container. A small plastic pitcher is easy to hang onto with one hand while you milk with the other.
- Pour the milk into another clean container before your pitcher gets full, doing it in two or three increments, so you don't risk getting it all spilled if the cow kicks or bumps you.
- Freeze the colostrum as soon as possible.
- Thaw colostrum in warm 110°F (43.3°C) water (water that feels hot but not burning). Never use direct heat on a stove or in a microwave, or you risk destroying antibodies. Immersion in boiling water will destroy protein antibodies, as will defrosting it in a microwave at settings above 60 percent power.
- When thawing a container full of colostrum in warm water or on low-power microwave settings, stir the ice hunk around in the thawing colostrum frequently, to make sure it thaws quickly and that parts of it don't get too warm. It's faster if you froze the colostrum in flat plastic zip bags; the frozen chunk is not as thick.
- Never heat colostrum to more than 104°F (40°C). It should feel warm to your touch but not hot. Feed it to the calf at his body temperature (101 to 102°F [38.3 to 38.8°C]).
- When you feed the colostrum outside on a cold day, start with it a little warmer than body temperature so it won't get too cool. Or put the bottle in an insulated jug of warm water until you feed the calf.

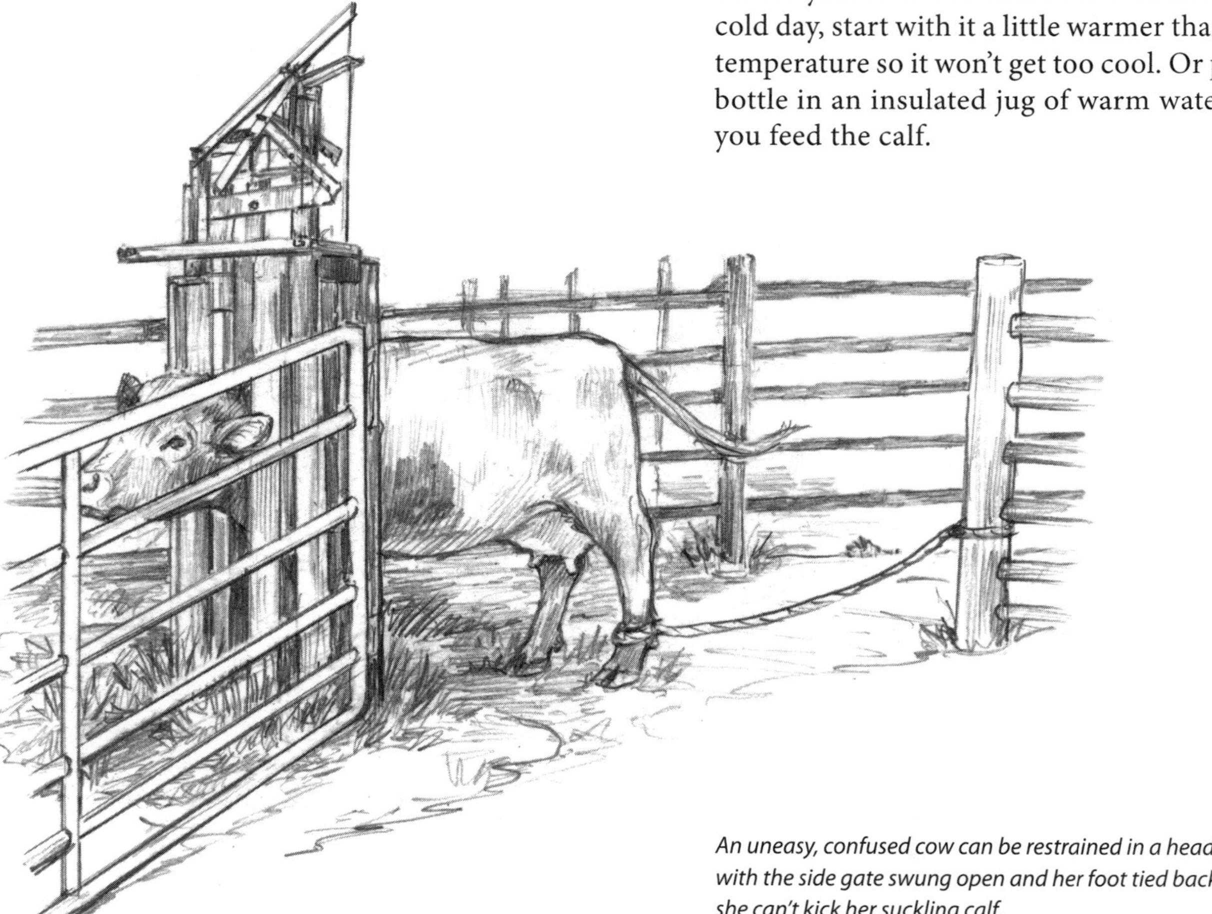

An uneasy, confused cow can be restrained in a head catcher with the side gate swung open and her foot tied back so that she can't kick her suckling calf.

- If you don't use colostrum you've thawed, don't refreeze it. It will keep a few days in the refrigerator in case you have another calf that might need it.

Getting Colostrum into a Calf That Hasn't Nursed

Make sure each calf nurses promptly after birth, especially in cold weather, before his mouth gets cold and he quits trying, or in hot weather, when he may quickly become stressed, lethargic, and dehydrated. If the calf is slow to nurse, help him.

When Udders Are Sore

Sometimes the cow or heifer is the reason a calf hasn't nursed. She might have a sore udder or frostbitten teats. A heifer may have some hard swelling *(cake)* in her udder, which causes it to be tender. If her calf tries to nurse, she kicks him. A heifer may be unsure about motherhood and won't stand still for the calf to catch up with a teat. If she's confused, she may bunt or kick him to keep him away from her udder. You'll have to restrain her to suckle the calf. Often, once the calf has nursed a confused heifer, she will mother him better and be less likely to kick; nursing stimulates production of hormones that encourage her to feel more motherly. If she continues to abuse her calf when he tries to nurse, keep her from hurting him until she accepts him (see chapter 8).

If a cow or heifer loves her calf but still kicks because of a sore udder, tie her to the stall or put her into a stanchion or head catcher to make it easier for the calf, or so you can help him figure out where dinner comes from. A head-catcher chute with a side or gate that opens will allow you to get the calf to her udder.

After the cow is restrained and you bring the calf up to her, she will often resign herself to standing still for nursing. If she continues to kick, tie her hind leg back on the side you are working. Put a double loop of rope around her leg, above the fetlock joint, using a half hitch. If you use only a single loop, or it gets below the joint, she may be able to kick out of it or shake the rope off. Tie the rope to something solid behind her and make sure there is enough slack that she can still put weight on that leg. Otherwise she'll keep kicking and fighting and may throw herself down and land on the calf or you. She needs enough slack to be able to stand comfortably but not enough that she can swing the leg far enough forward to kick you or the calf. After the first nursing, most cows will accept the calf. But if her udder is still sore, you'll probably need to hobble her until the udder is less tender.

Advantages of Sucking

When a calf nurses, the act of raising his head to the udder and sucking creates a reflexive action that makes a fold in the front part of the *reticulum* (the second stomach) that rolls over and forms a "tube." This becomes a temporary extension of the esophagus (the *esophageal groove*), which shunts milk directly into the *abomasum* (the fourth or true stomach) to be properly digested. If calves are given milk in ways that do not stimulate sucking action, the milk goes into the rumen, where, in an older calf with a functional rumen, much of the food value is lost because the rumen contains fermentation bacteria instead of the enzymes necessary for digesting milk. The rumen is designed for digesting forages, not milk.

One advantage to using an *esophageal feeder* probe rather than a stomach tube is that the latter tends to put the milk into the rumen. With an esophageal feeder, if you can hold the calf's head up in nursing position and stimulate a little sucking action with your finger in his mouth, the milk will go into the true stomach rather than the rumen. Colostrum can be given to a newborn calf using either method however, because the rumen in the young calf does not yet contain fermentation microbes that would hinder milk digestion.

Giving Substitute Colostrum

If the calf is unable to nurse because he's weak or cold, or his mouth and tongue are too swollen, give him warm colostrum via stomach tube or esophageal feeder. Use colostrum milked from his dam or from another source. This will give him the antibodies and nourishment he needs and will buy him some time for the swelling in his mouth to lessen.

Sometimes the calf's inability to nurse has more to do with the cow than the calf. An old cow or one with a hormone problem may not have milk, and you'll need to give the calf the colostrum he needs. A heifer might be flighty, and you don't want to upset her more by restraining her to milk her or suckle the calf, in case the calf might eventually catch up with her on his own after you feed him colostrum. By leaving the heifer alone, you won't interfere with bonding of Mama and baby. You can slip quietly into the pen or stall, feed the calf a bottle, and leave again; this won't upset the heifer as much as if you try to get colostrum from her. After drinking your bottle, the calf will have more energy and enthusiasm to keep trying to catch up with his mother to nurse.

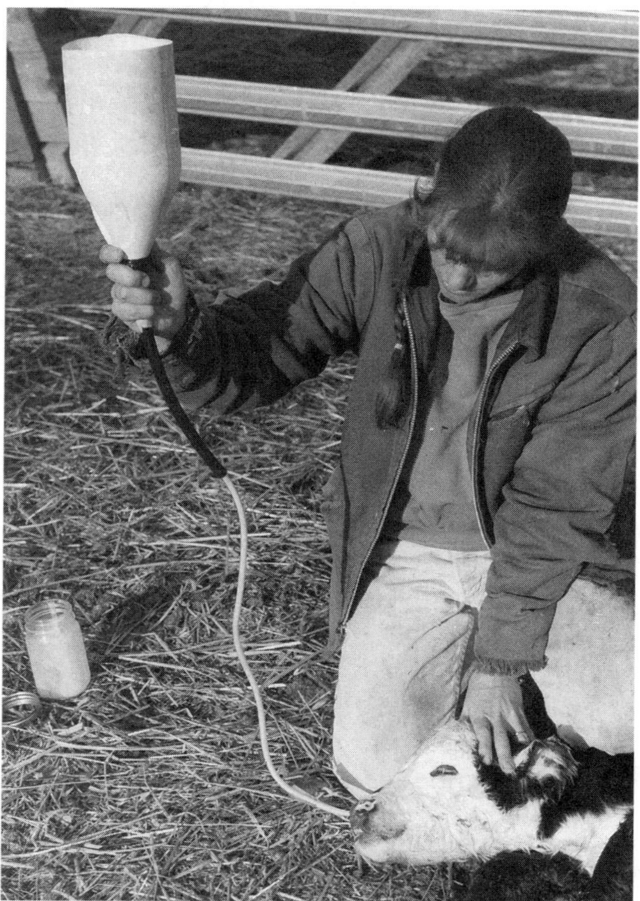

If a calf is weak, severely chilled, or unable to nurse his dam or suck a bottle for any other reason, give him colostrum via stomach tube or esophageal feeder.

Using a Stomach Tube

Substitute colostrum can be fed by nipple bottle, if the calf will suck, or with a *nasogastric stomach tube* or esophageal feeder. When using the nasogastric method, insert the long, flexible stomach tube into the calf's nostril five or six inches to the back of the throat, where it will be swallowed as you push it on down the esophagus and into the stomach. Make sure it goes into the stomach and not down the windpipe by blowing on your end of the tube. (For complete instructions, see chapter 11, page 240.) Attach a funnel to your end of the tube and pour in the colostrum. The nasogastric tube goes into the rumen and is ideal for giving fluids and medications to a scouring calf and getting gas out of a bloated calf but not as good for giving milk, which should not go into the rumen, where it cannot be digested. This is especially true for an older calf with a functional rumen but not as crucial for a newborn.

Using an Esophageal Feeder

An esophageal feeder is easier to use than a nasogastric tube. The feeder probe is a shorter, larger-diameter tube attached to a plastic container. The probe is put into the calf's mouth and moved to the back of his mouth, where he should swallow it as you gently put it on down his throat, into his esophagus.

There are several types of esophageal feeders available from your vet, feed store, or a mail-order supply catalog. They are made with a nonflexible hollow plastic or stainless steel tube (about ½ inch [1.25 cm] in diameter) with a larger-diameter (¾ to 1 inch [1.9 to 2.5 cm]) smooth bulb on the end that goes down the throat. A container for fluid is attached to the other end. Some feeders have a stopper or valve that keeps fluid in the container from entering the hollow feeding tube until you release it. Others have a container that hangs down until you are ready to administer the fluid; you raise it when you want fluid to go into the tube.

The rounded bulb on the end of the probe tube protects the mouth and throat tissues from being scraped or punctured, prevents backflow of fluids up the esophagus, and also helps the tube bypass the smaller opening into the windpipe as you are inserting it into the calf. The windpipe or trachea is below the opening into the esophagus. The latter is above

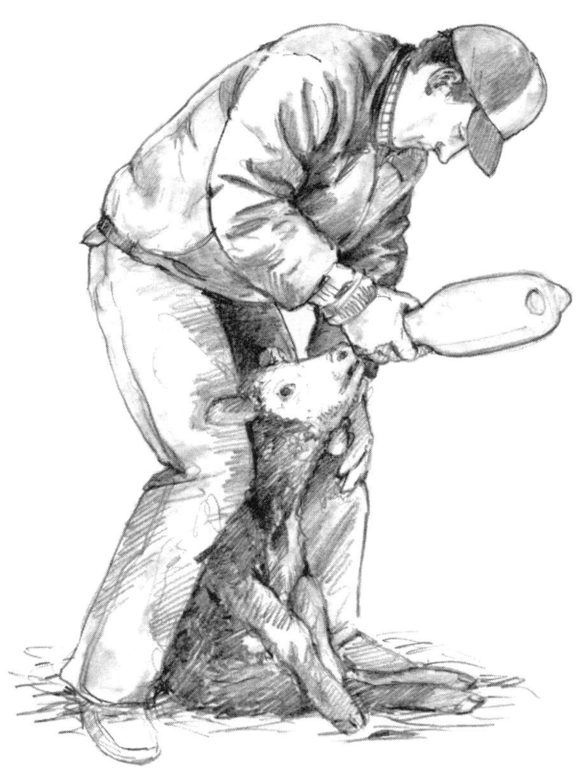

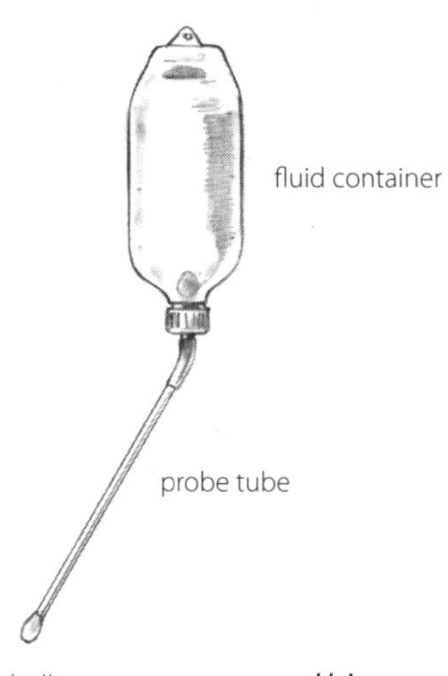

Using an esophageal feeder to force-feed colostrum to the calf. An esophageal feeder has a stainless-steel probe that you can move along the tongue to the back of the mouth where the calf will swallow it.

and slightly alongside the windpipe. You must not put any fluid into the windpipe or it will go into the lungs and drown the calf.

STEPS FOR USE

1. ***Make sure the esophageal feeder is clean;*** clean it thoroughly after each use and between calves.
2. ***Fill the holding container with colostrum*** or fluid (warmed to the body temperature of the calf).
3. ***If the calf is lying down,*** lift his head up to insert the tube.
4. ***If the calf struggles,*** restrain him by lifting the front of the calf up so he's sitting on his haunches.
5. ***Hold his head and neck between your legs*** (see illustration above). If the calf is standing, have someone hold his back end, or back the calf into a corner or against a fence or wall, step over his back, and pull his head up toward your body, with one hand under the lower jaw.
6. ***Gently put the feeder tube into the side of the calf's mouth*** — this is easier than trying to force it into the front of his mouth — and then slide it over the tongue to the back of the mouth and throat, where the calf should swallow it as you apply gentle pressure. You can feel and see the tube slip down the throat into the esophagus.
7. ***Stop pushing,*** and make sure it's in the esophagus by placing your hand over the front of the throat, where you should be able to feel the bulb end of the feeder through the calf's skin.
8. ***If you can see or feel the bulb in the throat,*** it is safe to continue pushing the feeder tube farther down. If you can't see or feel it, and the calf is coughing, it is probably in his windpipe instead of the esophagus. Take it out and start over.
9. ***Be sure it is in the esophagus*** and that the bulb end is down close to the stomach before you tip up the feeder container or release the fluid into the tube.
10. ***Hold the calf still and steady*** so that he can't struggle. You don't want to lose control of the calf, or the tube may come partway out and allow fluid to go accidentally into the windpipe and drown the calf.

When giving a newborn colostrum, give an adequate amount for the size of the calf (see box, page 152). A smaller amount can be used to stimulate the calf into getting up and nursing his mother or to make him more interested when you are trying to help him nurse his mother. Otherwise, give the full amount. Most normal calves have a strong suckle reflex soon after birth. If the weather is cold and you're not sure that the calf will nurse before he chills, you can give him a partial feeding just to make him eager for more and give him the energy to get up and go look for it. Giving him a bottle while he's still lying down does not confuse him nor interfere with his urge to seek the udder. He's not sure where that milk came from; he just knows he wants more — and he wants to find Mama.

Patience with First-Time Mamas

Sometimes a first-calf heifer is timid, confused, or not as motherly as an older cow. She may not lick her calf as quickly to dry him. In cold weather the calf may chill before he can nurse. We don't like to interfere with the bonding process of mother and calf with a first-time mama; rather than restrain her to get colostrum for her calf, we just feed him a bottle of colostrum before he gets up, then leave the pair alone so the heifer can finish mothering the calf.

Some heifers are unsure about this bumbling new baby "attacking" them. It takes a while for their mothering hormones to kick in.

The bottle-full allows the calf to take all the time he needs to get up and catch up with Mama's udder, and it gives him energy and antibodies he needs. It doesn't matter if it takes him a few more hours to get a complete nursing from mama. Some heifers are unsure about this bumbling new baby "attacking" them. It takes a while for their mothering hormones to kick in. Others are delighted and proud of their new baby and keep licking and licking, always facing the calf, never letting him get near the udder. Still others are sensitive about having the udder touched and keep moving away as the calf tries to nurse. Most calves persist and eventually zero in on a teat, especially if you've given them a bottle and they want more, and once the calf starts nursing, most heifers will settle down and stand still. Nursing triggers release of oxytocin, which stimulates maternal instincts and milk letdown.

Helping the Calf Find the Udder

If the weather is cold and we want to make sure a calf quickly accomplishes a complete nursing, we help him get to the udder. This is easiest with two people, especially with a timid heifer or a cow that might try to run off. One person can monitor the cow and keep her from moving away while the other person guides the calf. This doesn't work well in a large open area, where most cows or heifers will run off; only a gentle one that trusts you will stand patiently.

In a barn stall or small pen, however, one person can keep the cow in a corner by standing in front of her at a distance appropriate to keep her from running off but not so close that she feels trapped or threatened. A long stick or stock whip can be used as an extension of your arm, as a visual boundary to block her movements if she wants to move away. It can also be used to remind her to keep her attention on you if she thinks about becoming aggressive and bunting at the person who is helping her calf at the udder.

With quiet firmness, you can make almost any cow stand still while her calf is helped onto a teat, especially if she's a good mother and wants her calf to nurse. Her instinct is to get her calf nursing, to lick and point him at the udder. If the person helping the calf stays low and out of her main line of vision, keeping a mellow attitude — totally nonthreatening and not afraid, the cow won't worry too much. If you are the one helping the calf, keep him between you and the cow. Then when the cow turns her head to check what's going on at the udder, she sees and smells her calf; he's the closest thing, and she does not want to kick at him even if she'd like to kick you. If she gets no bad vibes from you, and you're not struggling with the calf or making her worry about him, she will accept what you are doing.

If she tries to smell you, raise your hand for her to sniff; it will be covered with the smell of her wet new calf, since you've been handling him. That will

A gentle cow will usually stand still and cooperate when you help guide her calf to a teat, since she wants her newborn baby to nurse. The cow usually won't protest or kick if you are quiet and keep a low profile, keeping her calf between you and her head, so she can smell him instead of you if she turns around to check on him.

usually satisfy her that you are not a threat. It's better to let her smell your hand, or jacket sleeve if it's covered with birth fluids, than some other portion of your body or clothing, which might worry her. Do *not* wear perfume, cologne, or a brand-new coat when working with cows, and do *not* have the smell of fried meat on your clothes or hair! As long as you smell familiar, like her calf, this puts her mind at ease. If the cow gets upset or tries to bunt you, the person watching her can draw her attention back with a slight movement of hand or stick.

Give a timid cow that's uncomfortable with having you that close or feels trapped in the corner a flake of alfalfa hay to eat while the calf is helped to nurse. This can settle her mind and give her something pleasant to do; she's more apt to tolerate the procedure and not run off. Keep everything quiet and calm, or you'll find it impossible to get her to cooperate. A gentle cow that knows you generally won't mind what you're doing and won't mind if you're talking, but with a timid cow or heifer, be completely quiet.

Handling Cranky Cows

An aggressively overprotective mother may not stand still and cooperate; she may be focused on chasing you out of the pen or stall. Decide whether you can safely make her behave using cow psychology or whether you should get colostrum into her calf another way. If he won't be able to nurse her before he gets cold or can't get on a teat because her teats are too large, figure out a way to feed him. In a pen or barn stall, you can grab the calf, with another person fending off the mean cow, and get him behind a fence or panel where you can safely feed him a bottle without the cow killing you. If he's out in a pasture, put him in the back of a pickup and feed him there.

Once he's had a good meal so that he won't get chilled, put him back with his mother, and he can nurse her next time he gets hungry. If the problem is big teats and he can't get on them, run the mean cow into a chute and restrain her while you help her calf nurse. Then be sure to sell her after she raises that calf.

The key to handling aggressive cows is to be dominant. They must respect you as they would a dominant herd member. We've had many aggressive cows but only a few that we had to sell because they were too dangerous. Most are smart enough to learn to let us handle their calves or help their calves nurse. To accomplish this you must have no fear of the cow. You also need a weapon; a stout stick to whack across her face if she tries to butt puts you in the position of "boss cow." All a dominant cow has to do to make another cow back off is shake her head and threaten. You don't need to use your weapon if a cow respects you as boss. Insist that she stand back while you iodine her calf or stand still and behave while her calf is helped to nurse.

HANDY HAME

WE LEARNED ABOUT AGGRESSIVE COWS in 1967 when we bought 40 pregnant Angus and crossbred heifers. Some were dangerous when they calved, especially as they got older and bolder with subsequent calves. It was a two-person job to iodine calves: one to iodine the calf and the other to beat off the cow with a stick.

Moosey had her third calf in the back stall of our old barn, which had been a garage/farm shop, with tools hanging on the wall. The amniotic sac didn't come off the calf as he was born. Lynn climbed over the partition into the stall to get the sac off so the calf could breathe, and to iodine the navel stump. Moosey lunged to her feet and charged before he could iodine the calf, pinning him against the wall. There was no way to escape; the back stall had three solid walls and a tall partition. She was pounding him with her head and might have killed him. Luckily there was an old hame — a metal "stay" from the collar of a work-horse harness — hanging on the wall above him. He reached up to grab it and whacked Moosey across the face with it. She backed off, and he got away.

From then on, we kept that hame handy and took it with us whenever we had to deal with an aggressive cow. The heavy metal hame was more effective than a stick; it could hit harder and never broke. It always changed a cow's mind if you hit her across the face or on a horn. It had a small metal ring on one end, and if you shook the hame at a cow, it rattled. We used it for many years as protection when handling aggressive mothers. Any mean cow we ever used it on knew the sound of that hame; all we had to do was rattle it, and she'd back off. It was our boss cow horn that gave us the psychological upper hand over wicked cows!

The person helping the calf at her udder must also be unafraid of the cow. If she senses fear, she'll turn around and try to butt that person. There is a fine line between firmness and excessive force. If you beat on a cow or yell, she'll become upset and will *not* stand still and may run over her calf. Quiet firmness works best. If a cow is totally unmanageable — on the fight, charging at you, and can't be handled when she calves — sell her. Some aggressive mothers become so overprotective that they lose their minds if you handle their calves and are a danger to anyone who comes near them. Some will actually trample their calves to charge at anyone who comes near.

Make sure that there are no dogs around when cows are calving or when you handle young calves. Cows instinctively want to chase away any canine to protect their calves. The presence of a dog, even some distance away, will disturb many cows and put them on the fight, making them so upset that they charge at you.

Tips for Helping a Calf Nurse

A calf's suckling reflex is strongest right after birth. If he doesn't nurse right away, he may lose that eager drive to nurse, making it more difficult to help him. If weather is cold and you want to make sure he nurses before his mouth gets cold, or it's hot and you want him to nurse before he becomes lethargic, feed him a little colostrum from a bottle even before he gets up, or very soon after, while he still has a strong instinct to nurse. If he's blundering around and hasn't found the udder yet (if he's going along the stall trying to suck on the wall or trying to suck the cow's brisket), aim him toward the udder and help him or stick a bottle in his mouth. Once he gets a few swallows he'll want more; it's easier to get him on a teat after he's had a taste.

Sooner Works Better than Later

A healthy calf will try to nurse on anything at first — your finger, a sleeve, whatever he can reach. This is the time to get him on the udder; don't wait until he gives up. If he's scared or stubborn when you try to guide him to the udder, or won't nurse when you stick a teat in his mouth because he's worried about what you're doing to him, milk a little from the cow into a bottle, with the calf standing by the udder so that the cow cooperates, and get him drinking from it. It's easier if he's reluctant to get some trickling down his throat with bottle and nipple than to force him onto a teat, especially if the cow is nervous.

Gently back him into a corner or have someone stand behind him and rub his back end while you get him sucking the bottle. Once he gets several swallows of colostrum, the lightbulb goes on in his brain — his stomach will tell him he needs more, and he'll want to nurse. After that, it's much easier to get him nursing a teat.

Don't Fight with Him

Some calves get distracted if you force them, or they get scared. Be very quiet and gentle. For a scared or reluctant calf, keep a low profile, and don't push him around. Take care how you get him to the udder; make it seem like his idea. If the cow is gentle and tolerates two people working with the calf, one can stay behind the calf to keep him from backing away from the udder, rubbing his butt (like Mama licking him). Vigorous rubbing of his back end, rather than pushing on him to hold him there, works best. Pushing against him just makes him instinctively back up even more. Rubbing his back end makes him think about nursing.

The person trying to get a teat in his mouth should not handle his head or mouth with too much forceful guidance, or he may resist. Just aim the teat into the mouth; slip it in with a finger. You want him thinking about milk, not defensive about what you are doing. Bull calves can be more frustrating and stubborn than heifers; they sometimes seem less "smart" — less eager and less focused on getting that first meal and surviving — so handle them carefully.

Fill Him Up

Make sure that the calf gets full. If he sucks one quarter and can't see how to get on another teat, slip another one into his mouth. Nature's plan is to have him ingest as much colostrum as he can hold for optimum antibody absorption and passive transfer of immunity. If necessary, help him get on each teat to suck, until he's no longer interested. A big bull calf, not generally as lively as a heifer, may get tired before he gets full; it could be hard for him to stand up that long. He may want to lie down partway through nursing and then will be hungry and more willing to try again after he's had a rest.

Even if you have to keep putting a teat into his mouth because he can't get back on it himself when he loses it, make sure you let him try on his own once he's had a taste. He must learn how to get on a teat by himself. A new calf's brain is like a sponge soaking up all new experiences; he learns very quickly by doing. He needs to learn how to maneuver his mouth and tongue to get hold of the teat. If you always stick it in his mouth when he loses it, he won't learn how to grab it — pick it up with his tongue — and get it into his mouth by himself. If the cow's teats are long or big, they can be hard for him to grab, but he must learn how to maneuver his tongue to get hold of them. Otherwise, you'll be helping him again the next time he tries to nurse. If the teats are big, however, help him get onto each one of them at least once, so they'll be a little smaller and easier to get into his mouth the next time.

MAKE SURE THE TEAT FLOWS

If the weather is cold, the end of the teat may be scabbed over. And sometimes the plug does not come out of the teat readily. You may have to give the teat a hard squeeze (and the cow may try to kick you!) to get it started so the calf can nurse.

Make Sure He Can Do It Himself

If the cow is uncooperative, or her teats are long or big (a pendulous udder low to the ground), or the calf is functionally slow for some reason, you'll probably have to help him nurse the first time. If you aren't sure he can get on teats by himself next time, check back in 6 to 8 hours. During his first days of life, a calf will nurse three to four times in 24 hours. If he's a big strong calf and nursed a lot the first time,

Help a Big Baby Nurse

This big, tall calf was clumsy and couldn't find the teats. The cow's udder is a little low and the teats are a little long, so the calf needed help to learn how to bend his head down.

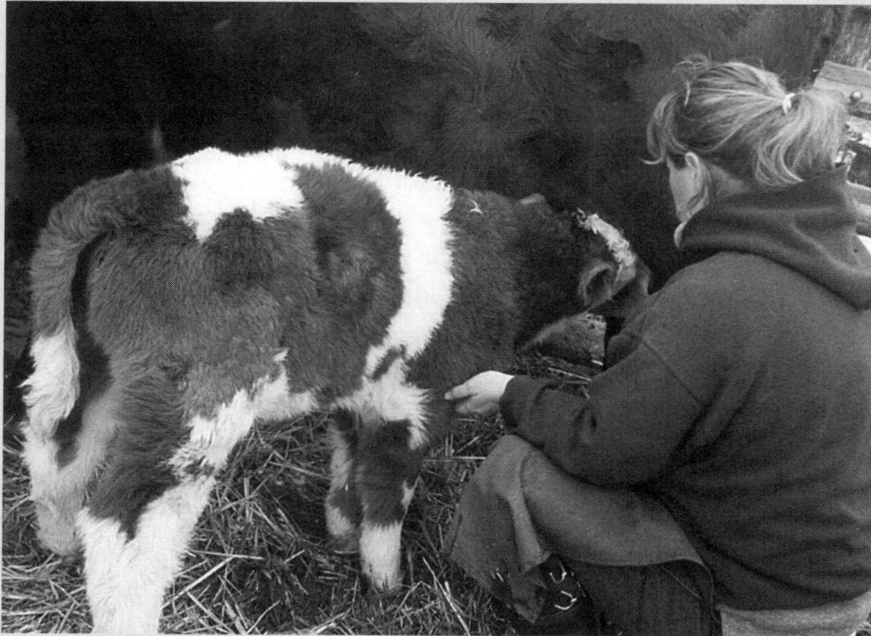

Gently guide a big, clumsy calf to the teat.

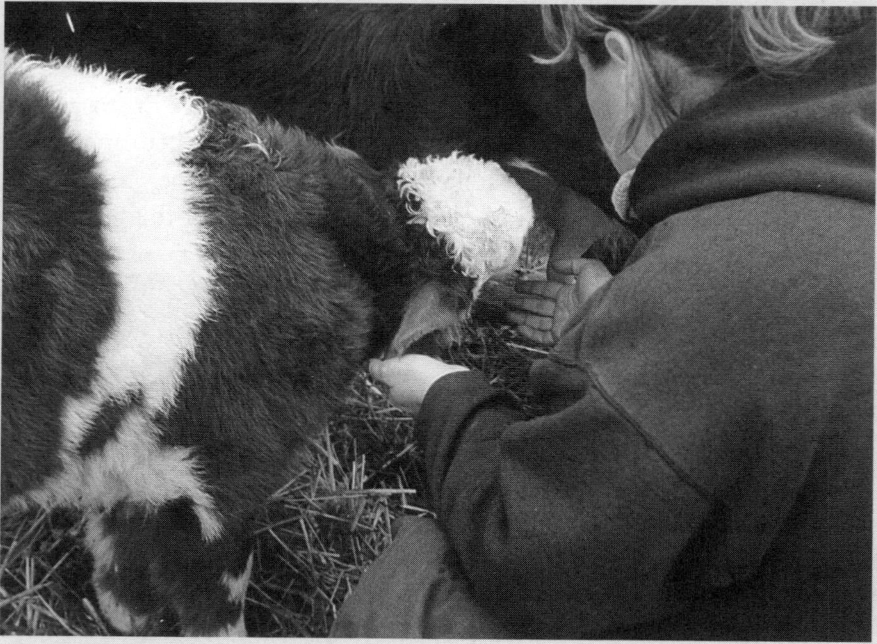

After he has had a taste of the colostrum, make sure the calf can get onto a teat by himself.

he may not be hungry again for 8 or 9 hours. But if he didn't get quite full, he'll be hungry sooner. If he got tired before he filled up, or the cow didn't have as much colostrum as he could hold, or he was only able to get on one or two quarters, he'll be trying again in a few hours. Observe him when he does, to see whether he can do it himself this time.

When you check, help him only if he's willing and hungry. It has to be his schedule, not yours. Wait until he's eager again or he won't be interested, and you'll be wasting your time and becoming frustrated by his lack of willingness. If he's lying down when you check on him and the cow has obviously not been nursed again (she has a full udder), and you're not sure whether he's hungry yet or not, get him up and aim him toward the cow. Stand back and watch for a moment, to see if he wants to nurse. He may have tried and given up when you weren't there, or he may not be hungry yet.

If he still can't get on teats himself and waits for your help, go ahead and help him, but let him "practice" after you get him started; see if he'll try to get on a teat by himself. If he can't, you'll have to keep putting the teats in his mouth to make sure he gets enough. After the second assisting, however, let him get hungrier before you offer to help him again. If he gets hungry enough and desperate enough, he'll be more determined and work at it more diligently — and finally figure how to get on the big or long teats himself. If a cow has a bad udder, decide whether to resign yourself to helping her calves every year, or sell her. Don't keep any heifer calves from her, because they may have bad udders, too! Never keep a bull calf from her; daughters of a bull tend to inherit his dam's udder characteristics.

Working with a Wild or Scared Calf

If the newborn calf is getting up for the first time when you help him nurse, he'll usually be cooperative because he isn't very frightened. Usually a calf accepts whatever he sees right after birth, bonding with you as he would his mother, although a few calves are "wild" and afraid of you from the start. If the first time he sees you is after he's an hour or two old, he may be afraid of you. Ideally, by then he will have nursed and bonded with his mother, and everything is fine. If you have to catch him to iodine his navel stump or do anything with him at that point, some calves are very wild; their instinct to escape predators has taken over, and they consider you a threat.

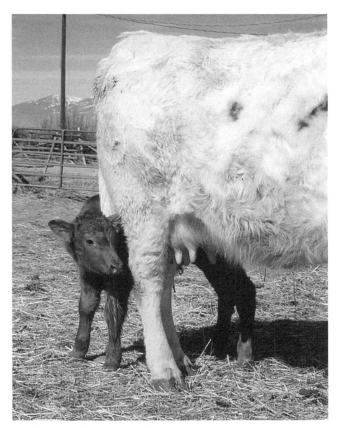

This newborn calf is looking for the udder but hasn't nursed yet; all four teats and quarters are still full.

Make Sure He Actually Nursed

Sometimes you come upon the cow and calf and aren't sure how old he is or if he's nursed. Ask yourself the following questions, and look for clues to help you make this determination.

Is the cow's udder still full? If all her quarters were full before calving, and one or more quarters are now slack and empty or the whole udder is empty, that's an obvious sign that the calf has nursed. The teat or teats he nursed should be smaller and maybe still damp and wrinkled. A full, dry, smooth teat has not been nursed.

If the cow is lying down when you check her, and you look at her udder as she gets up, it may be deceptive. The side she lay on may look smaller (teats shrunken) just because she was lying on them, and there was pressure against those teats or quarters. If you look at her again in a few minutes, it will be easier to tell if any quarters or teats are actually smaller; the teats that had the milk pressed out of them will have filled back up.

Some udders are hard to decipher, but if you're aware of what they looked like just before calving, you can usually tell if the calf has nursed. Make note, however, of any cow that has "lost" a quarter due to mastitis or some earlier problem. Otherwise you might think her calf has nursed because that quarter is slack and empty, when it actually had no milk to begin with.

Did he suck or just smack? On occasion when you observe a calf trying to nurse (when you peek into the barn to see if he got up and is doing okay), you'll hear "smacking" noises as the calf is busy at the udder, and you'll think he's nursing. This is usually a good sign, but on occasion it can also mean the calf is still learning how to handle his mouth and tongue, not sucking efficiently yet. He may be sucking his tongue or the side of a teat, making sucking sounds but not actually getting any milk from the udder.

Did he draw colostrum from the teat? If the weather is cold, the cow's teats may be sealed, with scabs from frostbite. Even if a calf sucks vigorously, he may not get the scab off or the plug out of the end of the teat; the quarter is still full even though the teat's been sucked. If he's actually getting milk, you should see evidence of that. There should be milk foam at his mouth or some milk dribbling down his chin and throat. If you watch closely, you'll see him rhythmically swallowing. Another clue is his tail wagging like a windshield wiper. A nursing calf has a happy, active tail. If you can't get close enough to see without disturbing the pair, or the calf is doing a lot of bunting or changing from teat to teat rather

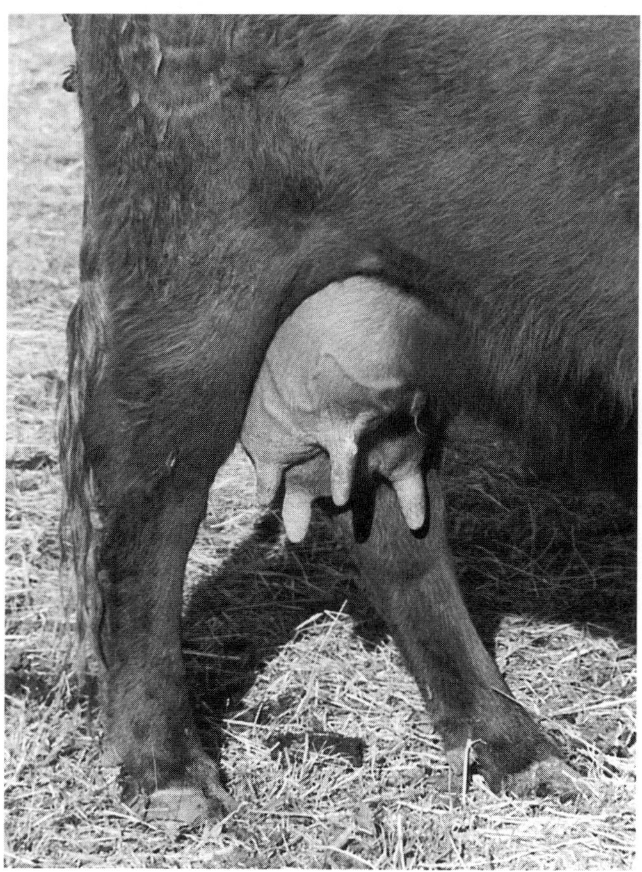

This udder shows evidence that the calf has not sampled the full quarters on the far side, where the teats are still big. He has suckled the teats and quarters on the near side; these teats are smaller and the quarters are empty.

Another Clue to Colostrum Consumption

Sometimes if we're not sure a calf has nursed, we try to give him a bottle. If he adamantly refuses, spitting out the milk like we're trying to poison him, this often means he's already had a taste from Mom and doesn't like the taste of ours. Even if it's colostrum that we got from her, he may not like the feel of a bottle nipple once he's been on the real thing.

The milk from Mama is the perfect temperature and the perfect taste, and the feel of Mama's teat in his mouth leaves an impression in his mind about what mealtime should be. The act of nursing has created a bond between cow and calf, and now that he knows what her udder is like, he is less apt to accept a substitute bottle.

Also, if he ingested a fair amount of colostrum from Mama, his hunger switch may be turned off and he won't be interested in any more food for a while. However, if he's still hungry and hasn't had much — or any — from Mama, he'll usually suck a bottle eagerly.

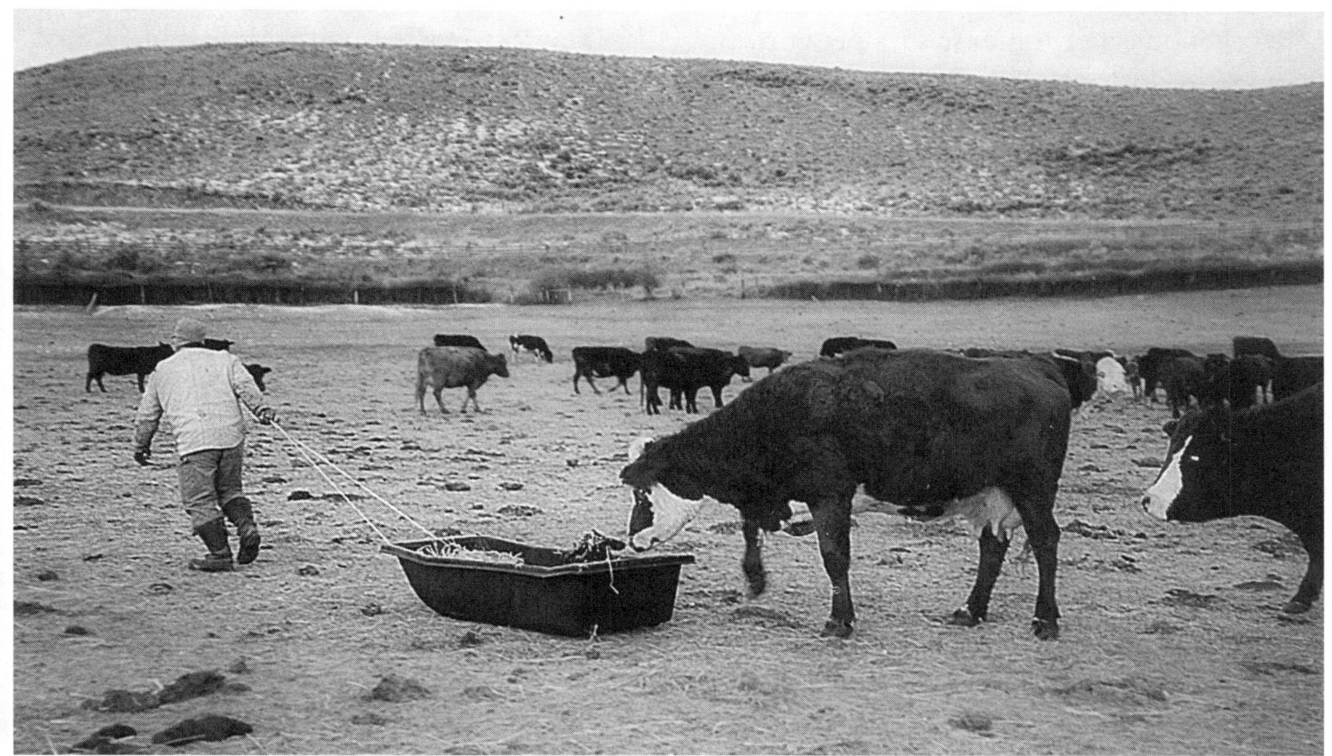

Bringing in a new calf from the field on a cold morning in a plastic calf sled, with the cow following, sniffing and licking him along the way.

than staying latched on, or the udder still seems full afterward, or the calf still seems hungry, check more closely.

Tips for Transporting Newborn Calves

If a calf is born in a field and you must bring him and Mama to a barn or pen, the cow will usually follow whether you are pushing and guiding a calf that can walk, or carrying a calf that can't walk. She may be confused, however, if you put him in the back of a pickup and may run back to where she had the calf. She follows her calf by scent rather than sight; smell is how she determines that it's her calf. If you carry her calf, most cows follow, but some will be confused because the calf is up off the ground. It's interesting to watch a cow following the person carrying her calf; the calf's scent seems to drop to the ground because many cows will come sniffing along behind, smelling the ground. If the cow is confused, however, you may have to put the calf down a few times so she can come up and smell him again, to know you have him.

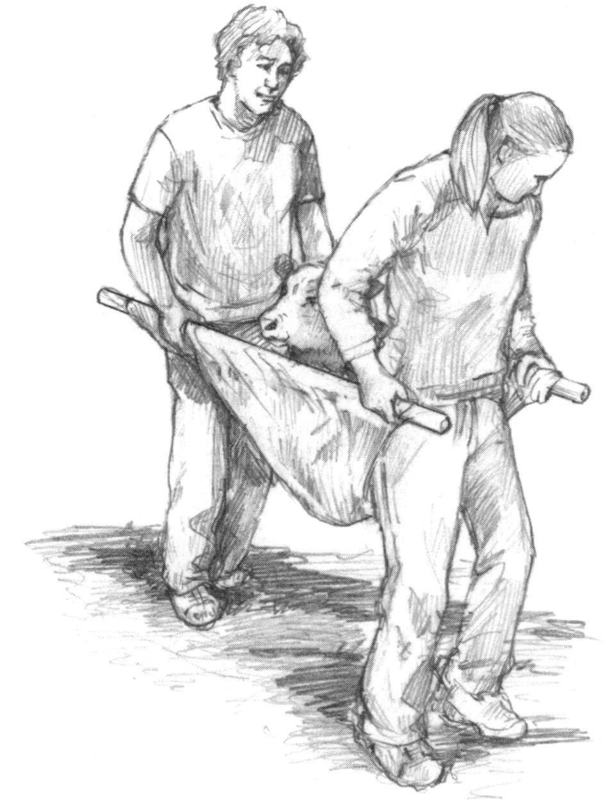

A calf sling is an easy way for two people to transport a newborn calf. Use a tarp, blanket, or rug folded over and tied to two broomsticks or shovel handles.

It's most effective to transport a newborn calf on a low sled or cart, pulled by hand or a four-wheeler, so the cow can follow and smell him. It rarely works to lift him off the ground to a pickup. Another way to carry a calf if you don't have a sled or cart is to make a stretcher with a rug, blanket, or tarp folded over small poles or shovel handles, carrying the calf between two people. If he's a big calf, this method is often easier than one person trying to carry him.

Cold-Weather Calving

If you calve in late winter or early spring, there are times Mother Nature makes it difficult. Even if your region usually has good weather, a freak storm may make your job harder or put newborn calves at risk. For instance, a multiday storm in late April put down two feet of snow one year in Nevada in a region where April is usually mild and ranchers calve without barns or shelters. But that year hundreds of newborn calves died. Ranchers put calving cows in every sheltered spot, such as haystack yards, for windbreaks but still lost many calves.

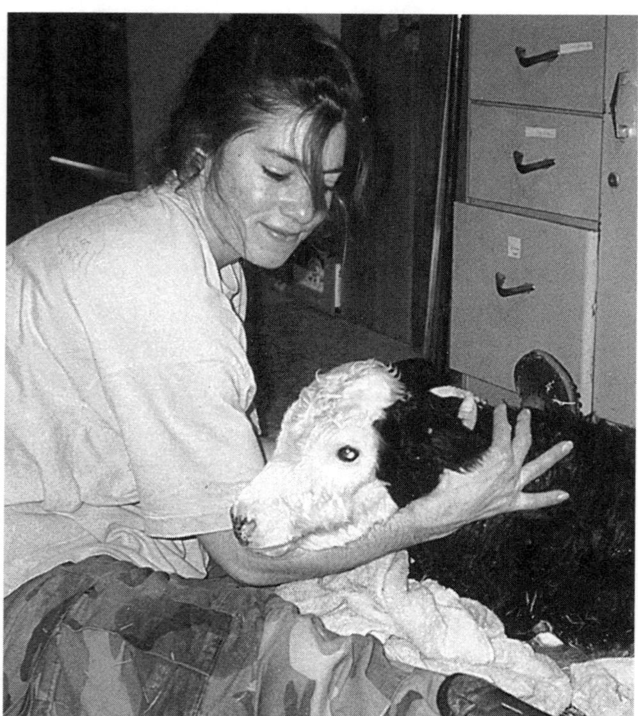

Daughter Andrea dries a newborn calf in our kitchen. Over the years we've dried many calves in our house during cold weather.

Lynn and I calved our herd in January for 35 years, with barns for calving cows, since it could be 30 below zero in our mountain region. It was labor-intensive, but we never lost a calf to freezing. Over the years, we saw many ranchers in our valley lose calves to cold weather during spring, when temperatures are generally milder, because they didn't have barns. A storm or cold spell in late February or March can wipe out many calves if it hits at the peak of someone's calving season and they don't have adequate shelter for new babies.

Over the years, we've taken care of thousands of calves during cold weather but haven't lost any to the cold, thanks to diligence and good facilities (see chapter 10). When we started on our ranch in 1967, the cows we bought calved in spring and summer. We shortened calving season to March and April, the traditional season in our part of the country because most ranchers have cows calved before they go to summer range on Bureau of Land Management (BLM) and Forest Service pastures in the mountains. But March and April are usually wet and muddy, triggering illness in young calves due to wet-weather stress and contaminated fields. We spent a lot of time doctoring sick calves those first years and lost some to scours until we learned how to be better calf doctors (see chapter 11).

So we decided to put the bulls in earlier and calve earlier — in January, when there are few wet storms and the ground usually stays frozen with temperatures that dip to 30 or 40 below zero Fahrenheit (–34.4 to –40°C). The calves stayed healthier, however, in the dry cold of January than in the wet mud of March. If you protect calves for a few hours after birth, they handle cold weather better than wet weather. Calves arriving in January have their winter coats — thick, long hair that gives good

TOTS CHILL FASTER

A small calf can freeze to death in cold weather more quickly than a larger one; body heat is lost faster from the smaller calf. A small body has more surface area per unit of body weight. In the larger calf it takes longer for internal temperature to cool to below viable limits.

protection against cold. Once they are dry and have nursed, they handle cold weather very well if they can get out of the wind.

We traded mud for cold. Labor-intensive calving (making sure that every calving cow was put into the barn, drying calves with towels if necessary) was preferable to labor-intensive doctoring. We cut our birth losses to almost zero by being there for every birth, able to help with any problems that might arise, and we eliminated losses from scours. We still treated a few sick calves, especially during wet years, but having the ground — and manure — frozen most of the time when calves were young dramatically cut down the incidence of sickness. Cold-weather calving has its challenges, however, and we brought many calves into the house to dry by the woodstove. One of the first times we brought a calf into the house to dry and warm him, we left the young mother, Grendel, in the calving pen near the house. She didn't like our stealing her baby and jumped into the yard to look in the window. We quickly ran outside to put her in the barn, so she wouldn't jump through the window and into the house!

We built another calving barn so that we'd have enough barn space for every calving cow: shelter for the first 12 to 24 hours of each calf's life, until the calf was dry and had nursed a few times.

As our cow numbers increased, we started putting cows into the barn to calve, checking them frequently to keep track of labor, to make sure we were present at births, rather than carrying new calves to the barn from the calving pens. We built another calving barn so that we'd have enough barn space for every calving cow: shelter for the first 12 to 24 hours of each calf's life, until the calf was dry and had nursed a few times.

For 20 years, we had no heat in our barns other than the body heat of the cows, which, in that enclosed area, always kept the barns at least 20 degrees warmer than outdoors. If it was subzero weather outside and only 5°F in the barn, we often dried a new calf with

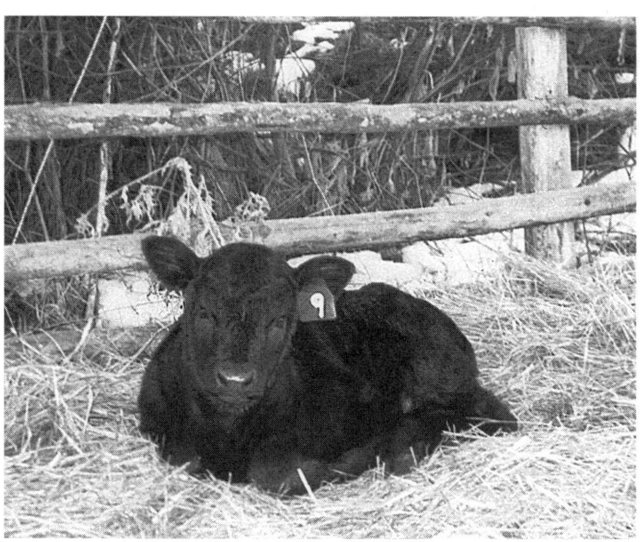

Once a new calf has nursed and is dry, he can handle cold, dry weather.

OUR CHOICE: COLD-WEATHER CALVING

MY FIRST EXPERIENCE with cold-weather calving was in March 1960, when I was in high school. My dad's cows were calving, and it was unusually cold that year. He drove into the fields at night, warming newborns in our old Jeep's cab with the heater going. We put calves in a shed to dry them before putting them back with their mothers. We put some of the calving cows into our haystack yard, out of the wind.

When we had to go to my grandfather's funeral in south Idaho that winter, a neighbor did our feeding and looked in on our herd for us. But he was busy with his own calving and couldn't spend nights at our place. Temperatures dipped to 30 below zero (–34.4°C). When we got home, four newborn calves had frozen to death. That tragedy stuck with me. I vowed that I'd never let that happen if someday I had cows of my own.

Here in central Idaho, weather is fickle. Though rare, we've had temperatures of 30 below zero in March, and three feet of new snow in April. My husband and I preferred calving early and being prepared for the worst rather than calving in the spring, in the fields with scanty protection for calving cows and their young calves.

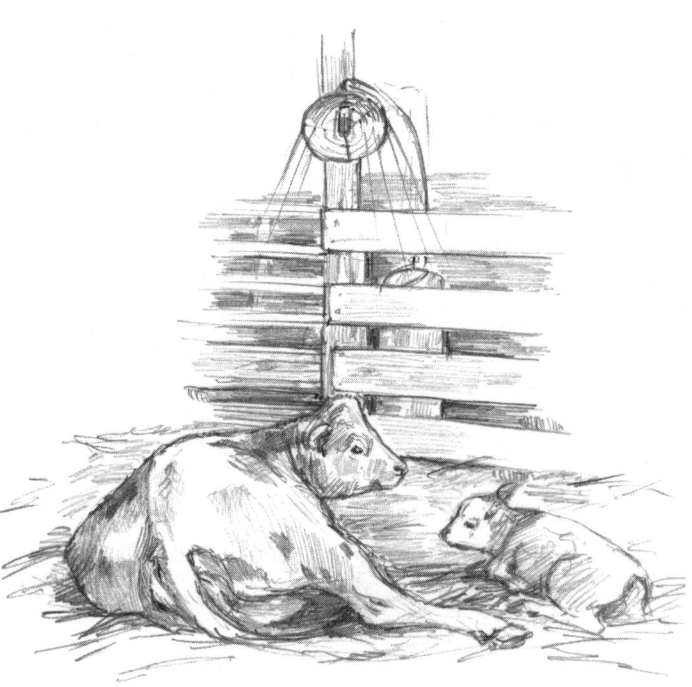

With caution, a propane space heater can be used in a barn stall to help warm and dry a newborn calf in cold weather.

towels. After one very cold winter (-40°F in January), we put a wood stove in each barn, but we used them only a few times.

There are many ways to dry and warm newborns: a stove in the barn, a space heater in a stall, makeshift thaw boxes with heat lamps, or commercial thaw boxes, which are often safer. You don't want a cow or calf knocking a heat lamp into the straw and burning down the barn.

Our son and his wife camp in an old trailer house at our place to calve their cows, and put chilled calves by the woodstove, where they dry them with towels and hair dryers. Frozen tails can be dipped into a jar of hot water. Frozen ears can be thawed instantly with a hot wet washcloth. Some people use a calf jacket and ear muffs made of insulating material that hold in the calf's own body heat. If no body heat escapes, the calf eventually warms up. However, immersion of all but the calf's head in hot water is the speediest way to warm a really cold calf and get his core temperature back up to normal quickly.

EMERGENCY THAW

SOMETIMES we don't get a cow into the barn in time and a calf is born outside, which necessitates intensive drying and thawing. Beautiful Eyes calved on ice by the creek, and we struggled to get the calf to the house on a sled. Lynn had broken his foot and was on crutches; he wasn't able to help except to defend me against the indignant cow. Beautiful Eyes was a purebred Hereford with lovely horns, and Lynn broke one of his crutches over her horns when she tried to halt our calf-snatching.

It was a challenge to get the calf out of the field. I pulled the sled and tried to keep the calf from flopping while Lynn beat on Beautiful Eyes with his crutch as she ran round and round us, trying to butt us with her horns. We finally got through the gate — had to slam it in her face — and dragged the calf into the house and bathtub, where we thawed him out.

We thawed a few calves in the bathtub in very warm water — the fastest way to warm a chilled calf. Quicksie also calved on ice by the creek on a cold night, and her calf was so cold that he had to go into the bathtub.

We overdid the bath on Freckles's calf, born at 40 below zero during the winter of 1978–79. It was so cold that the cows didn't lie down; they stood huddled together in the calving pen for warmth. We walked through them every 30 minutes to put any calving cows into the barn, but it was hard to tell when they were in labor since they didn't move much or lie down to calve until the very last minute.

Freckles showed no signs of labor at one check and had calved 30 minutes later; the new calf was freezing to the ground. We grabbed him and rushed him into the house and bathtub to thaw him out. His ears and tail were already frozen solid. But we bathed and toweled him dry so thoroughly before taking him out to the barn stall where we'd put his mother that we washed all his smell off. Though she had been a good mother to previous calves, she did not recognize this one as her own. We had to tie her up to make her stand still so that we could help him nurse. It was two days before she accepted him as hers.

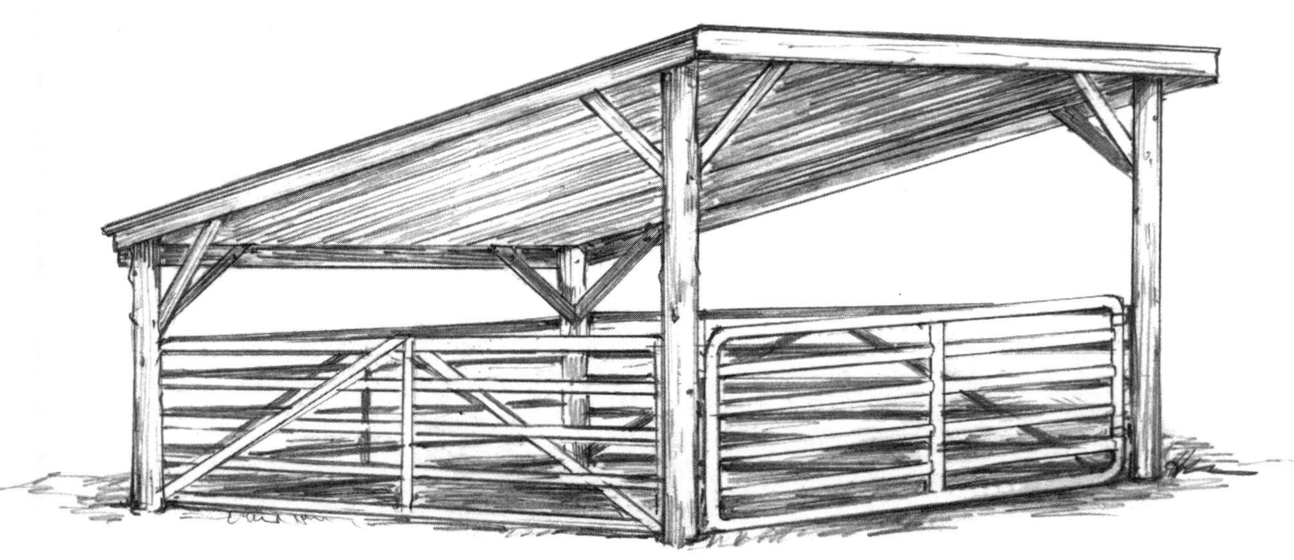

A calving shed for hot weather provides shade and also allows for ventilation.

Hot-Weather Calving

When calving in summer or early fall, a heat wave can be deadly for young calves. During the summer of 2006 in California, temperatures stayed over 100°F (38°C) for several weeks. Hundreds of dairy cows died, and many young calves succumbed to heat and dehydration. A newborn or young calf doesn't have the body mass and reserves of an older, larger animal and is very susceptible to dehydration. When it's hot, a calf doesn't feel like nursing and may not get the necessary colostrum or enough fluids to keep from being dehydrated. The problem is compounded if a calf is sick and losing fluid through diarrhea.

In hot weather, make sure calving cows and young calves have shade. Heat stress takes a severe toll on young calves. The color of a calf makes a difference. A black calf in a pasture with no shade and no breeze at 100°F (37.8°C) or higher may be unable to handle it.

Shade is just as important for warm-weather calving as shelter is in cold weather. Animals constantly exposed to sun get hotter than those with access to shade. If you don't have natural shade — brush and trees — make a series of shed roofs. The roof must be at least 10 feet (3 m) off the ground; 15 feet (4.6 m) is better, to allow plenty of airflow underneath so that a breeze can help to cool the animals.

Natural air movement under a roof is affected by the height, size, slope, and ease with which air can move through (no solid walls). Shade cloth has an advantage over a solid roof: Air passes through the material. A sloping roof provides better ventilation than a flat one. Solar radiation causes air directly under a roof to get hotter than surrounding air, and it rises. This air buoyancy creates air movement under a sloping roof by allowing the hot air to slide upward on the inside of the slope. As this air moves up, it drags cooler air in from the sides. The rate of upward movement depends on the slope of the roof and the smoothness of the material. A slope of 18 degrees works adequately on a small structure, and a 10- to 15-degree slope will have a similar effect in larger structures.

If it's extremely hot, a barn stall with fans can help to keep a calving cow or newborn calves from overheating. In a pen, you may have to find another way to cool cattle — put up shade or use sprinklers to spray them with a mist of water. For baby calves, heat stress can be just as deadly as cold stress.

INSULATE ROOFS FOR HOT WEATHER

A solid roof should be insulated, especially if it's metal or dark-colored, or it'll produce more radiant heat and become oven-like. A light-colored roof reflects sunlight and stays cooler underneath.

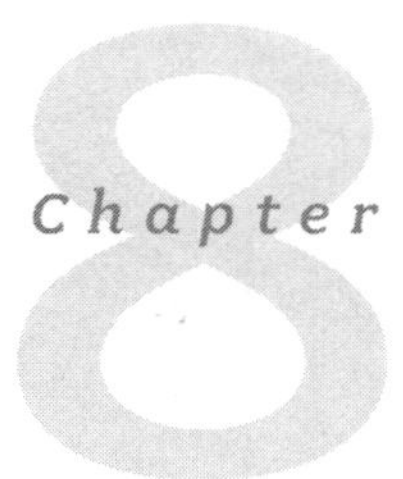

Chapter 8

Reluctant Mamas

Occasionally you encounter a cow or heifer that doesn't want her newborn calf. Usually it's a first-time mother. An experienced mama is generally a good mama, unless she was a poor mother the first time and her maternal instincts are once again slow to kick in. Most reluctant mamas change their minds in a day or so, start to love the calf, and are good mothers from then on. But a few seem to have a hormonal deficit. Even though you persuade them to mother the calf this year, they are just as stubborn with their fifth or sixth calf as they were with their first.

Nevertheless, learning to coax a cow or heifer to love and care for her baby right at the start will pay off in well-bonded, relaxed cow-and-calf pairs that are healthy and happy. And bonded pairs will take up less of your time and energy in the long run. If Mama will raise the baby, you won't have to bottle-feed him for the next four months!

Heifers Unsure about Motherhood

Some heifers are indifferent and hardly notice that they've calved. They may continue to lie there, not bothering to get up to lick the calf, or seem surprised to see these strange wiggling creature behind them. A heifer may walk away, ignoring the calf, or kick him when he gets up and staggers toward her.

If a heifer is not interested in her calf, help him to nurse her. The act of nursing tends to make her feel more motherly. If you can help the calf to nurse the indifferent heifer a time or two, she may decide that she likes him after all. You'll need to restrain her, at least the first time, so that she won't run off or kick the calf.

She's very interested in her calf; her instincts tell her that this is something important and that she must deal with him, but she's not sure how.

Heifers Strongly Opposed to Motherhood

If a heifer is stubborn about accepting her new calf or even viciously attacks him, you must keep her from killing or injuring him. If she's in a stall or pen, she may slam him into the wall or fence. In a big open field she may walk away from him, tired of rooting him around and knocking him down, but in a confined area she may just keep beating on him.

Sometimes it's hard to tell if a new mother is overly motherly or a calf-killer. She's very interested in her calf; her instincts tell her that this is something important and that she must deal with him, but she's not sure how. She smells him, starts bellowing and rooting him around — butting him if he moves or tries to get up. She may knock him down when he tries to stand. She's on the fight, ready to protect this new calf from anything and everything, but she's confused and focuses her aggression toward

EARLY EXPERIENCE WITH UNMOTHERLY COWS

THE 40 HEIFERS we bought in 1967 were Angus and crossbreds, and a high percentage were quite messed up about motherhood. They came from a feedlot, and we wondered if a growth stimulant had somehow hindered their hormones. Most behaved more normally the next year, but several did not improve whatsoever. At that time in our ranching career we didn't have the experience to know how to deal with them.

When one heifer tried to kill her calf, our vet suggested using tranquilizers, prompting us to name her Tranquiliza. She still kicked the calf; however, she just went about it a bit more slowly. We left her tied in the barn for several days and helped the calf nurse. She finally accepted him but was an indifferent mother the next three times she calved (we had to restrain her for nursing each time), so we sold her.

Even worse was Hilda, who tried to kill her calves three years in a row. We raised her first calf on a heifer that had lost her own. In our naive thinking we felt that we'd "messed her up" with too much human intervention, so we let her calve in a mountain pasture the next year. We never found the calf. We think that she either killed him or left him to die. The third year she calved in the corral, and we ran out there when we heard her bellowing. The only thing that saved the calf was that she pushed him under the fence where she couldn't reach him to kill him. We sold her and raised the calf on another cow.

him. Some breeds, including Angus, are notorious for bellowing and rooting their calves around when they give birth, especially the first time.

Usually, if you stay out of sight while you monitor the situation, the heifer will get it figured out. If she's furiously licking the calf and mooing at him even as she knocks him around a bit, she's going to be a good mother. She just needs a little time to transmit all of that motherly attitude in the right direction — to encourage him to the udder instead of rooting him around so harshly that he can't get up off the ground.

By contrast, if a heifer is *not* licking her calf and is knocking him around with her head, you must intervene. If she ignores him except when he moves, and then charges at him, there's a good chance that she's not going to mother him. If she knocks him into a fence or wall, she could injure or kill him, so you need to observe and be ready to rescue the calf if she continues this behavior. The heifer needs to be restrained so she can't hurt the calf — or you — while you help him to nurse.

After the calf nurses, the overly-aggressive heifer may simmer down and accept him, but it may take several supervised nursings with the calf in a penned-off area between nursings so she can't hurt him, until she changes her mind. You can usually get any nonmotherly heifer to raise her calf, but it may take two or three weeks of supervision and hobbles on the heifer (see page 176).

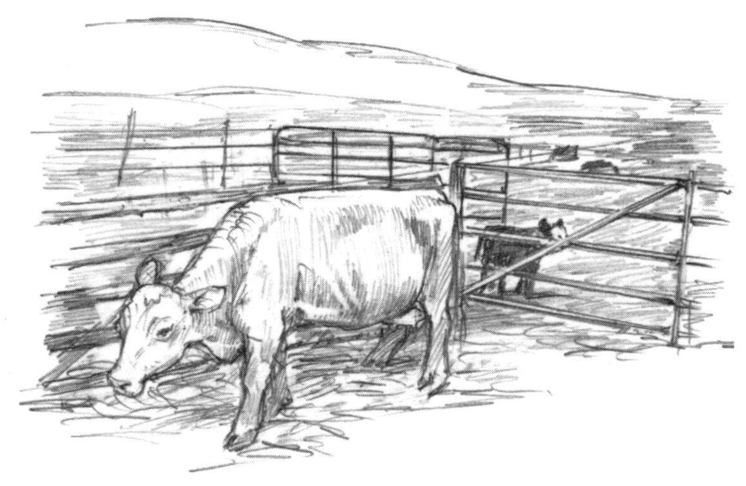

A cow and her calf can be kept in separate adjoining pens, so that the cow won't hurt the calf. Allow the calf to "visit" her twice a day to nurse — with supervision — until she accepts him.

ADOPTIVE MOMS SAVE MONEY

An orphan will do better on another cow than raised on a bottle. Though it might be labor-intensive for a few days while you convince a cow to accept the orphan, it saves time and money in the long run, because you don't have to buy milk replacer and feed the calf.

Cows with Hormonal Problems

On occasion, the normal hormonal sequence of calving doesn't occur. In the first group of heifers we bought, there was one whose cervix did not dilate when she went into labor; we hauled her to the vet for a c-section and named her Cearie. She was not interested in her calf and didn't have much milk, so we raised him on another cow. The next year she was fine. We suspected that the hormonal problem that caused failure of the cervix to dilate and lack of milk production had also affected her mothering instinct.

Another cow, Jancis, having her sixth calf, needed assistance to calve because her cervix didn't open fully. Our vet pulled the calf, but Jancis's milk never came in. We raised that calf on Prue, our pet cow with the cleft palate who often raised an extra calf along with her own. In more recent years, Cadillac's daughter Hot Rod had a hormone problem every time she calved — with little milk and no love for her calf until a week later. She had to be hobbled, and all nursings were supervised. We kept the calf in a separate pen between nursings so that she didn't kill him and fed him extra milk until he was a week old. At that point Hot Rod would produce more milk and become a good mother. After four years of this, we sold her.

Grafting a Calf onto a Different Mother

When a good cow loses her calf, you hate to sell her, but you can't afford to feed her for a year with no income to cover her expenses. One solution is to give her another calf to raise. He might be an orphan, a calf from a heifer who didn't want him, a twin whose mother didn't have enough milk or the desire to raise two, a calf from a cow with a bad udder or no milk, or an old cow's calf. Sometimes an older cow has poor milk production, and it's better to graft her calf onto a cow who can raise him better. The old, thin cow can then regain weight and be sold.

You might consider getting a day-old dairy calf to put on a cow that lost hers, if there are no suitable candidates in your own herd. But when bringing home a dairy calf, be careful that you don't bring home a new disease as well. Buy dairy calves directly from a farmer with a healthy herd, where you can also be sure that the calf had colostrum soon after birth. Don't buy calves from a sale barn, where you don't know their history. They may not have had any colostrum and may have been exposed to pathogens; if they get sick after you bring them home, your own herd becomes exposed.

HEIFER TOUGH ON TUFFY — AT FIRST

ONE OF OUR FIRST EXPERIENCES with an unmotherly heifer was Tuffy's mother. She calved quickly and easily in the corral, then got up and marched off, away from her baby. The calf bawled, and she looked back at him once to see what made that noise but just kept right on going.

Tuffy was not to be deserted so easily, however. He got to his feet and staggered after his departing mother, bawling plaintively. She kicked at him and kept going, so we brought the calf into the house and fed him a bottle. As I was drying the calf in the kitchen, my own young son needed a diaper change, so I left Tuffy lying on towels. He'd been enjoying the towel rubbing and when I got up he thought that I, too, was suddenly deserting him. He lurched to his feet and wobbled after me into the living room, where I diapered my baby with the help of a big, blundering, slobbery calf nose that I had to keep pushing away. Tuffy spent that night in the barn, after another bottle from us.

The next morning we were awakened by Tuffy's mother bellowing by the gate. Her full udder may have triggered latent maternal yearnings. Sometime during the night she realized that she had a baby that needed her. We brought Tuffy to her; she began licking and loving him, and he went to her udder to start nursing. As he slurped milk, she licked his little rear end quite roughly, as if to say, "Where ya been all this time, kid?" From that moment on, they were a bonded pair. She was a perfect example of delayed reaction to calving!

MIXED-UP MOTHERS

OVER THE YEARS, we've had several cows with a delayed response to calving. Some got better as time went on, like Gloria, one of the heifers we bought in 1967, who knocked her calf around for the first few hours. We had to tie her and help him nurse, and then she'd accept him. By her fifth calf we merely had to put a halter on her; one person could hold her while the other helped her calf to the udder. She became very gentle. She had 13 calves; the later ones she mothered without help.

Raspberry was similar: She needed restraint for her first several calves, but as she grew older, we just had to be there in the barn stall to help the calf nurse the first time, and she'd be a good mother. She had 12 calves, and the last 5 she mothered without supervision. By contrast, Ebony was a bad mother who did not improve. Although we tied and hobbled her and kept her calf in a separate pen for several weeks, and though she eventually mothered and raised her calves, she was just as hard on her third calf as her first. Not wanting to make that time commitment every year, we sold her.

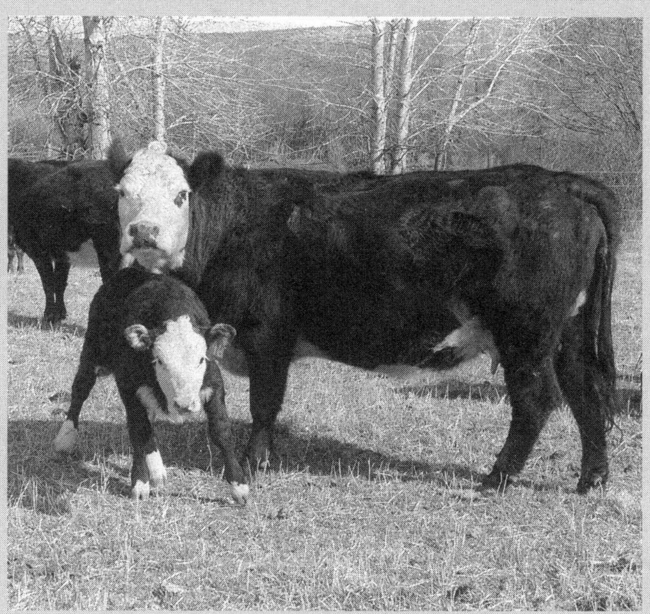

Gloria was a mixed-up mother who knocked her calves around at birth. She became more mellow with age and required less restraint and supervision with her later calves. She is shown here in 1974 with her eighth calf, Andromeda.

Convincing a cow to take a substitute calf can be quite a challenge. Sometimes it's easy, though, if it's a first-calf heifer who lost her calf at birth and wants to be a mother. Take her dead calf away, smear some of the birth mucus or her afterbirth on the substitute calf, then bring him to her stall or pen. If the calf is lively, he may startle and confuse her for a moment because her own calf was so still. If the bouncing baby scares her, tie him to the pen for a moment so he can't run around, and give her a chance to sniff him and become aquainted without being alarmed by his boisterous actions.

A cow that's already had calves is harder to fool. Some cows are so motherly that they'll accept another calf with minimal trickery. You can fool the cow by putting a commercial product on the calf that smells good, by pouring honey or molasses on the calf's back and hind end to encourage her to lick him, or by rubbing birth fluids from her dead calf onto the newcomer's back and hind end. Some cows will accept a substitute calf if you spray or smear a strong-smelling substance like cologne or mentholatum on the cow's nose and then on the calf, to confuse her sense of smell.

Using the Hide of Her Dead Calf

For a cow that's fussy about accepting a different calf, skinning her dead calf and putting the hide over the calf to be grafted is the most successful trick. The cow knows the smell of her own calf, even if he was dead at birth. If she had a chance to smell and lick him, then putting his hide over the adoptee will make the cow think he's hers by disguising the smell of the orphaned or rejected imposter. Her mothering instinct is strongest right after she calves; she is prepared physically and emotionally for a new baby and is more readily convinced to accept a foster calf. If her own calf dies when he's several days or weeks old, however, it's harder to trick her into taking a different one.

STEPS FOR TRICKING A COW WITH HER DEAD CALF'S HIDE

1. **If the cow lost her calf at birth or soon after** and is still in that same pen or barn stall, then leave her there, where she last saw her own calf.

2. **The dead calf should be skinned while fresh,** leaving the tail of the dead calf attached to the hide. The cow will smell and lick the calf's hind end, especially as he nurses, and you want the imposter to smell like her calf.

3. **Place hide over the replacement calf like a jacket.** Put the live calf's legs through the leg holes of the dead skin and the calf's head through the neck hole of the skin to hold the "jacket" in place. Or poke holes through the hide at strategic spots to put baling twine through, so you can tie the jacket legs around the calf's legs and the neck hide over the neck of the live calf (see diagram).

4. **Tie the hide under the belly and around the legs** to hold it in place. The hind part of the hide should drape over the hind end of the calf.

5. **When the replacement calf is hungry** and wanting to nurse, bring him to the cow in the pen or stall where she gave birth, as if you were bringing her baby back to her. This often works if she's been upset and worried about where her calf is and missing him. If you have moved the cow, put the substitute hide-covered calf into the stall where she last saw and smelled her own calf, and bring her back to that stall so she'll think that this is her calf.

6. **The sooner he nurses her, the better.** You want the calf to stimulate her motherliness before she becomes suspicious. If the substitute is several days old, however, he will be lively and running around; the cow may suspect that he's not her newborn calf. You may want to tie his legs together so that he remains lying down, until she sniffs him and starts licking him. A few smells of the jacket-wearing newcomer and most cows are convinced — or at least confused enough to let the calf nurse, especially if you supervise.

7. **Once the substitute calf has nursed a few times** and the cow is mothering him, it is safe to take off the old hide.

TO SKIN A DEAD CALF:

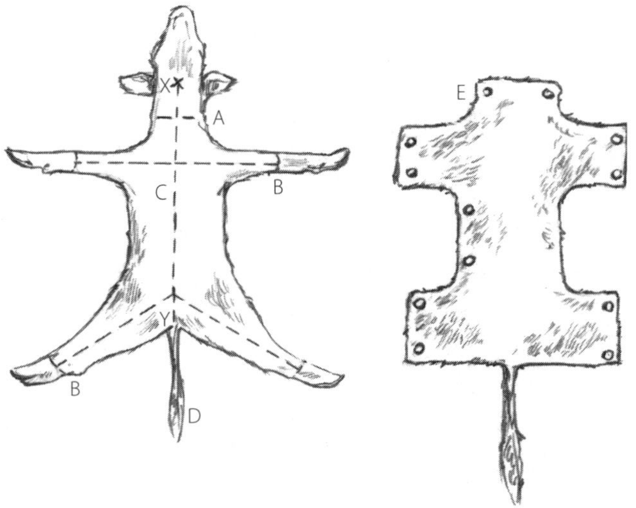

Lay the body on its back and slit the skin from throat (x) to rectum (y). Cut around the neck (a) and legs (b). Peel the skin from the body (c) after making slits down the underside of each leg. Leave the tail (d) attached to the hide. Poke holes (e) in the hide on either side of the neck, leg, and belly area so that it can be tied onto the live calf with twine.

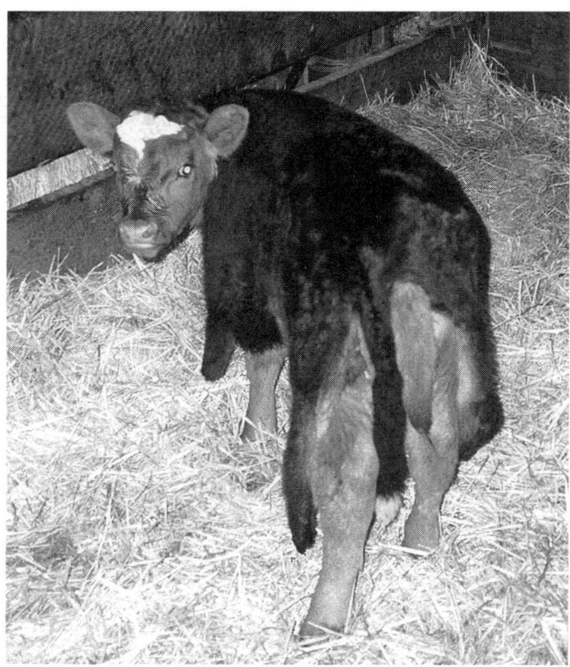

A substitute calf can be outfitted in the hide of the dead calf to trick the cow into adopting him.

Dog Trick

If a cow does not want to mother the substitute calf, you might kick-start her protective instincts and change her mind by bringing a dog into or near the pen. The urge to protect a calf from predators is so strong that a cow will become excited and upset about the dog and will want to protect the calf that she previously disdained. This may help her develop an interest in the calf, and she'll start to mother him. The dog trick sometimes works for a heifer that's indifferent about mothering her own new calf, too.

When Tricks Don't Work, Restrain the Reluctant Mother

Some cows can't be tricked and may still try to kick and bunt the calf. If hide-grafting and a dog fail to call up her maternal instincts, and she adamantly refuses to mother the calf, keep the pair in separate adjacent pens or stalls for a while so that the cow can't hurt the substitute calf. Tie hobbles on the cow's hind legs so that she can't kick him at nursing time (see page 176).

The urge to protect a calf from predators is so strong that a cow will become excited and upset about the dog and will want to protect the calf that she previously disdained.

If you don't have a separate stall or pen put a panel across a corner of the cow's stall or pen to make a small enclosure for the calf. Let him out with her three times a day for nursing, about every eight hours, until she accepts the newcomer and lets him nurse. (This strategy also works for heifers that won't mother their own calf.)

If the cow is hobbled so that she can't kick the calf and you give her some alfalfa hay or other good feed at nursing time, she'll usually stand still and won't try so hard to keep him from nursing. If she is still aggressively resentful, trying to butt him with her head or smash him into a fence or wall, restrain her during nursing time. A stanchion or head catcher works, but only if it's in or near her stall or pen. You can give her a little hay or grain to eat while she's restrained in it. If you don't have one available, put a halter on her and tie her while she eats hay and the calf gets dinner. If she's fed only at nursing time, she'll more willingly concentrate on food while the calf nurses and be less intent on attacking him.

If she's not gentle enough to halter easily, leave the halter on her. In a stall or small pen it's usually safe to let her drag a halter rope, if there's nothing for it to catch on. Then it's easy to tie her or hold the rope when the calf nurses, so that she can't move around, run off, or hit him with her head. Food helps her learn to tolerate the calf; most cows compromise and accept the trade-off of receiving food in exchange for letting the calf nurse.

Usually, after a couple of days of nursing the calf two or three times a day while restrained, even a stubborn cow will resign herself to letting the calf nurse, and you no longer have to tie her up at feeding time. You may still have to supervise nursings for a while, but the cow won't try to kill the calf; she realizes it's pointless, and she'll stand still. After a time you'll

COW FOOLED INTO ADOPTION

WHEN FREDDIE had a premature calf, we easily fooled her into adopting another calf. She took too long in early labor and expelled a bloody discharge that made us suspect that her placenta was detaching. We put her in the head catcher and checked her. The calf wasn't coming, so we pulled him. He was seven weeks early and very small, with short, velvety hair. He had a heartbeat, but we could not revive him.

In the next pen over were two calves without mothers that we'd been feeding on bottles. One was a three-week-old twin taken from her heifer mother because she didn't have enough milk for both calves. While Freddie was still in the head catcher, we smeared mucus from the dead calf on Bambi's back and hind end, and let her nurse Freddie. When we let the cow out of the head catcher, she turned around and licked Bambi, sure that this was her calf. They were bonded in that instant, and Freddie raised Bambi as if she were her own.

see little clues that she's tolerating him more or even starting to like him. You may find her standing next to his enclosure, content to be near him, rather than at the far corner of her pen, ignoring him.

Once she starts to show a change of heart, mooing at the calf in his enclosure, licking him a little while he nurses, or worrying about him when you put him back in his own pen after nursing, it's usually safe to leave them together. Watch them for a while to make sure she won't be mean to him. Even if you have to separate them again, it's only a matter of time before she accepts him. Once they can stay together, leave the hobbles on for a few days longer if you wish — to make sure she won't try to kick him — but once the cow begins to change her mind, you know your efforts were successful: Her hobbles can come off, and she will raise that calf.

Usually, after a couple of days of nursing the calf two or three times a day while restrained, even a stubborn cow will resign herself to letting the calf nurse . . .

Easy Hobbles from Baling Twine

Hobbles can be made from four strands of baling twine. Some cows are strong enough to break three strands if they kick hard or try to travel faster than the hobbles will allow. Choose twines that have been cut next to the knot, with the knot at the very end of the twine and not in the middle where it will interfere with making the hobbles. You don't want a knot in the way or in a location where it might rub on the cow's leg and create a sore.

Practice the following steps a few times by tying loops around some poles and making hobbles, perfecting your nonslip knots before you do it on a cow.

1. ***Tie 4 strands of twine together at knot ends.*** Restrain the cow in a head catcher with a side that you can move out of the way to give you room to work, so you can put the hobbles around her legs without being kicked.
2. ***Put a pole behind the cow*** to ensure that she will not keep moving forward or backward, or tie one of her legs back a little to anything sturdy behind her, with enough slack that she can put her weight on that foot to stand but not enough to bring it forward and kick you.
3. ***Situate the hobbles above the rope*** holding her leg, so that you can take the loop of rope off her leg and foot after you've made the hobbles.
4. ***Tie the first knot*** a few inches from the tied-together end of the twines so that there will be plenty of room to go around the cow's leg, then tie the twines in a loose loop around the leg. Make the loop only loose enough to get one or two fingers between the loop and her leg; if it's any looser than that she'll be able to pull the hobbles down over the joint and dewclaws when she tries to walk or kick, or she might get a toe of her other foot caught in the loop.
5. ***Double-tie all the knots so they cannot slip;*** if a loop tightens up and becomes smaller, it will cut off circulation to her foot.
6. ***Leave 8–12 inches (20.3–30.5 cm) of space between the leg loops,*** depending on the size of the cow. You want her to have enough slack to be able to walk but not enough to kick.
7. ***After you make the final knot*** to finish the second loop, make another double tie and extra knot, so that it cannot come undone. This ensures that your knots will stay in place.
8. ***Cut off the extra length of twine ends*** so that they don't drag on the ground, and your hobbles are finished.

Remember: Make sure that the loops are the right size around the cow's leg, neither too tight nor too loose, and the knots are secure and won't slip. If there's proper space between the loops to enable the cow to walk and to get up and down while hindering her ability to kick, the hobbles will serve their purpose.

To remove hobbles, cut the loop off one leg with a pocketknife or shears; the cow can't kick you very

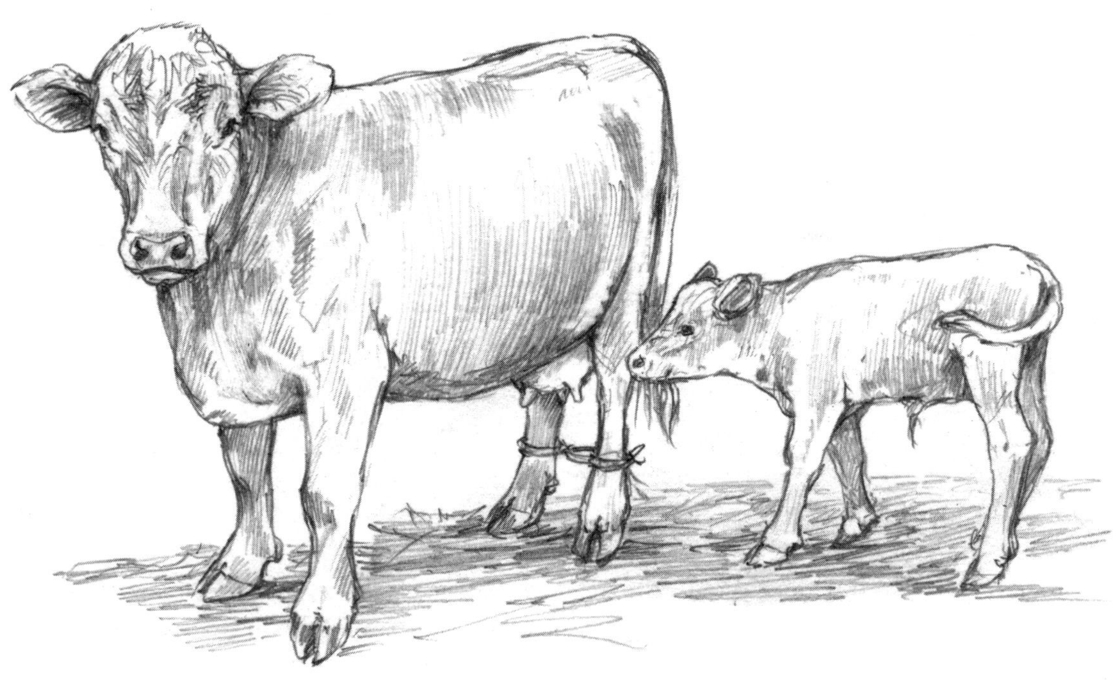

Cows may develop sore, cracked teats from cold, windy weather, and may not allow their calves to nurse. To resolve the problem, hobble a cow with chapped teats and put the pair into a small pen, so that the cow can't kick or run off when the calf tries to nurse. Then he can continue to nurse until the teats heal and the hobbles can be removed.

effectively. A gentle cow may let you snip off both loops, but if you don't trust her, clip the first loop, and then take her to a head catcher or chute (because now she can walk freely) to safely clip off the second leg loop.

Other Instances Where Hobbles Are Handy

Sometimes a cow loves her baby but her udder or teats are so sore that she still kicks when he tries to nurse. Injured or chapped teats may make her reluctant to let him suck. Windy, cold weather can make teats chap, crack, and bleed. When the calf nurses, the teats get wet with milk, and wind can chap the teats. Sunburned teats may also become sore. In severely cold weather, teats may have frostbite.

Chapped, cracked teats. If the cow kicks the calf when he nurses, he may be discouraged and not try again. The cow's udder gets full, and the teats are more swollen and sore, and it's a vicious cycle. Some calves are easily intimidated after being clobbered a few times. Others still try to nurse and will chase their mothers around. Sometimes they'll manage to nurse a little from behind — since the cow can't kick them very effectively in that position — but it's hard to get much milk if she is always running off. With this sort of behavior, the cow basically weans the calf, even if he's only a few weeks or months old.

Sometimes all that's necessary to prevent this is to put the pair into a small pen so that she can't run off when he tries to nurse. Even though she kicks or attempts to get away from him, it's easier for him to catch up with her or to nurse from behind. Since she still loves him (but just can't stand the pain when he nurses), she may resign herself to painful nursings because she can't really avoid the calf in this small area. After a few days her teats may heal enough, and you can let the pair out again.

When a cow won't allow the calf to suck. If necessary, put hobbles on the cow to wear while she's

MAKING HOBBLES FROM BALING TWINE

Inexpensive instant hobbles can be custom-fitted for any cow using discarded baling twine.

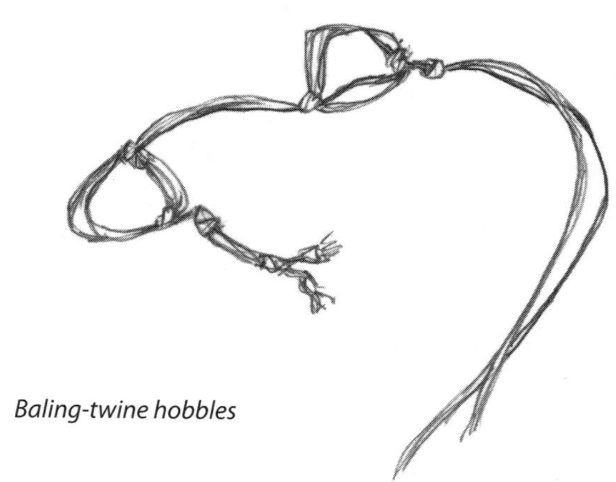

Baling-twine hobbles

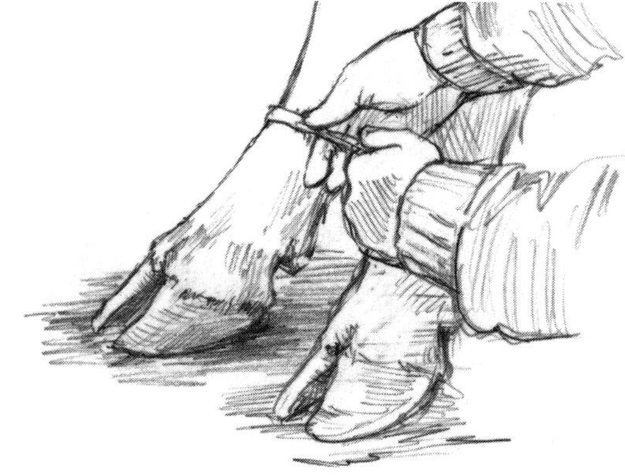

1. With the cow restrained, make the first loop around one leg loose enough to get two fingers between the loop and her leg.

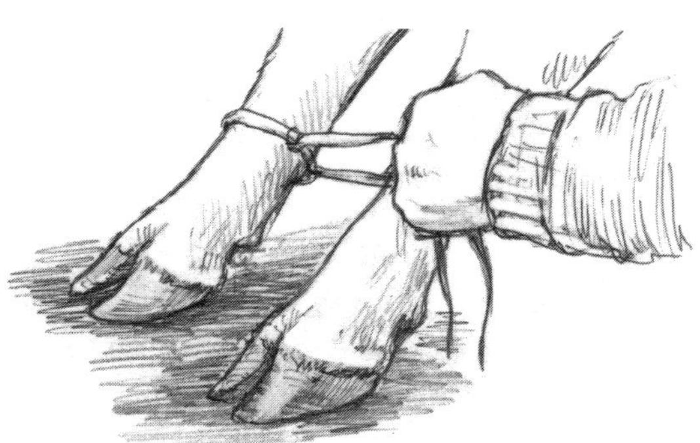

2. Leave 8 to 12 inches (20.3 to 30.5 cm) between the first loop and the next leg loop you are about to make.

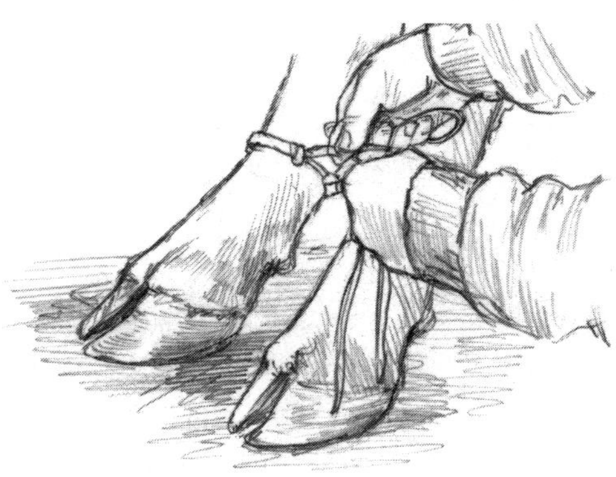

3. Make the nonslip knot and small loop that will become part of the big loop for the second leg.

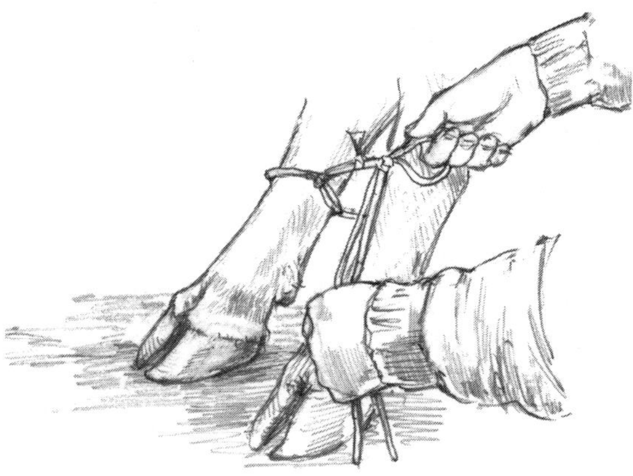

4. You are ready to go around the second leg and create the leg loop.

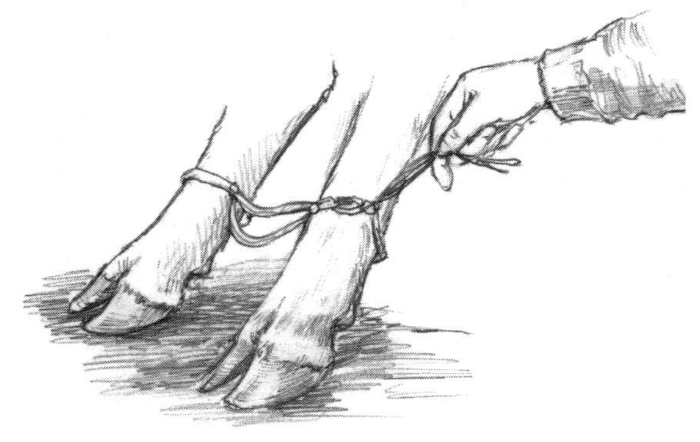

5. After making the loop around the second leg, the final knot is finished with a double tie and extra knot, to keep it from coming untied. The extra lengths of twine can be cut off.

HOBBLING IN EXTREME COLD

IN FEBRUARY 1989, after the Siberian Express blew in four days of -30°F (–34.4°C) temperatures, with strong winds that made the chill factor equal to 100 below zero (–73.3°C), we hobbled more cows than we ever have before or since. We didn't lose any calves to the cold, thanks to our calving barns, our efforts to dry every newborn calf in our house, and the calf shelters in every field. The calves in the fields spent all their time in those little houses, coming out only to nurse their mothers and then going right back inside. None of the calves lost ears or tails from freezing, but many cows lost their ear tips, and some had frozen teats.

Brushy windbreaks protected cows in three fields, but one field didn't have shelter; wind came from the wrong direction. All 50 cows in that field suffered frostbitten udders — the ends of their teats froze. After a few days the storm was over, but by then the dead skin was coming off of the ends of their raw and bleeding teats, and the cows were kicking their calves. Some calves were persistent, running after their mothers and nursing from behind whenever the cow stood still long enough for them to grab a teat. But 24 cows wouldn't let their calves nurse at all.

In desperation we brought those 24 pairs into the corral, put the cows through the chute and hobbled their hind legs with baling twine. We kept the hobbled cows in a small lot, where they didn't have to walk far to water (they had to walk slowly, with their hind legs hobbled) and where the calves could easily catch up with them.

The teats healed in three to four weeks, after the scabs came off and the raw ends healed. Then we snipped the hobbles off the cows and let the pairs go back to the big field again.

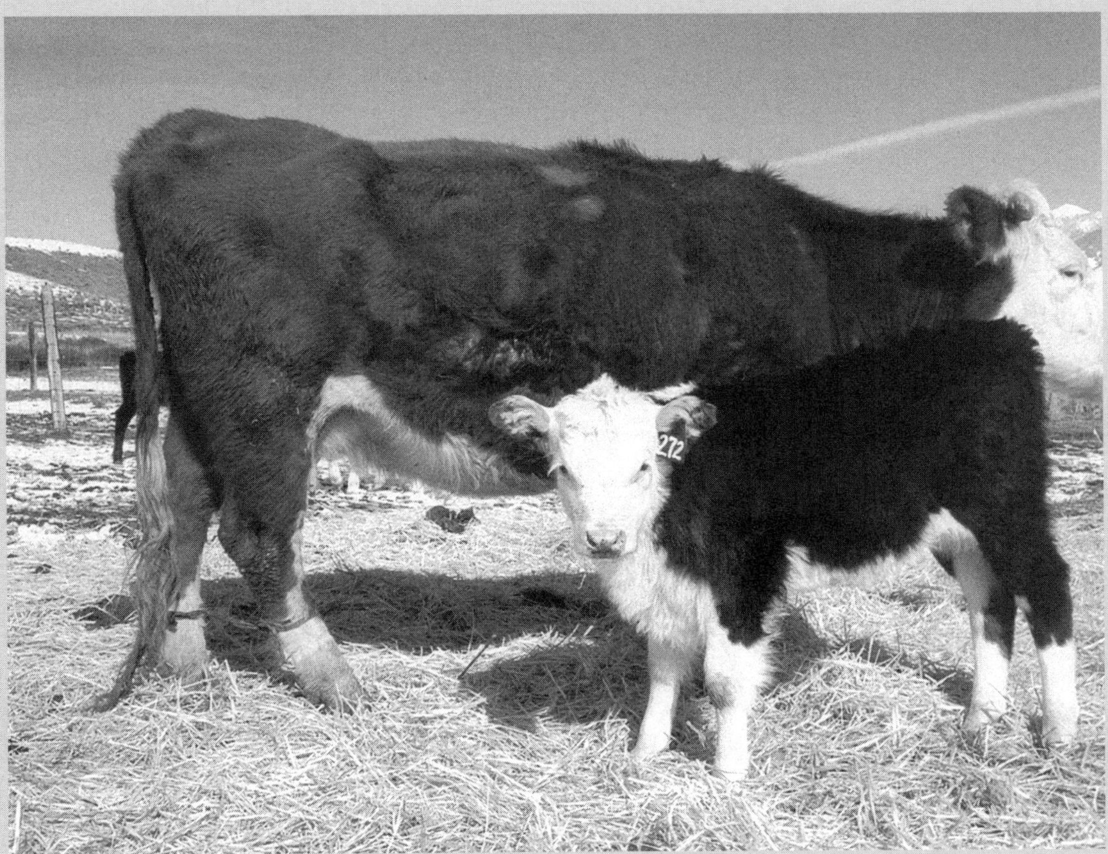

One of the 24 cows we hobbled in 1989 after the Siberian Express froze the ends of their teats stands with her calf. Hobbles must be the proper length between the legs, so that the cow can still walk but can't lift a leg high enough to kick her calf when he nurses.

HAIR THAT HURTS

THE FIRST CASE OF TEAT STRANGULATION we experienced was more than 30 years ago. I noticed Beatrick with one large teat, while driving along the feed trail after giving out the morning hay. I was checking udders as I always do, to see if any calves were sick and not nursing. We brought Beatrick and her calf into the corral and put her into the chute so that we could carefully cut off the hair ring. Fortunately, it had been encircling the teat only a short time; it had not yet cut into the skin. Once it was removed, we milked out the large teat, and she then allowed her calf to nurse it.

A newborn calf trying to find a teat may suck on a clump of hair and can ingest it if it pulls loose.

Since then, we've had several cases of teat strangulation. Some hair rings had cut into the teat by the time we saw the problem. The worst case occurred with a cow named Ruby in late spring, just before we were going to summer range. We were no longer feeding hay and therefore not observing the cows as closely; calves were big enough that scours was no longer a problem. They were on a large mountain pasture and doing well; we rode through them every few days to check on them.

Ruby's teat was nearly cut through the skin when I discovered it. We brought her down to the corral to remove the hair ring, and it took several days' treatment, milking her and applying ointment to the raw area after each milking, before it was healed enough for her to let her calf nurse.

Most of our cows don't have such long hair on their udders, but some do, like Ruby, who was half Shorthorn, and like some of our part-Angus cows, and we watch them closely. If there's matted hair hanging down from the udder at calving time, we pull the clumps of hair off to prevent problems. A newborn calf trying to find a teat may suck on a clump of hair and can ingest it if it pulls loose. Some ranchers clip hairy udders at calving time.

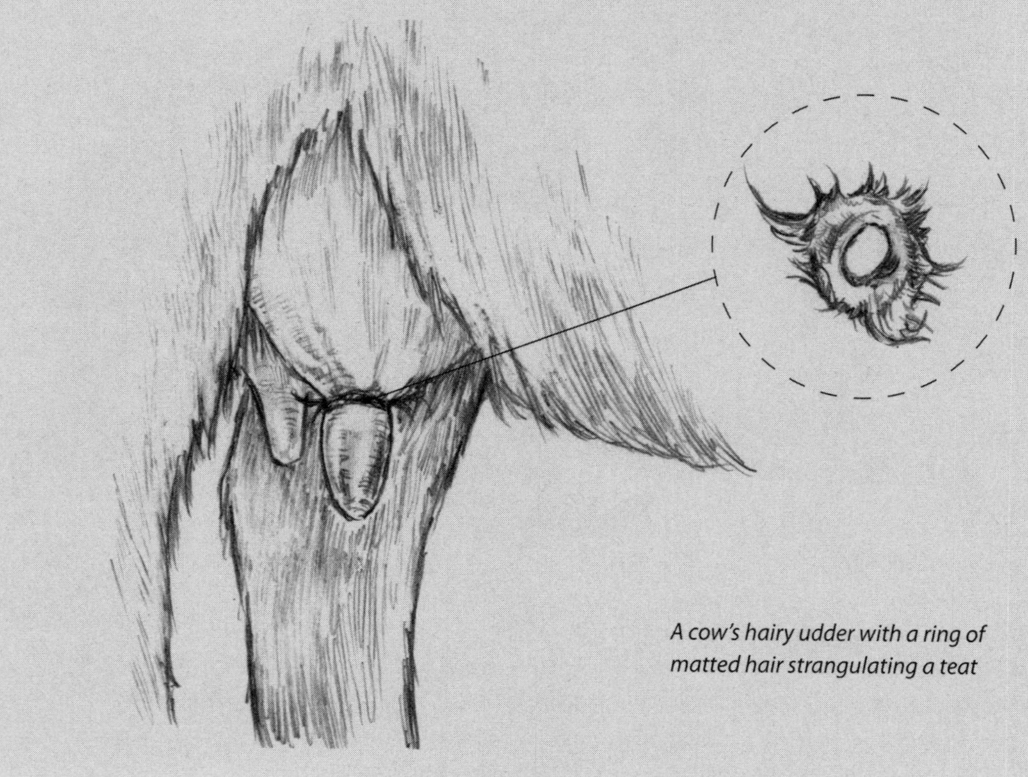

A cow's hairy udder with a ring of matted hair strangulating a teat

in a small pen, to keep her from hurting or discouraging the calf when he tries to nurse. Once he nurses the big, painful teats, they won't be so sore; he can keep up with her and keep her nursed out. Teats will heal faster when they are not so distended with milk. After she resigns herself to letting him nurse, and the teats are no longer sore, remove the hobbles.

Sore teats from injury. If a teat is injured (cut on barbed wire, for instance) and the cow won't let the calf nurse it, you may have to milk it a few times and treat it, or hobble the cow so that the calf can nurse it out. Some breeds and individuals have a lot of hair on the udder. This can help protect the cow's udder from sunburn or frostbite but is a disadvantage if her calf is nursing before she sheds the long hair, or when it sheds in clumps and matted snarls. A nursing calf may ingest a clump of hair and develop fatal blockage from a hairball (see chapter 15).

When a teat is strangulated. When cows have hairy udders, a more common problem is strangulation of a teat. As the calf nurses, the hair gets wet with milk and may get curled around the top of the teat. As the milky, matted hair dries, it may be entwined together in a strong, ropy wisp. More hair may mat to it with each nursing. If it completely encircles the teat and is matted back into itself, the loop gets tight and starts to cut into the skin as the udder fills with milk and the teat enlarges. The hair ring can't expand, so it constricts the teat.

If the hair ring is not noticed and removed, it cuts through the skin. That area becomes raw and sore, and the cow won't let her calf nurse. It's a vicious circle; the teat becomes larger and tighter because it's so full of milk, cutting off circulation as the hair ring puts more pressure on the swollen teat. It then becomes even more tender, and the cow more adamantly refuses to let her calf nurse. If neglected, the strangulated teat will die, and the cow will lose that quarter — or die, if she becomes seriously infected.

Chapter 9

When a Calf Needs Your Help

IF YOU RAISE MANY CATTLE or keep cattle for very many years, you'll definitely encounter tragedies and unusual situations in which the calf or cow has a problem, and survival of the calf depends on you. Being able to give intensive care to a compromised calf or feed substitute milk if something happens to Mama can determine whether that calf makes it to sale time, supplies meat for your table, or eventually takes his own place in the herd.

Some of our experiences with needy calves took a great deal of time and care, and we gained a lot of respect for their courage and will to live. Indeed, we enjoyed getting to know them intimately and having the opportunity to gain insight into their unique characters. This kind of interaction is what makes raising cattle much more than just a livelihood. There is great satisfaction in knowing that you helped an animal in the intense ways described in this chapter.

Care during Nursing and Milk Production Problems

Old cows may be in poor body condition because of loss of teeth and can't produce much colostrum or milk. Sometimes a cow does not have enough milk for her calf because of a hormone imbalance. But more often it's the calf that has the problem that hinders nursing. Most common is a swollen tongue due to pressure on the head from being in the birth canal too long, a problem that can be resolved by feeding the calf with a stomach tube or esophageal feeder until his tongue is back to its normal size and he can suck.

An old cow with no milk and other problems that threaten the health of calves creates problems that are often not so temporary. Sometimes to save a calf you must be in charge of feedings for a longer stretch of time and must strategize ways to keep the newborn alive.

When Mama Had No Milk

P.S. was our first calf "orphan." She was born to an old Hereford cow, one of a group of cows we leased when we first started raising cattle and were trying to build up our herd. The old cow was thin and didn't have much milk. The calf, named P.S. because she seemed like a postscript to the old cow's life, nursed almost continuously and was always hungry. I felt sorry for her and fed her a bottle of milk, which she sucked eagerly. We fed the old cow grain and alfalfa hay, hoping it might help her to produce more milk. After a few days, she seemed to be doing better, so we turned the pair out with the other cows. But the next day when we went to feed the cows, little P.S. came bawling to me, wanting some milk, and I realized she would starve if left with her mother, so we raised her on a bottle.

Some years later we had an eight-year-old cow, Jancis, with no milk at calving. She had all the signs of being in early labor but was dull and lethargic and did not progress. When we checked her, the calf's feet were trying to come through the cervix, but it wasn't dilating. We gave her and her cervix more time and checked again later because she was straining hard. All four feet were trying to come through, and the cervix was still not dilated. We called our veterinarian.

The vet pushed the hind feet back but was unable to pull the calf because his head could not come through the small opening. Finally, he was able to push the front feet back, bring the head through the tight cervix and then the calf's front feet one at a time into the birth canal alongside the head so he could pull the calf. Because the cervix and vulva were not relaxed enough, it was a *very* hard pull. The vulva tore as we pulled the calf out.

Jancis did not clean for several days and was lethargic and off feed. We gave her antibiotics, laxatives, and a magnet, in case she had hardware (see chapter 2), and she recovered but never came to her milk. We fed her calf some of our emergency supply of frozen colostrum, thawed and warmed, and raised him on a pet cow, Prue.

When a Cleft Palate Made Nursing Impossible

Prue was born on a cold January day in the calving pen. When we went out to iodine Hazel's calf we were startled by her face — her nose was not properly formed. We brought her into the house to dry by the stove and so that we could get a better look at her problem. She had a *cleft palate,* so we named her Prudence after a heroine with a harelip in the book by Mary Webb titled *Precious Bane* (E. P. Dutton, 1926). The calf's nostril on the right side was open at the bottom with nothing separating it from her mouth. There was no roof to her mouth for about 2 inches (5 cm) back, and the teeth in her misaligned bottom jaw were crooked.

We wondered what had caused this deformity, whether she would live, and if she could nurse. Would she drown if she tried to drink water? We learned that her condition can be caused by the cow's eating lupine in early pregnancy.

We decided to raise her in spite of her problem, feeding her on a nipple bucket instead of a bottle, since the nipple on the bucket was long enough to go past the hole in the top of her mouth. She nursed slowly, with foam bubbles coming out her nose, and she kept licking foam from her nose with her tongue.

Since it was cold, she spent her first five days in a box in our kitchen, until she jumped out while we were feeding cows. She wanted to play and chased our kids (ages two and four at the time) around the house. When we came back from feeding the cows, our son was standing on the couch banging on the window for us to hurry, and Andrea was hiding behind the couch. Prue had pooped in the toy box, climbed onto a chair, and from there hopped onto a bed. She was sound sleep on the pillow and had thoroughly wet the bed. After that we fixed a place for her outside.

Prue thrived on her nipple bucket with extra milk from our milk cow. She wore out nipples often; her crooked teeth chewed through them. She could never have nursed her mother. Hazel would not have tolerated the sharp chewing.

When we came back from feeding the cows, our son was standing on the couch banging on the window for us to hurry, and Andrea was hiding behind the couch. Prue had pooped in the toy box, climbed on a chair, and from there hopped onto a bed.

When Prue was two months old, we pulled one of her teeth with pliers. It was coming up through the roof of her mouth and was hitting the inside of her nostril, making it sore when she nursed and making her reluctant. After we removed the tooth — which was quite an effort, since it had a root on it 1.5 inches (3.8 cm) long, the raw spot healed, and she could suck her nipple bucket without pain.

We wondered if Prue would ever be able to drink water from any source other than her nipple bucket without getting water up her nostril. But when she was three months old, she sampled the water that was in a tub for the other "barn calves" we were raising on a dairy cow, and she learned to drink by putting her tongue over the hole in her nose. She made slurping, burbling sounds, and it took her twice as long to drink as other calves, but she had that problem solved. She was a pet by the time she grew up, so we kept her as a cow; she stayed in our herd until she was 15 years old, raising a number of extra calves along with her own. One year she raised three calves: Amos (Jancis's calf), Andy (her own), and Squeaky, an orphan heifer.

When a Calf Had a Broken Jaw

When a friend who knew that we were feeding several orphans with extra milk from our old milk cow wondered if we'd like another calf, we knew we'd have to be innovative. One of his cows had stepped on her newborn calf, breaking 2 inches (5 cm) off the lower jaw. The broken part was hanging there, held only by skin. Our friend didn't have time to try to save the calf, but he knew that we were softhearted and always tried to save even the most hopeless cases, so he gave us the calf; the kids and I held the calf on the back seat of our Volkswagen as we brought him home.

Upon inspecting him, we saw that the calf's broken jaw was dangling down and his tongue hanging out. There was a golf-ball-size, blood-filled bruise under the tongue. The calf, whom our son named Bozo, hadn't had much to eat. Our friend had forced a little milk down the calf's throat the night before, but the calf was very hungry. He was perky and strong. One thing we learned early, in our various experiences in dealing with sick and injured animals, is that the will to live is more than half the battle, and this calf certainly had good spirit.

When we started trying to fix his jaw, the blood-filled bruise under his tongue made it hard to get his mouth closed. I poked a sterile needle into the bulge in hopes of draining off fluid, but it had already solidified and would not drain out. So we left it that way, hoping the blood would reabsorb. The challenge was to get the broken part of the lower jaw back into proper place and hold it there while it healed. I used adhesive tape to tape his mouth shut while Lynn and the kids held the calf.

I could feel the broken, jagged ends of the bone under the skin and tried to line up the broken part with the rest of the jaw. When I got the jaw shut and in proper place, with the swollen tongue forced inside it, we put several layers of tape around his muzzle, back around his ears and behind his head to hold it in place, and one piece of tape up the middle of his face. The tape around his muzzle was tight, but he was able to breathe just fine.

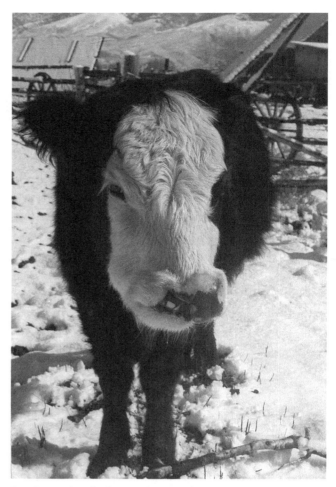

Prue learned to drink water from a tub despite her cleft palate, crooked jaw, and crooked teeth, but she could never suckle her mama.

We weren't sure how long it would take for the bones to knit, but we knew that young animals heal faster than adults; they have more bone-forming cells in their growing bones. We figured his jaw would knit in about a week, since a lamb with a broken leg will start walking on its splinted leg in four or five days. But to be safe, we left the tape on Bozo for two weeks.

To feed him we used a stomach tube, put into his nostril, so he didn't have to open his mouth while the jawbones were mending. As it turned out, we didn't have to tube him for the whole two weeks, which was good, because even though he wanted the milk, he didn't like the tube put into his nose three times a day; it was a hard job to feed him at mealtime. He greeted us with mixed emotions, not sure whether to run to us for dinner or away from us because he didn't like the tube. His reaction was comical.

After a few days, the tape around his jaw stretched enough so that he could stick his tongue in and out. He had complete control of the jaw (it all moved in once piece), so we knew that the bones were growing back together. The bruise under his tongue was gone; I poked my finger in his mouth, and it all felt normal. Since I could poke my finger in, we tried a nipple. He was six days old and had never sucked. We used a lamb nipple because it was small enough to fit through the small opening. He loved it! He did more chewing than sucking but by the third day was nursing well. After a few more days the tape stretched enough to allow a calf nipple.

When we took the tape off, we saw that he'd lost the hair under it, and he looked funny with his bald patches, but it soon grew back. The jaw looked beautiful! One side mended perfectly smooth, and the other had a small lump the size of a pea. Our repair job was a success.

Intensive Care for Weather-Stressed Calves

Because we calve in the winter, most of our intensive-care cases involve taking in severely chilled calves and giving them round-the-clock care until they are strong enough to return to their mamas.

When a Chilled Calf Needed Help

Bandit Eyes arrived on a cold December night in 1968. Her heifer mother Annie was in the barn and calved easily, but Annie didn't mother the calf and did not lick it. By the time we discovered Bandit Eyes, she was very cold; her ears and tail were frozen solid, and the inside of her mouth was cold. We brought her into the house and thawed her in our shower (we didn't have a bathtub yet) and dried her by the stove, but she was too chilled to nurse a bottle. We injected *dextrose* under her skin, since we did not yet know how to feed a calf with a stomach tube and didn't have one. In 20 minutes she showed interest in life and nursed the colostrum I thawed and warmed. She lay in front of the stove for several hours before she stopped shivering.

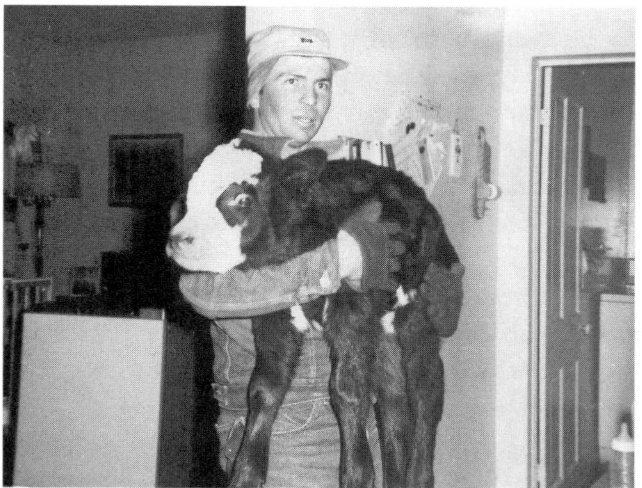

Bandit Eyes was the first calf that spent time in our house to get warm and dry. Her mother didn't want her and didn't lick her, and she nearly froze. She lived in our bathroom for a couple of days, until our Holstein heifer calved and was able to raise Bandit Eyes as well as her own calf.

When a Calf Had Frozen Feet

Brown Bug was born in February 1982. He got up and nursed his first-time mother Shulamit in the barn stall where he was born, and she loved him and licked him dry. The weather was cold the next morning, but we needed that stall for another calving cow, so we moved the pair to an old log barn. We were busy moving mamas and babies to different barns and sheds, and didn't take time to check on Brown Bug and his mother. We did not know he had developed diarrhea. That was the year a new "bug" hit our herd, and every one of the last 24 calves got sick before they were a day old (see chapter 11). Brown Bug was one of the first victims of that epidemic. He caught us off guard, and we nearly lost him.

When we went to move the pair to the field the next day, Brown Bug was weak and walking stiffly; his hind-leg joints were not bending. He had scours, and both hind legs were frozen solid, clear up past the hocks. His eyes were sunken, and his flanks were hollow and gaunt. So instead of putting him and his mama out to the field, we moved Shulamit to a pen near the house and carried Brown Bug into our kitchen, to fight for his life and his feet. Even though we hadn't finished our morning chores, we focused on this emergency, knowing that precious time had already been lost. Our immediate goal was to save this calf; the cows could wait for breakfast.

Dehydration from scours had lowered his body temperature and decreased circulation to his extremities, so both hind legs froze. We gave him two quarts (1.9 L) of electrolyte solution by stomach tube, then stood him in the kitchen in two buckets of hot water, one for each frozen hind leg. Our children helped steady him, kept him from moving around, and added hot water to the buckets as Lynn and I worked on the calf's feet, massaging them in hot water for two hours. It took that long before his feet began to feel warm instead of cold.

He got tired and wanted to lie down. After his feet finally thawed, we let him lie on a bed of towels next to the woodstove. We rubbed dimethyl sulfoxide (DMSO) liniment on his legs and around his hoofs, to increase any circulation he might still have, and hoped that we weren't too late. We massaged his feet whenever we were in the house. One foot had a little feeling and warmth; the other was numb and cold.

There might be a chance that only the outer layer of his legs had frozen and some deep circulation had kept his feet alive. A cow's lower leg has blood vessels between the bones. Unlike a horse, which has just one cannon bone in the lower leg, a cow has two toes instead of one, and a double leg bone. If we were lucky, Brown Bug's legs might not have frozen clear through to the center.

When we went to move the pair to the field the next day, Brown Bug was weak and walking stiffly; his hind-leg joints were not bending. He had scours, and both hind legs were frozen solid, clear up past the hocks.

We gave him fluids several times. He was so dehydrated it took more than 24 hours before he was able to urinate. He was too weak to go out to his mother to nurse, so we fed him with a bottle. To keep his mother from drying up, we tied her and milked her out and fed Brown Bug her milk. During the warmest part of his second day in the house, we carried him out to his mother, but he was too weak to nurse much. So we brought him back in, warmed his feet, and fed him a bottle; he could drink it lying down.

While cold weather lasted, we kept him in our kitchen, taking him once a day to nurse his mother, with socks on his feet to keep them warm. Three layers of old tube socks helped protect his feet from the cold and snow while he nursed. Once-a-day nursing was enough to keep his mother producing milk, and we fed Brown Bug bottles the rest of the time. Every day at noon we took him to Mama, and he became very excited whenever we started to put on his socks; he knew that it meant that he was going to her. He kicked in happy anticipation as Lynn carried him to his mother's pen. If we were late for his noon feeding, Shulamit would look toward the house and moo.

His feet became painful and swollen just above the hooves. He spent most of his time lying down, sometimes kicking his hind feet. He had a persistent fever, probably from all the tissue damage. We kept him on antibiotics for a long time. Eventually his feet were less sore, and he got too heavy to carry; we let him walk to his mother after putting

Sometimes Tubes Are the Right Choice

Be careful trying to bottle-feed a calf that doesn't have a strong willingness to suck. This may happen with a premature calf, a calf compromised by cold stress or heat stress, or one weak from a hard birth and oxygen shortage. A calf that's nearly comatose or impaired in any way may not have a good suckle reflex. The instinct to nurse is strongest right after birth, but if a calf is oxygen-deprived, he may not suck. If he's chilled, he may be shivering too hard to suck, or his mouth is cold and won't function properly. If his core temperature has dropped to the point where he can't shiver, he can't suck a bottle.

Feeding a calf with a poor suckle reflex risks getting milk into his windpipe because he can't swallow well, and this will lead to pneumonia. In these instances it is better to get colostrum into him via stomach tube or esophageal feeder and warm him if he's cold.

his socks on and helping him out the back door so he wouldn't slip on the linoleum floor. He could make it the rest of the way on his own, following us eagerly to his mother's pen. The weather moderated, and he could stay outside without refreezing his fragile feet with their poor circulation. We made a shelter in one corner of his mama's pen with three sides and a roof, straw for bedding, and a net-wire gate to keep him locked in except when he nursed, so he wouldn't stay out in the snow. We let him out three times a day to nurse. When the snow melted, we took the gate down.

He didn't lose his feet. Some of the hair and skin came off his pasterns, and he developed a crack at the top of one hoof, but it all healed. His pasterns grew wide, and his toes curled up on the ends, but he got over his lameness. He swung his legs wide in a unique waddle when he walked but enjoyed living with the rest of the herd that summer, running and bucking with the other calves.

I considered putting the tiny calf on my saddle and carrying him over the hill to the Jeep, but I wasn't sure if my young, skittish horse would tolerate such a novel passenger.

Intensive Care for Premature Calves

Over the past 40 years our kitchen has served as an intensive-care unit for many babies. Some needed only temporary warming or emergency treatment after a hard or traumatic birth in subzero weather, or during acute illness. Thirteen of the babies were premature calves that spent days, even weeks in the house — calves that were too fragile to live outdoors. Some of the calves arrived early for no apparent reason. In other cases the cow had a problem, and her body was getting rid of the fetus in an attempt to sustain her own life.

We've had calves born, or delivered by c-section because the cow was dying, as much as six weeks too early, yet they survived because we gave them the intensive care they needed.

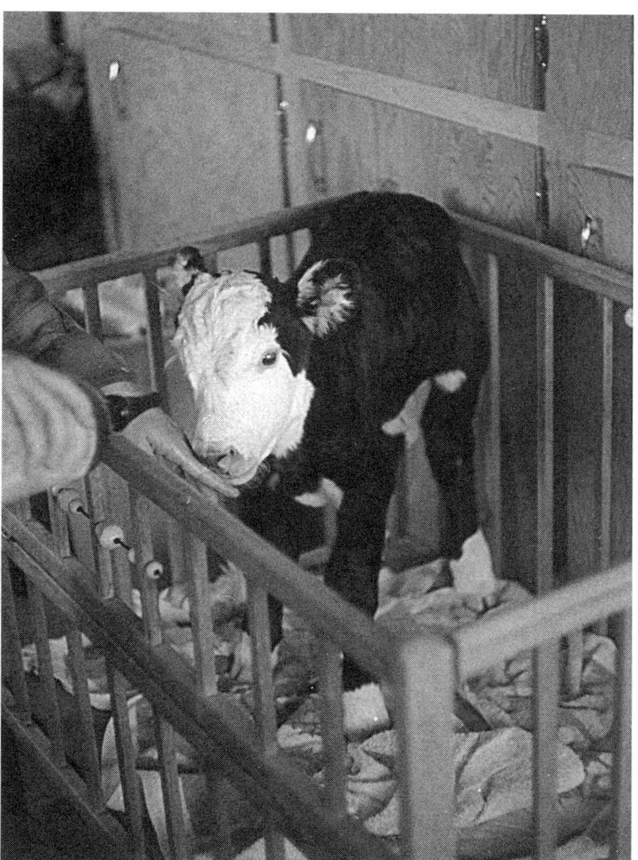

Rudolph was small enough for our daughter's old crib. He was the first premature calf who lived in the house.

When a Premature Calf Was Sick with Pneumonia

Rudolph was our first "preemie," born five weeks early. The cows were still on our mountain pasture that December, not due to start calving until January. After a snowstorm, we decided to bring them down to the fields, to feed them hay. Lynn drove our Jeep up the mountain to call the cows (they come when called, knowing they are moving to a better pasture or will be fed hay), and I rode my horse up another canyon to gather the farthest cows. In that far corner I found a cow with a tiny new calf. He weighed about 20 pounds (9 kg) — one-quarter the size he would have been at full term. His hair was short and fine, like velvet, and he was very cold.

I considered putting the tiny calf on my saddle and carrying him over the hill to the Jeep, but I wasn't sure if my young, skittish horse would tolerate such a novel passenger. So I went to get Lynn, who drove the Jeep as far up the canyon as he could,

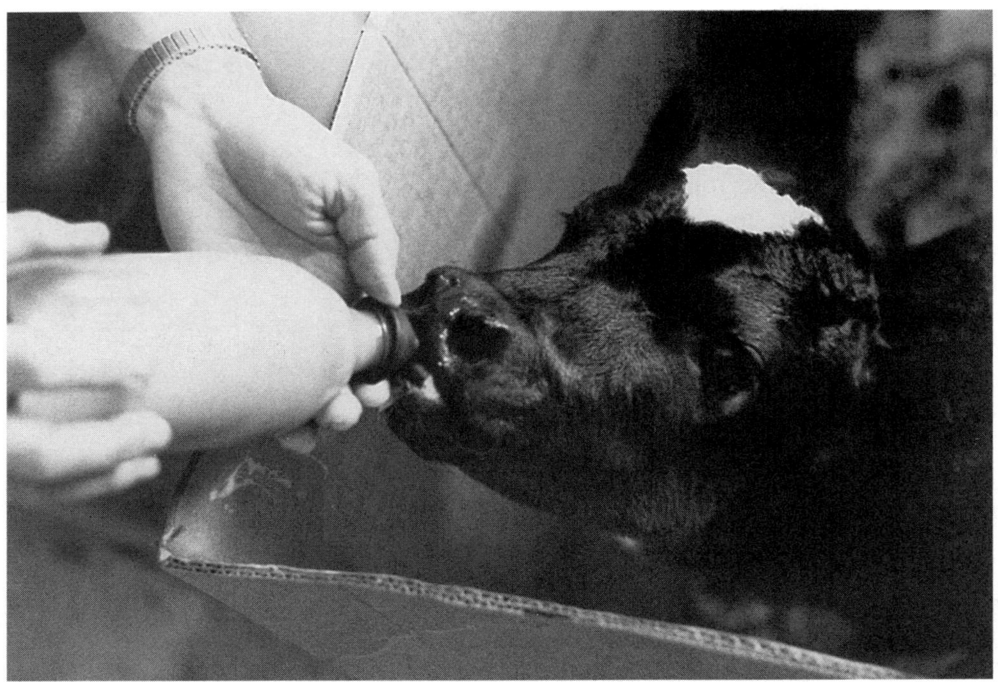

Boom Boom takes a bottle in his box.

then hiked the rest of the way through the snow. He carried the calf to the Jeep, with the cow following, while I herded the other cows. The calf rode on the Jeep seat the rest of the way home.

He was too frail to live with his mother in the barn; he was already showing signs of pneumonia after being chilled in the snow and was having difficulty breathing. We brought him into the house to warm him, gave him a bottle of colostrum, which he sucked, and injections of antibiotics. When our young children came home from school, they named him Rudolph because of his red, frostbitten nose. We kept him in the kitchen in our daughter's old crib; he was so small that he couldn't jump out. For several days we fed him every few hours and treated him for pneumonia around the clock. It was difficult for him to nurse a bottle because it took all of his energy and concentration just to breathe.

By Christmas, he was winning the battle. His fever was down and he was stronger, hopping around in the crib. He didn't have room for exercise, so we let him out every day for a few minutes to run and buck in the living room. His little feet had good traction on the carpet, better than on the slippery kitchen floor. Every time Lynn lifted him from the crib, Rudolph's little feet churned the air in eager anticipation, impatient to get down on the floor and run, taking off as soon as his feet touched the carpet. He'd go bucking and snorting around the room, and it took all four of us to guard the hot stove, the Christmas tree, and the archway to the dining room. If he zoomed out onto the linoleum, he was like the fawn Bambi on the ice pond in the movie, sliding out of control or doing splits. On the carpet, however, he could get up a lot of speed. He also enjoyed play-fighting with anyone who would get down on hands and knees.

After three weeks in our house, he outgrew the crib and tried to jump out. Even though he was not yet "full term" in size or time, we fixed a warm corner for him in a barn stall. He grew longer hair, and we raised him on a bottle with milk from our milk cow. He caught up in size and was sold with the other steers that fall.

When a Calf Was Six Weeks Early

One October, our children, ages 13 and 15, did chores while Lynn and I were gone for several days for a speaking engagement that I had at a cattlemen's meeting in Oregon. We regularly sold milk to neighbors because our cow gave more milk than our family could use, and the kids took milk to a neighbor whose cow was dry and due to calve in six weeks.

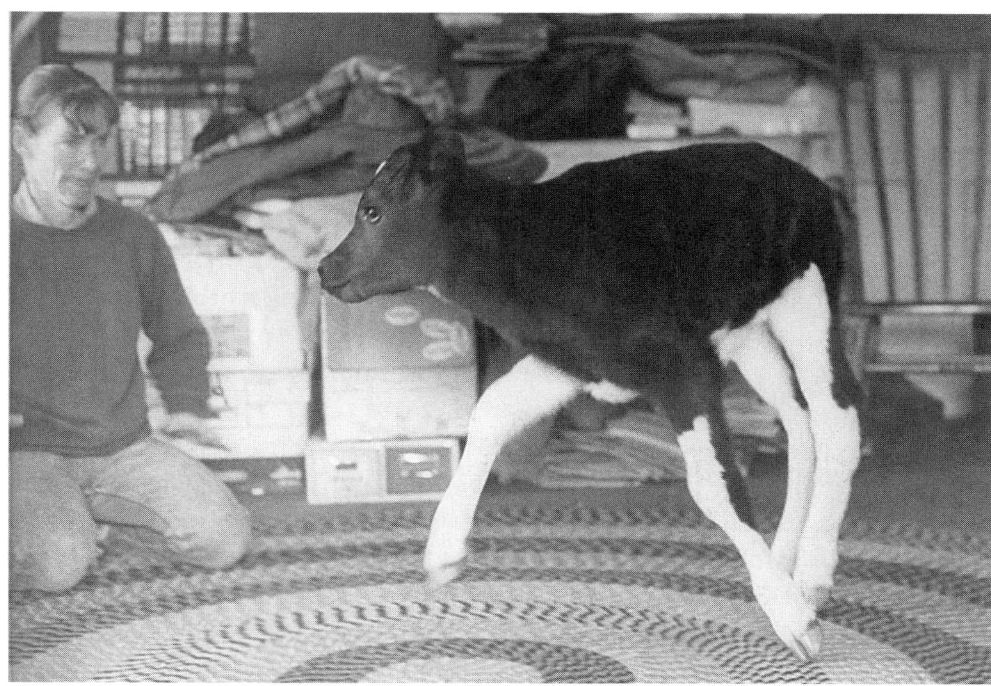

Boom Boom dances in the living room as part of his daily exercise routine.

When Michael and Andrea arrived at Jim's place, the vet was performing surgery on Jim's cow; she'd been sick and not eating. The vet suspected hardware disease (infection from eating a nail, wire, or other foreign object that penetrates the stomach lining) and was hoping to find the foreign object and remove it. But when he opened her up, he discovered that she had severe inflammation and infection in the abdominal cavity, and that there was no hope of saving her. Her calf was still alive, but Jim had no way to feed him and didn't want to take care of a premature calf. Our kids didn't want him to die, so Jim had the vet remove the calf and gave him to the kids.

It was a bull calf, tiny and frail. The wind was cold, so Jim lent them a blanket to wrap around the calf. Andrea held him on her lap in the Jeep cab as they drove home. They brought the calf into the house, and Andrea dried him with towels by the woodstove while Michael made an "incubator" from a large cardboard box, cutting a hole near the bottom so warmth from the stove could go in. They laid the calf on towels in the box, but he was still cold and shivering, so they put an electric heater nearby and blew warm air through the hole. They covered the box to keep the warm air in and put an electric heating pad on the calf.

We keep frozen colostrum in our freezer for emergencies, so Andrea thawed and warmed some in pans of hot water on the stove. She tried to get the calf to suck a bottle and lamb nipple, but he wouldn't. After a couple hours of trying, the kids called a ranch neighbor for help, since they didn't know how to use our stomach tube. The neighbor brought an esophageal feeder and force-fed the tiny calf.

He was weak and lethargic; the kids stayed up all night trying to get him warm. Andrea took his temperature, and it was subnormal most of the night. The colostrum they force-fed him gave him strength and energy, however, and by 2 AM he decided that he wanted to live. His first meal had worn off, and he was hungry. This time when Andrea offered him the bottle, he drank most of it.

By morning his temperature had come up to normal, but it didn't stop there. He soon had a high fever, breathing fast and shallow; they realized that he had pneumonia. The kids called us for advice on how to treat him. It would be a tough job to save him. At that stage of prematurity, his lungs were not fully developed, and pneumonia could quickly kill him. Andrea found the medications (antibiotics, an injectable expectorant to help break up congestion in his lungs, and anti-inflammatories to help bring down his fever). She filled the syringes, and Michael gave the injections. The calf was so small and skinny that it was hard to find enough muscle tissue to inject the medications, and he didn't like the needle prick.

When Lynn and I got home two days later and saw how tiny and frail he was (no bigger than a large cat), we were amazed that our kids had been able to keep him alive. He was just a fragile little hide stretched over tiny bones, with almost no hair. He still had a fever, but it was coming down. The kids were glad that we were home; they were worn out from staying up nights to feed and treat him. I took over night feedings; the tiny calf had to be fed every four hours to keep up his energy and fluids so that he wouldn't dehydrate.

With diligent treatment he got over the pneumonia and began jumping around in his box, kicking the sides and butting it with his head. He was so noisy the kids named him Boom Boom. He rammed the box so hard we feared that he might tip it over, so we fortified it with chairs, tying them around the box with a rope. Eventually we added plywood to make the sides of the box taller and stronger.

After he was a few weeks old, we gave him bigger feedings, reducing the number to four during a 24-hour period rather than six, and let him out of the box now and then for exercise. He loved to run and buck, chasing the kids and trying to butt heads with anyone who would play with him. He was still too small and frail to go outside in temperatures below zero. So he stayed in his box in the kitchen for four weeks, until he had more flesh on his bones and some hair. By Christmas, he was nearly the size that he should have been at birth, so we fixed him a place in the barn. We fed him milk from our old Holstein cow until another cow calved and had enough milk for two babies.

We were proud of our kids for saving him when his condition was critical and we weren't there to help. We kept Boom Boom until he was a big yearling. The kids were reluctant to sell him, even though they planned to convert him into savings for college. Raising him was a challenge that gave them much satisfaction and a sense of accomplishment, after nursing him into the world and saving his life.

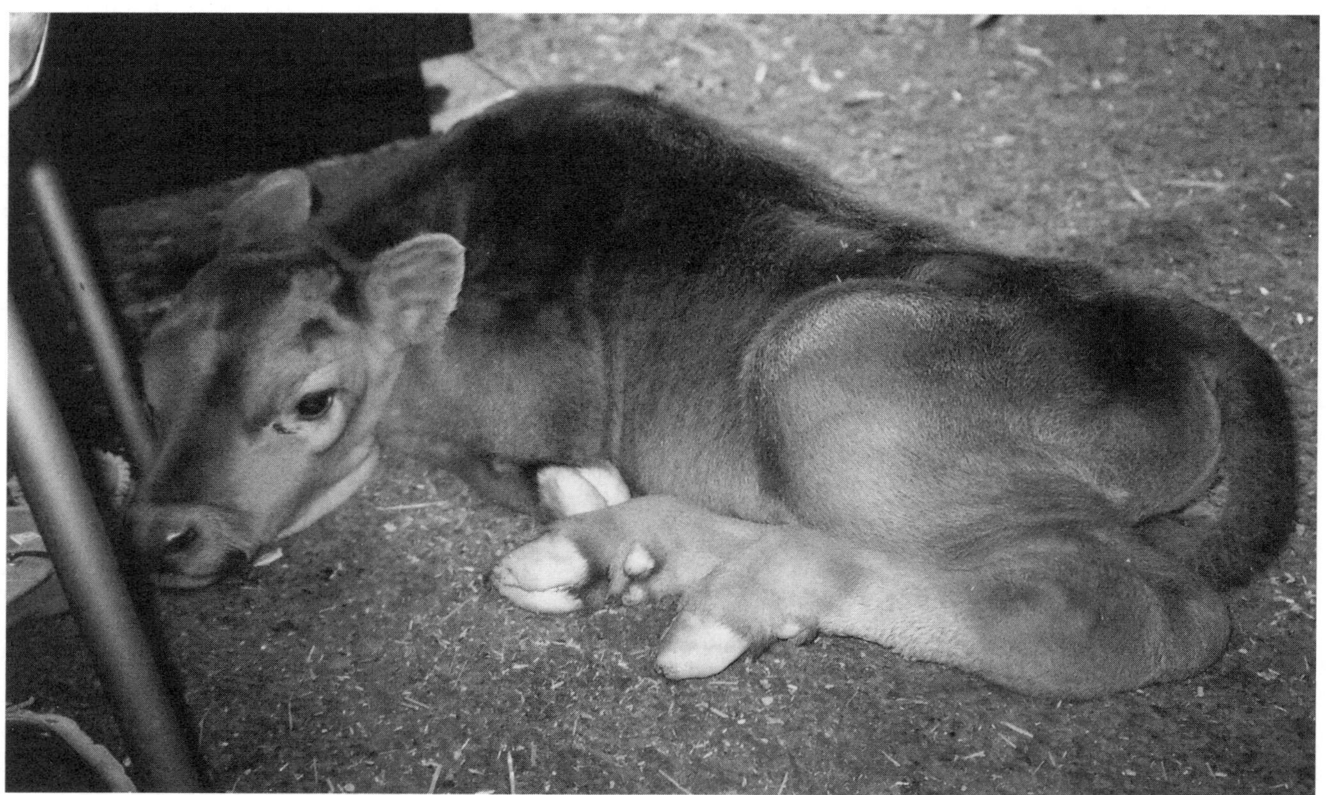

Little Red Chili Pepper, a premature twin, lies warming and drying by the woodstove in the trailer house on the night he was born. He was about seven weeks premature; he had very short, fine hair and was quite small.

Keep a Close Watch over Preemies

Most calves within six weeks of term can be saved with intensive care, by making sure they're immediately dried, kept warm, given colostrum, and fed small amounts very frequently through the first weeks. They must be in a clean environment, and the space where they're kept should not be too hot or cold, since their immature systems are not very good at regulating body temperature. Often the best situation is to keep the calf in the house at first, where you can monitor and feed him in a timely fashion, day and night.

Diligent health monitoring is crucial. A premature calf is vulnerable to illness and can die quickly if he gets sick. It's important to protect him from disease exposure and to start treatment immediately if he becomes ill. Pneumonia is always a risk because immature lungs are not very strong. The calf should be started on appropriate antibiotics immediately at any hint of respiratory illness (dullness, increased respiratory rate, difficult breathing, fever). Monitor temperature with a rectal thermometer. If it rises above 102.5°F (39°C), start him on antibiotics. A tiny calf can dehydrate quickly. If he won't nurse, he must be force-fed. Make sure you give an appropriate amount for his small size, taking care not to overdo it. Small amounts, given often, are safest.

When an Early Calf Was a Twin

Red Chili Pepper's brother was born first, limp and unconscious, and though he had a heartbeat we could not revive him with artificial respiration. Our son Michael, who helped us deliver the calf, reached into the cow to check for a twin but found nothing. So we grafted an orphan calf on the young cow, Freddie (see chapter 8). Eight hours later, Freddie gave birth to the second calf, which must have been in the other horn of the uterus.

Michael and his wife were checking cows at midnight, looked in on Freddie and Bambi to make sure the grafted pair were doing okay, and found Freddie licking a tiny new calf! This one was alive but had never gotten up. Fortunately the night was fairly warm, and Freddie had him licked dry. Michael and Carolyn woke us, and we put the tiny calf into their trailer house to warm him and feed him a bottle. He nursed, but the next time we tried to feed him, he refused. He had developed pneumonia. Thus began the battle to save his life; he needed round-the-clock intensive care.

It was spring break and our grandkids (ages 12 and 14) were out of school. They took the calf home to their house, and he lived in their basement for six weeks. The first few days were critical for saving his life. The calf was dull and lethargic and didn't want to nurse; he'd lost his will to live. So our granddaughter spent hours at a time sitting beside him, petting him, reading to him, singing, trying to get him to suck her finger. All the attention paid off. Eventually she got him nursing from a bottle, and from then on he made progress. Soon he was romping around the basement with our grandson. Since those kids were instrumental in saving him, we gave the calf to them and they named him Red Chili Pepper.

Our granddaughter spent hours at a time sitting beside him, petting him, reading to him, singing, trying to get him to suck her finger. All the attention paid off.

Dysmature Calves

Some calves have grown in their mother's wombs for the full term of pregnancy and yet are not quite ready to enter the world. This sometimes happens if there was a problem with placental attachments and the fetus did not receive adequate nutrients via the dam's bloodstream. It may also happen with twins. The calves may both be a little small, or one may be smaller and frailer than the other. Most *dysmature* calves can survive and be successfully raised, if cared for intensively for a while, like a premature calf.

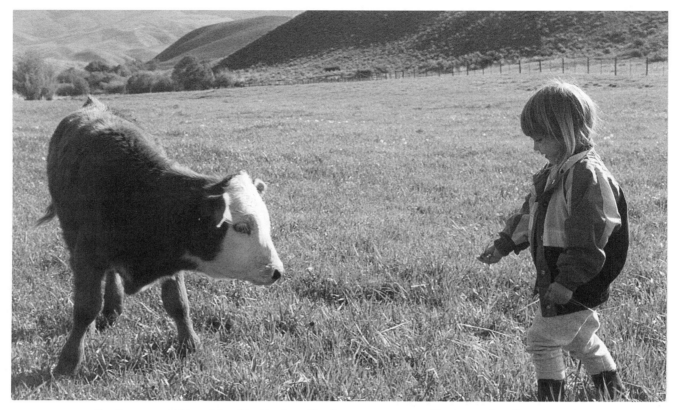

Our three-year-old granddaughter Heather offers Norman some grass. Norman preferred people to cows after spending a month in our home.

When a Calf Was Developmentally Delayed

Norman, born in 1994, was named for the calf in the Western movie comedy *City Slickers.* Her mother, Bohemian Barby (daughter of Yugoslavian Yentle and granddaughter of Swiss Miss), went into labor near her due date, but as the amnion sac emerged, part of the placenta appeared also. This meant trouble; the placenta was detaching too early, and the calf might die before delivery. So we quickly put Barby in the barn and tied her to the side of the stall to check her and assist the birth.

Lynn reached in and found tiny feet. Usually you can tell if a calf is still alive; when you grasp a foot, it usually jerks or moves if you pinch between the toes. This one did not. The calf was so tiny she was easy to pull out, and when she plopped down on the straw, we thought she was dead. The placenta came with the calf, and half of it looked rotten. Perhaps there'd been twins; Lynn felt an odd mass when reaching in again to check the uterus. Maybe a twin died earlier and mummified (see chapter 2).

Usually you can tell if a calf is still alive; when you grasp a foot, it usually jerks or moves if you pinch between the toes. This one did not. The calf was so tiny she was easy to pull out, and when she plopped down on the straw, we thought she was dead.

We were sure that this calf was dead until she surprised us and wiggled her head. We quickly got her breathing, and the young mama sniffed her calf and started licking her, but this calf was too tiny and frail to live in the barn. The longer she stayed out there, the greater the risk of pneumonia. So we whisked her into the house where we dried her by the stove with towels. Norman weighed only 34 pounds even though she was full term with a normal hair coat and erupted incisors. She was tiny but had a big attitude. She was soon on her feet, trying to wander around the house. We fed her colostrum and put her into a cardboard box. She was so small that she lived in a toilet-paper box (14 by 24 inches) until one of us could make a trip to town and bring home a big freezer box. She lived in a cut-down freezer box for four weeks.

We put towels in the box for bedding, changing them a couple of times a day. She urinated regularly but passed feces only once every 24 hours, usually during the night shift when our daughter and son-in-law were checking the calving cows and giving Norman her midnight bottle, so it was easy to keep her bed clean. She was so tiny that we gave her just a pint of milk (half a liter) every four hours.

Andrea and Jim often let Norman out to gallop around the back room. Lynn and I were supposedly asleep so I could get up at 2 AM to take over the early-morning calving shift, but I'd hear the clatter of little hoofs as Norman raced around the back room. She always tried to go into the dining room, but Jim, who was sitting in the doorway on a stool reading a book between trips to the barn, would stick out his leg to stop her. Most other times of day we were all too busy to let her out of her box, but she entertained herself by chewing on her bed towels and shaking them, as a dog would. Even after she grew up, she loved to chew on cloth; she'd grab our sleeves or pant legs with her mouth and nibble away.

She finally got to live outside when she was a month old and had grown from 34 pounds to 70 (15.4 kg to 31.8). Another first calver, Margot, had lost her three-week-old calf to acute gut infection (see chapter 11). The calf was in shock by the time we discovered that he was sick, and though we gave him IVs, we could not save him — one of the few calves we've ever lost. This was our chance to give Norman a real mother, since her own mother had long since dried up her milk.

Margot wasn't happy about the substitute; we hobbled her to keep her from kicking Norman when we put them together in a small pen. Norman was excited to have room to run and was more interested in zooming around the pen than in her new mother. We had to teach her to nurse the cow. Margot finally accepted the substitute child, but Norman was very independent and did not consider herself a bovine.

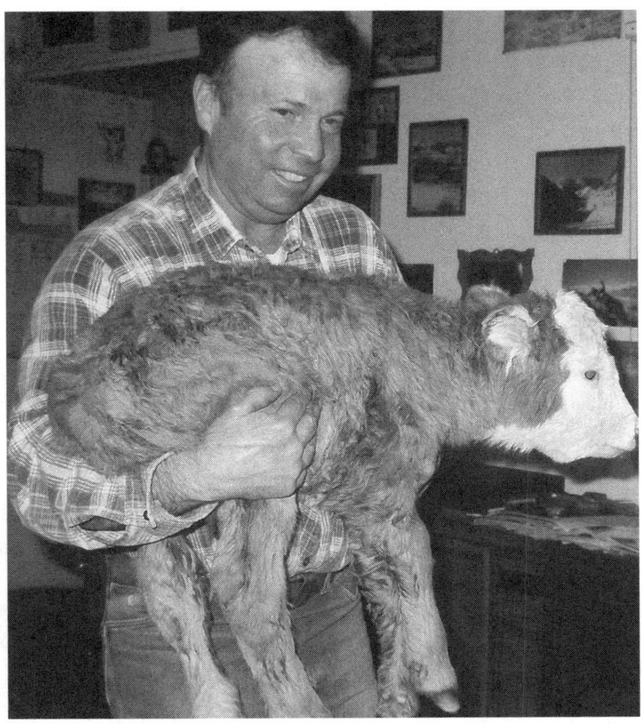

Lynn brought full-term but tiny Norman into the house to dry her.

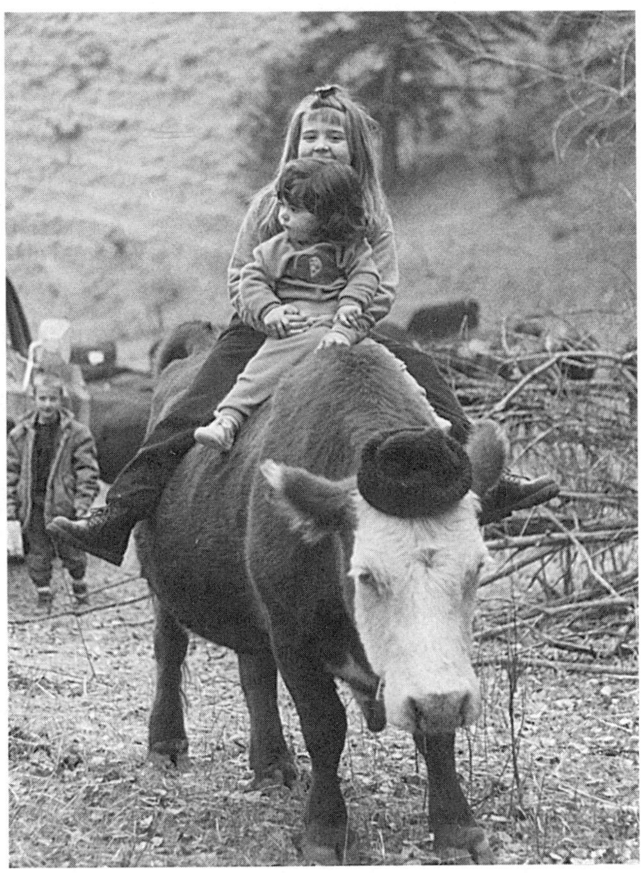

Our two granddaughters, Heather, age seven, and Emily, age one and a half, ride gentle and tolerant Norman.

IF YOU CAN'T CAST A BROKEN LEG, TRY A SPLINT

In most cases of a broken leg bone, the vet will need to fit a cast. However, if the leg is broken between hock and stifle, there is no way to immobilize the bone. Using a dog splint is one way to heal the leg. There are several sizes of dog splints. Be sure to use a splint that fits the calf. Below is what we did when one of our calf's legs were broken.

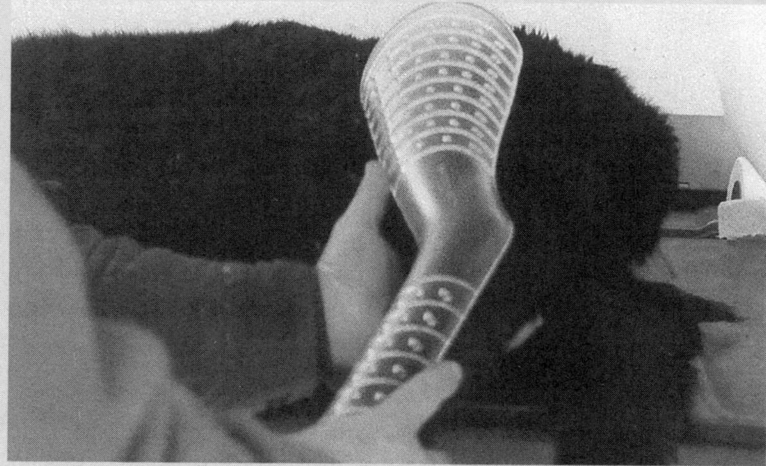

1. Find a splint that fits the calf's leg.

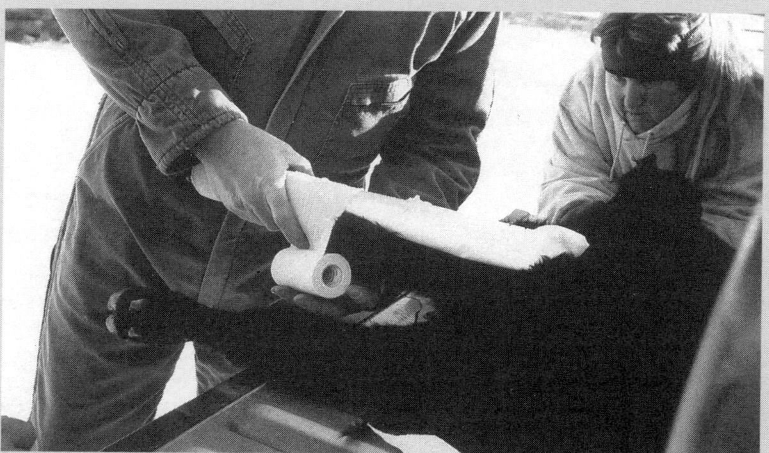

2. Pad the splint and affix it to the leg by wrapping it as high up the leg as possible.

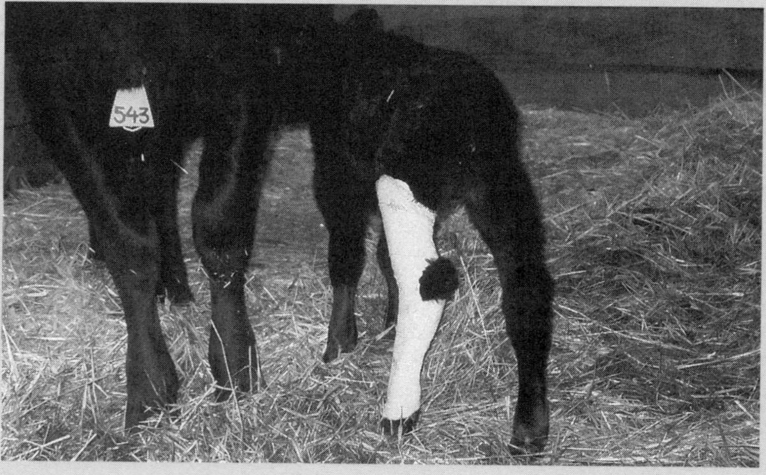

3. Adjust the splint as the leg grows. When our calf's leg was broken in this spot, we had to slit the old tape and retape the splint once, to adjust for the growth of the calf's leg. At four weeks of age, the calf was still wearing the splint but would soon have it removed.

She preferred to associate with people. Even when she grew up and had calves of her own, she always wanted us to scratch her ears or under her chin. Whenever we rode range and came across Norman, she expected us to get off of our horses and pet her. In later years, she even tolerated our grandkids riding her around the pasture.

Intensive Care for Wounded and Post-op Calves

Although he moves and lives in a herd, each calf is an individual that experiences life differently from all the others. With these individual experiences come unique challenges for the calves that may include injuries, wounds, and medical interventions.

When a Calf Was Stepped On

A few years ago Rishira stepped on her calf's hind leg after she was born and before the calf had a chance to get up and nurse. Rishira was worried about a calf bouncing around in the next pen and didn't pay attention where she was stepping. We saw that her calf couldn't get up and realized that she had a broken leg. Lynn held the calf's hind end up while I helped her nurse. We named her Peggy Sue. We tried to make a splint, but our homemade contraption wasn't sturdy enough, so we called one of our vets to help us to put a cast on her. With proper support for her leg, she was able to walk around, nurse her mother, and even buck a little.

We put the pair in the barn, since the cast could not get wet. We let them have three stalls and lots of bedding to make sure the cast stayed clean and dry. We didn't leave a water tub in the stall, since calves love to run through their mama's tubs or play in them; we watered Rishira twice a day, taking the tubs out afterward. After a couple of weeks, we slit the cast down one side and taped it together, to give the growing leg bone more room. After two more weeks, we took it off completely, and the leg had healed perfectly.

Two years later we had a similar case, but this time a newborn calf's hind leg was broken higher up and in a location impossible to cast. Like Rishira, this day-old calf's mother stepped on him. She broke the calf's bone on the upper hind leg midway between hock and stifle. Because there is no way to completely immobilize the bone between these two joints with a cast, we used a dog splint. We affixed the padded splint to the leg by wrapping it in place with adhesive tape as high up the leg as we could go. We had to slit the old tape and retape the splint once, to adjust for growth of the leg. We were able to remove the splint when the calf was one month old. The bone healed and the calf fully recovered.

When I got back to look at Dixie she lay unconscious, barely breathing, with her eyes rolled back in her head. I took her temperature, but she was so cold it wouldn't register on the thermometer. A phone call to the vet confirmed our suspicions: The calf was in shock.

When a Calf Had Abdominal Surgery

Dixie was a month old when she became constipated and unable to pass any feces at all. We gave her mineral oil, then castor oil, but nothing came through. We took her to town in our car, and our vet surgically opened her abdomen and found that a piece of small intestine had died, perhaps from the trauma of being stepped on by a cow. He cut out a 4-inch (10 cm) section and sewed it back together. We brought Dixie home and put her in the kitchen by our stove. She was still groggy from the anesthetic and lay there quietly on towels. We hurried with evening chores, and when I got back to look at Dixie she lay unconscious, barely breathing, with her eyes rolled back in her head. I took her temperature, but she was so cold it wouldn't register on the thermometer. A phone call to the vet confirmed our suspicions: The calf was in shock.

Her circulatory system was failing; we needed to increase her blood volume, quickly. We warmed a bottle of sterile electrolyte solution and dextrose on the stove, and we gave her an injection of *adrenaline,* which acts as a stimulant and also constricts the small blood vessels, halting further loss of fluid

DIXIE'S CLOSE CALL

When **month-old Dixie** became constipated and several days' treatment with fluids and oil did not resolve her problem, we took her to our vet for surgery. He located and removed a 4-inch section of small intestine that had died, possibly from bruising and lack of blood flow. The dead intestine was acting as a blockage; the blockage and necrotic tissue soon would have killed the calf. The surgery was a success, and we brought the unconscious calf home again, but Dixie slipped into shock instead of coming out from under the effects of the anesthetic. It took heroic emergency efforts at home in our kitchen to reverse this condition and save her. Then followed a lengthy recovery, during which she lived in our kitchen but was taken to the barn once a day to nurse her mother. Our children, age 6 and 8 then, enjoyed having a pet calf in the kitchen for 10 days.

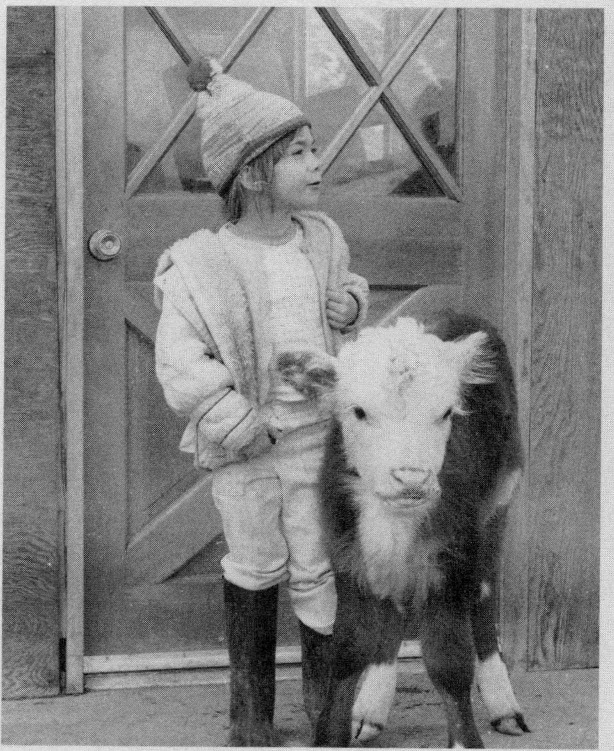

Our 6-year-old daughter Andrea helped guide Dixie down the back porch steps to go across the driveway and into the barn for her once-a-day reunion with Mama.

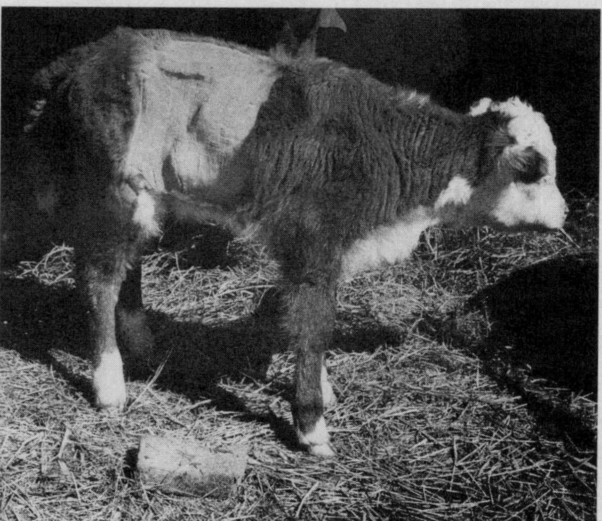

A week after her surgery, Dixie is enjoying the sunshine by the barn door after nursing with Mama.

from the capillaries. If the treatment is given in time, IV fluid and injection of adrenaline and steroids prevent irreversible damage from lack of oxygen to the tissues.

It was difficult to give her the IV fluid; she had such low blood pressure we couldn't find her jugular vein until we shaved her neck with our hair clippers. We finally got the fluid into her vein and tried to warm her up, propping her limp body with towels, with an electric heating pad over her, covering her with towels and jackets, with only her face sticking out. Her temperature was still too low to register, and her respiration was slow and shallow. We were afraid she'd be dead by morning. We went to bed but looked in on her periodically whenever we got up to check on the calving cows. There was no change in the mound of towels and jackets.

Then at 2 AM, she raised her head when Lynn walked through the kitchen. I got out of bed to see the miracle myself. She was indeed awake and looking at us with awareness. I prepared to take her temperature and found she'd passed a great quantity of loose feces with all the castor oil that had been in there for several days! The surgery was a success. Her temperature was up to 96°F (35.5°C) — not yet normal (101.5°F [38.6°C]), but definitely better. We almost danced with joy as we mixed a feeding for her, which included a drug our vet gave us to keep her bowels soft while the intestine healed, and gave it to her via stomach tube. We fed her fluids every six hours and milked her mother Drusilla to add milk to the mix. Dixie was passing lots of feces and kept me busy putting fresh towels under her and washing messy ones. It was like having baby diapers again.

The next day she was stronger and able to stand. We made a jacket from an old sweatshirt and took her to the barn a couple of times to nurse her mother. It was a happy reunion; Drusilla was glad to see her calf and didn't worry about the red coat Dixie was wearing to keep her shaved side warm. By evening, she was doing so well that we left her in the barn with her mother, wearing her jacket.

But we were rushing things. Though we gave her more feedings of extra fluid, it wasn't enough. Two days later we brought her back into the house because she was constipated and her temperature was dropping. Back in the kitchen, we gave her more fluid, castor oil, and several enemas to soften the hard balls of feces and help with fluid intake. The large colon can absorb liquid, and especially a saltwater solution. For the next two days we fed her by stomach tube every six hours and took her to nurse her mother just once a day because she was so weak. She passed no bowel movements at all. We had houseguests, and Dixie got lots of attention from extra kids who thought it exciting to have a calf in the house. It was nice to have no mess while that family was staying with us, but I longed for a big mess: Two days with no bowel movements was an ominous sign. The morning after our company left, Dixie passed manure. Once again, I was washing messy towels but rejoicing as I did it.

Dixie had adjusted to life as a house calf. She lay content on her towels, perky and interested in everything going on around her. We got her up and turned her over several times a day and took her to the barn to nurse her mother. In the house she was quiet and resigned to lying there; the few times she tried to get up and walk she found the kitchen floor too slippery. But when we took her out to the barn she became eager and active, not wanting us to catch her when she finished nursing. After we carried her back to the house, however, she would lie peacefully on her towels, a house calf again. We kept her in the kitchen for 10 days. Those last days we didn't have to carry her back and forth; she'd run down the back steps and over to the barn to her mama. She recovered fully.

Chapter 10

Preventive Care

A SUCCESSFUL, HEALTHY CALVING SEASON takes planning. If you have easy-calving cows and large, clean areas for birth, you typically can let Mother Nature oversee the health and well-being of the cows and their babies. In other circumstances, Nature needs your help to make sure calves are born safely and not exposed to illness or severe weather. If you have limited space, or confine cows in calving pastures or small lots to be watched closely, risks for contamination and infection are increased. Plenty of uncrowded grassy pasture or adequate bedding for newborns in barns or pens, and minimal stress are keys to raising healthy calves.

With crowding comes greater exposure to infection, and increased social stress. The results of crowding are Nature's way of controlling animal populations. People who raise livestock must build management practices around ways to minimize crowding, stress, and contamination to reduce incidence of illness. When there are too many animals in one area, they get sick and die. The risk for disease is especially high in newborns. Preventing illness in young calves should be a priority.

There is a growing movement toward raising natural beef and organic beef, with minimal or no artificial additives, like drugs. This can be accomplished only if you work diligently at keeping the animals healthy — which means a good vaccination program and clean, uncrowded conditions. There are times, however, that circumstances prevent optimum conditions, and baby calves become ill. In these instances you often have to rely on antibiotics to save them.

The environment that the calf is born into is one that we've created. We are responsible for trying to prevent or treat any illness that might result from the conditions of that environment. Early detection and prompt treatment with an appropriate drug can make a big difference in whether the animal recovers or dies.

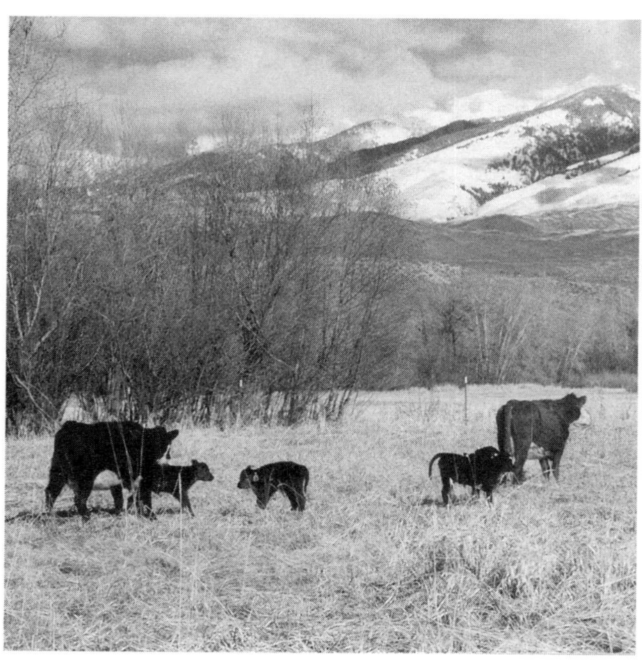

The best protection against disease in baby calves is a clean environment. Keep newborns in a new, clean area without mud or manure and away from the calving cows.

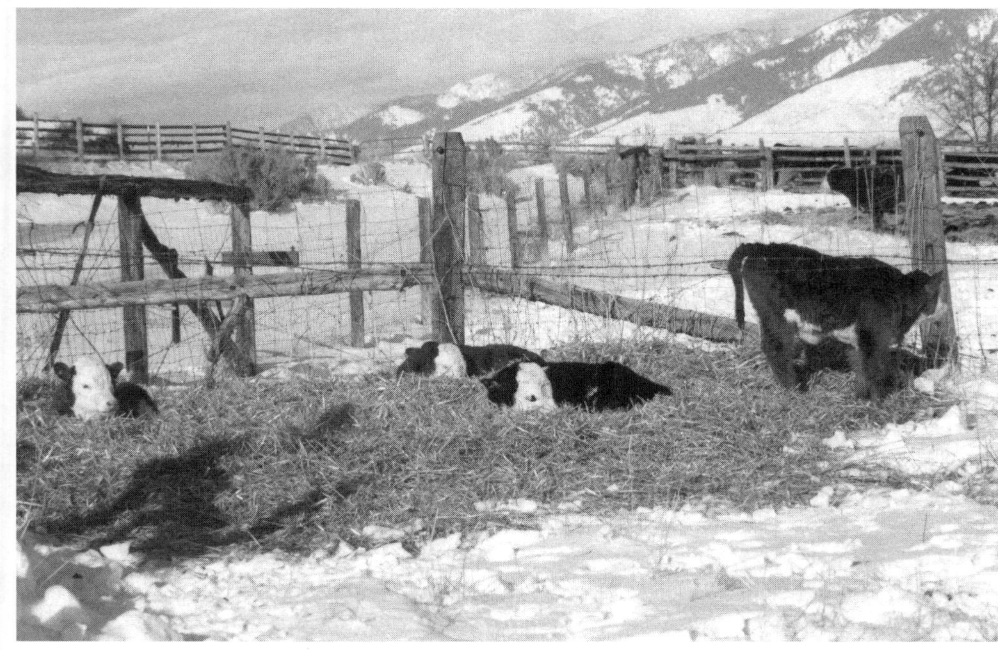

If the weather is wet or cold, provide clean bedding in every field where there are baby calves so that they always have a clean, dry place to sleep.

Every herd, ranch, and farm is different and has its own problems and solutions to those problems. What works well for your neighbor may not work as well for you. Each stockman works at solving his own unique issues of disease, but often methods helpful in other herds can be used to advantage in yours. Together with providing each calf an adequate amount of high-quality colostrum soon after birth, the best protection against calf loss is a conscientious effort that includes good nutrition, proper sanitation, and a sheltering program.

Clean Conditions for Calving

The best protection against disease in baby calves — and cows, at calving time — is a clean environment. Incidence of scours (diarrhea) in a herd is not related only to calves' levels of immunity via colostrum antibodies, but also to their level of exposure to infectious organisms, which is highest in areas (outdoors or inside) where animals are too densely congregated. If calving cows must be confined, extra steps must be taken to, among other things, provide fresh bedding daily, move them to new locations periodically, if possible, and move cow and calf pairs to a new pasture away from the cows that haven't calved yet. A disastrous incidence of calf sickness and death can occur in baby calves if management methods are not adequate.

Minimize Contamination

Providing clean, unused calving and feeding areas and not introducing new animals into the herd provide maximum protection against any new "bug." Scours is primarily a problem of contamination; the young calf becomes sick because he comes into contact with another calf with scours, or bacteria from manure, or infected discharges from cows in the mud, in manure, on the cow's udder, or elsewhere. If sick cattle and calves in earlier years inhabited a pen, pasture, calf shed, or barn, these pathogens may still be viable under certain conditions.

During wet weather, if cows are grouped in feeding areas and have mud and manure on their teats, calves ingest high levels of pathogens. Feeding large, round bales puts calves at high risk unless the bales or bale feeders are frequently moved to clean ground, because cows congregate around the bales, making a quagmire of mud and manure where they stand and eat. The same problem happens when cattle are fed silage or other feed in bunks or any single area. Access to the feed is often through deep mud and manure if cattle are constantly walking to and from that spot. If a calf must nurse mud and manure off the udder, he may get sick.

If cows are confined for calving, provide ample clean bedding as often as needed when old bedding gets soiled by manure or wet from weather. In every field where baby calves are contained, put out bedding during bad weather unless they have places out of the wind that stay clean and dry. Even if calves are using calf houses with new clean bedding put in periodically, the cows also need a clean place to lie down so that their udders won't get dirty.

If snow is deep when you start or during calving, remove it with a tractor and blade or make sure there are adequate areas of bedding so pairs won't have to lie in snow. Snow itself is clean (though it can chill a newborn or young calf or frostbite cows' teats), but melting snow creates a dirty environment. If a calf is born in mud or nurses a muddy udder, he may ingest pathogens before he gets any protective colostrum.

During wet weather, if cows are grouped in feeding areas and have mud and manure on their teats, calves ingest high levels of pathogens.

Snow Tip

If you calve when the ground is still snow-covered, sometimes it's better to leave the snow rather than remove it. As long as you have adequate bedding areas that are dry, leaving snow on fields and pastures creates cleaner conditions than blading it off and having bare, muddy ground while calves are young and likely to eat mud and dirt.

We have better luck preventing scours by putting out straw for cows to bed on and widening our feed trail every day so that they are eating in clean areas that have not been tromped on. When we put hay on clean snow, cows and calves also waste less hay by not trampling it into the mud. If you have to feed on ground that is already contaminated with feces, calves are more likely to pick up pathogens from manure.

Reducing Exposure to Pathogens

Management techniques that help to reduce the calves' level of exposure to pathogens include:

1. ***Washing the teats of any cow*** or heifer you have to restrain to assist in delivering a calf.
2. ***Thoroughly washing all equipment,*** especially an esophageal feeder or stomach tube, between calves when administering colostrum to a newborn or fluids to a sick calf.
3. ***Keeping calving stalls and pens*** clean and dry.
4. ***Moving pairs to clean pastures*** as soon as possible.

First-calf heifers need special consideration and redoubled efforts on your part. They are more often confined at calving than are older cows, because they may need assistance. Nevertheless, their calves are more susceptible to disease, due to fewer antibodies in the heifers' colostrum compared to that of mature cows, and this may increase risk for disease. You should therefore put calving heifers in your cleanest area and change bedding often enough that they never get dirty udders. And remove any sick calves and their mamas from the group immediately for treatment of the calves, so that they won't spread disease to the other calves.

Don't Let Calves Eat Twine or Dirt

Calves often gobble down dirt and mud, especially if they're born in the winter when there's not much green grass. Young calves are curious, like little children who put everything into their mouths. Calves have to sample everything. They chew on baling twine, which can be dangerous: A balled-up wad of twine in the stomach can plug the digestive tract, causing fatal blockage. Similarly, licking hair off fences or bushes where cows rubbed off shedding hair can create a hairball blockage (see chapter 15). Don't leave baling twines where calves can reach them, and gather wads of hair off fences if cows rub while shedding.

Calves eat mud and dirt if there's no green grass, partly because it's fun and partly because there's nothing to graze. Unlike green grass, hay and supplements don't meet their complete nutritional needs for certain vitamins and minerals. Feeding a mineral supplement can reduce dirt-eating but rarely stops it completely. They often eat dirt even if salt and other minerals are available.

Unfortunately, dirt and mud contain bacteria, including clostridia, that can create acute and toxic gut infections. Dirt and mud also quite often irritate the gut lining, enabling infection to gain entrance to raw tissues. Some calves eat so much dirt at once that they develop fatal blockage (see chapter 15). For winter calving we fenced off creeks, ditches, and gravel bars and watered the cows in troughs rather than give their calves access to the dirt and gravel that they love to nibble.

KEEP YOUR CHUTE AND HEAD-CATCHER AREAS CLEAN

If you put a cow in a chute or head catcher to help with a calving problem, wash the chute or head catcher afterward. If the cow or heifer lies down while you are pulling the calf and gets manure on her sides and udder from the last cow you assisted, her calf may pick up pathogens from his dirty mother. Having clean straw underfoot before you start helping her is always a good idea.

WEATHER MAKES A DIFFERENCE

IN THE SPRING OF 1993, some ranchers in eastern Idaho lost 50 percent of their calves due to weather-related scours. We had a high incidence of scours on our ranch when we calved in March and April during the late 1960s. One year, every calf on the ranch got sick by the time he was two weeks old. We spent 8 to 10 hours a day just doctoring calves! We couldn't change to summer calving because our cows were on public-range pastures in mountainous areas during summer, which makes it impossible to check on them sufficiently. We decided to calve in January — when the ground, mud, and manure are frozen — and have done so for 35 years, greatly reducing scours. We have less sickness in cold, dry weather than in wet springtime.

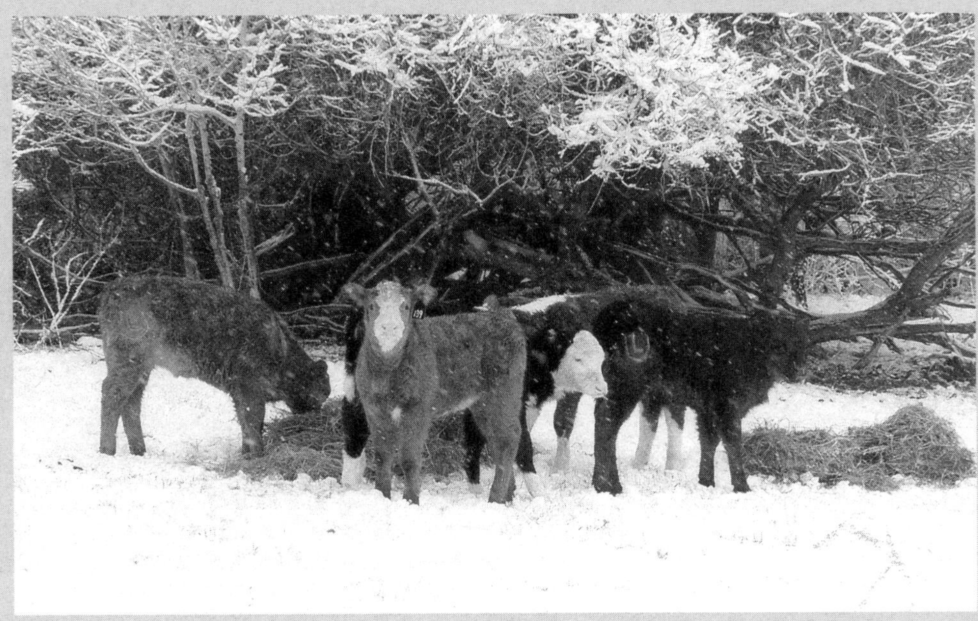

Dry cold is healthier for calves than wet weather. They don't chill as readily, and all the manure stays frozen, keeping the environment cleaner.

Weather

Pathogens are always present in pens and pastures that cattle have previously inhabited but are more accessible if the ground is wet. Calves pick up pathogens when they drink from puddles or nibble dirt or mud. Cows get dirty udders when confined during wet weather. You can cut down on scours if you change your season of calving to a time of year when the ground is not muddy. This may mean calving earlier — when the ground stays frozen, manure freezes quickly — or later, after spring thaw, when the ground is dry and pastures are grassy, not muddy.

Calving Facilities

If you calve in late spring, early summer, or early fall in a climate where the weather is mild but dry, there is little need for any shelter but a windbreak. If you have occasional hard rains, however, you'll want some kind of barn or shelter where you could put a calving cow during a deluge.

Make sure calving pastures are on high, well-drained ground where there won't be water flowing through or accumulating. A calving cow might lie in water and drown her calf as he is born. Sudden flooding during spring thaw or a hard rain may also put newborns at risk. The cow may choose a dry place to lie down when she goes into labor, but by the time the calf emerges, he may be headfirst in a puddle or stream.

Keep wind chill in mind. If there's wind, the cooling effect on a wet calf can be dangerous. For instance, if it's 30°F (–1°C) and wind is 40 miles per hour (64.4 kph), this is equivalent to 13°F (–11°C). A 30°F windy day is much harder on a newborn calf and chills him more quickly than a still, sunny 20°F (–6°C) day.

Calving Pens

If you want to keep an eye on heifers, or on all the cows in case of inclement weather, you'll need small pastures or pens to put them into as they get close to calving. Have an adequate supply of bedding (straw, wood shavings, or whatever is available in your region) so that you can periodically put out new bedding to keep the cows clean — and warmer in cold weather.

HOW COLD IS IT REALLY?

	Temperature (°F)																	
Calm	**40**	**35**	**30**	**25**	**20**	**15**	**10**	**5**	**0**	**-5**	**-10**	**-15**	**-20**	**-25**	**-30**	**-35**	**-40**	**-45**
Wind (mph) 5	36	31	25	19	13	7	1	-5	-11	-16	-22	-28	-34	-40	-46	-52	-57	-63
10	34	27	21	15	9	3	-4	-10	-16	-22	-28	-35	-41	-47	-53	-59	-66	-72
15	32	25	19	13	6	0	-7	-13	-19	-26	-32	-39	-45	-51	-58	-64	-71	-77
20	30	24	17	11	4	-2	-9	-15	-22	-29	-35	-42	-48	-55	-61	-68	-74	-81
25	29	23	16	9	3	-4	-11	-17	-24	-31	-37	-44	-51	-58	-64	-71	-78	-84
30	28	22	15	8	1	-5	-12	-19	-26	-33	-39	-46	-53	-60	-67	-73	-80	-87
35	28	21	14	7	0	-7	-14	-21	-27	-34	-41	-48	-55	-62	-69	-76	-82	-89
40	27	20	13	6	-1	-8	-15	-22	-29	-36	-43	-50	-57	-64	-71	-78	-84	-91
45	26	19	12	5	-2	-9	-16	-23	-30	-37	-44	-51	-58	-65	-72	-79	-86	-93
50	26	19	12	4	-3	-10	-17	-24	-31	-38	-45	-52	-60	-67	-74	-81	-88	-95
55	25	18	11	4	-3	-11	-18	-25	-32	-39	-46	-54	-61	-68	-75	-82	-89	-97
60	25	17	10	3	-4	-11	-19	-26	-33	-40	-48	-55	-62	-69	-76	-84	-91	-98

Frostbite Times 30 minutes | 10 minutes | 5 minutes

Wind increases the amount of heat lost from the body surface. The combined effect of wind and temperature is expressed as "equivalent temperature." For instance, 20°F (–6.5°C) with a 20-mile-per-hour (32 kph) wind would have the same effect on exposed flesh as minus 9°F (–22.7°C) with no wind.

Familiarize Young Mamas-to-Be with the Calving Shelter

It's frustrating to you and stressful to the animal if you have to run her around to make her go into a barn to give birth. Each new group of heifers that uses our calving pens or barn gets some training ahead of time. Though our heifers calve at the same time as our cows, we bring the heifers into the calving area a couple of weeks ahead, not only because heifer due dates are more unpredictable — they sometimes calve as much as two to three weeks ahead of schedule — but also because this gives us a chance to gentle them.

We walk through them several times a day and night. This gets the flighty heifers accustomed to us. After a few days, they no longer jump up when we walk through them but continue to lie there unconcerned. Once a day we put part of their hay into a smaller calving pen that serves as the entrance for going to the barn, so that they get used to going through that gate. Thus they are willing to be herded in when they are in labor. We also use a babysitter cow to lead them into the barn.

Another aid for making sure heifers are always easy to handle at calving is to halter-break them as calves. Doing this at weaning time works, though it's even easier if you can halter-break them younger and smaller, when they are easier to handle. This is a very beneficial practice, especially for the small farmer with only a few cows and no squeeze chute or head catcher (and a job off the farm and not much help, to boot). A calf never forgets her tying-up lessons. If you ever have to restrain her later in life, having her halter-trained saves time, frustration, and risk of injury. You can often handle a problem by yourself — and anywhere the cow or heifer happens to be — if you can tie her up.

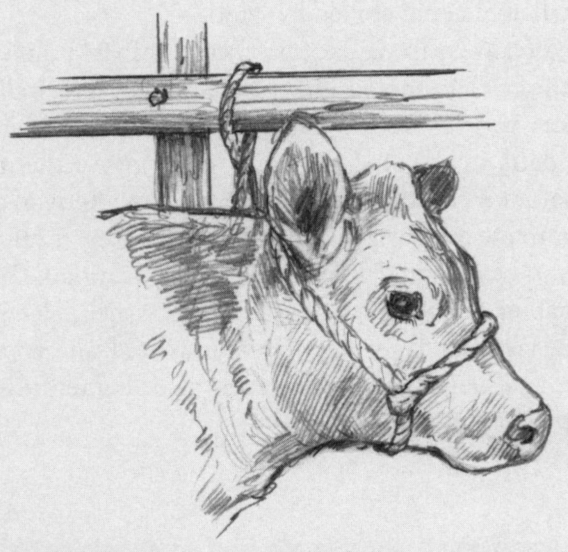

Halter-breaking heifers as calves makes them much easier to handle or restrain later.

If they may need to go into a barn or smaller pen for calving or to be restrained for assistance with a calving problem, get them acquainted with the facility. Older cows that have been through the routine before will know where the gates are, but a heifer with no prior experience may be difficult to bring into the small pen or barn alley some dark night. Design your pens so gates are in the most convenient place to gently herd an animal from the larger pen into the smaller one. Gates should be located in corners rather than along a straight fence line, so that you can funnel the animal toward it, with no chance of her running past it.

Strategically located yard lights can illuminate calving pens and barn entranceways and other areas on dark nights. Yard lights in the large holding pens are easier than using a flashlight to get an overview of the group and to know what each cow is doing. Our "maternity ward" is close to the house, on a gentle slope, so we have a good view of everything in it. Cows at the top, far end are higher on the slope, making our view of them unobstructed by cows in front. With yard lights illuminating the area, we watch them with binoculars from windows in the house and don't have to go out unless a cow is observed in labor or we can't quite see all the cows and need to check more closely.

Calving Barns

If you calve when weather may be fickle, it's very helpful to have a barn or shed, even if you only need it part of the time. Shelter for cold nights, cold or windy spells, or storms with driving snow or rain, will more than pay for itself over time; you'll have less sickness, spend less money for medications, spend less time and effort doctoring, and have fewer calf deaths. Using a barn stall, you can make sure each cow has a clean, dry place to calve, with no risk of lying in a puddle or a snowbank, or of the new calf immediately being chilled by wind.

If you always move each pair out within 24 hours, after the calf has nursed and is dry and the pair is well bonded, you can keep a barn free of disease. Never leave pairs in the stall for long; if you move them out before a calf has a chance to get sick, he won't contaminate the barn with pathogens. Make it a rule not to use calving facilities to shelter sick animals. If sick babies need shelter, use a different shed. Keep calving facilities clean and uncontaminated, and you won't have newborns getting sick from something they picked up in the barn.

If weather is adverse when pairs need to come out of the barn, put them into pastures with windbreaks, well-bedded pens with windbreak corners, or a shed-type shelter where they can spend another day or two, if necessary, before going out to big pastures.

The Benefits of Barns

In our region, where many ranchers calve in late winter or early spring before cows go to summer range in the mountains, the old notion that barns are a haven for disease is well refuted. Many ranchers calve all of their cows in a barn. This eliminates finding a calf dead in a ditch or frozen in the snow. Before we started winter calving, we averaged a 4 percent annual death loss calving out in the fields. We cut that loss down to less than 1 percent when we changed to winter calving, in barns, and were present for every birth.

Barn calving enables you to better manage calving cows because you're more likely to see problems faster; it allows you to vaccinate or treat calves at birth, thereby reducing scours during the first

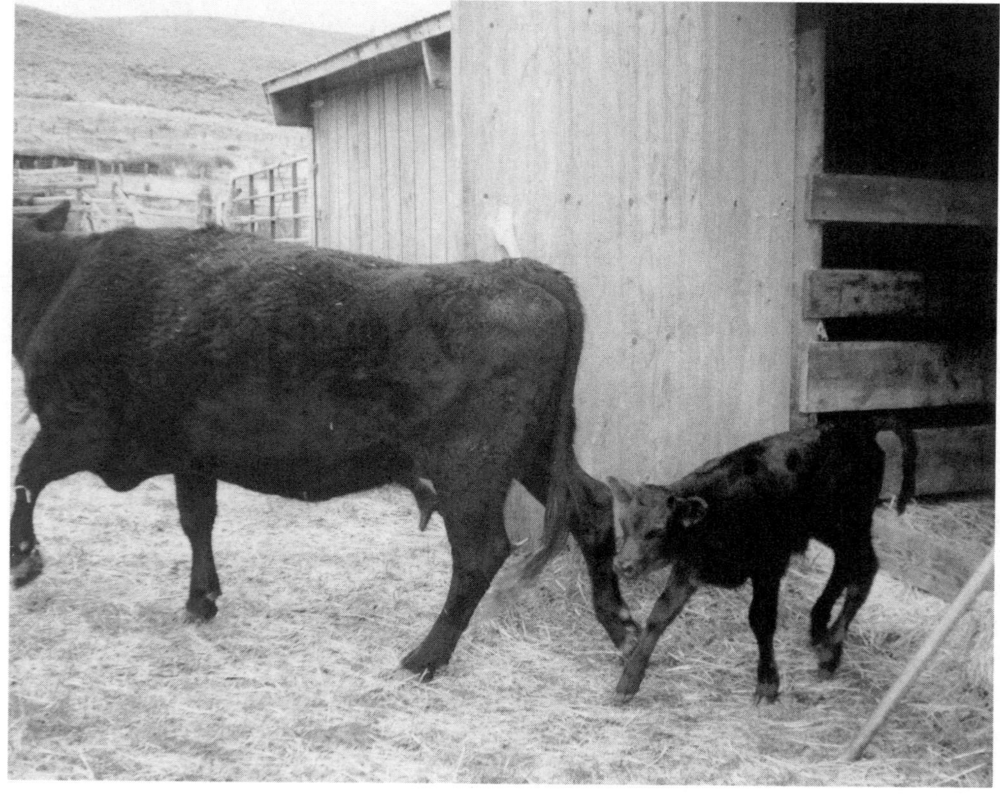

If you always move each pair out of the barn as soon as the calf is dry and has nursed and the pair is well bonded, the barn won't become contaminated with pathogens from sick calves.

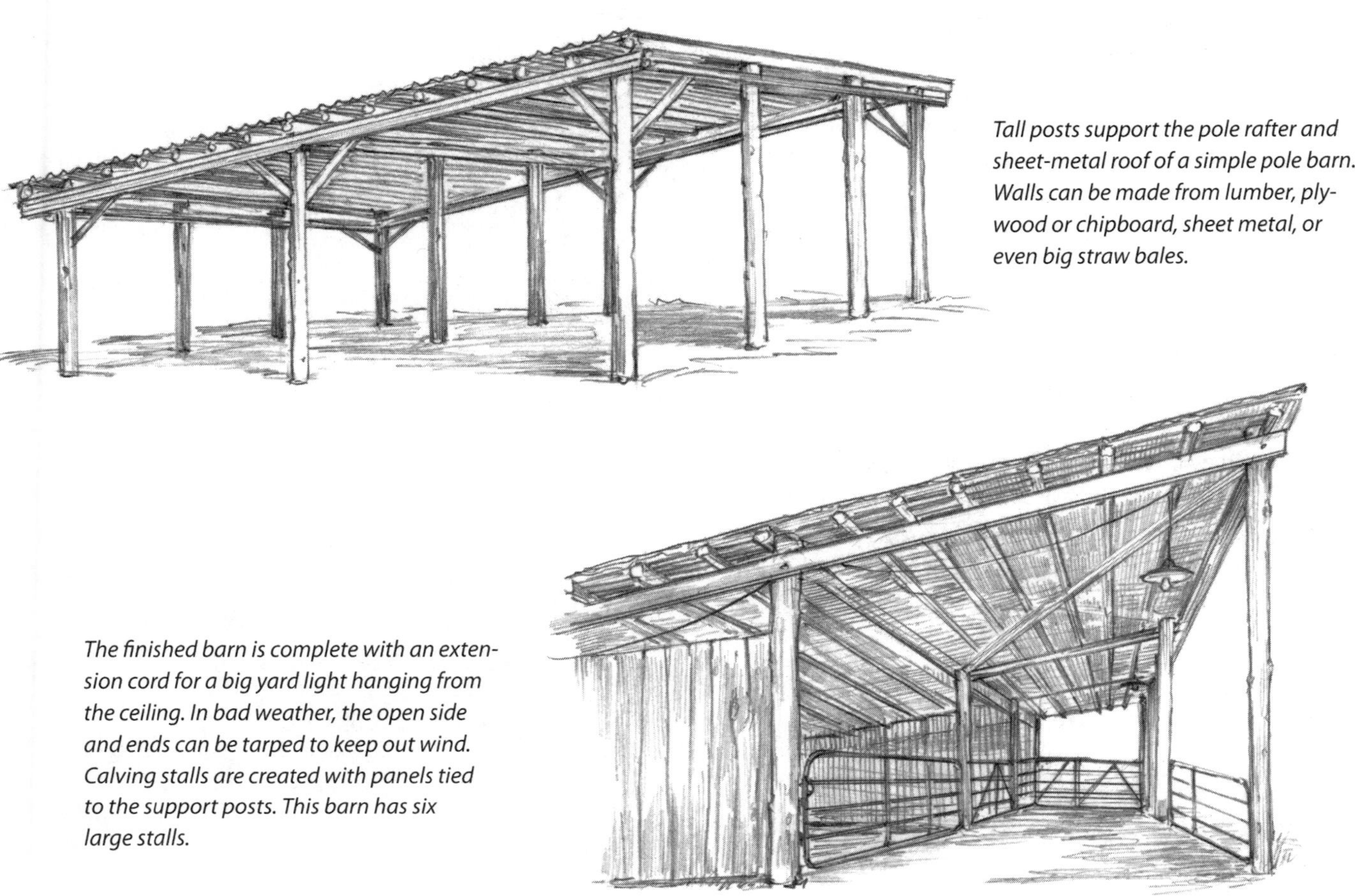

Tall posts support the pole rafter and sheet-metal roof of a simple pole barn. Walls can be made from lumber, plywood or chipboard, sheet metal, or even big straw bales.

The finished barn is complete with an extension cord for a big yard light hanging from the ceiling. In bad weather, the open side and ends can be tarped to keep out wind. Calving stalls are created with panels tied to the support posts. This barn has six large stalls.

weeks of life; and it makes it easier to help a heifer calve or suckle a calf. Many aspects of care and solutions to problems are more feasible, and you're more apt to attempt them, if cows or heifers are in the barn to calve instead of in a big pasture where it's hard to catch up with them. You can also keep a cow and calf by themselves for a few hours without interference from other cows, which can be crucial for heifer mothers.

Calving-Barn Designs

There are many ideas and designs for calving barns. You can adapt innovative and helpful tips from many sources, to create or improve your own facilities and to fit your space and purposes. Following are some simple designs:

A simple pole barn uses tall posts as supports for a metal roof, with metal or boards for walls. Upright posts can be set into the ground and well tamped, or anchored to a buried beam. For an insulated roof, use plywood, on pole or board rafters, covered with a sheet of plastic or tarp. Spread wood shavings over the plastic and cover them with metal sheeting. Outside walls can be insulated, or an insulated "thaw" box can be situated in a corner for warming calves.

Note: You need a warm place for chilled calves, but don't have the barn itself too warm. It needs ventilation to make sure air is fresh and dry, not laden with bedding dust or ammonia fumes from soiled bedding. Airtight, humid barns can lead to pneumonia.

An old garage or farm shop can be easily turned into a barn. We used our three-aisle garage shed as our first calving barn by dividing it into six or nine stalls with pole panels. That wasn't enough space, however, when we were calving 10 to 20 cows per day, so we built another barn behind it, with a pen area between them.

A bigger barn was built inexpensively with tall posts set deep in the ground, using rough lumber for walls, and a metal roof. The roof slopes forward in front, with a higher but longer slope to the rear, and a row of windows between the two slopes lets in sunshine. We made the doorways large enough to get a tractor through for easier cleaning. Inside partitions and moveable panels are made of strong, 2-inch(5 cm)-thick boards. There's no wasted space; rather than having an alley, each row of stalls is itself an alley. Rather than hinged, the panels are tied in place with doubled baling twine, which can be cut easily with a pocketknife when, in an emergency, we want to make a stall larger or smaller quickly, or move or swing a panel when a cow is calving.

An impromptu barn can be made inexpensively by using big straw bales for walls and insulation and poles or metal panels on the inside to keep the cows from eating them. Tall posts can support a solid tin or board roof that will keep snow out better than a tarp. The front can be enclosed with panels and a durable tarp that can be rolled down to keep out wind or rolled up to let in sunshine.

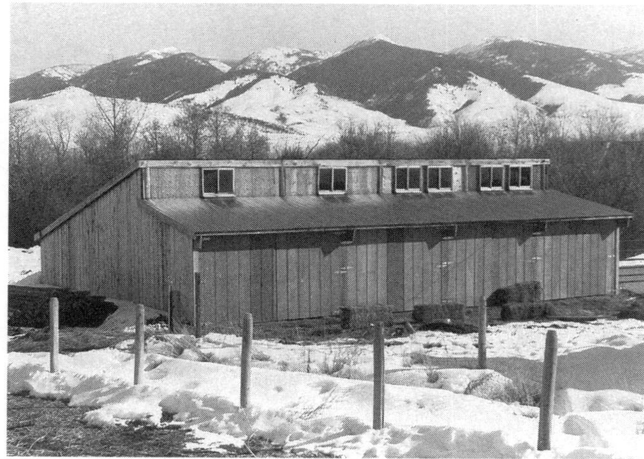

Our big calving barn, before the pens were built around it, has windows that let in sunshine for light and warmth.

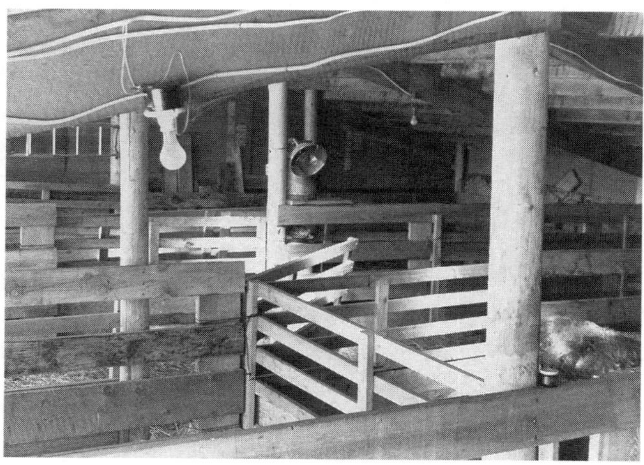

The barn has four aisles, each one divided by moveable board panels into several stalls.

Adjustable Barn Stalls

It's handy to have posts for anchoring moveable wooden or metal panels that make individual stalls larger or smaller as needed. If the walls of each stall are moveable, you can make more stalls if necessary, or move a panel to allow room to maneuver a calf puller or keep a cow from smashing her calf into the side of a stall if she's lying against it as she calves and won't get up. Sometimes it's impossible to get a cow or heifer up when the calf is partway out; it's better to move the panel out of the way if she's lying against it. Moveable panels are handier and safer than a solid aisle and stall walls; you can adjust them to fit the situation.

In our big barn, we have four rows of stalls; the barn is four wide aisles divided into stalls with moveable board panels. They are solid on the bottom half so that a calf can't stick his head through and get bashed by a cow in the next stall. There's a side panel in each aisle, so that we can shuttle a calving cow or a pair into another row of stalls if necessary. When we empty the barn, all pairs usually go out at the same time, but if for some reason there's one that should stay in longer and she's in front of a cow that should come out, we can bring the outgoing cow through

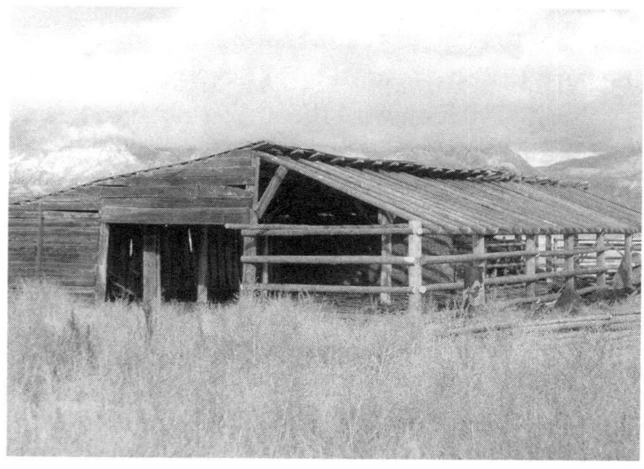

This instant, inexpensive barn can be created using an old three-sided shed. Expand it by setting posts out in front to create a fence or wall that supports more roofing. Metal sheeting can be added for an additional roof, and tarps or straw bales can make a windproof wall around the outside.

the side panel into the next row without disturbing the pair that stays in.

A head catcher can be situated in the barn to restrain a cow while you assist her during labor or as she suckles her calf. In our barn, we restrain a cow behind any panel, tied to a sturdy post in the solid aisle partition, by pushing the panel tight against her, with a rope behind her holding the panel, so she can't back out of this makeshift "chute." Then we don't have to tie her or move her to another part of the barn or out to our head catcher. When she's sandwiched between the panel and the sturdy aisle partition, we can correct a malpresentation or pull her calf and swing the panel away when we are finished or if she lies down. If she goes down, she's not cramped as she would be in a chute; we can move the panel away.

If a heifer is too wild or flighty to restrain easily for correcting a calving problem, or helping her calf nurse, we use a head catcher located in the pen between the two barns. It's handy for use in conjunction with outdoor pens as well.

A head catcher can be situated in the barn to restrain a cow while you assist her during labor or as she suckles her calf.

Calving-Barn Sanitation

Barn calving can be very clean and disease-free, but only if you make sure that each cow has clean, dry bedding, that manure and wet bedding don't build up to create ammonia fumes, and that no pairs are left in the barn for too long after calving. Keep it clean and move them out: That's the key to avoiding sickness.

- In mild weather, clean each stall between cows, and put in new bedding for each new occupant so there won't be manure, wet bedding, old rotting afterbirth, and the like.
- In severely cold weather, you can allow straw bedding to build up, removing only the wet and dirty areas daily and covering each stall floor with enough new straw to be clean for each calving cow. Buildup of straw and manure generates heat and can make the barn warmer. Cold weather will keep manure frozen, and it won't get sloppy or fill the air with ammonia fumes.
- Clean a small area with a pitchfork and a wheelbarrow. For quick and easy cleanup of a large barn, use a tractor and blade.

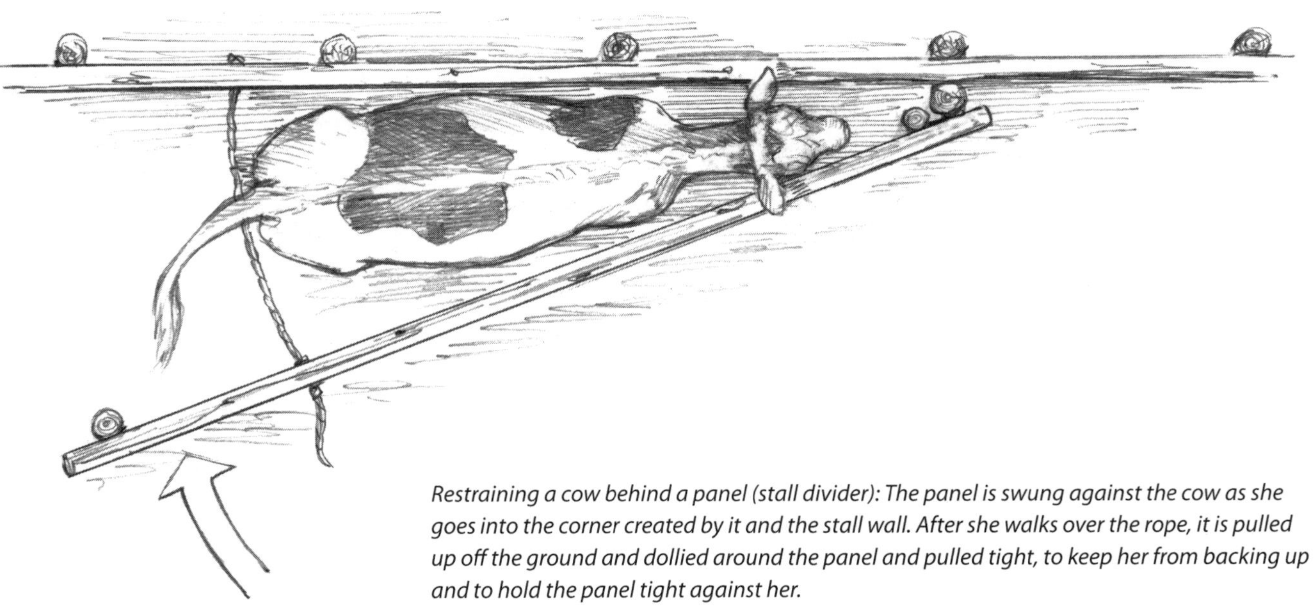

Restraining a cow behind a panel (stall divider): The panel is swung against the cow as she goes into the corner created by it and the stall wall. After she walks over the rope, it is pulled up off the ground and dollied around the panel and pulled tight, to keep her from backing up and to hold the panel tight against her.

Tips for Getting Cows into the Barn

If Bessie won't budge at the barn door, try the following methods for coaxing her along.

- Create a small holding area next to the barn to keep cows from running off when you're trying to put them inside.
- If heifers have never been in a barn, they can be hard to get inside. Take time to lure them into the holding pen with feed a few times before they calve. If you wish, you can leave the barn doors open, put feed inside, and let them go in and out of the barn a few times before calving season starts. Be sure to clean the barn thoroughly after a training program.

> COW BODY LANGUAGE
>
> Cows never forget a bad situation, but if they weren't stressed in previous attempts to put them in, cows will associate the barn with calving; many will want to go in there to calve, especially during bad weather. Some of our cows give us a clue that they're in early labor by coming to stand by the gate to the barn pen, waiting to go into the barn where they have previously calved.

- Once the cows have been in a barn to calve, they usually go in readily the next year — if they didn't have a traumatic experience being chased in there during previous seasons.
- Use a babysitter cow to lead a heifer into the barn. When a heifer goes into labor, bring a gentle cow with her into the holding area. Open the barn door, let the cow go in, and the heifer will usually follow if you gently encourage her from behind. Heifers are timid and suspicious, and there's no point in trying to force one to do what she's afraid to do. Cattle are herd animals and take their cues from other herd members. If the older cow goes willingly into the barn without giving off warning signals that it's scary, the heifer will follow.

Portable Calving Sheds

Portable calving stalls can be made with welded pipes for the frame (2.5-inch steel pipe or 2.25-inch drill stem pipe). The skids can be 2 by 8 boards, logs, rough-cut lumber, or anything else that's sturdy enough. Use 2 by 6 boards for uprights. Walls can be plywood or boards, old siding, or whatever you have available, with metal sheeting for the roof. This portable shed can have two or three stalls, each with a built-in pipe head catcher (dairy-stanchion style)

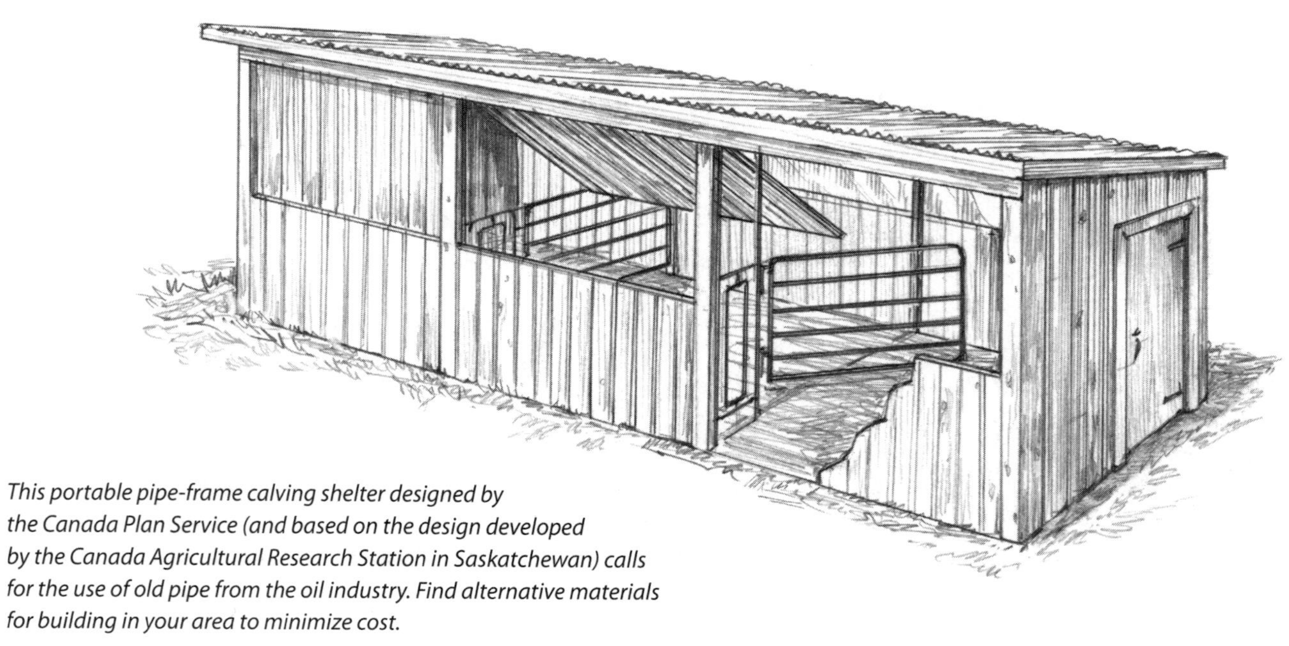

This portable pipe-frame calving shelter designed by the Canada Plan Service (and based on the design developed by the Canada Agricultural Research Station in Saskatchewan) calls for the use of old pipe from the oil industry. Find alternative materials for building in your area to minimize cost.

and a crowding gate to put the cow into the head catcher. A heat lamp can be situated in the corner of each stall, if you wish, behind a protective barrier so that it can't be bumped. Propane heaters can be used if there is no electricity. The Canada Agriculture Research Station at Melfort, Saskatchewan, created this design for portable calving sheds about 30 years ago, and their program has used them ever since.

The advantage to a portable shed is that you can pull it to any field that you use for calving. Portable panels can create an alleyway leading to the shed, for bringing a calving cow or heifer into a stall. If you situate it next to an existing fence, you can create a small catch pen in front of the shed. If you feed the cows or heifers near it, it's usually easy to get an animal into the pen, and from there into the shed. Feed a little hay in the catch pen, to get animals used to going in there, so that it won't be a challenge to put one in when she's calving.

If you construct the shed doors with a top and bottom, the top part of the door to each stall can be swung upward in mild weather to let in sunshine for warmth. The bottom can be open when the calving stalls are no longer needed, allowing calves to use the facility as a shelter or calf *creep* (an area where calves can go in to eat, but cows cannot). These sheds can be moved to wherever you need them. Two can be located face to face to create a small barn with an alleyway between the two sets of stalls.

Head Catchers

Whether you calve in a barn or outside, a means for restraining a calving cow or an uncooperative mama, to let the calf nurse, is helpful. Gentle cows

STAR BARN COW

OVER THE YEARS, we've used several babysitter cows, but the one who did it longest was Rhinestone "Rhiney" Rhonda, who started when she was 3 and led heifers into the barn until she was 17 and toothless. She almost always calved toward the end of calving season, which worked nicely, since she could lead most of the heifers in before she herself calved and went to another pasture. Altogether, she led more than 500 heifers into the barn and took her job very seriously. Even if she was comfortably bedded down for the night, if a heifer started calving, all we had to do was call her name, and Rhiney would get up and go to the gate, leading the heifer in from the big maternity pen as we gently herded her. Then Rhiney marched to the barn, and we'd herd the heifer along behind her. Once they were both inside, Rhiney would turn around and come back out as we shut the door on the heifer and march back to the small pen, where she got her reward — a flake of alfalfa hay. She dutifully performed her job in anticipation of her alfalfa "cookie."

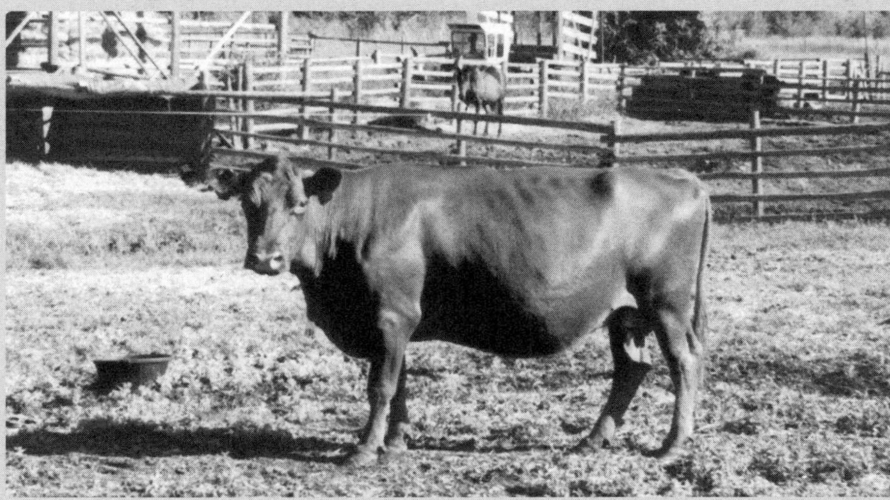

During her long career as babysitter cow, Rhiney, shown at age 16½, led more than 500 heifers into our barns.

How to Make a Head Catcher

Oregon State University (OSU) published a design in the 1980s for making a simple, inexpensive, wooden calving stall and head catcher outside or in a barn. The OSU plans call for the use of a pad of rough concrete under the stall or head catcher to keep the floor from getting slippery or muddy, while providing good footing. It can be kept clean and dry by sweeping it between cows. In a barn you can install a floor drain to remove liquid.

Put the head catcher between two stout posts. Mount hinge holders for 8- to 10-foot-long (2.4 to 3 m) metal gates on these posts. Attach hinged swing-away or metal gates on both sides of the head catcher. Hinge a second set of gates to the back wall of the barn, or opposite side of the pen if it's an outdoor calving pen, making a chute or alley for putting the heifer into the head catcher. Once you catch her head, the gates can all be swung away so that she can lie down during the birth and give you maximum room for helping her or using a calf puller. In an outdoor pen, these swinging panels also form part of a small pen to later hold the heifer and calf until they are well bonded.

To corral and catch the heifer, close and chain one set of side panels to create the small pen. Use the second set of gates to guide a heifer into the head catcher. The panels will confine her adequately and reduce your chance of being kicked. Stabilize the panels with an angled foot brace on both sides to keep them from swinging when you want them stationary. You can fasten a chain behind the heifer once she is caught.

After a birth using a head catcher, don't let the heifer go forward when you release her. Encourage the heifer to back out of the head catcher so that she can pivot around and smell and lick her calf as she would if she were giving birth without a restraint. Taking a few minutes to do this can save a lot of problems later. She needs to know that she's had a calf, and that this baby is hers. If she walks forward out of the head catcher, and you move her to a new location before she smells the calf, the bonding process is disrupted. This really confuses some heifers, and they are less likely to mother the calf.

To accommodate a c-section or help a calf nurse in the head catcher, the OSU plans call for remodeling the left-hand gate. Cut the gate in half to allow the top section to swing down and out of the way for a c-section, and allow the lower portion to open up for suckling a calf, while the top part still confines the heifer. Another way to suckle a calf is to just swing one of the gates clear away and tie the heifer's leg back on that side, so that she can't kick you or the calf as you help him to nurse (see chapter 8).

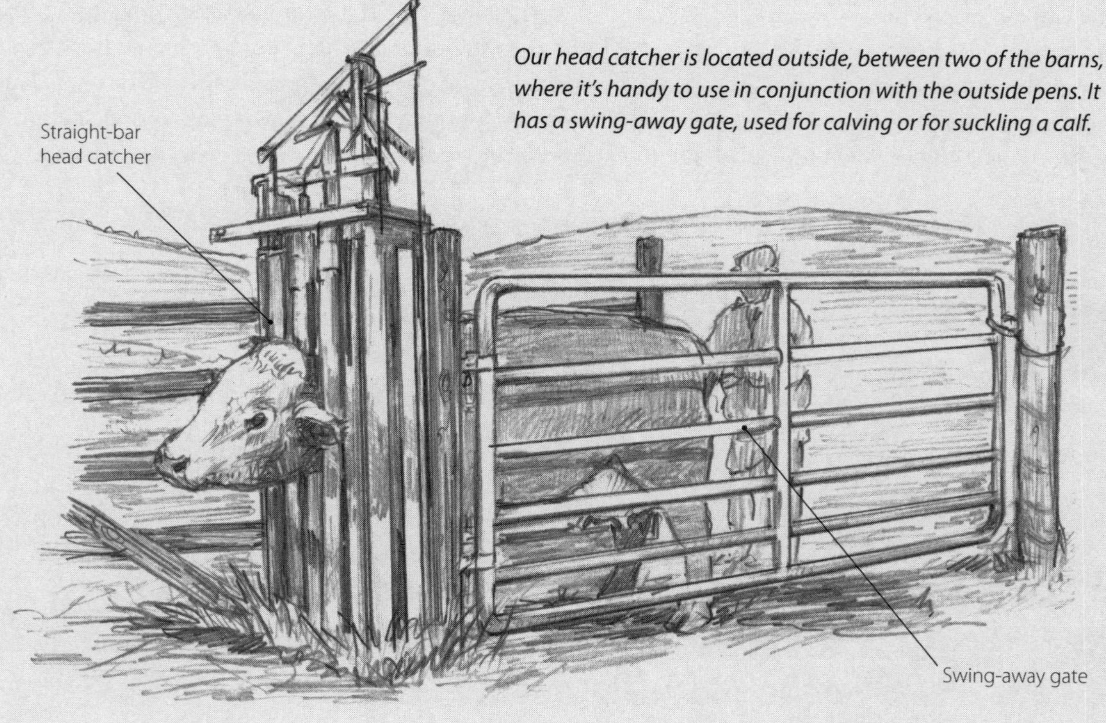

Our head catcher is located outside, between two of the barns, where it's handy to use in conjunction with the outside pens. It has a swing-away gate, used for calving or for suckling a calf.

can be haltered and tied, but flighty cows and heifers are more easily restrained in a head catcher.

A simple head catcher or stanchion is better than a squeeze chute for calving problems. The latter can get you in trouble because the cow will often lie down during delivery. Even if she doesn't, you may need more room for applying traction in the proper direction. If you have to use a calf puller, you may not have room to move it appropriately. If a cow goes down on her belly in a squeeze chute, she is stuck and can't be rolled onto her side.

If the head catcher is placed outside in a small catch pen or a calving stall, it should be located where you are feeding your cows or heifers, so that they are familiar with it and will go into the stall more readily. A commercial head catcher will work for a calving stall or catch pen if it opens to the floor with straight sidebars, so that the cow can lie down without choking. For calving, you must modify a curved head catcher by welding a straight pipe in place of the curved section.

The head catcher should have a rope so that you can pull it shut from the rear or side of the animal. The area in front should be open and well lit so that the animal will put her head through without balking, thinking she can walk on through. If it's dark or looks like a trap, she won't put her head through. A floodlight above and behind it for night calving enables her to see her way through and illuminates the area for pulling a calf, doing a c-section, or suckling a calf on a reluctant heifer.

Windbreaks

If your place has no natural windbreaks, such as a mountain canyon, a sheltered draw, or areas with trees and brush, one can be made from large straw bales in a row, rough-cut boards or plywood attached to a fence, heavy-duty tarps fastened to a fence, or even high mounds of snow.

A Wall of Snow

One rancher I know always makes a snow windbreak for his calving area before his cows start calving. Using a four-wheel-drive tractor and blade, he heaps up snow to create a horseshoe-shaped ridge of snow 6 to 8 feet (1.8 to 2.4 m) high, around part of his 30-acre calving pasture. Then he readjusts the blade and cuts a sharp up-and-down edge in the leeward side of the horseshoe, like a wall. With straw bedding inside the horseshoe next to the wall, it makes a good shelter. With the snow scraped off a grassy area that's well sodded and won't get muddy, this gives the cows access to forage and a bedding area next to the windbreak. They have a warm place to lie and don't suffer the loss of body heat they would if sleeping on frozen ground.

"Second-Day Pens"

Windbreaks in small pens next to your barn, where cows with new calves can be sheltered for a second day before sending them out to a big field, can be created by putting tarps or plywood on the fences. If you have bad rain or snow, you can create a small

A windbreak can be made of large straw bales and used to protect the animals in the nearby barn during a severe winter.

roof over the corner of each pen, using plywood or tarps. Calves can lie in the straw in windbreak corners in the sunshine and be very warm, even on a severely cold day.

We use these "second-day pens" when we take cows and calves out of the barn. This makes it possible to get pairs out of the barn quickly, to make room in the barn for new occupants and ensure there's never any sickness in the barn, yet still provide shelter for the young calves. A new calf, even after he's dry, has an immature "thermostat" for a while and may have trouble maintaining body temperature in cold weather; he's more easily chilled and stressed than a slightly older calf.

Often, if you put a cow with a new calf out in a field, she'll take him to a far corner and hide him somewhere away from predators and inquisitive and interfering herd mates. Unless there are brushy patches in those hideout areas, she's apt to stash him in mud or a snowbank. If a pair can spend a day in a shelter pen with windbreak and dry bedding, the calf is another day older and wiser by the time you put him out in the field; he's more apt to bed on straw or in a calf house rather than let his mother park him in a snowdrift. He'll remember the straw he snuggled into earlier and will stay at the bedground or come back to it, where he knows it's warm and dry.

Often if you put a cow with a new calf out in a field, she'll take him to a far corner and hide him somewhere away from predators and inquisitive and interfering herd mates.

Our shelter pens have a windbreak in each corner, and calves quickly learn to use these sunny, sheltered areas bedded with straw. On a cold night, the calves bed in these corners, and the cow usually lies in front of her calf, keeping him warm, tucked between her and the corner.

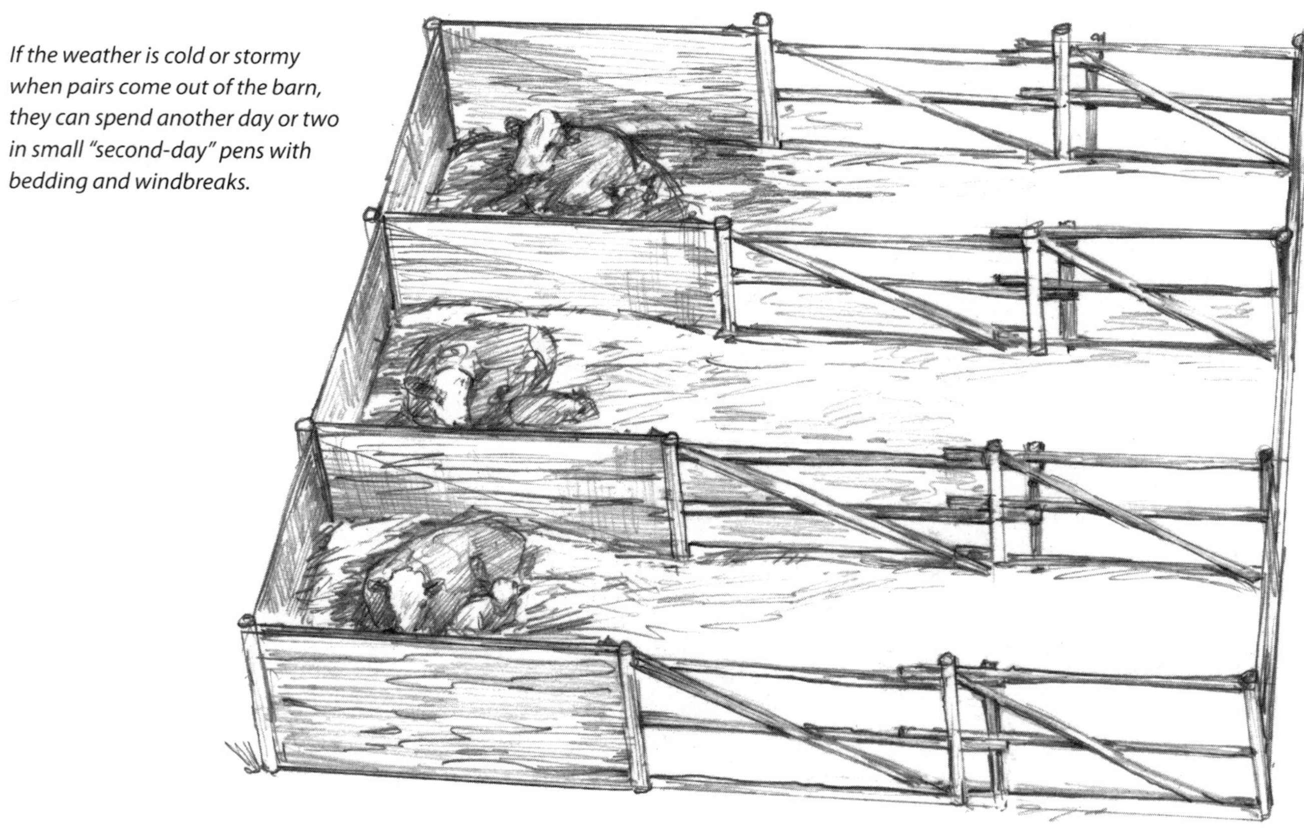

If the weather is cold or stormy when pairs come out of the barn, they can spend another day or two in small "second-day" pens with bedding and windbreaks.

Isolate Pairs to Encourage Bonding

Individual pens are best for some cows, especially first-calf heifers, until they are well bonded. Heifers sometimes get confused and mother any new calf, or let another cow's calf nurse. It helps to keep pairs in separate pens until calves and young mamas figure things out. It also helps with older cows. Some are very aggressive and mean to other cows' calves — bunting them or crushing them into the fence.

In nature, a cow goes off by herself to calve, so that her new calf will bond to her and not be confused by other cows. The first day or so of his life, the cow may hide him where she calved and leave him there while she goes to graze or find water. By the time she brings him back to the herd, he knows who his mother is and is not as likely to try to nurse the wrong cow and get kicked or bunted. Even if he makes a mistake, he's older and agile enough to get away from a cranky cow. But in a small pen the young calf may try to nurse any cow that approaches him and may not be wise enough to avoid getting hurt. Keep each pair separate until you can put them in a larger pasture.

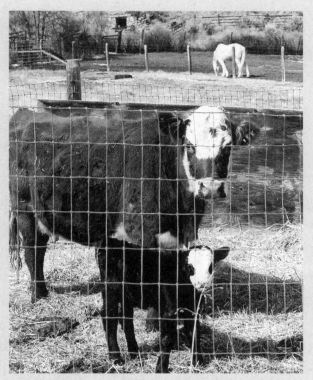

If new pairs are confined and can't be out in a big pasture, keeping them in an individual pen until they are well bonded is a good idea. That way, the calves won't try to nurse the wrong cow, and aggressive cows won't hurt another cow's calf.

Calf Shelters

With adequate shelter, calves suffer less stress and illness. Windbreaks and brush are not always adequate during a severe storm; we also have calf shelters in every field. Harsh weather can be hard on calves if they have no dry place to sleep. The stress of being constantly wet and cold lowers their resistance to disease. If the only place a calf can sleep is in a puddle or on a sheet of ice, he can't fight off scours when he's using all his energy just to stay warm.

If you plan to move a calf shelter, put a few small boards under the runners. Then you can pry the runners loose from frozen ground with a bar when you hook your rope or chain onto the house to pull it. Otherwise, the runners freeze solid to the ground.

Shelter and protection from bad weather outweigh any problems caused by congregating calves in a calf house. With shelter, our calves all did fine during the winter of 1978–79. That year it was 42° below zero (–41°C) when we started calving, and it stayed at 30° below zero (–34.4°C) for three weeks. The calves also stayed healthy the winter of 1983–84 when it was subzero all through January, and the year we were visited by the Siberian Express in early February — when wind chills were 100° below zero (–73.3°C) for five days.

Our Calf Houses

Lynn designed our first calf house in 1968 and later built many more for all of the fields where we had young calves. Each house is 16 by 8 feet (4.9 by 2.4 m), long and narrow so that it can be pulled through a gate. It has a slatted wooden floor and a sloping metal roof that's higher in front and is built on runners so that it can be pulled by a pickup or tractor. Up to 25 calves fit comfortably in each house. The floor makes the house heavy and sturdy, keeps it from being tipped by strong wind, and keeps the calves out of mud and melting snow.

We situate houses with the opening away from prevailing winds. The front is partly closed; the small opening reduces air movement inside the house, keeping it warmer. In cold or windy weather, calves stay inside the houses, coming out only to nurse. It is amazing how warm it is inside, with the body heat of several calves. They quickly learn that the calf house is the driest, warmest place in the field.

With pole panels or an electric wire, we keep our cows away from the front of the house, making a yard where only calves can lie in the straw. The cows can't eat the straw bedding or accidentally lie on any calves that lounge in front of the houses in the sun. We used to think we should move houses periodically to prevent contamination, but over the years we found that putting fresh bedding in periodically is more important than moving them. They've been in permanent locations on our ranch for the last 30 years.

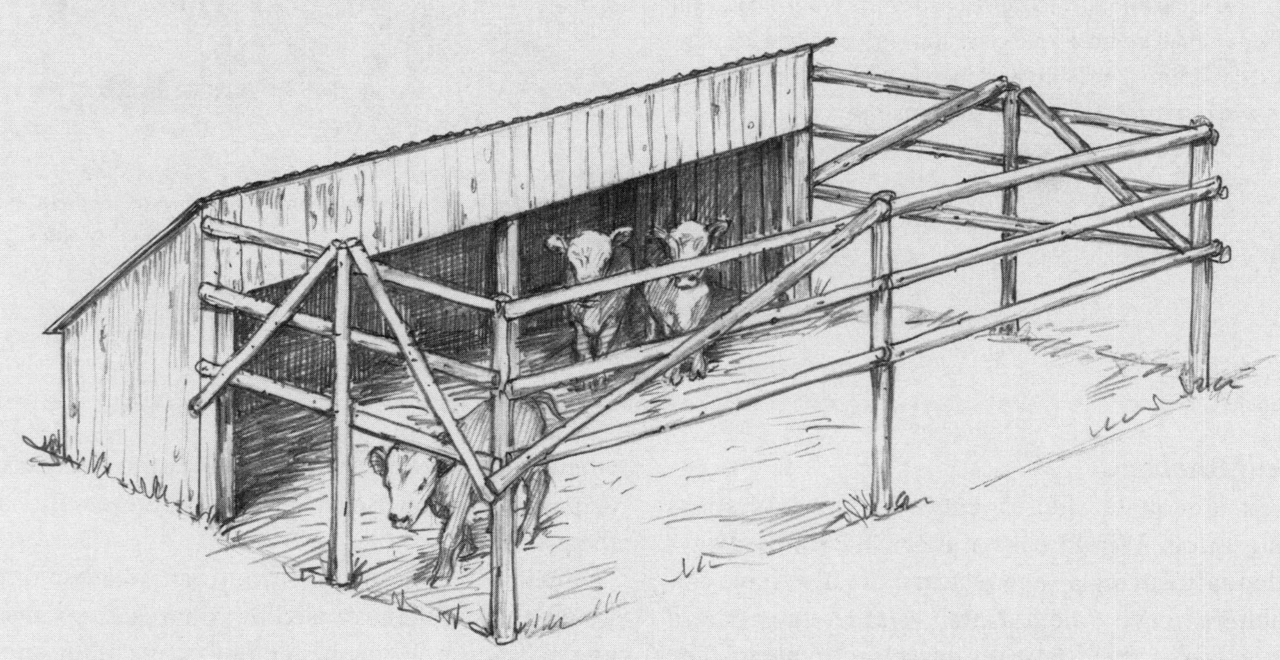

Wooden calf houses can be fitted with an electric wire or pole panels around the "front yard," so that the calves can slip under the front wire or pole but the cows are kept out.

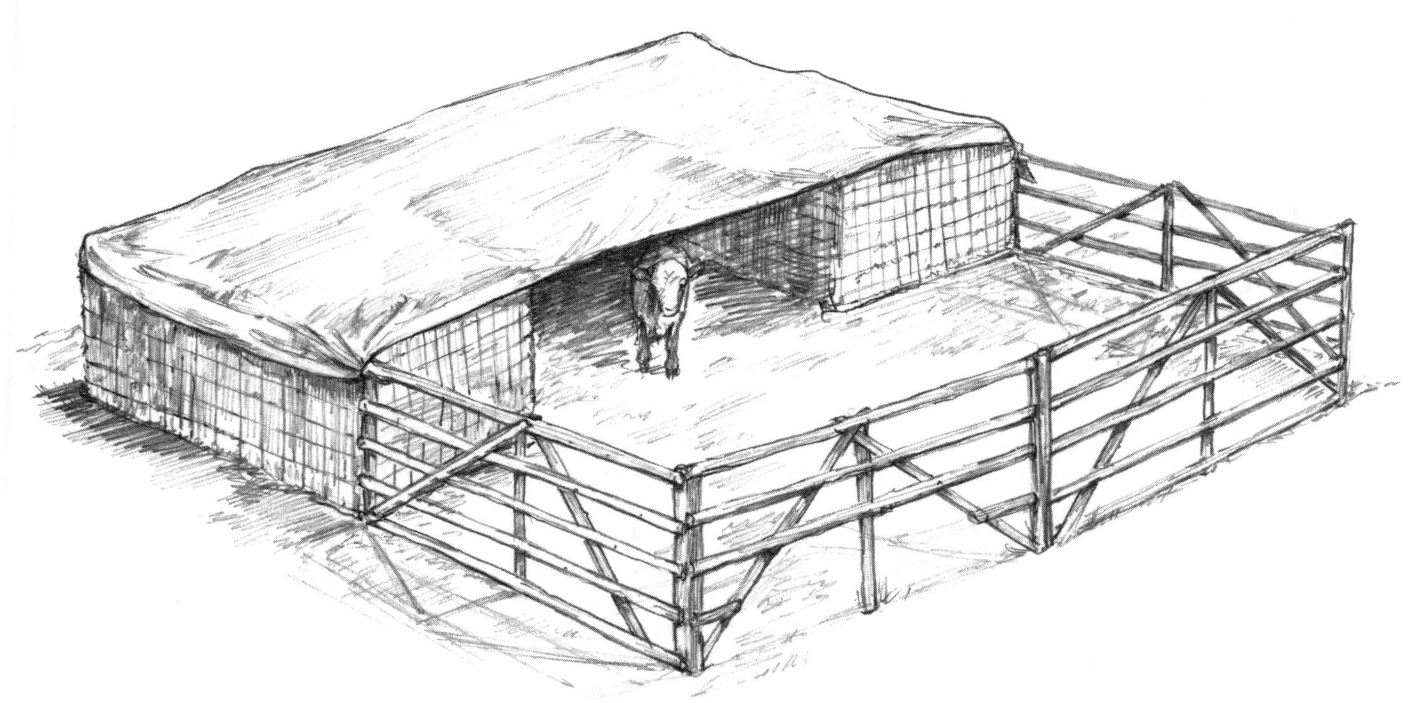

This instant calf house uses big straw bales for the three walls and mesh "hog panels" around the outside of the straw bales to keep the cows from eating them, pole panels to keep the cows out and the calves free to come and go, and poles across the top as rafters to hold up the tarp roof.

Calf-House Designs

There are many designs for calf houses and many ways to build shelters inexpensively. Following are just a few ideas.

A small hut, 8 by 8 feet, with open bottom and front is the finished product of a University of Idaho design piloted on six Idaho ranches in 1985 (13 years after we started making our own). It's 4 feet high in front, 3.6 feet high in back, with a 2 by 6 board nailed across the front, high enough to let calves go in and keep cows out.

Large straw bales, or small bales piled on one another, can be used as walls for instant calf shelters. A tarp will work as a roof over the top if you use several poles to prop it up and keep it from sagging. Straw walls make good insulation. Panels or net wire along the outside of the bales keep cows from eating the walls, and a panel in front keeps cows out of the shelter.

An old metal silo, among other materials, can be used to create an inexpensive calf shelter. The silo can be converted into several houses by cutting it apart, bending the sections, and making miniature Quonset huts. A 45-foot-high, 25-foot-diameter silo will make 20 calf houses. They can be mounted on treated poles for skids and cross-braced with poles or planks across the bottom.

There are many ways to create winter shelter. What you create for your situation will depend on materials available, the severity of the weather, and how you handle your cattle. Ideas can be adapted to fit your conditions. The goal is to have adequate shelter for young calves during bad weather and a good place to work with calving cows that need assistance. There's nothing more frustrating than losing a calf just because you don't have a place to help the cow calve, or losing calves to bad weather or stress-related sickness.

Disease Prevention

Digestive-tract infection is a major cause of death in young calves and one of the biggest calving-season headaches for stockmen. Finding ways to prevent losses and minimize the number of calves you must treat for scours (diarrhea) is crucial. Even if they are born safely, you may still lose them to disease; your risk and worry do not end with a healthy calf's live birth but continue until he is past the critical age for scours.

Scrape and haul off all manure and bedding following the calving season, so that the ground has a chance to dry out in the sun all summer. Start a calving season with a clean area and a clean barn. As soon as calving is over, clean out all bedding so barn stalls can dry out. If there were any sick calves in that barn, wash the walls and floor. Let it go empty — with access to sunlight if possible — until next calving season.

Scrape and haul off all manure and bedding following the calving season, so that the ground has a chance to dry out in the sun all summer.

Calve in a clean area, and not where cows spent fall and winter. Some cows carry pathogens and shed them in manure; a wintering area will be contaminated. If you can move all the pregnant cows or just the soon-to-calve cows to a clean field before calving or even sort out daily the cows that are getting close to calving to a clean field, calves won't be as exposed to pathogens when they are born.

Peer Groups

We group calves as they arrive and never have more than 30 to 50 pairs in one field, and fewer is better. Crowding adds to stress and contamination. Each group of calves is about the same age. The two-year-old cows with their first calves are in separate pastures from the older-cow pairs. First calvers need better feed, chances to eat without bossy older cows eating more than their share, and your close monitoring of their calves. These calves are more vulnerable to disease, as heifers' colostrum is not as rich in antibodies as that of older cows. We watch heifers' calves closely and treat them at the first hint of any illness.

Move Pairs out of the Calving Area

Keep pregnant cows in a clean area. Never leave calved cows with pregnant cows, or you run a risk of having pregnant cows' udders contaminated with bacteria from lying in a bedding area where a calf scoured or a calved-out cow left drainage or pus. Dirty udders lead to disaster; the newborn calf ingests pathogens with his first nursing, and the antibodies from colostrum may not protect him in time. If you bring calving cows into the barn or calving pen to calve, put them in a new field after they calve. If cows calve at pasture, move pairs to a new field after the calf is up and nursing and the pair has bonded.

Once calves are a few days or weeks old, some may become ill and contaminate the area, setting the stage for an epidemic of scours among later newborns, unless you sort off cows as they calve and put them in a new place. Although this requires that you provide more small pastures, when cows and calves are moved to clean ground in small groups, there's less risk for disease. If you get an outbreak of scours, you can contain it in one small group rather than dealing with the whole herd. A disease-carrying cow may give a bug to her calf, but if you have removed them from the calving area, the sick calf will at least be in an area where the calves are a little older and stronger and more able to handle the bug (see chapter 11). A sick calf excretes a thousand times more bugs than a carrier cow does. One sick calf will spread more disease than your whole adult herd, so move the calves out.

It's easy to move a cow and young calf, even if you have to put the calf in the back of your pickup and have someone follow with the cow or put the calf in a little sled or wagon pulled by a four-wheeler and have Mama follow you to the next field. Any calf more

MOVING COWS WITH YOUNG CALVES TO A NEW FIELD

Whether your cows calve in a barn, calving pen, or pasture, they should be moved to a new clean field as soon as possible. Usually within 24 hours the pair is well bonded, the calf has nursed a few times, and he is able to travel with Mama. Some very young calves will readily follow Mama at that age. Others get tired or confused and may need a little help, especially if you are moving several pairs at once and some of the cows go on ahead. The calf may not know where Mama is and will want to run back to where he last saw her. If you are moving several pairs at once you'll need helpers. When escorting one pair a good distance, it's often easier to transport the calf, and let Mama follow.

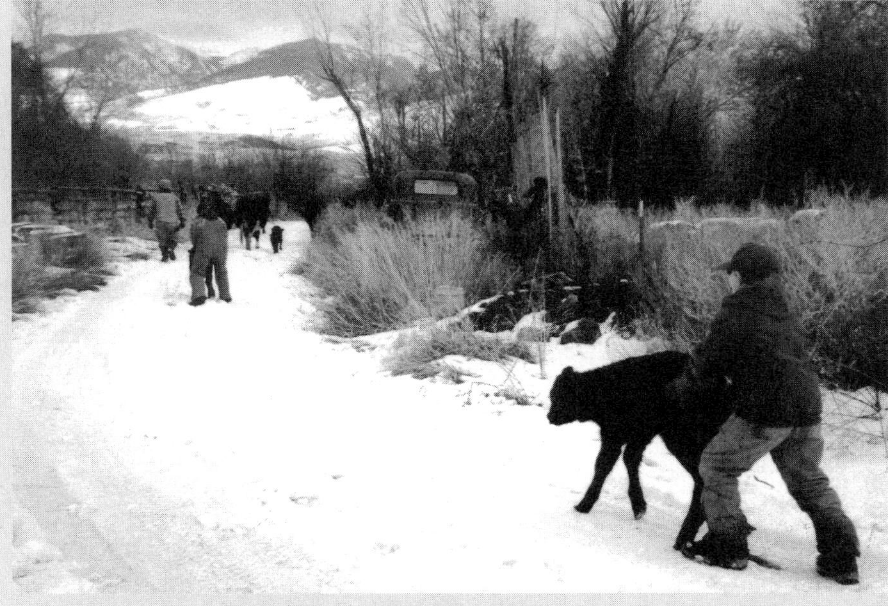

When moving several pairs at once, calves may get left behind if they are not yet accustomed to following their mothers, and it may take two or three people to bring the stragglers. In this group, our grandkids are helping to push the confused calves.

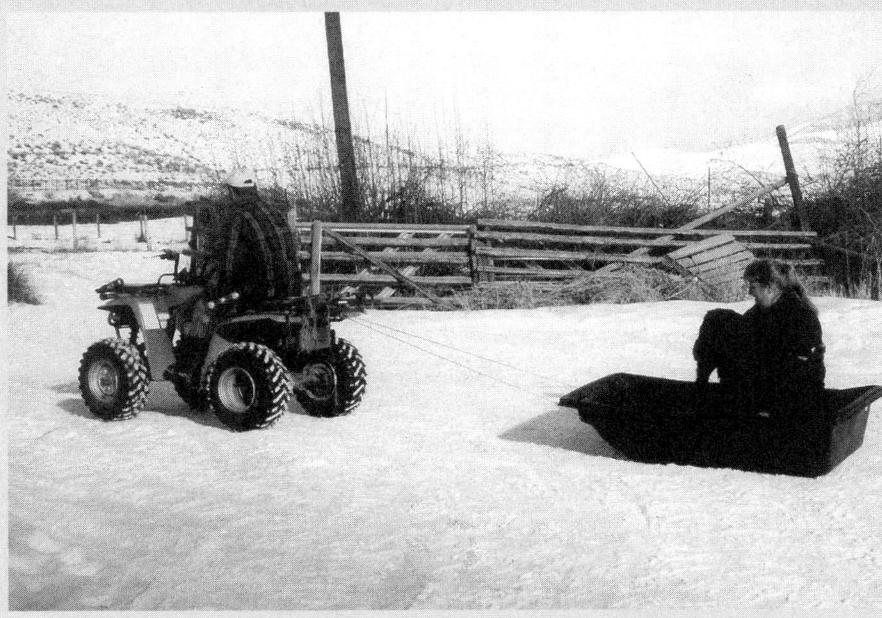

Our son Michael and his wife Carolyn bring a calf to the field from a calving pen. When you have to transport a calf in this manner, the cow will usually follow if she can see her calf.

than a day old can walk and will instinctively follow his mother once you get them "lined out" and going. You can herd the pair, or several at a time, to the new pasture. This often works best with at least two people, however, in case some of the calves are slow to catch on or get left behind by speedy mamas.

Group Calves According to Age

Scours can be prevented by grouping calves by age in clean pastures. Don't put new babies with older calves that may have been sick; the bugs can quickly overwhelm the defenses of the younger calves. Put them in a separate group in a new, clean place, and they'll have a better chance of getting past the critical first three or four weeks without getting sick. If you have many cattle, plan on using several different pastures as you move through calving season. Put the first calves and their mothers in one pasture; one to two weeks later, start a new group in a new pasture, making sure there's not much more than a week or two in age difference between the oldest and youngest calves in any pasture.

Late-season calves are much more likely to get scours than calves born earlier. Pathogens become more prolific, and levels of contamination rise dramatically after calves have been sick. The bugs become more virulent, multiplying in a sick calf. Weather is also a factor. If first calves come when ground is snow covered or frozen — or dry in a fall calving program — pathogens are not as accessible or as prolific. Then, as thawing or wet weather creates mud, the later calves not only have high levels of bacteria waiting in the mud, but wetter weather to stress them. In a fall calving situation, the later calves may face miserable weather as winter approaches.

Late-season calves are much more likely to get scours than calves born earlier. Pathogens become more prolific, and levels of contamination rise dramatically after calves have been sick.

Monitor Young Calves Closely

Since our calves are born before the greening of the grass, we feed hay to each group in the early morning and late afternoon. Twice daily is more efficient for hay consumption, as less is wasted, and each cow is more likely to get her share. We also feel that it's essential to check calves twice a day and spot problems early, before they become life-threatening. Once a day is not often enough. Some types of scours and pneumonia can be fatal after just a few hours. A calf may be fine one morning and dead the next morning. But if you see him again in the evening, you have a chance to notice that he's sick and treat him.

While Lynn feeds hay, I drive the truck in a loop so that I can see every cow and look at every udder and every calf as I pass by them. I count calves or mark off their numbers in a notebook as I see them at each feeding time to make sure I see them all. I look for evidence of dullness or scours and make sure that there are no calves lying in the bushes or calf houses.

It's just as important to check udders. If a cow has a full udder, I go looking for her calf by number or take a closer look at him if he's with the group. We enjoy our cattle and name them all (even when we had 180 cows, we named every cow and every calf) and know them each by sight. But with numbers there's no mistake — which is vital when they need treatment.

Identifying Calves

An identification system is crucial to management of the herd. Tagging calves with individual numbers is especially important on any farm where one person does the feeding and monitors for signs of sickness and another doctors the babies. The feeder can tell the doctoring person the numbers of the calves that are sick or not nursing. Unless you know which calf is which, your treatment program will fail.

It also helps to have calves tagged with the same number as their mamas. If a cow has an ear

Tagging, Banding, and Dehorning

The best time to tag a calf is when he's about a day old, before he becomes more fleet and hard to catch. If you tag him during the first day of life, however, wait until after he has nursed and bonded with mama.

There are many types of ear tags, and most of them require a special tool for inserting or punching them through the ear. Most tags are blank, so that you can write the desired numbers on them with a special marking pen. Situate the tag centrally, not too deep into the ear nor too close to the outer edge. Place it between the ribs of cartilage.

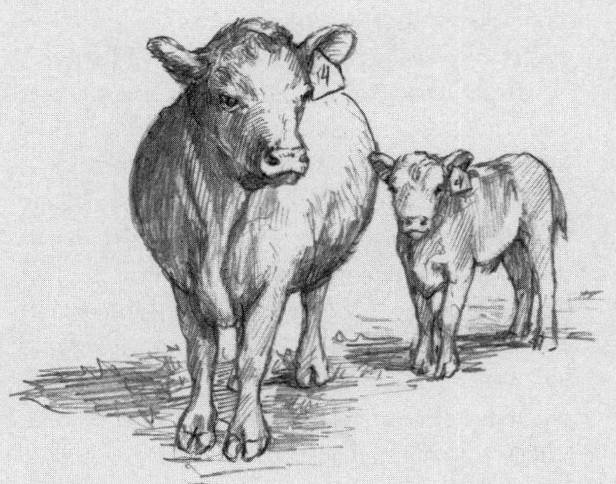

An individual identification system is crucial to good management.

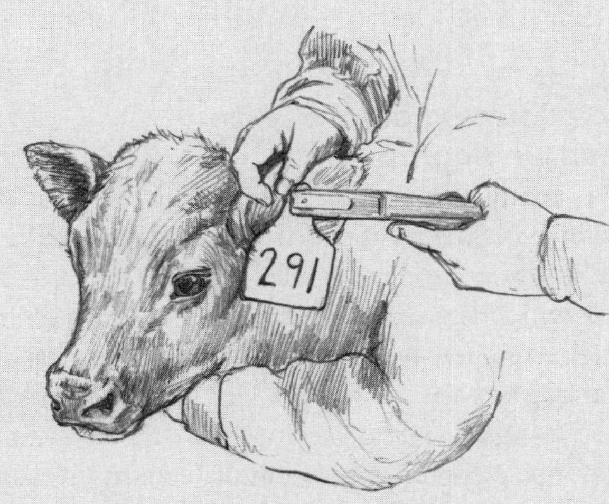

You'll need a tagging tool to attach an identifying number to a calf.

While bull calves are restrained for tagging, it is also a good time to band the bull calves to castrate them. Using a band is simplest at this time and much easier on the calf than waiting until he is bigger. The testicles of a young calf are small and don't have a very large blood supply.

TO BAND (CASTRATE) A BULL CALF

1. One person holds the calf on the ground and keeps him from kicking or standing up.
2. A second person applies a strong, thick rubber band (the size of a cheerios breakfast cereal piece) above the testicles with a banding tool that stretches the rubber band for placement.
3. Remove the tool and the band is left above the testicles tightly encircling the top of the scrotal sac and cutting off the blood supply.
4. The testicles die, shrivel up, and fall off within a few weeks.

This method is bloodless and it's painless after the initial application. There is less risk for infection, which can be a problem with surgical castration. Ranchers who don't handle calves at birth (that is, when cows calve in large pastures, unattended) usually remove the testicles surgically at branding time, slitting the scrotum with a clean, sharp knife, sliding each testicle out and cutting it off.

TO DEHORN A CALF

Calves of horned breeds should be dehorned at an early age. The smaller the horn buds, the easier it is to dehorn them and the less stress there is for the calf. Calves can be dehorned at the same time that you tag and band them, using a dehorning paste, or a battery-operated dehorner designed for very young calves, to burn a circle around the horn bud, which severs the blood vessels and nerves. Another option is a standard electric dehorner, which is used when calves are a few weeks to a few months old, whenever they are handled for vaccinating and branding. Do not wait until weaning age; by then the horns are larger and there is more risk for serious bleeding, and much more pain and stress for the calf.

or brisket tag or a freeze-brand number 125, her calf should have ear-tag number 125. Then if that cow has a full udder or her calf is missing, you can look for calf number 125, to see what's wrong with him. Later, after a heifer calf grows up, she can receive her own permanent number if you decide to keep her as a cow. The simplest, most effective ID system is to have calves tagged with their mothers' numbers.

Catching Problems Early

Whenever you see a calf with any hint of sickness, catch and treat him as soon as possible. Early detection and treatment is crucial for swift recovery, and with some illnesses can make the difference between life and death. It's easiest to catch and treat sick calves at feeding time, when they are in among the eating cows. If they are accustomed to you, the cows don't mind if you walk through them while they're eating. They are concentrating on eating and less apt to run to their calf and take off with him. If you are tricky, a cow may not even know that you are sneaking up on her calf to catch and treat him.

If you are diligent in your efforts to observe and check the calves twice a day and catch and treat any calf as soon as you discover that he's sick, you can usually halt scours before the calf is dehydrated . . . and in need of intensive care.

If a calf is ill or has loose feces, treat and halt the diarrhea before the calf spreads it all over the pasture. Isolate the calf, if possible. Bring the cow and calf in from the field to a doctoring pen or sick barn — *not* your calving barn — for shelter and treatment until the calf has recovered. If you are diligent in your efforts to observe and check the calves twice a day and catch and treat any calf as soon as you discover that he's sick, you can usually halt scours before the calf is dehydrated or in shock and in need of intensive care (see chapter 9).

Calfhood Vaccination

All calves should be vaccinated for *blackleg* at some point in their first few months to give lifelong immunity against this highly fatal clostridial disease. Blackleg is included in a seven- or eight-way clostridial vaccine that also protects against *C. perfringens.*

Other vaccines, such as IBR/BVD, and vitamin and mineral injections can also be given at this time if your veterinarian recommends them for your calves. IBR and BVD are serious viral diseases by themselves, but they also stress the immune system, making calves more vulnerable to other diseases. If you've ever had cases of IBR or BVD or problems with respiratory disease in calves on your farm, this vaccination should be given to calves as young as eight weeks.

Keep in mind that any calf that you vaccinate that early should be revaccinated a few weeks or months later for optimum immunity. Most calfhood vaccinations should be repeated by the time the calf is six months old or soon after, such as at weaning time or a few weeks before weaning. For instance, the first dose of blackleg is usually given between two and four months of age (though it can be given earlier if you have a problem with this disease on your farm) and repeated in a booster at weaning time. In some instances, and in certain states, all heifer calves must be vaccinated by your veterinarian against Bang's disease (brucellosis) between four and ten months of age.

Vaccinating before Calving Season Begins

On many farms, vaccination of cows can help reduce incidence of diseases that cause diarrhea in calves. If your calves suffer from a type of scours for which there's a specific vaccination, vaccinate the cows a few weeks or months before the start of calving season.

There are several vaccines that can be given to a cow during pregnancy to stimulate immunity so that she'll produce antibodies in her colostrum. Some are solely for *E. coli,* and some are combination vaccines against *E. coli,* rotavirus, and coronavirus. Vaccinating the pregnant cow is cheaper, and usually works better, than trying to vaccinate calves at birth. If the calf ingests antibodies from colostrum, he has instant passive immunity to protect him.

Some herds have *clostridial* infections in young calves. These bacteria *(Clostridium perfringens)* produce toxins that shut down intestinal function, a condition called *enterotoxemia.* The toxins seep into the bloodstream when the gut shuts down, causing a general toxemia that damages internal organs. The calf goes into shock and dies quickly unless this condition can be reversed (see chapter 11). A calf can be protected, however, by vaccinating the cow to make sure the antibody level in her colostrum is high. Most beef cows are protected if they get a seven-way or eight-way clostridial vaccination annually or semiannually. Antibodies in colostrum protect the calf if he nurses soon after birth. If your herd has problems with *C. perfringens* in older calves — that is, if you are losing calves at two to three months of age, after passive immunity from maternal antibodies has diminished — calves can be vaccinated at one to two months of age, at branding time.

Vaccination Not a Magic Bullet

Vaccination won't protect against all kinds of scours. For instance, there are more than one hundred types of *E. coli* bacteria, some of which are not pathogenic, and *E. coli* vaccines protect against only a few. But vaccination may help in certain situations. Sometimes your vet can identify the specific infectious agent behind a scours outbreak, and sometimes pathogens are never identified. Just "shooting in the dark" and vaccinating cows could be a waste of time and money. Most vets recommend a certain vaccine only after evaluating herd history and management, disease risk, cost of vaccine, and accessibility of cows for giving precalving vaccinations. Vaccination is not a cure-all. Vaccination alone is rarely enough to prevent scours; it must go hand in hand with good management and a clean environment.

Assisting Immunity in the Calf

If you vaccinate calves for *C. perfringens,* it can be done at any time during the first weeks of life, but you need to give a booster later. Calves don't build strong immunity at an early age, and the vaccination needs to be repeated. Discuss this vaccine and schedule with your vet.

There are oral products to give calves protection from *E. coli* scours, and these are fairly effective if given immediately after birth. This works well in a dairy but may not be practical in a beef operation unless you are handling every calf at birth. It doesn't do much good to give the calf an oral vaccine several hours after birth; the pathogens may already have been ingested.

Calving Seasons

The time of year you calve can make a difference in calf health. You hope to calve when conditions are optimal for grass and you'll need less purchased feed, since a cow's highest nutrient requirements occur during lactation, but also when weather conditions are favorable to calf health. There is no ideal time of year to calve, since conditions vary from one region to another, and even one farm to another. You have to figure out what schedule works best for you and your cattle.

Calving in April is traditional, when cows can take advantage of green grass while lactating. But in a hot climate, if this puts breeding season during the peak heat of July and August, cows and bulls may have weather-related fertility problems. Calving in May and June may mean heat stress on baby calves and breeding problems if weather is hot in August and September. Calving during February and March puts breeding season at a more optimal time, ahead of hot weather, and cows still have green grass during peak lactation. But adverse wet-weather conditions stress young calves and can lead to muddy, contaminated pastures and outbreaks of scours and pneumonia.

Calving in September and October works in some areas, if winters are minimally wet and fairly mild, and cows have a lot of fall and winter pasture that does not snow under. Calving in late winter — January and February— in a climate where ground

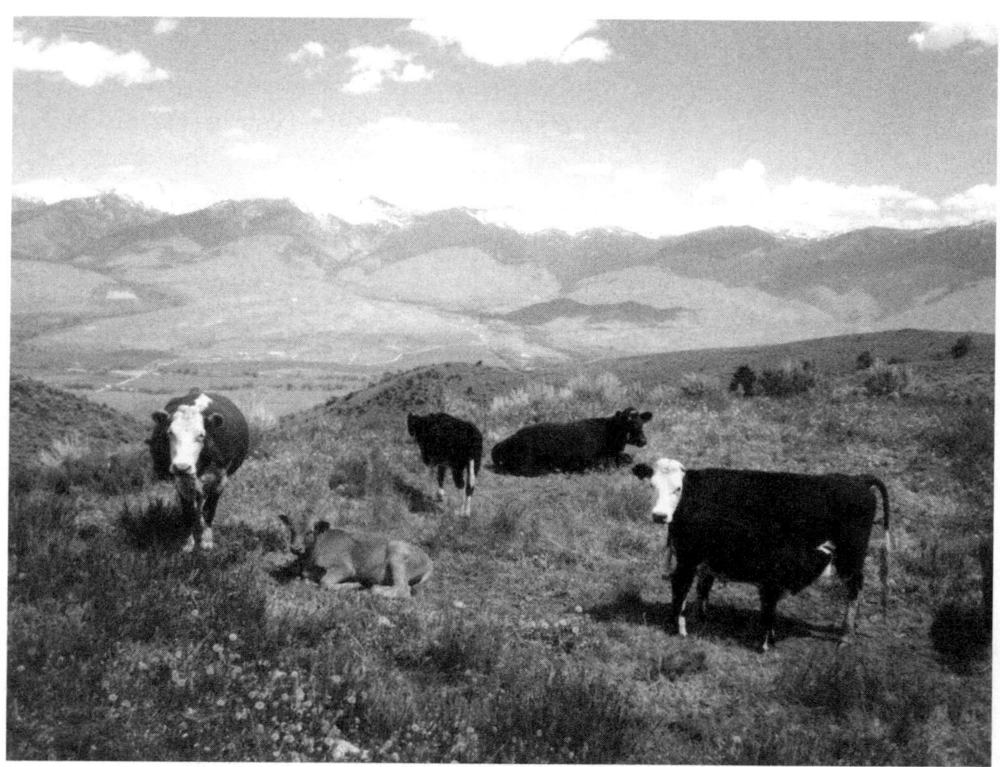

Cattle on rangeland are often spread over thousands of acres of mountains and canyons. This is not ideal for getting all the cows bred in a short time. It takes more bulls, and some cows may still be missed and end up being bred late.

stays frozen that time of year can reduce sickness, especially if cattle are congregated for calving, because there is no mud that will stick to them and their manure stays frozen. But cold-weather calving is labor-intensive if cows must be put into a barn to calve. Calving and breeding this early requires that you have more hay for lactating cows.

Some western ranchers calve this early, not only because of reduced illness in calves, but also to have cows bred in their home pastures before they go to public ranges. They can breed their cows to their own bulls, at home, and specifically select the bulls, such as choosing a different bull for heifers than for older cows.

On public ranges, all cattle run together. Most range pastures are large and in mountainous terrain. When cattle are spread over these huge pastures, it's a challenge to get them all bred quickly; bulls must do a lot of traveling, and some cows get missed. Range breeding means a strung-out calving season and some late-born calves, unless you cull late calvers, which can cut deeply into herd numbers. Most ranchers don't like late calves that are too small to sell in the fall. They must be wintered and fed hay that might be needed for the cow herd, then sold as yearlings the next spring.

There are always trade-offs to consider when it comes to deciding when to calve. Each stockman must weigh the advantages and disadvantages of each season and choose a time that works best for his or her own situation. This means taking everything into consideration: climate; feed resources; number of cows that breed on time, compared to number of open or late cows; facilities and labor availability; and the expense of raising the calves until sale time. The best plan is one that pencils out to cost the least, including the cost of time involved during calving, time and money spent on treating sick calves, and the loss of any animals due to calving problems or illness.

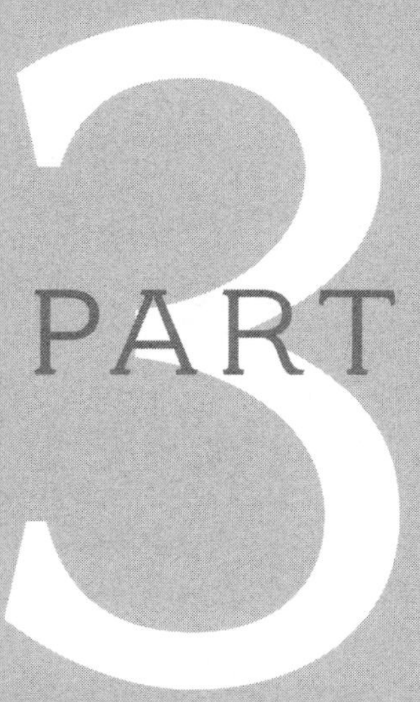

PART 3 Managing Calfhood Illness

Chapter 11

Viral and Bacterial Scours

SCOURS IS DIARRHEA — the most common symptom of intestinal infection in calves. It is the top killer of baby calves because of the acid-base/electrolyte imbalance and dehydration that accompany it.

Other kinds of intestinal infection are so acute that they kill a calf before diarrhea even begins. Enterotoxemia caused by *Clostridium perfringens,* and certain strains of *E. coli,* among other types of acute bacterial infection, can produce toxins that go through the gut lining and into the bloodstream, causing the calf to go into shock and die before there's evidence of diarrhea.

Digestive-tract infections can be due to protozoa, viral pathogens such as rotavirus or coronavirus, or certain kinds of pathogenic bacteria. Some of the cases that are the most damaging and hardest to treat, with high risk for fatal complications, are caused by bacteria.

How Scours Kills

Dehydration is often the actual killer when a calf dies of scours. He is losing electrolytes and body fluids faster than he can replace them; the damaged gut can't absorb fluid. In early or mild cases, a calf is still relatively strong and lively. As dehydration progresses, he becomes dull, his mouth is dry and his skin less elastic, his eyes are sunken, and his legs are cold. Body systems can no longer function. Without treatment to replace fluids and body salts to reverse this condition, the calf becomes too weak to stand or nurse, his temperature drops to subnormal, and he becomes comatose and dies. The best way to help the calf is to replace the fluids and salts he is losing — at the first sign of diarrhea, before he gets weak.

Many cases of diarrhea are caused by a combination of viruses and bacteria, and some are complicated by protozoa (see chapter 12). Some stockmen feel that they can tell the type of scours by looking at the color and consistency of the feces, but feces can be deceptive. Some cases are not typical, and many are caused by multiple agents. Few instances of diarrhea in young calves are simple infections; it can be difficult to tell whether you are dealing with viral or bacterial scours because symptoms are the same: profuse, watery diarrhea and progressive dehydration. Finding a pathogenic virus in a lab test may not mean much, as these viruses are often present in normal animals. Just because a test detects a virus does not necessarily mean that it is the cause, or the only cause, of the diarrhea.

Many bacteria can also be isolated in culture tests, but illness may be complicated by more than one organism. Keep in mind that there are human health concerns when dealing with salmonella (a bacterium) or cryptosporidium (a protozoan). *E. coli* can also affect humans, but the *E. coli* strain that's a concern in contaminated meat and other foods is not the one that affects baby calves.

When dealing with diarrhea, proper antibiotics can help a calf fight bacterial scours but are of little value against viruses or protozoa. Giving sick calves fluid is the most important treatment in most cases.

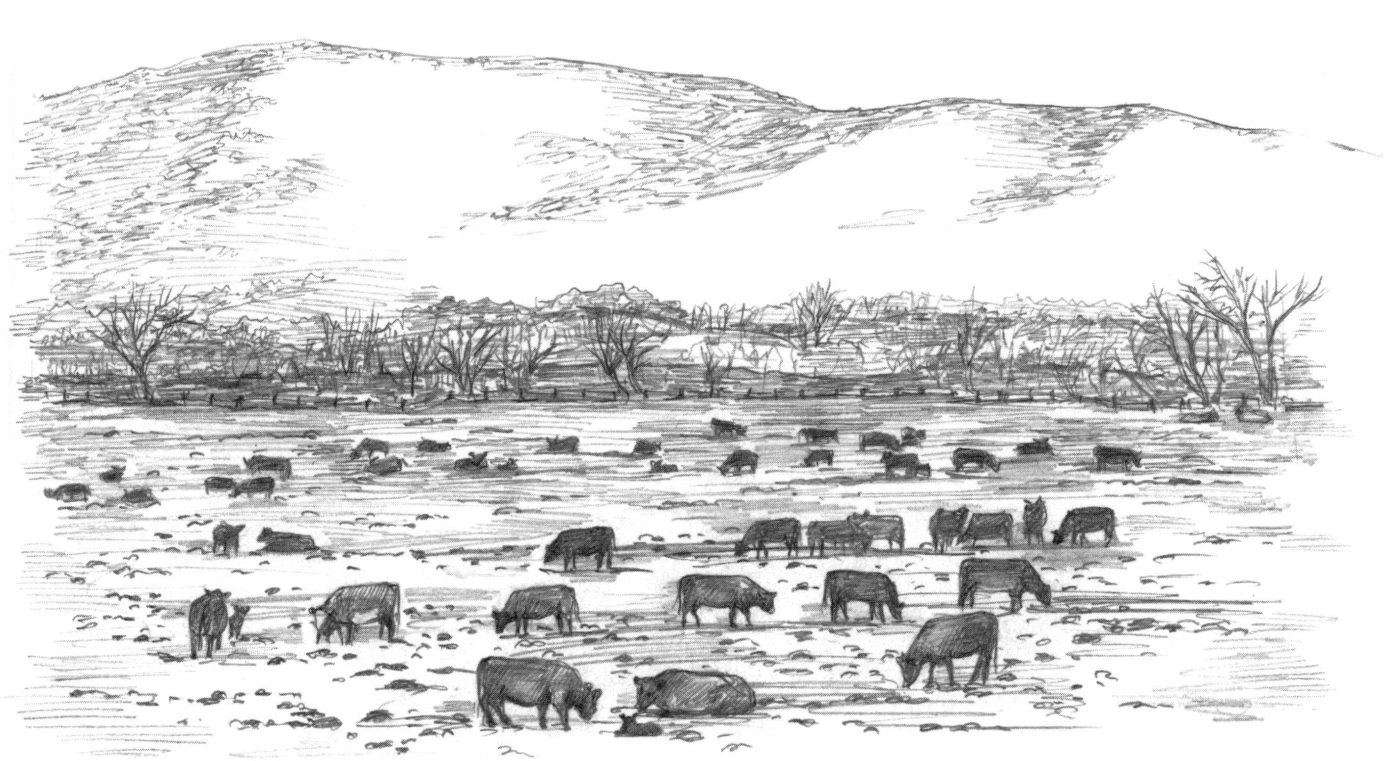

If calves are in a contaminated environment, such as where the herd of pregnant cows spent the winter, they are at higher risk for illness.

Consider the Age of the Calf

The younger the calf, the more rapidly he will dehydrate; thus, he needs fluids more often. Except for acute toxin-forming infections that cause toxemia or septicemia, most scours are deadliest in the first weeks of life. A calf becomes more resistant to pathogens as he grows older; a young calf is more likely to die unless intensively treated. He has fewer reserves, so is more vulnerable to dehydration, and his intestinal lining is less able to regenerate quickly after being damaged — lengthening his recovery time, especially if he's younger than 17 days.

The same kind of infection that's a life-or-death emergency in a two- or three-day-old calf is usually not as serious in a three-week-old calf. The latter may still need treatment, but he's more able to fight off infection without as much gut damage and risk of serious dehydration. Any calf that scours at under two weeks of age should be treated as an emergency case — given fluid and medication immediately — whereas an older calf is more likely to handle it with minimal treatment. If he is strong and hard to catch, and continues to nurse his mother, he may get over diarrhea quickly with just one treatment, or even without treatment. But if he's dull and not nursing, he needs treatment.

Defeat Diarrhea Daily

Scours prevention includes keeping your cow herd healthy and well-nourished and maintaining up-to-date vaccinations. Include bovine virus diarrhea (BVD) vaccination in your regimen; a persistently infected BVD calf has a compromised immune system, making him both difficult to treat and susceptible to all kind of scours.

Diagnosis, to learn which bug you are dealing with, can be helpful in determining the best treatment, but management factors to prevent contamination (see chapter 10) are much more important than diagnostics, treatment, or vaccination. Vaccines will work if used appropriately and in combination with good management, but none will be effective in the face of an outbreak caused by poor management.

Factors That Make Calves More Vulnerable to Scours

Many complex factors determine whether a calf will get diarrhea during his first weeks of life. These include health and immune status, environmental factors such as weather, and pathogens present in his environment. If a calf is a little premature, has had a difficult birth that compromised him with oxygen shortage and resultant acidosis, which interferes with his ability to absorb antibodies, or does not obtain adequate levels of antibodies from his dam's colostrum, then he is at higher risk of developing diarrhea at an early age.

If pastures are contaminated, many calves start to scour at three to four weeks, when antibodies from colostrum are no longer protecting them and temporary immunity is wearing off. This may happen sooner if a calf did not nurse promptly or get enough colostrum. Once this temporary immunity is gone, the calf must build his own immunity as he comes into contact with various pathogens.

Age and health of the dam make a difference in effectiveness of passive transfer of antibodies. First-calf heifers generally don't have as many antibodies in colostrum as does an adult cow. Risk of diarrhea in young calves born to heifers is four times greater than in calves born to older cows. A very old cow, however, may also have poor colostrum. If any cow is undernourished during pregnancy, her calf may not be vigorous and her colostrum may be lower in antibodies, making him doubly vulnerable to diarrhea pathogens. Anything that interferes with the cow's immune system — inadequate calories, protein, or trace minerals in diet, BVD infection, etc. — can keep her from providing a protective level of antibodies in her colostrum.

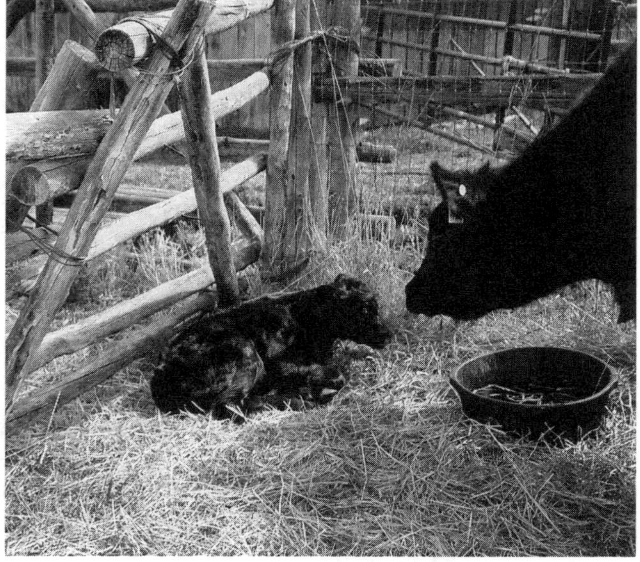

If a calf becomes sick, remove him and his mother from the herd to a pen by themselves for treatment, so that he won't spread pathogens all over the pasture.

Animal Density

With many types of scours (viral, bacterial, protozoal), nearly every calf may encounter the pathogen in the first month of life but not get sick if he has good passive transfer of antibodies from his mother, or gets a low dose of pathogens when first exposed. A low dose may enable him to start building immunity. He may get an infection, but not enough to damage the intestine and cause diarrhea, since it takes the pathogens a while to multiply and do severe damage. If his first exposure is high, however, he's likely to become sick. If you have one scouring calf in a 15-acre pasture, the exposure level for other calves is much less than with one scouring calf per 50 square feet.

Certain weather and environmental conditions contribute to epidemics of scours in young calves. Cold, wet, windy weather or hot weather, or temperature changes from one extreme to another can be stressful and can lower immune defenses of calves. In bad weather, stockmen often congregate calving cows to watch them more closely or to provide shelter, resulting in more contamination and more risk of diarrhea in calves. Calves born late in calving season are more at risk for scours than calves born earlier. The environment for the later calves is already contaminated with feces from calves that have been sick. The larger the herd size, the greater the chance for disease spread. Calfhood diarrhea is less common in a small group of cattle than in a larger group.

The primary source of infection is the feces of infected animals, but healthy cows and calves are also known to spread disease, since most pathogens can exist in healthy animals without causing illness. Many bugs that cause scours in calves are carried by adult cows; if any of these organisms get into a calf, however, his immune system may not be able to handle it. Calves that develop diarrhea act as colonizers for pathogens. Because they spread exponentially more organisms in their feces, a sick calf and his mother must be immediately removed from the other cows in the herd for treatment, or an outbreak is imminent.

Salmonella and E. coli *bacteria can live for a long time in the environment — even from year to year in a damp place like a calving barn.*

Since pathogens are present in feces of healthy animals, any place where there is a high density of cows (calving grounds and pens) or that has many cows passing through (a calving barn during a calving season) will have an increased population of pathogens, especially bacteria like *E. coli,* through calving season. Unless a barn or pen is regularly cleaned out and disinfected or left vacant for a period, calves exposed to that environment will be at high risk for scours.

Salmonella and *E. coli* bacteria can live for a long time in the environment — even from year to year in a damp place like a calving barn. Sunshine helps, as does cleaning out all of the old manure. Letting the barn sit empty, dry, and open all summer after you clean out the manure helps minimize bugs during the next calving season.

Scours Caused By Viruses

Viral scours tend to strike during the first two weeks of life, whereas bacterial scours attack calves at any age. Viral scours won't respond to antibiotics, but you can help the calf by giving fluid and electrolytes, along with gut-soothing, diarrhea-slowing medications like Kaopectate (keolin and pectin). Antibiotics are of value only in halting possible secondary bacterial invaders.

Rotavirus

Rotaviruses are a primary cause of diarrhea in calves and are found on many farms. Once this virus is introduced to a farm, brought in by a new animal or on a person's contaminated feet or clothing, it is hard to eliminate. It remains stable in cattle feces for a long time, as well as in the air and on any surfaces it touches, and is resistant to most disinfectants. Adult cattle serve as a source of infection for newborn calves, even though adults rarely become ill.

Once established, rotavirus usually persists indefinitely on a farm. It can lurk in the barnyard, in barns, and on pastures. The resultant diarrhea in calves is very contagious and can spread to an entire group of calves by fecal contamination of feed, bedding, water, dirty udders, and human hands, among other things. Even when cattle are in large pastures, the virus spreads rapidly; calves can be infected soon after birth by the dam's feces or from contact with infected calves. Newborns are protected only during the first few days of life, while they still have some colostral antibodies active within their gut.

The rotavirus is tough and aggressive and can attack a calf's intestinal lining even though there may be no prior damage to the lining. Some viruses invade only after an animal's resistance has been lowered by stress, or his tissues have been weakened

First Calves Born to Heifers Have More Scours

Not only do heifers have lower levels of antibodies in their colostrum than cows, but they can be more prolific carriers of scour pathogens, shedding more bugs in their feces. They are still young and responding to all sorts of antigens. Even if you vaccinate them, they don't respond to the vaccine as well as an adult cow does; they don't have as much immune experience. A heifer that had a hard birth may be slow to mother her calf, and the calf may be slow to get up and acidotic if he became short on oxygen. The calf may not suckle promptly and may not absorb enough antibodies. If you have to give him colostrum, use colostrum from an older cow.

by something else. The rotavirus, however, marches right in and starts the attack on its own, though it's common to see a mixed infection of viruses and bacteria — making the diarrhea more deadly and harder to treat.

Protection via Colostrum

Cows with antibodies in colostrum give their calves protection from rotavirus for as long as there are antibodies in the calf's intestine. Even though the calf may still excrete rotavirus in his feces if he becomes infected, he won't develop diarrhea while protected. Many calves are infected with rotavirus on farms where it exists, but not all will develop diarrhea; some just shed the virus in their feces.

The main protection against rotavirus in the first week of life does not come from antibodies absorbed into the bloodstream (IgG antibodies) but from a different type of antibody (IgA) that remains in the gut. This protection lasts only as long as there are antibodies present in the intestine itself, explaining why rotavirus diarrhea occurs most commonly after five to seven days of age, when there is no longer colostrum in the cow's milk. Calves are susceptible between one and three weeks of age; however, diarrhea can hit as early as two days of age if a calf did not get much colostrum or if the antibody level in the colostrum was low. If the calf got a high level of antibodies, both absorbed and remaining in the gut, he has a much better chance of survival.

Cause and Effect

Factors that influence the severity of diarrhea include the age of the infected calf, amount of antibodies ingested at birth, weather and temperature, and whether the infection is complicated with the presence of other pathogens, such as coronavirus, bacteria, or protozoa. The highest mortality rates are among the youngest calves that did not receive adequate colostrum, especially if they're subjected to weather stress. Some of the most serious cases are also infected with *E. coli.*

The incubation period for rotavirus infection is 18 to 24 hours. When the calf becomes sick, he may have fever and be noticeably dull for a few hours, then break with diarrhea. The runny feces may be

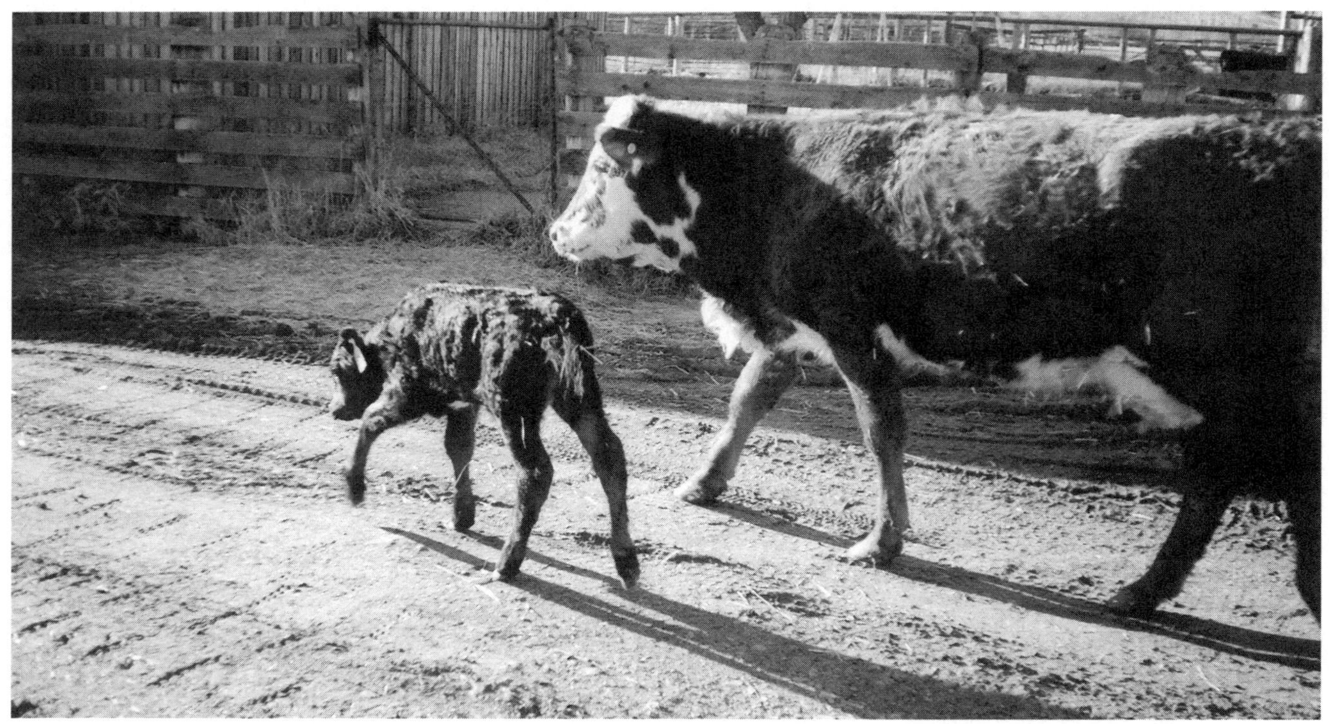

Rotavirus diarrhea usually hits calves when they are only a few days old — after there are no longer any IgA antibodies from colostrum in the cow's milk to give local protection in the gut. Calves from heifers like this first calver may not get as high a level of antibodies; heifers' colostrum is not as rich as that from an older cow.

very watery and yellow-green to gray in color. In mild cases, the calf may just be off feed for a day or two, but in severe cases with explosive watery diarrhea, he will dehydrate quickly and need good supportive care and fluids given orally if gut damage is not severe, or intravenously if his gut cannot absorb the fluids. Care and treatment of sick calves is covered later in this chapter.

Coronavirus

Coronaviruses cause acute diarrhea in calves that are from one day to three months of age, most commonly between one and two weeks old, and hit calves most frequently during winter, in a cool, moist environment. Many cattle herds are infected; most adult cattle have come into contact with coronaviruses at some point in their lives. A high percentage of cows shed the virus in manure, especially during winter and at calving. Calves born to these "carrier" cows are at high risk of developing diarrhea. Coronavirus can also cause mild respiratory infection, especially in calves two weeks to four months old.

Protection via Vaccine

Vaccinating pregnant cows with a combination vaccine containing rotavirus, coronavirus and *E. coli* can reduce scours in newborn calves. It won't reduce cows' seasonal shedding of the virus during winter but does reduce shedding at calving time. The bacterial vaccines for *E. coli* and the C and D toxoids against *Clostridium perfringens* work well to create a good immune response and high antibody level in the cow. The viral vaccines for rotavirus and coronavirus are less dependable but do seem to help in some herds.

ORAL ANTIBODIES: ANOTHER OPTION

If vaccinating the cows has not helped, there's an oral antibody product, given to calves immediately after birth, that contains *E. coli* antibodies and coronavirus antibodies. This can be used if you choose not to vaccinate the cows. You can't do both, however. If you vaccinate the cows ahead of calving, the maternal antibodies in the colostrum will counteract the oral antibodies you give to the calf.

Preventive Medicine

The prevention of rotavirus diarrhea depends on clean conditions and on vaccination of cows in late pregnancy. If you have rotavirus on your farm, vaccinating cows ahead of calving to ensure high level of antibodies in colostrum can help reduce the incidence and severity of diarrhea in calves. Your vet can advise you on what vaccines to use and at what stage in gestation they'll be most effective for development of peak antibody levels in colostrum by calving time. Rotavirus vaccine must generally be given within 40 days of calving; if it's given before then, the cow won't have a high level of antibodies in her colostrum. Know the calving dates of cows and vaccinate accordingly.

There are several different *serotypes* (types of microorganisms) of coronavirus and also some corona-like viruses. If the vaccine works in your herd, you may be dealing with a virus similar to that used in the vaccine; if vaccine doesn't seem to help, your herd may be affected by another strain altogether.

Why Vaccines Don't Always Work

One reason the vaccine against rotavirus and coronavirus is often not effective is that neither virus stimulates a strong immune response from cows, either naturally or with vaccine. This is why cows carry these viruses in their bodies year after year. The levels of antibodies produced in response to vaccination of cows are somewhat protective against the low number of viruses ordinarily shed by mature cows. But if a calf becomes sick with rotavirus or coronavirus, he'll shed millions of virus particles in every squirt of diarrhea. Immunity conferred by vaccinating cows in passing antibodies to the calf can be completely overwhelmed in the face of this kind of exposure. Even calves that had good colostrum consumption when they were first born may get sick, if they're in pastures where other calves have been scouring. Thus, it is important to make sure *every* calf gets sufficient colostrum, to keep an outbreak from starting.

Watch for Illness

It's important to check calves often enough to know whether one is getting sick. A calf with diarrhea should be removed from the herd and put with his mother into a "sick pen" or barn for intensive treatment so that he'll recover more quickly and won't contaminate the pasture.

It's hard to know what makes the difference between a good year and a bad year when there are so many factors in the healthy-calf equation.

Some years are worse for scours than other years, whether or not you vaccinate. The weather — amount and timing of rain or snow, wind chill, mud or dry ground — plays a big role in the health of the calves. After a year with lots of diarrhea, some stockmen might start a vaccination program. The next year there are fewer cases of scours, convincing stockmen that the vaccine has worked — but the weather is better, too. It's hard to know what makes the difference between a good year and a bad year when there are so many factors in the healthy-calf equation.

Keep Equipment Clean

If you put a heifer in a chute to help her calve, or in a pen or stall afterward to make sure she mothers the calf, and then the calf starts scouring, the whole area is contaminated. It is important to keep the chute area and stalls clean. It's also crucial to keep clean whatever you use to give colostrum to a new calf, or fluid to a sick one. It's best if you never use the same tube for a newborn calf that you've used for a sick calf. Always clean the equipment between calves and keep spare tubes or esophageal feeders on hand. Then if one develops a leak or breaks, you always have a spare one. Throw away the one you used last year; start with a new one for each calving season.

Scours Caused by *E. Coli* Bacteria

There are many strains of *E. coli.* Only a few are *pathogenic* (causing disease), and these strains don't all affect calves the same way. Some cause *septicemia* (infection throughout the body) by damaging the intestinal lining enough to pass through it and into the bloodstream. Their powerful toxins cause toxic shock; without prompt treatment, the calf succumbs to the infection and dies.

Other types remain in the gut, causing diarrhea and dehydration. They are *enterotoxigenic,* meaning that they produce or contain a toxin that affects cells of the intestinal lining. This enterotoxigenic type is the most common *E. coli* infection in very young calves. These strains cause diarrhea by adhering to the wall of the small intestine, where they multiply and release *enterotoxins* that damage the gut, rendering it unable to absorb fluid and nutrients. Production of enterotoxins also results in fluid and electrolytes being drawn from the bloodstream into the intestine.

Critical First Few Days

E. coli infections can strike a calf at any age, with youngest calves usually most susceptible and most adversely affected. Some types of *E. coli* cause scours soon after birth, if pathogens are ingested ahead of or at about the same time as colostrum. If a calf nuzzles a dirty cow or sucks a dirty udder, he may pick up bacteria. This pathogen is often one of the first encountered by a newborn calf and may even be transferred from the dam to the calf as she licks him. It is most common in calves younger than three days and may appear as early as 10 or 12 hours of age, especially if calves don't get enough antibodies from colostrum.

Studies in beef and dairy calves have shown that 80 percent of infections with the K99 strain of *E. coli* occur in calves younger than four days of age. As the calf gets older, the cells of the small intestine's lining become more resistant to colonization by these bacteria. The critical time is during the first few days, when the enterotoxic strains of *E. coli* are most able to establish themselves in the small intestine and multiply, producing toxins that draw fluid into the intestine and create diarrhea.

Prevention via Oral Vaccine

When every calf breaks with watery diarrhea at one or two days of age, it's usually an epidemic due to enterotoxic *E. coli.* If you didn't vaccinate cows ahead of time, oral vaccine can be given to each calf immediately after birth. These products contain concentrated antibodies for K99 *E. coli* and act as a colostrum substitute, but you must get them into the calf before he gets sick. They work for prevention, but not for treatment. If calves get loose feces within a few hours after birth, if you're not quick enough about giving them oral vaccine, you can treat them with an oral antibiotic used for *E. coli* scours in newborn piglets.

Some types of *E. coli* scours can't be prevented by vaccine given to the cows ahead of calving or to calves orally right after birth because vaccine protects against only four of the K99 subtypes, and there are hundreds of strains of *E. coli.* In this instance, all you can do is use the oral piglet antibiotic soon after birth. This will halt the incidence of deadly scours.

If a calf older than three or four days develops diarrhea from *E. coli,* there are usually multiple infections involving a virus. These multiple infections are common in calves one to two weeks of age and are more serious than single infections. Calves with a rotavirus infection during the first two weeks of life are more vulnerable to *E. coli* because the damage done by rotavirus enables the bacteria to colonize the intestine of the older calf.

How to Check Levels of Dehydration

A calf that is only mildly dehydrated still has warm feet, and if you pull up a pinch of skin on his neck and let go, the skin quickly springs back into place. To check for the level of dehydration, observe how long it takes for the pinched skin to return to normal.

- **At 2 to 5 percent of body weight in fluid loss** (dehydration), it takes three to five seconds for the skin to sink back into place. His gums will be dry instead of moist.
- **At 8 percent dehydrated,** it takes five to eight seconds for the skin fold to return. His legs and feet will be cold, and his eyes will seem sunken.
- **At 9 to 12 percent dehydrated,** it will take more than eight seconds for his skin pinch to sink back. His eyes are quite sunken.
- **At more than 12 percent dehydrated,** it will take longer than 10 seconds for skin to go back; his eyes are very sunken, and his gums are white. By this stage he is in shock and near death.

Fighting Dehydration

Young calves dehydrate quickly, making any *E. coli* diarrhea that strikes young calves potentially deadly. To obtain protection, calves must ingest colostrum immediately after birth or be given oral vaccine or the pig antibiotic. To be fully protected by their dams' colostrum, they need to continue nursing regularly, every six to eight hours, as most healthy calves do, during the first days of life, since the remainder of the cow's colostrum, though diluted by incoming milk, still contains antibodies that have a protective effect within the gut. Nursing twice a day may not be adequate, because ingested antibodies are already absorbed or digested from the gut 12 hours later, though the antibodies that entered the bloodstream and were absorbed early on can still give passive protection. Calves living with their mothers will nurse more often than twice a day. If you are feeding an orphan calf a bottle, be sure that you feed him every six to eight hours while he is young.

Sources of Infection

Infected animals, healthy or sick, are the main source of infection for enterotoxigenic *E. coli;* their feces contaminate the environment. Passage of bacteria through an animal creates a multiplier effect because each infected cow or calf excretes many more bacteria than originally ingested. Calves with diarrhea are the greatest multipliers, excreting huge numbers of bacteria in their liquid feces. Recovered calves continue to shed high numbers of bacteria for several weeks following the outbreak.

AN EXTREME CHALLENGE

ON OUR RANCH we never had scours in calves less than a week of age until 1982. We were almost done calving (only 24 cows left out of 170) when our vet came out to do a c-section on a heifer. He'd been to ranches all over the valley that season and inadvertently carried a pathogen into our barn. From that point on, we had the bug. All 24 of the remaining cows' calves got sick soon after birth. We almost lost the first one because we weren't expecting it. By the time he was 12 hours old, he had severe diarrhea and was too weak to nurse. We moved him and his mother to our sick barn and gave him fluids and medication. When we went back six hours later to give him more fluid, he was even more dehydrated. We realized that we were dealing with a diarrhea problem more deadly than we'd seen before and that newborns were much more fragile than week-old calves.

If you ever experience an epidemic in newborns, and standard antibiotics do not halt the acute infection, have your vet do a fecal culture on a calf that has not been treated and some antibiotic sensitivity tests to find out what type of drug might be helpful.

In spite of the fluid we'd given that calf six hours earlier, he was wobbly and almost too weak to stand. His condition had deteriorated almost to the point of needing IV fluids, and his diarrhea was worse; he was squirting colored water. Even though we were extremely busy attending calving cows — checking the maternity pen often and putting any calving cows into the barn because the weather was very cold — we knew that we had to double our efforts to save this calf.

We gave the calf 1½ quarts (1.4 L) of electrolyte solution every three hours for a couple of days. This turned his health around, and we saved him. The rest of the calves all got sick very soon after they were born, but we watched them closely and started each one on fluids and medication at the first hint of diarrhea, and repeated the fluid treatments every 2½ to 3 hours. With this intensive care, they all recovered more swiftly than the first case because they didn't get quite as dehydrated before we started treatment. We were glad that there were only 24 of them. This labor-intensive treatment would be impossible for a full calving season with 170 calves! Our neighbors were having similar problems, and vaccination against K99 E. coli did not protect against this bug; it was probably a different strain. Commonly used scour antibiotics — neomycin, tetracyclines, sulfas — also didn't halt the infection. We talked to our vet, and he suggested that next time we squirt into the calves' mouths an oral antibiotic (Furazoladone, which has now been replaced by trimethoprim-sulfa) used for E. coli scours in baby pigs.

The next calving season we tried the pig medication. We made sure that every calf was up and nursing before he was an hour old, helping if necessary, and immediately followed nursing with a dose of the oral antibiotic. This was labor-intensive, too, but not as difficult as treating every calf repeatedly during his first days of life. A few calves started getting loose feces at 12 to 24 hours of age, sometimes with their very first bowel movement, in spite of the antibiotic. But a second dose at the first hint of loose feces stopped the diarrhea.

We hoped that the bug would die out over the summer or might be present only in our calving barn. But even a calf born on grass pasture in August got loose feces. That's when we realized that the bug had colonized in the herd. Some years, we got by without treating the first few calves born, but soon into calving season the problem cropped up again. So we stuck with our pig-medicine treatment and didn't have any sick calves.

In recent years we've finally been able to dispense with giving every calf an oral dose of pig medicine, possibly because newer scour vaccines are more protective. The vaccines that we are using now, given to our cows a couple months before they calve, seems to augment their colostrum with antibodies against this pathogen and provide their calves with some immunity to this particular type of infection, if they nurse immediately after they are born. We have only an occasional calf that needs the oral pig antibiotic on his first day. If you ever experience an epidemic in newborns, and standard antibiotics do not halt the acute infection, have your vet do a fecal culture on a calf that has not been treated and some antibiotic sensitivity tests to find out what type of drug might be helpful.

Some healthy animals shed bacteria for an unknown length of time. These carriers serve as reservoirs of infection. *Carrier* animals introduced into an uninfected herd are thought to be a major cause of outbreaks in herds that previously had no problems with *E. coli* scours. Human visitors can also bring bacteria from an infected farm.

Septicemia

Some types of *E. coli* infections cause septicemia and very rapid death due to endotoxic shock that affects multiple body systems. If a calf survives the septicemia, he may have permanent damage in joints or infection in certain internal organs, depending on where the infection settled. Evidence of these complications usually appears a week later. The calf may become lame or may develop meningitis or pneumonia.

This type of septicemic *E. coli* infection comes on suddenly, and the calf usually hasn't had time to develop diarrhea; he is depressed and weak and may not be able to stand up. His legs are cold, and though he may have had a fever briefly at the beginning, his temperature soon falls to subnormal levels as he goes into shock. A calf with this type of infection can be difficult to save unless you begin treatment immediately. Often the illness comes on so quickly that unless you are checking calves frequently you don't realize the calf is sick until it's too late.

Like other gram-negative bacteria, *E. coli* may contain poisons within their cell walls. When the bacteria die and decompose, the *endotoxins* are released. Once the toxins get into the bloodstream, which they do as soon as they damage the gut lining, they cause poisoning throughout the body. The result is a general toxemia and damage to vital organs as the calf goes into shock. Or the toxins may create a sudden and severe weakness similar to food poisoning in humans; the calf becomes wobbly and is soon too weak to stand up, even though he is not yet severely dehydrated.

These types of *E. coli* are very diverse, and it has not been possible to create a vaccine against them. Septicemic strains of *E. coli* can attack calves less than five days old, and vaccines that protect against other strains that cause diarrhea aren't effective. Giving the sick calf an antiserum or *antitoxin* for *E. coli* may help treat an acute case, since these products are not as strain-specific as the vaccines; ask your vet about the possibility of using this for treatment. Cows may have protective antibodies in their colostrum, however, if they themselves had earlier exposure, they may be able to protect calves from septicemia even if the calves develop diarrhea. Once passive transfer of antibodies from colostrum wanes, however, calves are vulnerable.

Vaccine

Vaccinating cows before calving season can help reduce the incidence and severity of certain types of *E. coli* scours in young calves. Vaccines are directed against a specific antigen that is part of a bacterium. The most common *E. coli* bacterium that affects calves soon after birth needs a specific antigen, the K99 antigen pillus, to bind to the small intestine. *Pilli* are minute appendages of certain bacteria that are associated with antigenic properties and that can stick to the small intestine. Once there, the antigen can be destructive, but if it can't bind, it is harmless.

The vaccine creates antibodies in the cow, passed on via colostrum or via an *E. coli* vaccine given orally immediately after birth. This vaccine is effective for preventing diarrhea but does not seem to protect against strains of *E. coli* that cause toxemia and sudden death due to release of endotoxins.

Treatment

If begun in the early stages while infection is still confined to the small intestine, treatment is usually effective for *E. coli* diarrhea. An oral antibiotic and supportive therapy including fluids and electrolytes will usually reverse dehydration and halt the infection (see page 231). If the calf dies, it's usually from dehydration, acidosis, and electrolyte imbalance. Extreme metabolic changes can occur in a calf with severe diarrhea, and if too much fluid is lost from the body, he goes into shock. Very young calves tend to dehydrate more rapidly and severely than calves older than a week. Any one- to three-day-old calf must have very aggressive treatment — oral fluids given every few hours, or IVs, if oral fluids were not begun soon enough — in order to save him.

Enterotoxemia (Clostridial Infections)

Enterotoxemia is simply the presence of toxins in the bloodstream from bacteria that are normally found in the intestines. This is a potentially fatal condition that can be caused by several different types of bacteria, but the term as used by stockmen most commonly refers to infection with *Clostridium perfringens,* types B, C, or D.

Toxic Release

The *exotoxins* created by *C. perfringens* bacteria are different from the endotoxins produced by *E. coli.* The latter are produced as the bacteria die, releasing the toxin from the cell wall. Exotoxins are created while the *C. perfringens* bacteria are still alive, produced as they multiply.

Prevention

This disease can be prevented by vaccinating cows before calving season to stimulate development of antibodies (see chapter 10) or by vaccinating the calf soon after birth. It can also be prevented in epidemic situations by giving each calf a dose of antitoxin at birth for more immediate, temporary protection. Antitoxin is much more expensive than the vaccine, however. It's cheaper to vaccinate the cow ahead of calving and to make sure that her calf nurses immediately after birth to get the passive transfer of antibodies.

Some stockmen, trying for ultimate protection, vaccinate the cow and also vaccinate the calf after he's born, but this is a waste of money. If you vaccinate the cow ahead of calving, it won't do you any good to vaccinate the calf soon after birth because antibodies in the cow's colostrum interfere with the calf's ability to produce an active immunity; his body already has the antibodies from the colostrum he just ingested. The antigens in the vaccine are neutralized by maternal antibodies and can't stimulate the calf's body to mount an immune response, thus interfering with the calf's ability to produce an active immunity. You must choose whether to vaccinate the cows or the calves; it doesn't work to do both.

The key to this decision is noting the time frame when calves on your place become ill with enterotoxemia. If you usually have problems with this disease in very young calves, you should vaccinate the cows a few weeks before calving or give the calves antitoxin at birth to give immediate protection. If you have problems in several-week-old calves, you are better off to vaccinate the calves at birth and not vaccinate the cows before calving season. On many farms the typical age for enterotoxemia is one to three months — after passive transfer from colostrum has worn off. In these situations it's best to vaccinate the calves rather than the cows so that they can be building their own immunity.

An injection of C and D vaccines (*toxoid,* modified or inactivated bacterial toxins, used to stimulate immunity) shortly after birth will protect most calves, producing active immunity within a few days. If this isn't enough protection, if you experience the disease in very young calves before the toxoid has a chance to stimulate immunity, you should either vaccinate the cows ahead of calving or give the calves both toxoid and antitoxin, which are two different products. These can be injected in opposite sides of the neck within a few hours after birth, according to one of our veterinarians.

Antitoxin is like the protection a calf gains from colostrum; it produces instant passive immunity to protect a calf immediately, but only temporarily. Passive immunity, gained either through colostrum, from vaccination of the cow ahead of calving, or through antitoxin, lasts only about three weeks. After that the calf must depend on a direct vaccination.

Cause and Effect

Bacteria that cause enterotoxemia are usually present in the intestines of calves, picked up from the environment, but are generally in the form of dormant spores. They cause disease only if they change into an active multiplying form, which they do under certain conditions. Once they are no longer dormant, they multiply rapidly and produce toxins that compromise the gut lining and leak through it into the bloodstream. The deadly toxins not only shut down the gut, causing extreme pain and colic (the calf kicks at his belly or lies on the ground thrashing his legs), but can also quickly compromise other body organs, and the calf goes into shock. In a short time he slips into a coma and dies, unless given massive doses of antitoxin. This type of infection can kill calves so quickly that you may not see them sick; you just find them dead.

The type of exotoxin produced by *C. perfringens* depends on the nutrients available in the calf's digestive tract. Concentrations of protein or carbohydrates are what determine whether type C or D toxin is produced. This problem has been called *overeating disease* because it often hits calves whose mothers milk well, especially if a calf goes off feed for some reason and then loads up on milk afterward. The sudden milk overload creates ideal conditions for the bacteria to multiply. Milk is high in both protein and carbohydrates, so the bacteria in a calf may produce either type of toxin. When vaccinating calves to protect them against enterotoxemia, use a vaccine containing both C and D toxoids.

Colicky Bloat

The calf has acute gut pain. He is kicking at his belly, thrashing on the ground, and staggering around; he goes into shock within a few hours and dies swiftly unless treated immediately. Although it may appear to be *C. perfringens,* there are other toxin-producing bacteria that cause illness and similar symptoms. Many calves show no signs other than severe gut pain before going into shock; they do not have time to develop diarrhea. Others become dull and bloated, then go into shock and die. For want of a better term to describe this disease, on our ranch we call it "*colicky bloat.*" Some of the calves become colicky without bloat, while others become dull and bloated, but we suspect that it's the same bug in each situation and we use the same treatment in these cases to reverse the condition.

Switch Treatments

If any calf suffering from symptoms of enterotoxemia does not respond to administration of *C. perfringens* antitoxin, he should be treated with castor oil and neomycin if he's not yet in shock, or large amounts of IV fluids if he's already going into shock.

Saving Calves from Colicky Bloat

Our pastures have been used intensively for cattle for more than 120 years — that's 120 years of contamination with pathogens that cause diarrhea in calves. When Lynn and I began ranching here in 1967, we had to become good calf doctors to keep from losing calves. We learned to treat diarrhea diligently, and to check calves vigilantly to halt scour cases early. We've lost only one calf to scours since 1969.

Colicky bloat is another type of gut infection that continues to haunt us, however, not only because our vets have not figured out the cause, but also because it can kill a calf in a few hours. He may be fine at one check and dying of shock — and sometimes bloat — five or six hours later. This acute gut infection can be fatal three to twelve hours after the first signs appear. We always save these calves, however, if we find them before they go into shock. That's why it's crucial to check them often.

Colicky bloat is another type of gut infection that continues to haunt us, however, not only because our vets have not figured out the cause, but also because it can kill a calf in a few hours.

Since this type of infection can affect calves up to three months of age while they're on wet fields in early spring, we don't relax our vigilance even after they are past the critical age for scours. We feed cows twice a day, splitting the hay ration into two portions, primarily so that we can check the herd morning and evening to be sure to discover any sick calves in time to treat them. The problem stops when they leave the fields and go to mountain pasture.

Some years the bug is worse; infections seem more acute, and we get more cases. During the wet spring of 1995, when we had an early thaw and flooded fields, we had many emergency cases. The worst six lived in our kitchen for a while, in intensive care. We increased our diligence, walking through the calves at midday between feedings and twice in the night until fields dried out and the epidemic eased. Spring of 1996 was also bad; we treated more than 30 calves for colicky bloat and had to take one, Witsi, to our vet for IV fluids.

There is no vaccination against the pathogen that causes this highly fatal condition, and the antitoxin product for enterotoxemia due to *C. perfringens* has no effect. Many calves in our valley die from this problem every spring. Veterinarians and lab tests have not identified the pathogen. Our vet thinks it might be a type of *E. coli* (see page 233), of which there are several hundred serotypes.

This pathogen, whatever it is, strikes calves most commonly at three weeks to three months of age, when passive transfer from maternal antibodies wanes. This suggests that cows growing up on our place have encountered it and have antibodies against it to protect their calves through colostrum intake. The fact that heifers' calves tend to get it sometimes as young as two to three weeks of age shows that antibodies in colostrum are protective, but that immunity gained from passive transfer is generally not as strong and long-lasting in heifers' calves. Frustratingly, this acute infection can swiftly kill big healthy calves that are well past the "risky" age for scours.

Wet weather and mud create ideal conditions for colicky bloat. Each wet spring we have as many as 15 to 30 cases of this acute bacterial infection in our herd of 170 cows. Our vet thinks that the bacteria live in the soil: When calves eat mud or dirt, nurse a dirty udder, or drink muddy water, they ingest pathogens, which may multiply rapidly in the gut under certain conditions and produce toxins that damage the lining. If not treated quickly, toxins leak through the damaged lining into the bloodstream, creating general toxemia and shock, which can swiftly kill the calf. The calf's blood pressure and temperature drop, mouth and legs become cold, lungs and kidneys fail, and he soon dies.

When a calf is sick with colicky bloat, there's usually no time to develop diarrhea, or even feel sick for very long. His mother is usually completely nursed out. He feels fine until he's hit suddenly by severe gut pain. You might be watching a bunch of calves out on the bedground or at feeding time, and one will sud-

WITSI'S STORY

THE LAST WEEK OF JANUARY 1996 was stormy and cold — 10 below zero with a wind chill equivalent to 45 below. When I went out at daylight to feed horses, I heard a cow bawling and hiked through new snow to the field above the house to see what the problem was. Witsi's mother was bawling and her calf was not in the calf houses or along the fence where we'd put straw for bedding. Finally I saw a lump in the snow along the far fence; Witsi was lying flat, covered with two inches of snow, looking dead. As I brushed snow off her head, I heard a slow, wheezing breath. I ran to get Lynn and the Jeep.

Witsi was big, almost a month old, and we could barely lift her into the Jeep. Her temperature was very low, so we brought her into the house to warm her up, gave her an injection of dexamethasone to try to reverse shock, and tried to give her an IV. Her blood pressure was so low that her veins were collapsed; we managed to give her only one liter of fluid and couldn't get an IV needle or catheter to stay in a vein, so we loaded her into the back of a covered pickup, put warm towels over her for the 12-mile trip to town, and took her to our vet. He got a catheter into her jugular vein and gave her several more liters of fluid.

By evening she'd regained consciousness and could hold up her head, so we brought her home, keeping her in our kitchen and dosing her with fluid and electrolytes by stomach tube; she now had diarrhea. After she became strong enough to stand, we took her to the barn, putting her and her mother into a stall next to a stove. We saved her, but bacteria and toxins circulating in her bloodstream while she was in shock affected her joints. She developed septic arthritis, like a calf with joint ill from navel infection (see chapter 14). This required a long follow-up treatment with antibiotics to eliminate the joint infection.

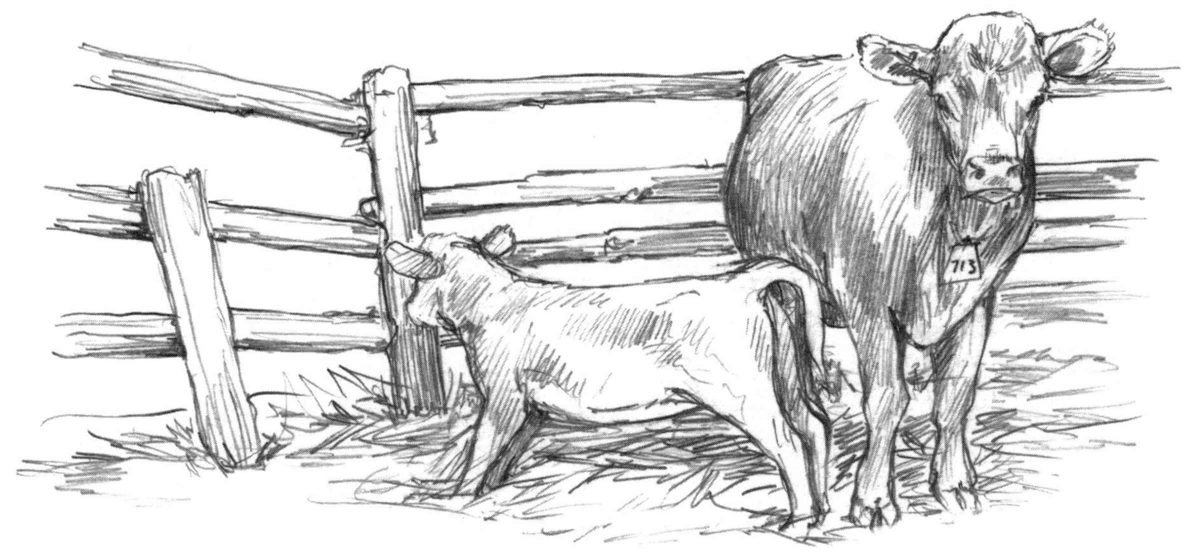

A calf with "colicky bloat" may stretch swaybacked, kick at his belly, and throw himself onto the ground.

denly lie down, then get up again, only to lie down or start kicking his belly or show other signs of pain.

He may lie flat on the ground, thrashing and kicking, or stand in an odd position, stretched and swaybacked, kicking. Some calves run wildly, trying to get away from pain, then lie down and get up repeatedly, or throw themselves onto the ground, only to get up and run again. The calf may stagger as he walks, with legs buckling, sinking to the ground. If you try to herd him, he may want to lie down. Or he may be bloated and dull, reluctant to move.

Treatment

The only way to save these calves is to find them soon after they become sick and treat them in time to reverse the conditions that are causing shutdown of the gut. Whenever we see a calf kicking at his belly, or staggering around, or dull and bloated, we consider it an extreme emergency; we halt what we're doing and walk the calf and his mother in from the field if the calf can walk, or put him into the feed truck and take him to the barnyard with Mama following. If he is critically ill, we rush him straight to the barn, or the house if the weather is bad, for intensive care, or bring medication to the field to treat him on the spot. Our son and his wife carry a doctoring kit with them in their tractor or feed truck containing a thermos of warm water for giving fluids to a calf with diarrhea or for mixing with castor oil to treat colicky bloat. Colicky bloat is not a situation where you wait to see if they'll get better.

If a calf is not yet in shock, shake 4 to 6 ounces of castor oil with an equal amount of hot water, and add a proper dose of the oral antibiotic neomycin sulfate solution. Give the calf the mix by stomach tube or esophageal feeder (see page 240) to stimulate movement in the shut-down gut, so that toxins won't just stay there and leak into the bloodstream. The liquid neomycin sulfate solution combats the bacteria and the castor oil relieves the pain and or bloat. Our first vet recommended the combination of neomycin sulfate solution (which alone combats many bacterial gut infections) and castor oil to us when we initially encountered this problem in 1968. The

CHOOSE CASTOR OIL

Mineral oil will not help a calf with colic or bloat caused by bacteria that are creating toxins and shutting down the gut. Mineral oil merely lubricates, soothes the gut lining, and breaks up gas. It does not stimulate the tract to move nor absorb toxins. You must get the gut working again, and castor oil is best for this.

newer treatments have not worked any better, and most don't work at all for this problem. Without castor oil, these calves soon go into toxic shock.

The castor oil not only helps relieve pain by relieving the blockage, stopping bloat, moving toxic material on through the gut, and halting damage to the gut lining, but it also binds and neutralizes the toxins, rendering them harmless. They can then be digested along with the castor oil, with no ill effects on the calf.

We don't give oral fluids or electrolytes to these calves; they are not dehydrated because they have not had diarrhea. If they are going into shock, they need fluids intravenously, not orally. If they are bloated, there is no room in the gut for fluids — only for the castor oil. Get the oil and neomycin into the calf soon enough, and he won't need emergency fluids.

The liquid neomycin sulfate solution combats the bacterial infection, getting to the site of the problem quicker than pills, which don't dissolve readily if the gut isn't working. If you give a calf castor oil and neomycin before he goes into shock, recovery is swift and dramatic. He feels better within an hour or so, and if he was bloated, that condition is resolved as well. If necessary, we repeat the castor oil treatment a couple of hours later to get the gut moving if the calf is still in pain or bloated. If he is experiencing extreme pain and thrashing on the ground, we give him an injection of the colicky-horse remedy, Banamine, to ease his pain more quickly (appropriate dosage depends on the size of the calf).

If the calf is bloated, however, near suffocation because the distended rumen is putting pressure on his lungs, and more dull than colicky, you don't have time to give oil and neomycin. You must first relieve the bloat so that he can breathe. The quickest way to relieve bloat is to stick the distended rumen with a big sterile needle (see chapter 15). Let the gas out so that he won't suffocate, and then give the castor oil and neomycin. It may be necessary to stick him again and let more air out if he continues to bloat, until the castor oil has time to work. If he's in a far pasture when you find him with serious bloat and there isn't time to get a sterile needle, you can stick him with the tip of a sharp pocketknife.

COLD-WEATHER TUBE TIP

A stomach tube is easier to put into the calf if it is very flexible. In cold or windy weather, it's quite possible that the plastic tube may become stiff. In this case we put the tube into a thermos jug of hot water when taking it outdoors to treat a calf, blowing the water out of it just before inserting it into his nostril.

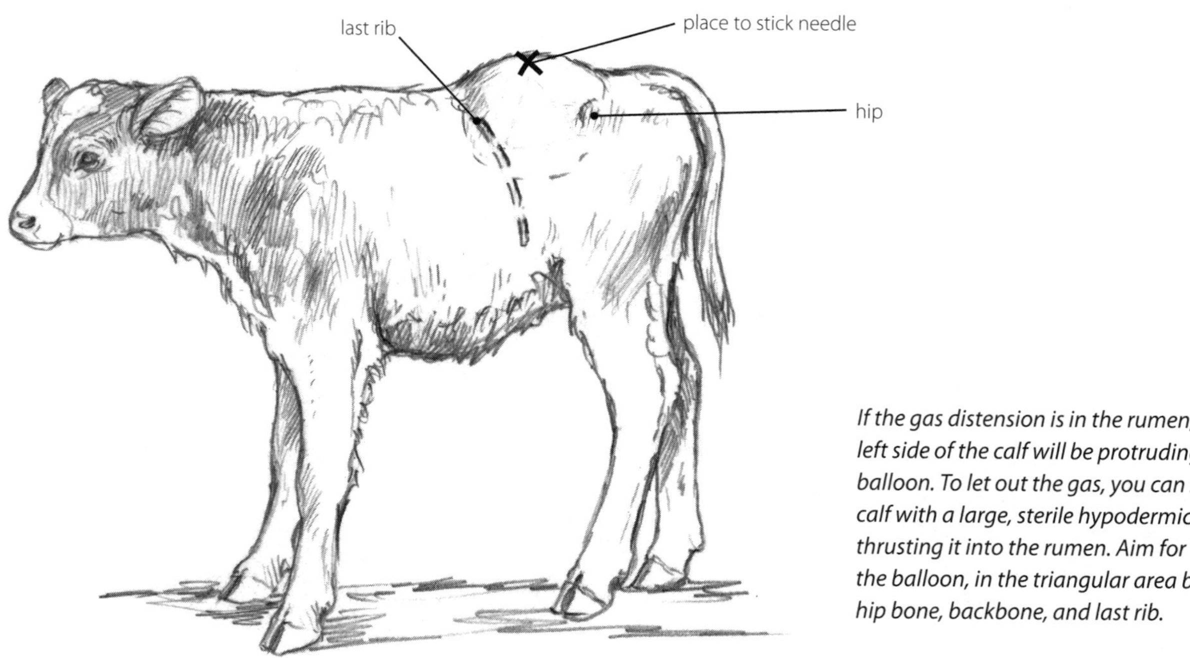

If the gas distension is in the rumen, the left side of the calf will be protruding like a balloon. To let out the gas, you can stick the calf with a large, sterile hypodermic needle, thrusting it into the rumen. Aim for the top of the balloon, in the triangular area between hip bone, backbone, and last rib.

OUR MOST EXTREME CASE OF BLOAT

BOULDER WAS BORN JANUARY 15, 1994. At one month of age she suddenly developed colicky bloat. I heard her mama bawling that afternoon, and hiked up into the field to see what was wrong. We always pay attention whenever we hear a cow bawling, since this is a clue that she's worried about her calf. I found Boulder dull and bloated, so I slowly herded her and her mama down through the field and into a corral. She needed treatment immediately, but Lynn was in town to get our mail and groceries and Boulder was too big for me to handle by myself. I called our daughter, who lived close by, and she came to help me. We backed the calf into a corner and gave her castor oil and neomycin by stomach tube.

Three weeks later, she bloated again. The bloat subsided after another treatment, but within a few hours it was serious again. Another round of castor oil resolved it. Four days later, she was bloated so badly that she could hardly breathe, and we stuck her rumen with a needle to let out the gas and keep her from suffocating while we put castor oil into her. We checked her again an hour later and her rumen was still tight and full, so we stuck her again, released more gas, and gave her more oil.

She was the first case that did not respond fully to two doses of castor oil (usually one dose is enough); we gave her more oil at midnight and several more times the next day, along with fluids, because she was dull and not nursing. She had not passed any bowel movements, even though she'd been given more than 30 ounces (887 mL) of castor oil in just over 24 hours — much more than we'd ever given any other calf.

We continued to treat with oil, fluid, Karo syrup for energy, and probiotics (products containing the microorganisms needed for proper digestion: "good bugs") to try to get her rumen functioning again. We were afraid to give her any milk yet, in case she had a complete blockage. After a massive dose of castor oil the fourth day, she finally passed a small amount of loose manure, full of mucus and gut lining. She would not nurse; she probably had a sore gut from damage done by toxins and raw spots where the gut lining had sloughed away. After six days of continual treatment with castor oil and fluids, she finally nursed her mother and passed firm balls of manure.

Full recovery took all summer. We'd put the pair out, only to get them in again a few days or a week later to treat the calf again. Boulder was never as sick again, but she was occasionally bloated so badly that she needed castor oil. She was fine within a few hours after treatment and would go a week or more before the next episode. We were afraid she'd be a bloater the rest of her life.

Her mother, Beller, became very cooperative and was our best ally, though she was normally very independent. She'd bawl every time Boulder got bloated or dull. Whenever we heard that cow bawling, we knew we had to bring them to the corral and tube the calf with oil. Beller would hover over us, wanting us to hurry up and fix her calf; she seemed to know that we were helping.

Boulder became very gentle. It would have been impossible otherwise for two people to back a four-hundred-pound calf into a corral corner and put a stomach tube down her nose. She resigned herself to the ordeal and stood still, without a fight. By late summer she finally outgrew the bloating episodes. Whatever damage had been done to her rumen by the infection must have healed. We had so much time and effort invested in her that we figured the only way to come out ahead was keep her. She became a good cow and never bloated again. She's had a calf every year — Pebbles, Rocky Feller, Granite, and others — and is still in the herd at this writing, ready to have her twelfth calf!

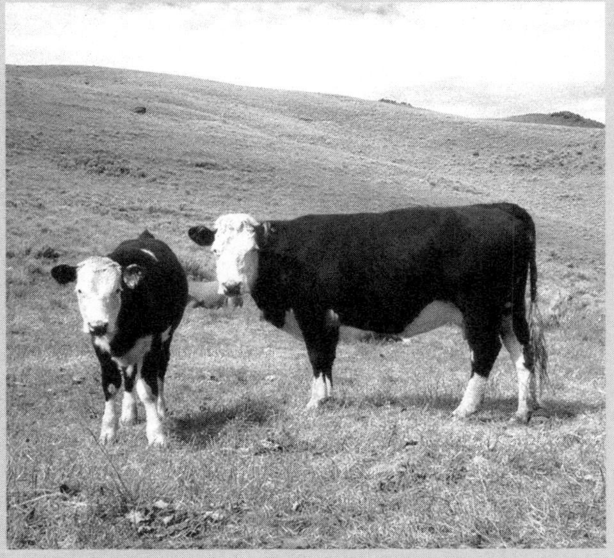

Boulder, pictured here as a five-year-old cow with her calf, survived many bloating episodes as a calf and extensive treatment to save her.

HOW TO ADMINISTER CASTOR OIL AND NEOMYCIN

Use a flexible plastic or nylon stomach tube 4 feet (1.2 m) long, ¼ inch (.64 cm) in diameter, smoothed or beveled on one end with a knife, sander, or grinder so it won't scrape the nasal passage and throat.

1. Set aside a large (140 cc) syringe used to force oil down the tube once it's inserted.
2. Before inserting the tube, tuck the calf's nose downward toward his chest rather than up in the air. If his head and neck are stretched out, with nose up, the tube is more likely to go into the windpipe instead of into the esophagus, where it can be swallowed.
3. Put the smoothed end into one nostril, inserting quickly before the calf resists by clamping the inner part of his nostril shut, thereby making insertion more difficult and harder on the sensitive tissues.
4. Once the tube is in the nostril, push it to the back of the throat, where the calf must swallow it down into his stomach. If the calf fails to swallow the tube and it starts back out the other nostril as you are putting it in, pull it out and start over.
5. Keep pushing the tube in, but make sure he swallows it; otherwise, it will go into his windpipe.
6. Make sure the tube is in the stomach, not the windpipe, or you'll drown the calf when you give him fluid or oil. Usually he will cough if the tube starts into the windpipe; if he coughs, take it out and start over. If the tube goes down easily and quite a way (at least 2 feet [.6 m]), it's in the stomach. If it's in the windpipe it can't go as far: The windpipe branches into two smaller bronchial tubes.
7. Check to be sure that the tube is in the stomach by blowing on your end. If you hear burbling noises or smell stomach gas coming out, it is in the stomach. If your blowing makes the calf cough, it's in the windpipe, and you must take it out.
8. If you hit a gas pocket when you insert the tube into the stomach, gas will come rushing out your end. If the calf is bloated, this helps relieve the pressure. If you hit gas, don't put the tube in farther until you have let out all the gas that will come. Once it stops rushing out, put the tube in a little farther, and give the oil.
9. In a container, shake 4 to 6 ounces (118 mL to 177 mL) of castor oil (amount depending on the size of the calf) with an equal amount of hot water (hotter than body temperature, but not so hot that it would burn the calf), and a proper dose of neomycin sulfate solution (appropriate to the size of the calf). Suck the mix into the syringe by pulling the plunger back to create a vacuum in the syringe. Oil and water will quickly separate in your container — make sure you get some of each into the syringe. Bring an extra jar of hot water to suck into the syringe if needed, to keep the oil mix warm. It takes several full syringes to give the full dose of oil/water mix.

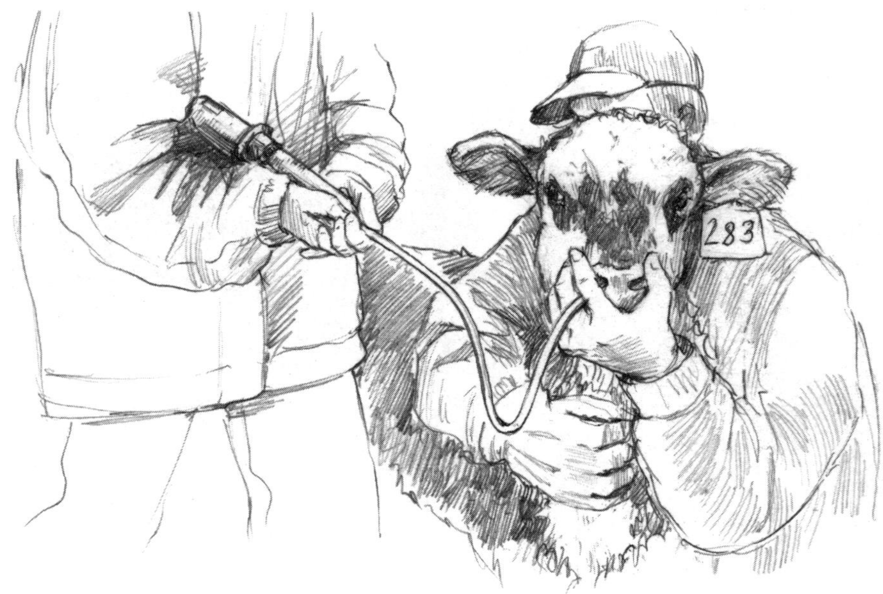

Forcing the thick castor oil down the tube with a large syringe calls for a helper to hold the calf steady.

Inserting a Stomach Tube

Sometimes when you put a stomach tube into a calf to administer castor oil, you can release gas. For this reason, a nasogastric stomach tube that goes into the nostril, down the throat, and into the stomach is better than an esophageal feeder when treating colicky bloat. It's impossible to get gas out through the feeder's probe; it doesn't go into the stomach. The longer stomach tube can hit a pocket of gas. If you don't have a stomach tube, use an esophageal feeder to administer oil. And be sure to give plenty of warm oil, because castor oil is thick, and much of it will stay in the probe, coating the sides.

Follow-up Treatment

If the calf is not yet in shock when you give castor oil and neomycin, recovery is dramatic; in an hour or so, he feels better. Bloat is gone if he was bloated, and there is no more gut pain. If you catch the problem early, he won't develop diarrhea. But every case should be watched closely for several days after treatment. Some calves have so much gut damage from the acute infection that part of the lining sloughs away a few days later, leaving painful raw spots. There's usually mucus and membrane in the feces.

Some of these calves go off feed completely a few days after recovering from colic or bloat, and become dull. They may pick at hay or grass and drink water but refuse to nurse. They may fiddle at the udder but won't actually suck. The cow has a full udder. The calf may be off feed only a day or two, or remain dull and not nurse for a week or more, until the raw spots heal. Some will starve to death unless force-fed.

You may have to feed the calf twice a day for a few days if he's not nursing at all, or sporadically for a week or so until he nurses his mother regularly. This may mean milking the cow periodically to keep her from drying up. We tube the calf with mineral oil to soothe the raw gut lining and give him milk by tube on days when he won't nurse. Some calves become thin because they don't nurse their mothers enough to sustain themselves. They often grind their teeth because of discomfort in the gut and drool from chewing. We keep tubing them with milk, and this often gives them strength and incentive to try to nurse. Some calves need probiotics added to their feeding or given as a paste or pill (obtained from your vet) to aid proper digestion.

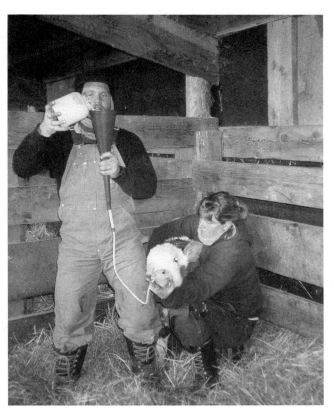

My son Michael and his wife Carolyn feed Quasi some milk via stomach tube. After recovering from the life-threatening crisis of acute gut infection, some calves like Quasi go off feed a few days later due to the discomfort of shedding the damaged intestinal lining. The sloughing intestinal lining leaves raw ulcers, and the calf must be force-fed until the gut heals and he starts nursing again.

Emergency Treatment for Bloat

One spring, when we had several emergency cases and severely bloated calves, I tried something different on the calves that we had to stick with a needle. After getting as much gas as possible out through the needle, I attached a syringe to the inserted needle still poking into the rumen, and directly injected a dose of neomycin sulfate solution. This put the antibiotic right where it was needed to halt the multiplying bacteria creating gas and deadly toxins, and worked faster to halt further bloating than neomycin given by stomach tube (though the calves still need the castor oil via tube). There was no further bloating in calves directly injected with neomycin, and we didn't have to stick them again.

Toxemia and Shock

If the calf is already in shock when you find him, he needs intravenous fluids and intensive care. If the weather is cold, we put him by a stove or heater, with heating pads over his body, as we administer fluids. The only way to save him is by giving 4 to 5 liters (1 to 1.3 gal) of IV fluids and medication to help reverse shock and restore proper circulation. He's suffering from toxemia and shock; the bacterial toxins attack all his body organs, causing massive shutdown. His circulation fails; blood pressure drops; mouth and extremities become cold (his temperature may drop too low to register on a rectal thermometer); kidneys start to fail; his lungs, liver, and brain are damaged. At this point he soon dies. But if kidneys and other internal organs are not yet too damaged by the toxins in the bloodstream, the calf will survive if given fluids intravenously.

Halt toxemia and reverse shock by giving adrenaline (epinephrine, which can be given IM, SQ, or IV), an IV injection of dexamethasone (a steroid, used for reducing pain, inflammation, swelling, and fever), and 4 or 5 liters (1 to 1.3 gal) of IV fluids to restore circulating blood volume, dilute the concentration of toxins in his bloodstream, and keep his kidneys working. But if there is already too much damage to lungs, kidneys, and other vital organs, he will die, no matter how heroic your efforts. Once his kidneys fail, you will lose him.

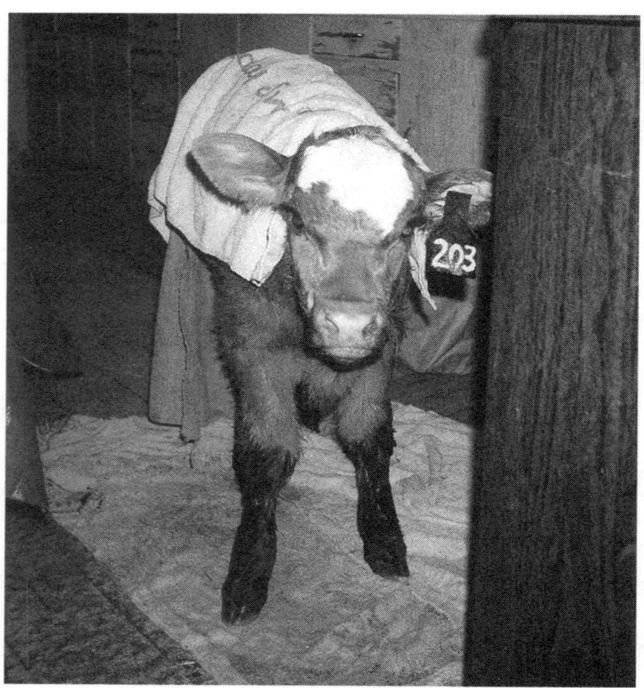

A month-old calf is recovering from severe colic and bloat caused by acute toxin-forming gut infection. We brought him into the house to treat him for shock and warm him up.

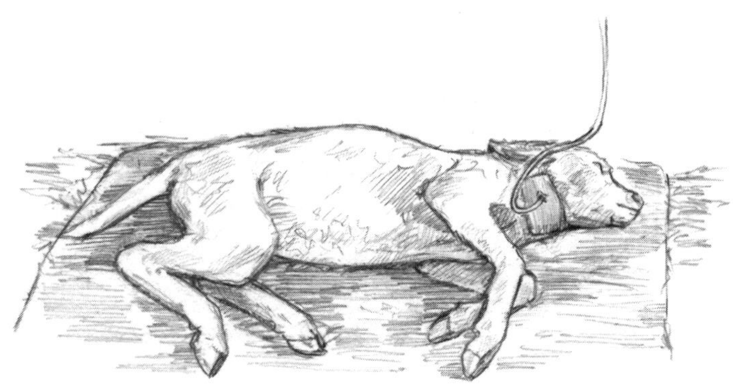

Administer IV fluid to an unconscious calf that's deep in shock. Sometimes it's necessary to shave the calf's neck to locate a collapsed jugular vein.

The kidneys and liver are the body's best detoxification systems. If they shut down, this creates a snowball effect: Toxins build up more quickly in the body. If kidneys keep working, then once they begin to excrete the fluid you're putting in, they begin to remove toxins from the bloodstream. If the calf starts producing urine while you are giving IV fluids, there's a good chance that he will recover; our vet says that recovery rate in these instances is about 90 percent.

Many commercial IV solutions work well for treating a calf with toxemia. The exact makeup of the solution does not matter, as long as it is *isotonic,* meaning that its electrolyte concentration is the same as that in body tissues. Any solutions that are too concentrated, such as 50 percent dextrose, will force the body to draw water from body tissues to try to equalize and dilute, making the problem worse. You want to restore body fluid, not deplete it.

If you are not experienced at giving IV fluids, and the calf is in shock, get the calf to your vet *fast.* If you have many cases that you are unable to treat with castor oil before they go into shock, ask your vet to show you how to give IV fluids. Finding the jugular vein is the toughest challenge on calves that are already in shock, with low blood pressure: The vein may be collapsed.

Salmonella

This disease severely afflicts many dairy herds and some beef herds. The more than 2,200 serotypes of salmonella bacteria are categorized into three main groups: those that affect only humans, types affecting only animals, and a group that causes disease in both humans and animals. One of the most common serotypes that cause disease in humans and animals, including cattle, is spread by cats, birds, infected cattle, and other domestic animals. Another type that can infect cattle can live in the mammary glands of cows' udders and is excreted in milk — one reason not to use colostrum from a dairy farm.

Young calves exposed to feces containing salmonella are highly susceptible. The mortality rate may be high in calves less than three months old unless treated. Bacteria are spread by direct contact and by feed, water, and bedding contaminated with feces from an infected animal. Introduction of an infected or carrier animal into the herd can be the source of an outbreak. This pathogen can survive for 14 months or longer in a contaminated pen or barn and may live for up to six years in dried feces.

The disease is most deadly in newborns, and survival depends on the degree of exposure, antibody levels in their colostrum intake, and stress. The disease may exist on certain farms, with outbreaks in calves due to a contaminated environment. Some adult cattle shed more pathogens at calving time due to the stress of giving birth. Wet conditions increase spread of disease, as does concentration of too many animals in small areas.

Some animals become carriers, shedding the organism either continually or periodically, such as during periods of stress, even if they show no signs of illness. Stress can result from weather changes, change in diet, transportation, vaccination that produces a systemic reaction (fever, etc.), calving, and many other factors.

Treatment

Care for a salmonella-infected animal consists of fluids, electrolytes, and an appropriate antibiotic. Use of antibiotics for salmonella is controversial because of development of resistance to antibiotics in some strains. That problem stems more from overuse of antibiotics, such as mass-medicating groups of calves that have been in contact with a sick one, than from treating individual sick animals.

Treating the calf early with an approved antibiotic is often successful, but if much of the intestine is damaged by the time treatment is begun (24 to 48 hours after onset of diarrhea), chances for saving the calf are slimmer. Your vet can diagnose salmonella and advise you on treatment. Trimethoprim-sulfadoxine can be given orally to young calves, but give older calves (with a functioning rumen) an injection of the drug. Some drugs that were most effective against salmonella are now banned in food animals.

There is vaccine available to be given to cows ahead of calving to increase the level of antibodies in colostrum. Calves themselves can be vaccinated at one to three weeks of age, but the best protection is to vaccinate the cows during late pregnancy and make sure calves get adequate colostrum; this gives them proection for about six weeks. After that, the calves can be vaccinated if they are still at risk. A combination program of vaccination, good management (keeping the environment as clean as possible), and not introducing new animals into the herd can control the disease.

AGE OF CALVES WHEN PATHOGENS STRIKE

Pathogen Type	Age of Calf
Clostridium perfringens (types B and C)	5 to 15 days
Clostridium perfringens (type D)	1 to 4 months
Coccidiosis (protozoa)	older than 21 days
"Colicky bloat"	3 weeks to 3 months
Coronavirus	5 to 30 days
Cryptosporidium (protozoa)	5 to 35 days
E. coli (enterotoxigenic types)	under 3 days
E. coli (attaching types)	15 to 30 days
Rotavirus	2 to 15 days
Salmonella	5 to 42 days
Other viruses (including BVD)	2 to 4+ weeks

Using Fecal Samples or Necropsies to Aid Diagnosis

Sometimes a vet might take a fecal sample from a sick calf or send a dead calf to a diagnostic lab for a *necropsy* to try to find the cause of infection, especially if there's a large number of sick calves. Cryptosporidia and coccidiosis can often be detected by looking at fecal samples under a microscope. A culture may show growth of certain bacteria, or a vet may use an electron microscope to detect rotavirus and coronavirus. Take a fecal sample from a calf that has not yet been treated, and transport it in a sterile container, untouched. If the calf has already received antibiotics, it may be difficult to culture the organism.

The same is true of a necropsy: Send a dead calf that has not been treated. This may mean sacrificing a sick calf that hasn't died. Most stockmen are reluctant to do that, thinking that the calf might have a chance to survive, and would prefer to send to the lab one that looks the worst after being treated with several different drugs, or one that died in spite of treatment. But you can't learn much from those.

In a herd epidemic, it may be beneficial to sacrifice one calf in order to discover the cause of infection and be able to treat the remaining calves more effectively. Sometimes it's possible to do lots of fecal-sample tests without having to do a necropsy, but it may be cheaper to do a necropsy. If a stockman has several hundred calves, sacrificing one calf to do a necropsy may save many others.

Keep Them Nursing

Do not withhold milk from a scouring calf that's still strong enough to nurse. In years past, veterinarians recommended taking the calf away from the cow for 24 hours, giving fluids every 6 to 8 hours instead of milk, but milk does more good than harm. Milk may keep the damaged gut irritated longer, but the calf needs the nutrients that milk provides. A calf that continues to nurse is stronger. If he can stay with his dam, he'll recover faster, not only because he won't be as weak if he can nurse but also because he needs the comfort and security he gets from Mama. You don't want to create more stress by separating them.

If he's too sick to nurse, force-feed him about 10 percent of his body weight daily in milk or milk replacer, divided into four to six feedings. Give fluids and electrolytes between those feedings if the electrolytes contain bicarbonate. The problem of bicarbonate interfering with proper digestion of milk is minimized if you alternate the milk and electrolyte feedings (see pages 245 and 246).

What's Needed in an Oral Solution

Oral solutions for a calf that is weak and dehydrated should supply four things:

1. Enough sodium to replace what's been lost by the body, to help normalize fluid volumes in the tissues
2. Agents that facilitate absorption of sodium and water from the intestine: glucose, acetate, propionate or glycine
3. An alkalizing agent (acetate, propionate or *bicarbonate*) to correct metabolic acidosis
4. Energy

Treating Diarrhea

In our herd of 170-plus cows, we've always had scour problems, but intensive treatment has been successful. In 40 years of raising calves, and more than 7,000 calves born, we have treated at least 1,500 for scours. Since 1969 we've lost only one to diarrhea. By contrast, from 1966 to 1969 we lost a dozen. In 1969 every calf on the ranch had scours by the time he was two weeks old; we spent most of each day treating calves. That was the year our vet showed us how to use a stomach tube — before esophageal feeders were invented. From that point on we were able to effectively halt dehydration. We stopped using pills and began using neomycin sulfate solution and had better luck with this liquid antibiotic. Each stockman must figure out which medications work best for the pathogens on his or her place.

Even though drugs to combat pathogens — antibiotics aimed at bacteria — are often given to scouring calves, most important is to combat fluid and electrolyte (essential body salts) loss. Standard treatment to prevent or reverse dehydration is to administer oral electrolyte solutions when a calf starts scouring. In serious infections, this can make a difference in whether he lives or dies.

If a calf is still strong enough to stand, oral solutions via stomach tube or esophageal feeder are adequate to maintain hydration, but once he becomes too weak to stand, oral fluids are not absorbed well in the gut. If a calf is down, especially if he's too weak to hold his head up, he needs intravenous fluids. A calf that's going into shock also needs intravenous support, because he can't absorb fluids from a shutdown gut and because only IV fluid can reverse falling blood pressure and restore circulating blood volume. If this is the case, administer the antibiotic intravenously in order for it to be adequately absorbed and to combat septicemia.

ONE DOSE AT A TIME

When using any kind of electrolyte solution, mix with water only the amount you'll use at one time. It doesn't keep if it sits too long before use.

Giving Oral Fluids

If a calf is still strong and able to absorb fluids orally, give him 1 to 2 quarts (.95 to 1.9 L) of warm water, with electrolyte powder added every six to eight hours, or more often for a very young calf with serious diarrhea. Use commercial products — single-dose packets or a container from which you use a certain amount each time — or a homemade mix. There are many good commercial electrolyte products. Check with your vet for a recommendation. One that works well for weak calves is D-Lyte H20-K, which contains a microencapsulated potassium chloride that is released gradually over 8 to 10 hours. This isn't needed for a calf that is not yet weak but can be helpful for one that's weak or unable to stand.

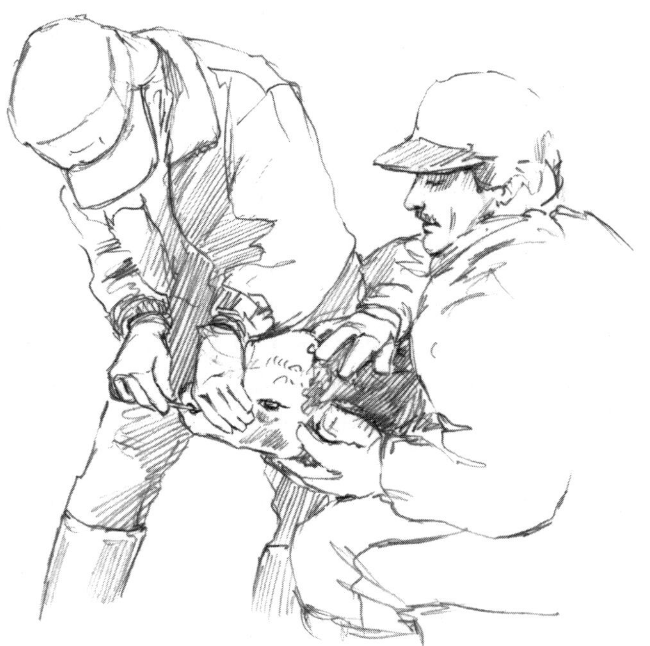

Insert a stomach tube via the nostril to administer fluid and electrolytes to a scouring calf.

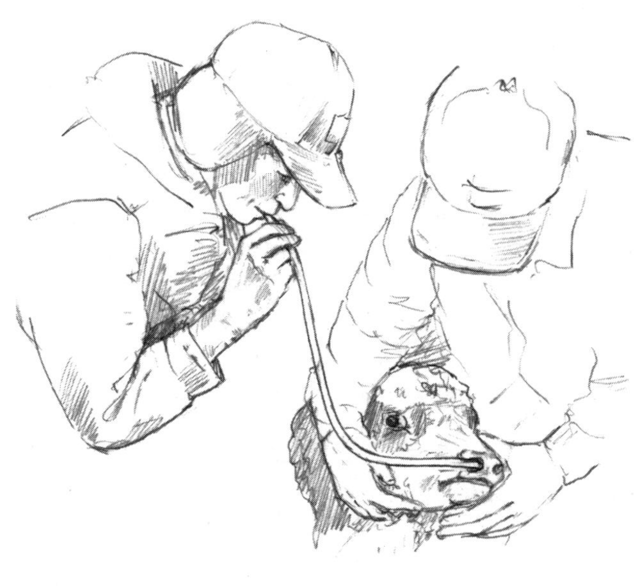

Blow on the tube to make sure that it's in the stomach and not the windpipe before pouring in the fluid.

Oral or IV Fluids?

You waste time and money giving fluid and medications orally if the calf needs IVs. If he is very dehydrated, blood supply to the tissues decreases, and he starts to go into shock. He shunts whatever fluid is still circulating in his bloodstream to the most critical organs, such as the heart and brain; everything else has to go without, including the gut. If he's that dehydrated, there's not much blood supply to the gut, and he can't absorb oral fluid.

You can easily tell if a calf needs an IV. If his blood supply is not servicing the gut, it won't service his skeletal muscles, either; he can't walk, and his legs will be cold and clammy. A calf that can still absorb oral fluids may be very dull and depressed but still strong. A calf whose health lies somewhere in between can be helped by subcutaneous fluids (injected under areas of loose skin over the shoulders), but he can absorb it there only if he has blood supply to these tissues. *Remember:* If he can't walk, then he needs an IV.

Recipe for an Electrolyte Solution

Try the following for a homemade, inexpensive electrolyte solution that is just as effective as a commercial product and does not contain bicarbonate and energy that the calf may not need:

If the calf is strong and not severely dehydrated, mix ½ teaspoon (2.46 mL) of regular salt (sodium chloride) and ¼ teaspoon (1.23 mL) of "lite" salt (a mix of sodium chloride and potassium chloride) in 2 quarts (1.9 L) of warm water. You need only water and simple electrolytes to prevent dehydration.

If the calf is severely ill, weak, and dehydrated, add ¼ teaspoon (1.23 mL) of baking soda as an alkalizing agent to neutralize acidity (acidosis), which can lead to coma and death. After a couple of days of treatment, leave out the baking soda if the calf is improving, or change to a commercial product that does not contain bicarbonate. You don't want to overbalance the body pH.

Giving IV Fluids

Once a calf is too weak to raise his head, the only way you'll save him is with IV fluids. You can usually get him on his feet again with fluid containing bicarbonate. If you know how to give an IV and have the appropriate IV tubing and needle, you can make your own IV fluid using a gallon of distilled water from a grocery store and baking soda. Fill a plastic syringe cover (the case for a 20-cc syringe is just the right size) to the top with baking soda and dump that into the gallon of water.

Insert the sharp tip of the IV tube, which is designed to penetrate an IV bag, into the bottom of the plastic gallon jug of distilled water, which has been warmed to body temperature. Once you get a needle into the jugular vein of the calf, open the open/shut flow-regulating valve on the tube, and let the tube fill with water to get all the air out of the tube, then attach it to the needle that's inserted into the jugular vein. The size of the needle is what determines rate of flow; a 20-gauge needle in the vein will keep the flow at a safe speed. But for a calf with very low blood pressure — flat out, severely dehydrated and acidotic — you can run fluid into his vein fairly quickly without danger, using a larger-diameter needle.

Most calves get up after you give them a gallon of this fluid by IV. This doesn't mean they won't go down again if they are seriously scouring, but you can repeat the IV treatment (another gallon of distilled water and baking soda) if they get weak again. If they're still scouring after they get up after the IV treatment, you can use oral electrolyte fluid containing potassium to replace what they lost due to acidosis. If they can't get up, however, or don't look at all improved, their problem is more complex than simple scours (possibly septicemia), and you might not be able to save them; consult your veterinarian.

Other Medications for Scouring Calves

If the calf still has a functioning gut, include gut-soothing medications along with oral electrolyte fluids. Products such as kaolin/pectin or bismuth subsalicylate can protect and soothe the gut while helping to slow its contents. Add Kaopectate or Pepto-Bismol to each mix of electrolyte solution given orally. An oral antibiotic can be added to the mix once a day or as often as your vet recommends.

USING A SIMPLE IV

If a calf is weak and dehydrated, you can usually get him on his feet again with a simple IV, using a gallon of distilled water with baking soda added. Any medication that needs to be added to the IV can be put into the jug of distilled water. Gently but firmly hold the calf still as the warmed fluid runs into his jugular vein.

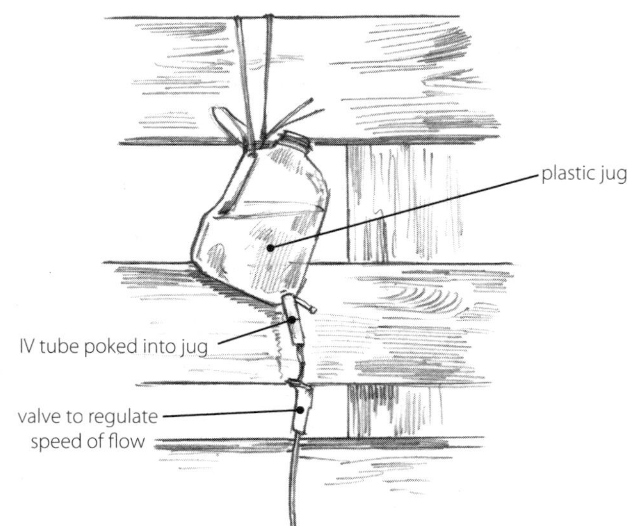

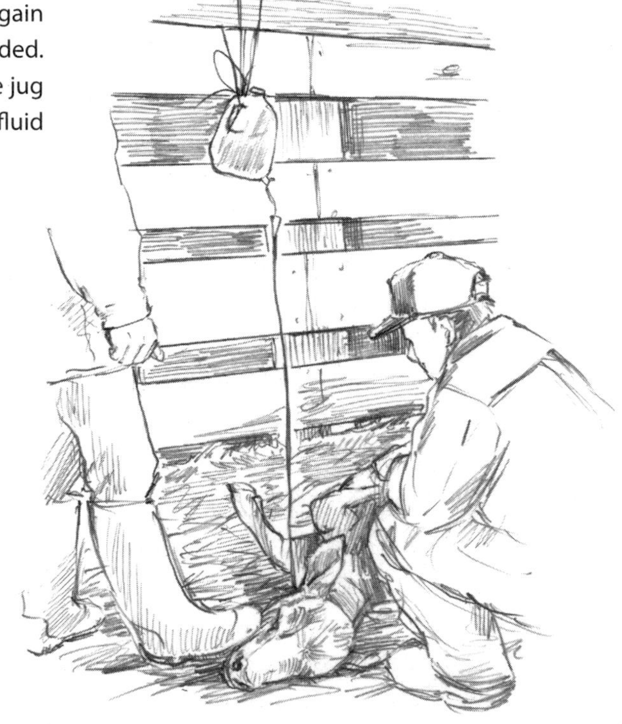

Antibiotics

If bacteria cause diarrhea, or if a viral infection is complicated by bacteria, an oral antibiotic is helpful. Antibiotics won't deter viruses but will help to control bacterial invaders. For instance, rotavirus, the mildest of viral scour infections, causes temporary diarrhea that may affect calves one to three days old. These calves respond well to antibiotic and fluid therapy because bacteria often complicate the viral infection. The antibiotic may quickly control secondary invaders, so the problem appears to be resolved by antibiotics, even though virus caused the initial infection. Coronavirus, in contrast, is more deadly, often affecting calves seven to ten days old, and does not respond to antibiotics. Fluid therapy is the most beneficial treatment. Your vet may be able to determine whether the calf is fighting viral or bacterial scours (or protozoal infection; see chapter 12) and prescribe an appropriate drug.

When Choosing Medication

Use the following list for tips when considering scours medications and the behaviors of the particular infection:

- Have your vet culture the bacteria and see which antibiotics work best against it, or find a drug that works through trial and error — and then stick with that drug.
- Certain drugs work well on one farm but not on another, or work for certain types of scours but not others.
- Products commonly used include neomycin sulfate, tetracyclines, sulfonamides, trimethoprim-sulfonamide mixtures (effective against several of the more common soil-borne pathogens), and ampicillin. Cephalosporin derivatives such as Baytril and Naxcel are also used.
- Neomycin liquid, a drug that is not absorbed into the body but rather stays in the gut where it does the most good, can be added to oral fluids and gets to the site of the problem more quickly than pills.
- When using an antibiotic for scours, give it just once a day, unless otherwise recommended by your vet, and don't use it for more than three

days in a row unless your vet recommends it, or you may eliminate the normal intestinal flora. Some of the newer antibiotics have longer-lasting action, and one dose lasts for several days.

- A few drugs work well in combination (such as trimethoprim and sulfa), but some counteract the effects of others, and some don't work for intestinal infections, so consult your vet.
- After any long-term antibiotic therapy, the calf may need probiotics to repopulate the normal intestinal bacteria essential for proper digestion and to keep opportunistic pathogens at bay. If normal gut flora is wiped out by antibiotics, there's a risk of pathogenic fungi or drug-resistant bacteria taking their place.
- Give the gut antibiotic as a liquid once a day, added to one of the three or four oral electrolyte feedings, rather than as pills or an injection. A liquid preparation gets to the site of the problem faster and is more effective than pills or an injection. Many scour medications come in pills or boluses, but studies have shown that they don't dissolve readily in a gut that's compromised by infection. Necropsies of calves that died of scours often reveal pills given several days earlier, still in the stomach and not fully dissolved.
- If your vet prescribes an antibiotic that comes only in pill form, crush the pills and dissolve them in a little water.
- If the infection is one that stays in the gut, use an oral antibiotic that targets the gut. But if a calf has fever, sore joints, or signs of any other problem besides diarrhea, he needs systemic antibiotics, too; the infection is not in the gut alone. A calf with septicemia as well as diarrhea needs injectable antibiotics, since most oral medications don't get beyond the gut efficiently. Your vet can prescribe a broad-spectrum product that won't hurt the kidneys, such as the cephalosporins Naxcel and Excenel.
- If a calf is dehydrated, don't use sulfa. When using any type of sulfa, you must maintain good hydration; a high concentration of sulfa in the bloodstream can crystalize in the kidneys and cause irreversible kidney damage, killing the calf.

Disadvantages of Bicarbonate

Most electrolyte products in North America contain bicarbonate or *acetate,* alkalizing agents to help reverse the symptoms of severe acidosis. When a calf is severely ill with scours, the body pH changes, becoming too acidic, which leads to organ damage and eventual organ failure, shock, coma, and death. The calf needs a product containing an alkalizing agent, such as sodium bicarbonate (baking soda). But bicarbonate has drawbacks. It interferes with the calf's milk digestion and curd formation. If a calf is drinking milk, this can aggravate diarrhea and interfere with his ability to absorb energy. Bicarbonate also alkalizes the abomasum, the fourth or true stomach, interfering with the calf's natural defenses against bacterial proliferation. A normal, healthy calf has a low stomach pH, which helps to inhibit growth of pathogenic bacteria such as *E. coli* and salmonella.

In Europe, it's common to use acetate as the alkalizing agent. Acetate works just as well and doesn't alkalize the abomasum. Unlike bicarbonate, acetate stimulates sodium and water absorption in the small intestine and produces energy when metabolized. A seriously ill calf that is unable to nurse can be given bicarbonate, but don't give it to a calf that's still nursing or at the same time that he's given milk or milk replacer. Wait two to three hours after a milk feeding before giving fluid or electrolytes containing bicarbonate. If you use a commercial electrolyte product, check ingredients. A few contain acetate; Calf-Lyte, produced in Canada, and Hydra-Lyte, from the United States, both contain acetate instead of bicarbonate.

Neomycin Sulfate Solution for Early Treatment

On our ranch, where scours in one- to three- week-old calves is caused by bacteria that respond to neomycin sulfate, we've cut down on the number of cases needing fluid and electrolyte therapy by treating every calf with neomycin at the first hint of sickness.

In earlier years, we added liquid oral antibiotic to the warm water and electrolytes that we gave each sick calf via stomach tube. Eventually we realized that some of the calves in very early stages of scours were not yet dehydrated and didn't need the fluid. We wondered if we might be able to halt the infection before they got dehydrated by giving the oral medication very soon after they got sick.

In 1988, we started putting the neomycin solution into small pumper bottles and just squirting it into the calves' mouths. I measured how many squirts for a dose (1 cc per 40 pounds [18 kg], or 2 to 3 cc for a young calf, equals seven squirts from the pumper bottle). I carry the bottle in my coat pocket when we feed cows morning and evening, and we catch and treat any calf in early stages of scours. This halts the infection before it damages the gut and causes dehydration, and we rarely have to give fluids. In a typical calving season, we might treat one-third of the calves with neomycin for early scours but have to give fluid and electrolytes to only two or three. For instance, in 1993 (a bad year, when some of our neighbors lost 30 to 50 percent of their calves to scours), we treated 63 calves in our herd of 170 with neomycin, gave follow-up treatment with fluid and electrolytes to three calves, and did not lose any.

We used to buy several gallons of Kaopectate products a year, but now a gallon lasts several years. The key is early detection and treatment. With effective treatment we save more calves and spend less money on medications, reducing the number of cases that must be treated intensively or hauled to a vet. The extra time taken to check young calves often and treat any in the early stages of illness saves time and effort later, when they would otherwise be weak and dehydrated or in shock.

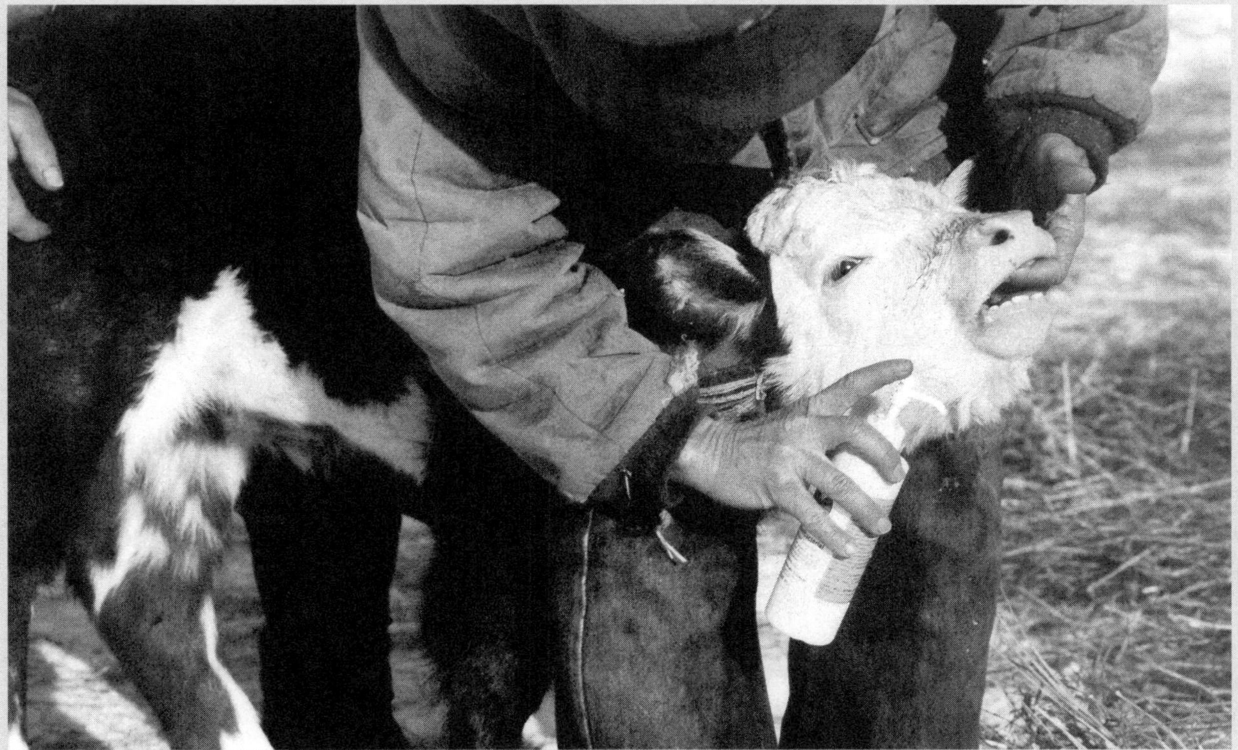

Early treatment with neomycin sulfate solution at the first hint of bacterial scours will usually halt the infection. If you squirt neomycin sulfate solution from a pumper bottle into the back of the calf's mouth, make sure that he swallows it.

Tips on Catching Calves for Treatment

Sometimes a calf is so ill by the time you discover his problem that he's not hard to catch for treatment; however, it's best to find him much sooner, while he's still strong and a challenge to catch. Some stockmen feel that if a calf is hard to catch, he isn't sick enough to treat. But from my perspective, if he's easy to catch, you are a little late.

> **CHECK THAT TEMP**
>
> Some veterinarians recommend carrying and using your animal thermometer when checking calves, since signs of diarrhea may be a day behind a rise in temperature. A calf's normal temperature is 101 to 102°F (38.3 to 38.8°C), so any reading over 102.5°F (39.2°C) justifies on-the-spot treatment with antibiotic. If a calf is not nursing, check him.

Watch Out for Mama

It can be challenging to catch a calf that's not very sick and to deal with protective mamas. You want cows to be good mothers, but some are aggressive when their calves are young and dangerous to anyone handling the calves. In our herd we deal with both cows and calves at calving time — to iodine navels, tag ears, put rubber bands on the little bulls' testicles, and move cows into and out of the barn. Our cows must be manageable. We respect a protective mother, but we also demand that she respect us. Any cow that can't be safely handled is sold. A cow that is smart enough to respect us if we have a stick, not charging over us if we are working with her calf, can stay in the herd.

Lynn and I work as a team handling newborns or catching sick calves to treat. Most cows are not as aggressive if there are two people, because they're outnumbered and because they sense that we are confident. If you're not afraid of a cow, she knows. But if you are afraid, she senses it and quickly takes

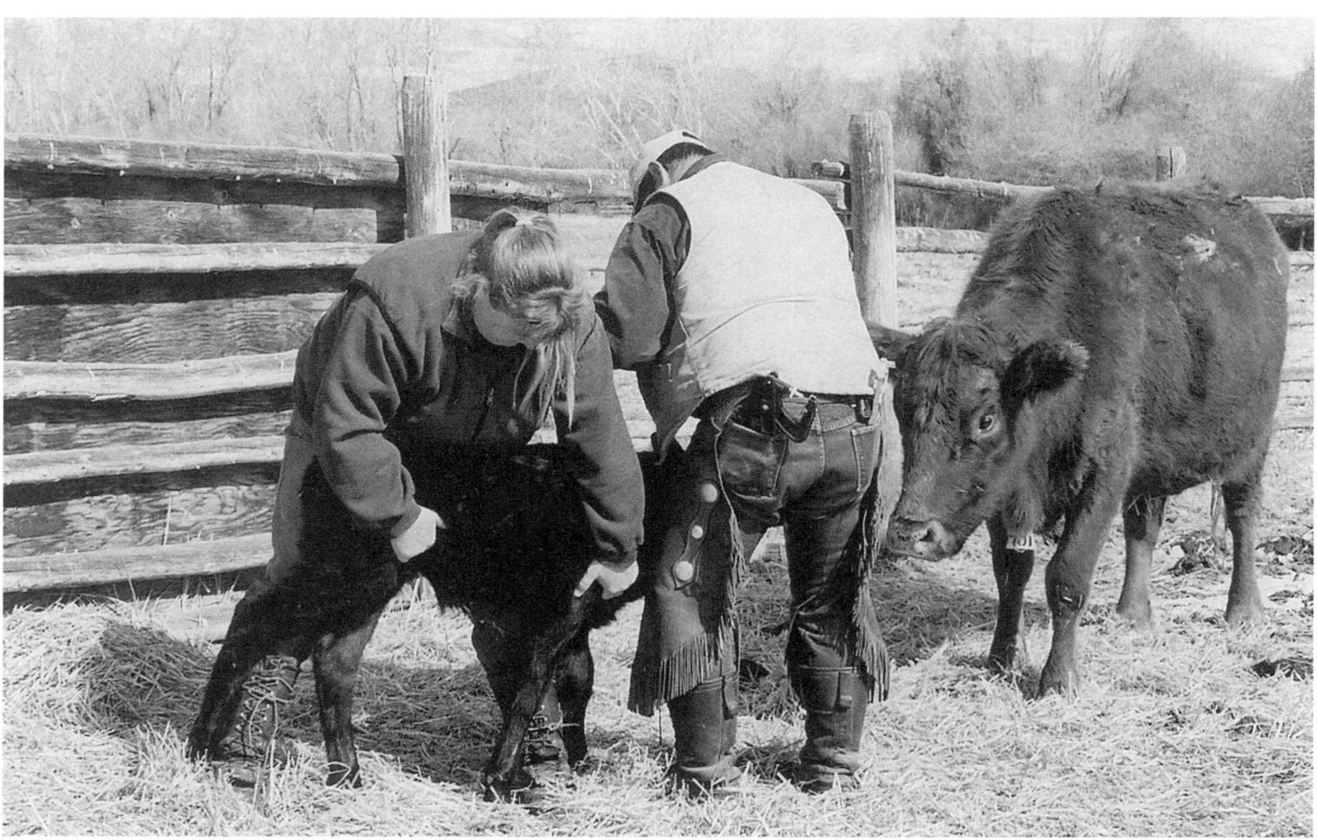

When you are treating a calf, the cow may be worried about him and may try to protect him, but she needs to know that she must respect you.

advantage of you. Never take your eyes off of an aggressive cow. When handling cattle, you must act like the dominant "herd boss." It's easier to be confident, however, if you have someone with you to hold the calf and stare down the cow while you treat the calf quickly and properly.

The person keeping the cow away should have a weapon. Cows are smart enough to know when you are defenseless, and they know when you are prepared to hold your ground with a stick for whacking them across the nose. There've been instances in which Lynn and I were treating calves out in a pasture and were saved from being trampled only by quick action — like the time he quickly pulled off his belt and whacked the charging cow in the face with the belt buckle, or when the only thing we had for a weapon was the ear-tagging tool in my coat pocket, a 5-inch-long (12.7 cm) small metal tube with a sharp point on the end, which I poked into the cow's nose as she started butting me.

When handling cattle, you must act like the dominant "herd boss." It's easier to be confident if you have someone with you to hold the calf and stare down the cow.

Most cows will halt if you have a weapon they respect, just as they would halt and not threaten a dominant cow. The tender nose is a good target. Hitting the bridge of the nose or face works best if you have a stout stick. Don't hit a cow on top of the head, which could seriously injure or kill her. Don't flail wildly with a whip, or you may injure an eye. If you have no weapon and she's butting you, she'll usually back off if you grab an ear and twist it hard, or poke her eye with your finger, but we don't like the cow to get that close. If we must catch a calf that has a mean mama, we have a stout stick. You want something that's easy to carry and hold while doctoring a calf, that you can use at close range, and that's sturdy enough to give a good rap across the cow's face without breaking.

The most important rule to remember when working with cows and babies is "no dogs." The presence of a dog in the background or in your pickup (even if he doesn't bark) can upset a cow enough to put her on the fight, even before you get anywhere near her calf.

Little Things Count

Make sure that a sick calf has access to water and salt if he's up and around. If given an opportunity, a calf with diarrhea will drink water to replenish fluids. If you isolate a cow and her sick calf in a doctoring pen, make sure that the water source is within reach of the calf. He'll often sip water even when he doesn't feel well enough to nurse his mother.

If the calves are out in a field or pasture, remember that they need water as well as milk from Mama, especially as they get older and when the weather is warm. Provide a tub of clean, fresh water in the calf creep or calf house yard or make sure troughs are low enough for calves to reach the water. They will drink from puddles otherwise and pick up more pathogens.

A scouring calf will also eat salt to help replace what's lost through diarrhea. If the salt for cows is in a mineral mix, provide an additional source that's just plain salt so that calves can help themselves to it when they crave without overloading on other minerals. You can also mix one-third potassium chloride with two-thirds regular loose salt, and put it into tubs for calves in their calf-house area. This makes a self-feeding electrolyte mix that they eat readily if they need it. Potassium chloride should never constitute more than one-third of the salt mix, though, or it will be bitter and calves won't eat it.

Getting Your Hands on Baby

If a calf is dull, you can sneak up behind him and grab him before he gets away. If he's lying down, grab or tackle him around the neck, from behind, so that he won't see you coming. If he's standing, grab a hind leg. If he sees you, he'll run off. We do a two-person sneak to catch a lively calf before he realizes what's happening (see photos on next page). This usually works for a calf that's not been caught before. After that, he'll be suspicious, and you'll have a harder time catching him a second time.

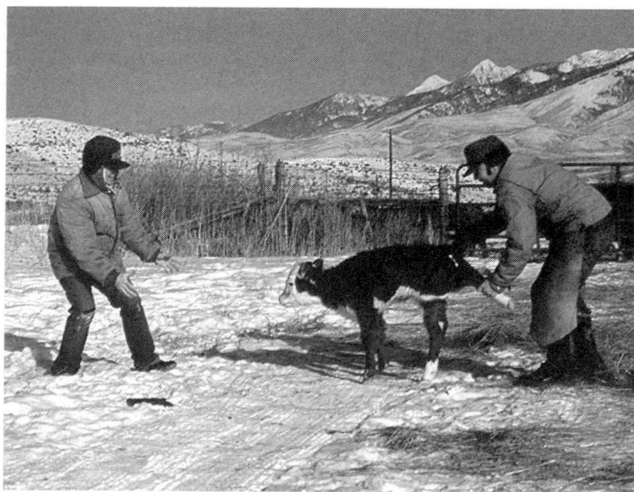

I distract the calf while Lynn sneaks up behind and grabs a hind leg.

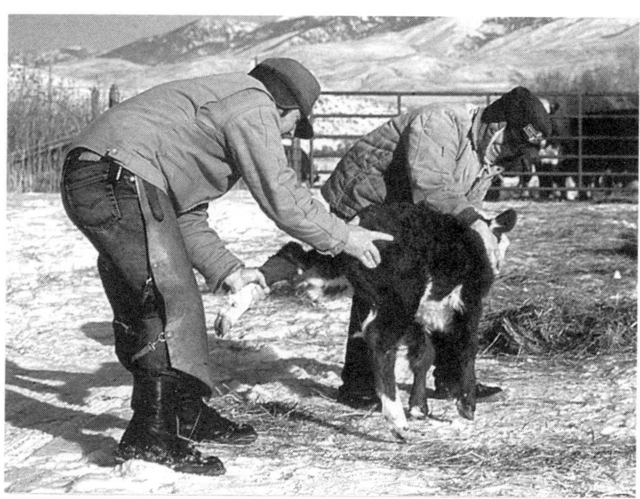

After Lynn grabs a hind leg, I grab the calf's head.

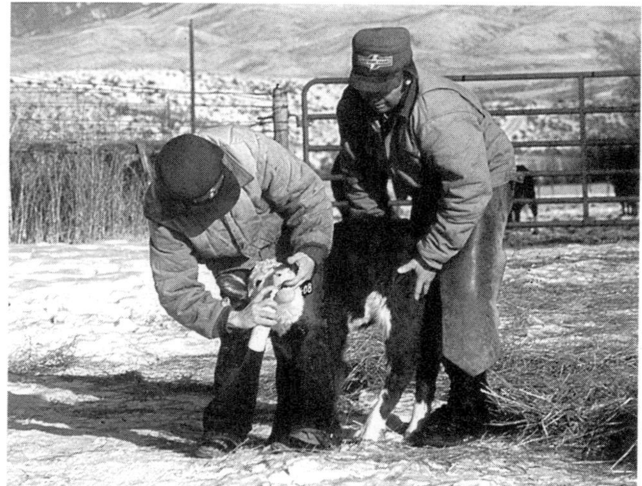

With Lynn holding the back end of the calf, I straddle the calf's neck to hold his head steady and squirt the medication into the back of his mouth.

The Song-and-Dance Trap

To catch a calf that needs treatment, one of us walks in front of him at a nonthreatening distance. That person distracts the calf to keep his attention — sings or makes funny noises and movements, not as much to startle him as to arouse his curiosity. This might mean hopping or waving your arms while the other person sneaks up quietly behind the entranced calf in his blind spot as he's looking forward at the "entertainer," and grabs a hind leg. The front person then comes swiftly to grab the head, and the calf is caught. One of us gets a good hold on him, and the other treats the calf. You can often be finished before Mama knows about it if the cows are busy eating hay. But if the calf bellows when you grab him and all the mamas come running, be prepared to fend them off.

By Crook

If a calf is too big to catch or suspicious because he was caught before, we take the pair to a smaller pen where we can corner the calf. If a calf is far from a corral and you don't want to bring him and Mama home when all he needs is one treatment, there are ways to capture him even if he won't let you sneak up to him. One method is a *sheep hook* or shepherd's crook (see next page). We put a longer handle on it so we can snag a calf's hind leg without having to get too close. A calf is less wary at a certain distance. Unless he is wild or you've caught him before, this distance is short enough to get within range with a long-handled hook before he is alarmed.

A small calf that's too wild or suspicious to grab by hand can usually be caught with the hook.

The two-person decoy distraction works, allowing the calf-snagger a chance to get into position to catch a hind leg with the hook. A small calf that's too wild or suspicious to grab by hand can usually be caught with the hook. It takes strength to hang onto a big calf with the hook, and some may kick out of it. There are catching hooks made for calves that include a leg-locking mechanism that makes kicking free impossible.

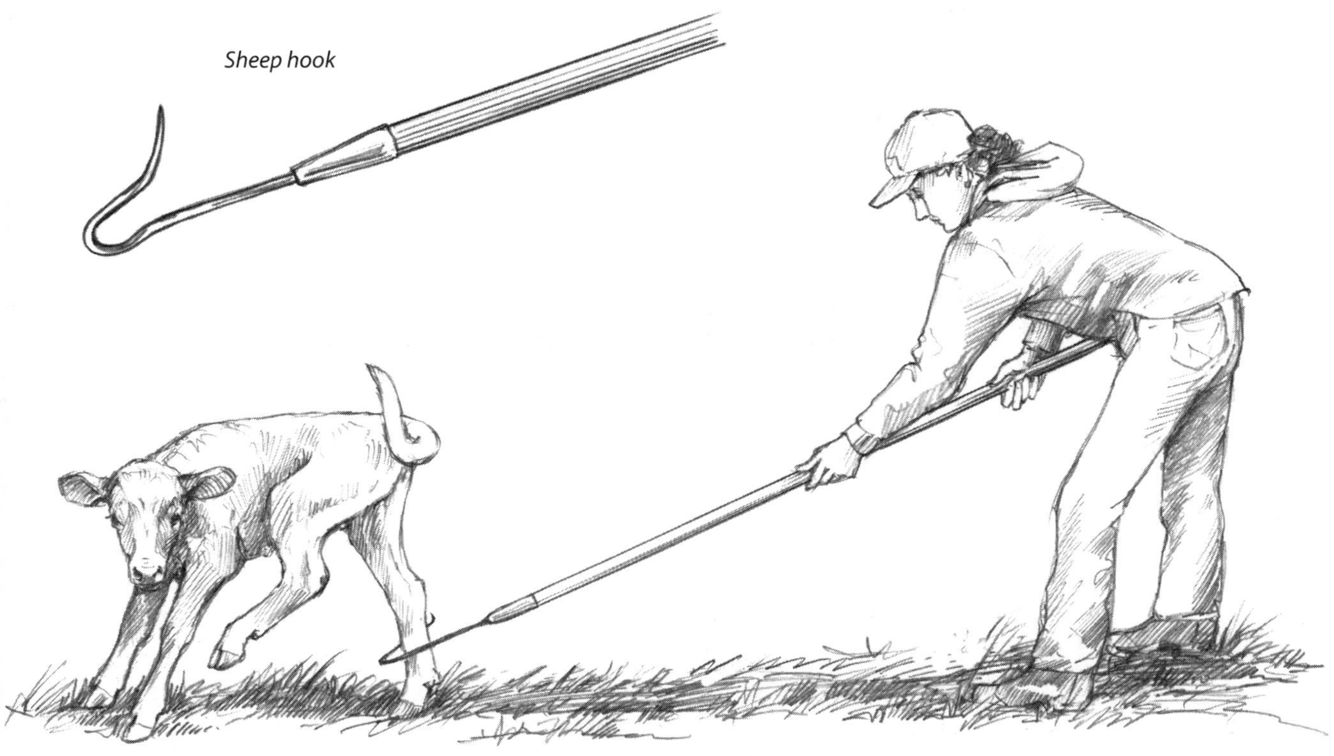

Use the sheep hook to grab a calf's hind leg.

Chute Catch

Another way to catch an elusive calf is to make an instant chute, easing him behind a solid gate if there's one available, and catching him in the narrow *V* made by the gate and the fence. If there is no sturdy gate handy, we herd the calf between a fence and the feed truck, after parking the truck against the fence at an angle, and then walk the calf along the fence and into this trap. A net wire fence or pole fence makes the best trap. A calf can shimmy through barbed wire unless it is very tight and has a lot of stays between the posts, holding the wires in place.

The trap trick works best when you are feeding hay, stringing hay close to the fence so that all the cows and calves are close by. A calf won't get as suspicious and wild if he's with the herd, close to other cattle. Gently ease him through the herd along the fence, and, if you are patient and tricky, he'll be in the trap made by the fence and the pickup before he knows it. A sneaky catch by a hind leg or herding him into a trap to grab him is easier on him (and you) than chasing him around.

Once you've treated him, assess his condition and decide if one treatment will be adequate. If there's any question, bring him and Mama to a pen so that you can get hold of him more easily for continuing treatment. Many calves relapse because they weren't given the correct number of doses at first. After you've had a lot of experience, you'll have a better idea about whether a one-time treatment early in the course of the illness will be enough, or if you should bring the pair to a pen for multiple treatments.

LEAVE YOUR ROPE AT HOME

Someone who ropes a lot can catch a calf with a lariat, but don't try this unless you are good at it. You must catch the calf on the first try. If you miss, you alarm him and ruin your chances of sneaking up on him; he won't let you get that close again. Avoid stress when working with sick calves; running one around trying to rope him is very detrimental.

Protozoal Infections

SOME TYPES OF INTESTINAL INFECTION and diarrhea are caused by one-celled animals called *protozoa*. The two most common types of protozoal infection in calves are *cryptosporidiosis* and *coccidiosis*. Both can be debilitating and sometimes fatal.

Coccidiosis

All cattle are infected by *coccidia* protozoa, one-celled parasites that live in the intestine. There are many kinds of coccidia; at least 13 species live in cattle. Only two of these are pathogenic. Calves tend to develop immunity to these after being infected, but immunity against one type of pathogenic coccidia does not protect against the other, so a calf could suffer more than one bout of coccidiosis while growing up. There is no vaccine; the only way a calf gains immunity is by being infected.

Since a few coccidia are passed in feces of healthy animals, these pathogens are almost always present in a calf's environment. By the time calves are six months old, they have all been exposed, though only 2 to 5 percent of them show symptoms of infection.

Adult cattle have developed immunity and rarely become ill with coccidiosis unless they are stressed enough to have a hindered immune system. Though they don't usually become ill themselves, they continue to pass a few of the parasitic eggs *(oocysts)* in their manure, thus serving as a continual source of infection for calves. Young animals have not yet gained enough immunity to withstand the parasite and may become ill with diarrhea if environmental conditions are right. The best defense against coccidiosis is good management, preventing buildup of contamination to infective levels.

Life Cycle of the Bug

In the gut, an oocyst hatches into eight sporozoites. Each sporozoite invades a cell in the intestinal lining, destroying that cell as the sporozoite forms a packet of new oocysts, which ruptures and releases more than 100,000 new oocysts. Theoretically, each oocyst can eventually develop into 28 million new organisms, and the disease can quickly become an epidemic among confined calves. Ingestion of about 125 sporulated oocysts can cause destruction of more than 12 billion intestinal cells, interfering with digestion and absorption of food nutrients and causing bloody diarrhea. The incubation period from the time the calf ingests oocysts until he breaks with diarrhea is 16 days or longer. At first the coccidia stay in the small intestine, and the calf looks normal. On about day 16, parasites move into the large intestine and produce male and female cells to create and fertilize more oocysts. When these new eggs develop and mature, they rupture through the intestinal cell lining. By day 18 or 19 the calf has diarrhea, and there may be blood in the runny feces. By day 21 there will be oocysts in the manure.

The Disease

Coccidiosis causes diarrhea, weight loss, and lowered resistance to other diseases. It can be serious in baby calves who have not yet developed immunity. The intestinal lining, damaged by the multiplying coccidia, is much more susceptible to bacterial and viral infections. There is often more than one pathogen involved, such as bacteria or viruses, when baby calves have coccidiosis, making illness and diarrhea much worse. Even mild cases can have an adverse affect on calves, however. Calves showing no symptoms can still have their growth rates affected.

Coccidiosis can cause blood in the feces, anemia, and emaciation. This disease occurs wherever there are cattle, but often without symptoms if cattle are healthy and not congregated. Illness may occur only when cattle are confined in small areas, allowing oocysts passed in manure to build up to infective levels. These parasites usually cause trouble only when animals are stressed or ingesting overwhelming numbers of protozoa.

Stress — bad weather, drought, weaning, disease — can inhibit the immune response, and the parasites can then overcome the calf's resistance. Stress weakens the calf's immune system and enables the protozoa to divide more rapidly and move through more life cycles before the calf can start building immunity. This causes greater damage to the intestinal lining.

In an outbreak, most calves in a group become infected, but usually only a few show signs of disease. In a serious outbreak, however, up to 80 percent of calves may develop visible illness. Among those that show symptoms, mortality rate can be as high as 10 to 15 percent unless they are treated in early stages. In calves that don't show symptoms, *subclinical* (not obvious) infection may reduce weight gains until the intestines heal.

Mortality rates can be high in calves that haven't had a great deal of previous exposure when they are suddenly introduced to a high level of infection. This can happen when wet, warm weather "brings to life" oocysts in old manure around feeding or watering areas where cattle congregate, or when calves are gathered into corrals where there's lots of manure. Many outbreaks of coccidiosis occur during the first 30 days in a weaning pen, especially in spring or fall, if wet conditions stimulate development of oocysts that were shed in manure. Oocysts can survive in old manure for more than a year.

Oocysts enter a susceptible calf through contaminated feed or by a calf lying in manure and then licking his hair coat. Once swallowed, the parasites develop and multiply rapidly in intestinal tissues, destroying the lining and releasing millions of oocysts that then pass out of the body with manure to further contaminate soil, feed, and water; thus, the cycle begins again.

Since coccidia are common in a calf's environment, most calves are thoroughly exposed in the first year of life. Protozoa build up wherever cattle are crowded (corrals, calving areas, intensive pasture-rotation systems). It is impossible to eliminate them from the soil; disinfectant won't kill them. Oocysts survive on the ground for months or years; all they need are heat, moisture, and oxygen to become infective.

A *spore* is the reproductive element of fungi, protozoa, and algae. Oocysts sporulate (liberate spores as part of the multiplication process) in moderate

Subclinical Cases

When an animal has a subclinical illness, the animal has an infection, but it is so mild that no symptoms are obvious. When an animal has a clinical case of illness, there are signs of the illness. Subclinical cases can still be a cause of disease transmission and future outbreaks, however, since even these seemingly healthy animals can spread the infection.

In a group of calves exposed to coccidiosis, almost all are affected to some degree, but not all show signs of illness. Most of these cases have a brief illness. The digestive tract is upset, interfering with food absorption for two to three weeks. By then the calf builds immunity and can protect himself from further infection, but he still harbors coccidia in the intestine, shedding a few oocysts in his manure for the rest of his life. This is why most adult cattle continually shed a few oocysts, and even though they don't get sick, they contaminate the environment if kept in a small area where manure builds up.

temperatures; 53 to 90°F (11.6 to 32.2°C) is ideal. High temperatures and dryness impede *sporulation*. Oocysts can survive freezing (down to 18°F [–7.7°C]) for a couple of months, but temperatures lower than minus 22°F (–30°C) usually kill them. They sporulate in winter on hair coats of cattle dirty with manure, even if it is too cold for sporulation on the ground. When cattle lick themselves or each other, they ingest parasites.

Coccidiosis often shows up in calves during times of stress — at weaning, when young calves are grouped with their mothers in small feeding areas, after prolonged weather stress, or during weather changes. Infection is common when cattle are fed hay on the fecally contaminated ground, and, if the same feeding ground is used repeatedly, infection rates rise drastically. If cattle are fed in bale feeders and cows stand in the same areas to eat, they get mud and manure on their udders, and calves get a heavy load of oocysts when they nurse. Outbreaks occur in calves on pasture when cattle gather at water sources, feeding areas, mineral boxes, etc. The source of contamination is always the manure of infected cattle or carrier animals.

Large numbers of sporulated oocysts must be ingested before signs of coccidiosis occur. This can happen with continual reinfection and contamination buildup whenever cattle are crowded. Some farms have coccidiosis in young calves, especially if cattle are in the same fields, pastures, or pens during calving each year, and especially during wet weather. Other farms struggle with the problem in older calves, at weaning during a wet fall, or when overwintering replacement heifers (calves kept to replace culled or old cows sold) are being fed.

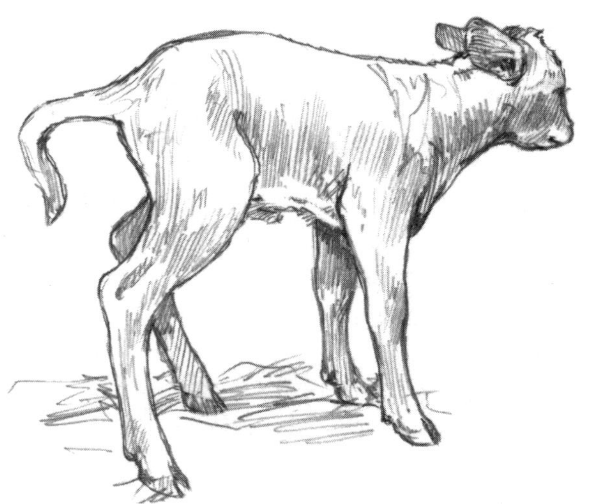

A common sign of coccidiosis is frequent straining, due to the irritated intestine and rectum, as the calf tries to pass feces.

Duration of Illness

If he's not reinfected and there is only one cycle of multiplying oocytes, the disease is self-limiting; it runs its course. But if the calf is still in a contaminated environment, he can be reinfected. There will be parasites within that calf at various life-cycle stages until the immune system builds some resistance. If a calf is sick for a long time, this may mean that he has concurrent infection with bacteria or viruses, or that he may simply have extensive gut damage that takes a long time to heal.

Symptoms

Rupture of cells in the intestinal lining during the protozoa's swift multiplication results in diarrhea, although a calf may be sick for a while before you realize it. The following are symptoms and signs of coccidiosis:

- Fever in the early stages
- Sudden onset of severe diarrhea, with foul-smelling watery feces, often brown in color, containing blood or mucus
- Rear end, hind legs, and tail covered with loose feces
- Calf straining continually to pass feces with or without passing any
- Rectal prolapse in severe cases, due to all the straining
- Calf going off feed or not nursing
- Anemia, if the calf has lost much blood; pale mucous membranes; weakness and staggering
- Occasionally, brain damage in acute coccidiosis, resulting in muscle tremors, lack of coordination, convulsions, collapse, or coma

After coccidia stop multiplying and the calf's intestinal lining heals, bowel movements firm up again, but this may take a while if the calf is constantly reinfected by contaminated fecal material. Even though damage to the gut is already done by the time you see diarrhea, it's still worth treating the calf. In most cases the disease is ongoing: All coccidia in the gut are not developed and multiplying at the same time. You can't halt damage that is already in progress, but treatment may kill coccidia more recently ingested and in earlier life stages. Although the calf has probably started to develop immunity, you should still treat him because of the risk for *secondary infection* — potentially serious because of his lowered resistance — and also to limit further contamination of the environment.

Mild Cases of Coccidiosis

A calf may have brown diarrhea and slow growth for a while but no blood in the feces if the illness is mild. Some have persistent diarrhea but are never very sick; these calves continue to nurse their mothers and don't go off feed but have loose feces off and on for a long time. Diarrhea may persist for as long as it takes the intestine to heal. The calf is unable to absorb normal amounts of fluids and nutrients and loses weight or fails to grow. His hair coat becomes rough, and he may be dull, with no energy. Without good care and supportive treatment, he may become susceptible to other types of scours or pneumonia.

Treating a Prolapsed Rectum

If a calf prolapses, the rectum should be gently washed with warm water and mild disinfectant, well rinsed, and pushed back in. The opening should be stitched, or his continual straining will push it right back out. Two or three stitches of *umbilical tape* (a wide, soft cotton "string") anchored in the thick skin around the rectal opening will be adequate. Stitches can be removed after the calf recovers.

DON'T LET THEM STOP EATING

We've had several severe cases of coccidiosis in which calves needed supportive treatment — shelter, fluids, gut soothers, milk when they didn't nurse their mothers enough — just to keep them going. This made a big difference in their recovery.

Preventive Management and Treatment

Young calves are very susceptible to coccidiosis because they have no immunity. Cows don't pass much immunity to their calves via colostrum because they don't create many antibodies against protozoal infections. There is no vaccine against this disease, so the best way to prevent it in baby calves is to limit exposure to high numbers of oocysts.

Assess your situation, and strategize ways to minimize buildup of manure in calving areas or pastures. A farm or ranch with no winter grazing areas, where hay is fed from December through March or later, has ideal conditions for coccidiosis to infect baby calves if cattle are grouped in feeding areas or congregate around bale feeders or big round bales.

If you use only a few acres as a hay-feeding area in winter or have to reuse the same feeding spots for round bales or to accommodate a feed truck without getting stuck in the mud, those places become as dirty as a corral. The cows are continually passing a few oocysts, which may stay dormant in manure if the weather is cold. When it warms up and the oocysts become infective, the baby calves, who lie on manure and then lick themselves, or nurse dirty udders, are exposed to high levels of infection.

A fall-calving herd can get caught by coccidiosis if you start feeding hay early when pastures run short or snow covers grass. If weather is mild, or warm days enable oocysts to sporulate, they have suitable conditions to cause infection: Calves develop coccidiosis in moist warm weather. Calves over three weeks old are susceptible because they are eating hay by then and may eat contaminated feed.

If coccidiosis shows up in a group of baby calves, isolate sick calves and their mothers, and treat the calves so they won't keep shedding oocysts into the environment. Treatment includes medications to

Tips for Reducing Exposure in Young Calves

All management practices should focus on cleanliness and avoidance of stress and overcrowding. Use the following as a checklist to minimize coccidiosis.

- Don't feed hay on the ground unless you can spread it in a clean area.
- Change feeding areas and move bale feeders often to new locations where cattle have not been fed before.
- Calf shelters should be kept clean and moved if calves get diarrhea.
- Keep group size small.
- Group calves according to age. New calves and mamas should be separate from older calves that may be shedding millions of oocysts.
- If coccidiosis appears, isolate sick calves so that they won't spread oocysts.
- Pens or feeding areas where cattle are congregated should be kept clean and dry, with new bedding put out periodically and old bedding hauled off, so oocysts won't have time to sporulate and become infective, and dirty bedding won't soil hair coats or cows' udders.
- Have cattle spread out on good pasture or keep changing feeding areas, so cattle are scattering the oocysts passed in manure over a larger area. Calves then encounter the parasite and begin to build immunity but don't ingest enough oocysts to develop disease.
- If early-spring calving areas and pastures are quite contaminated from winter hay feeding, consider fall calving as long as weather and feed conditions stay favorable and cattle aren't grouped.

halt development of protozoa, fluids, electrolytes, and gut soothers to ease the diarrhea and its effects on the body. Move the other calf-and-cow pairs to a new, clean pasture or feed in a different area. If you can't move the herd to clean ground in wet weather, or they must stay in a pen or small pasture, protect calves with medicated feed.

Using Coccidia-Inhibiting Drugs

When calves are grouped and confined, keep group size small, and use medicated feed or water to inhibit coccidia. A group of weaned calves can be treated with medicated water, but while calves are small and still nursing their mothers, a medicated creep feed works best. Deccox can be added to salt or water, but young calves don't always use salt, and when they are nursing they may not drink much water, especially in cool weather. Adding Deccox or some other product to a calf creep feed (a grain mix fed to the calves in an enclosure or "creep" where calves can get in but cows can't) by the time they're three weeks old can keep calves from getting sick. If healthy calves start to eat 3 to 4 ounces (88.7 to 118.3 mL) of the feed daily at that age, they'll get a full dose of the medicine, and that will prevent coccidiosis until you can get them spread out and away from contamination. Sick calves won't eat well and won't consume enough of the drug to hinder coccidia.

Deccox (decoquinate) is the best drug for baby calves. When calves are older (weaning age), you can keep coccidia in check with ionophores (monensin, lasolocid), which have a mild coccidiostatic effect; that is, they inhibit multiplication of coccidia. These drugs can keep healthy calves from getting sick if the environment is not too contaminated. But for stressed calves or young calves, Deccox or amprolium are safer; monensin can have toxic effects on baby calves if they overeat it.

Feeding calves Deccox when they must be confined can prevent outbreaks of coccidiosis and debilitating diarrhea. The cows may be passing a small number of oocysts, but if a young animal gets diarrhea it spreads thousands. In outbreaks of coccidiosis in confined calves, all calves in a group should be treated with a coccidia-inhibiting drug even if they're not all sick. It is always better to try to prevent coccidiosis than to have to treat it when you have an epidemic to deal with.

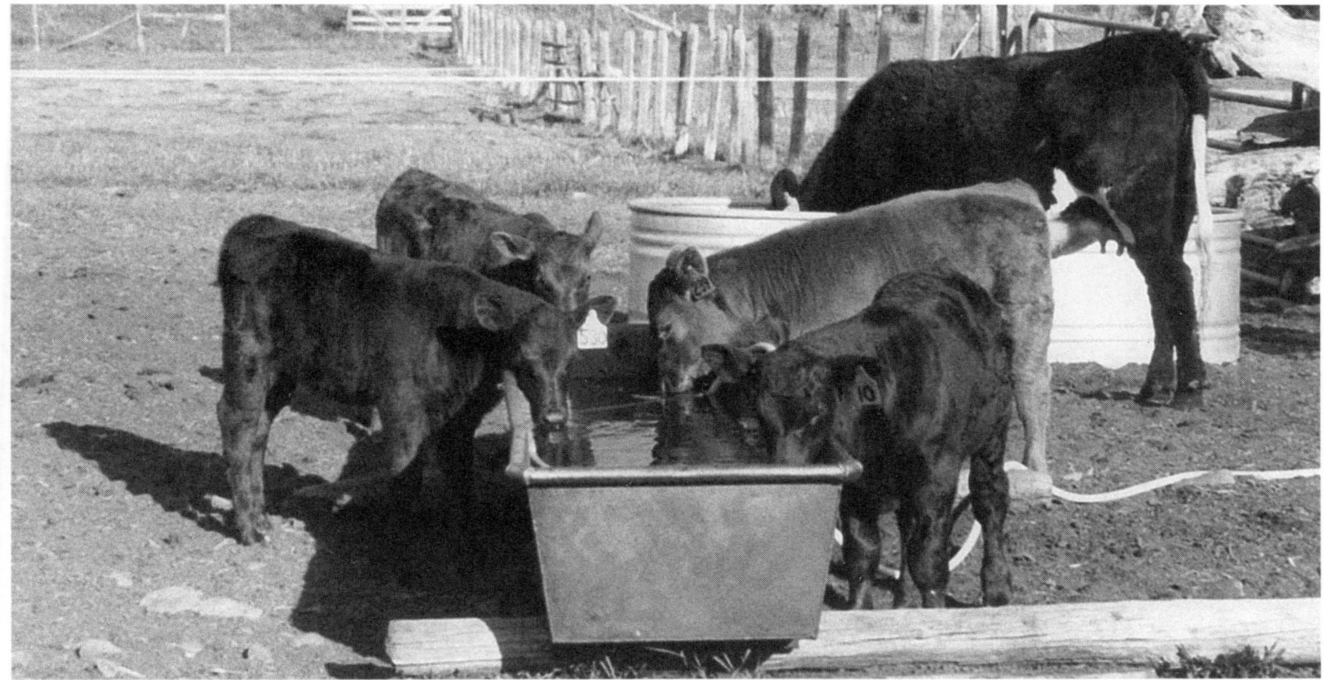

If calves have access to clean water, and don't have to drink out of puddles that may be contaminated with feces, they are less likely to pick up coccidia.

Treatment Once Calves Are Ill

Several drugs are effective against coccidiosis if given early before signs appear; they're less effective after a calf is sick. At that point additional supportive treatment (such as administering fluid and gut soothers) may be needed to save him.

To treat a sick calf, use amprolium (Corid) or a sulfa. Your vet may recommend something else as well, depending on the situation and how sick the calf is, especially with possibilities of a secondary infection. Always consult your vet.

If a calf is very sick and has lost a lot of blood due to diarrhea, he may become *anemic* (short on red blood cells) and very weak. Injections of vitamin B may help him to build more red blood cells quickly. Fluid by stomach tube, esophageal feeder, or IV feedings are needed to prevent dehydration and death (see chapter 11). Most calves go off feed for a while or eat poorly, so oral supportive fluids should include nutrients (milk or milk replacer) until he nurses his mother regularly again.

When a calf is constantly straining with diarrhea, rectal prolapse (the pushing out of the rectum) can occur. It may be necessary to apply anesthetic ointment to the rectal tissues to reduce pain and straining or to take stitches across the anal opening to allow for the passage of feces but prevent rectal prolapse (see page 257).

Acute coccidiosis may affect the brain; calves develop nervous signs (muscle tremors, lack of coordination, convulsions), or they collapse and can't get up. These calves have a high mortality rate in spite of good treatment. Affected calves may die within 24 hours after onset of bloody diarrhea and nervous signs, or they may linger for several days in a coma.

A Difficult Diagnosis

Proper diagnosis isn't always easy. Mild cases go undetected, since the calf does not seem sick and may not have blood in the feces. Some stockmen don't think coccidiosis can occur during good weather, but if calves have access to a lot of manure, they can get coccidiosis at any time. If you suspect coccidiosis, a vet can check fecal material under a microscope to look for oocysts, but it won't be a conclusive finding. A calf may shed a few oocysts in feces, since many calves encounter coccidia at a few weeks old, but the infection-causing diarrhea may be due to something else. On top of that, oocysts may not show up in a fecal sample if you're checking feces

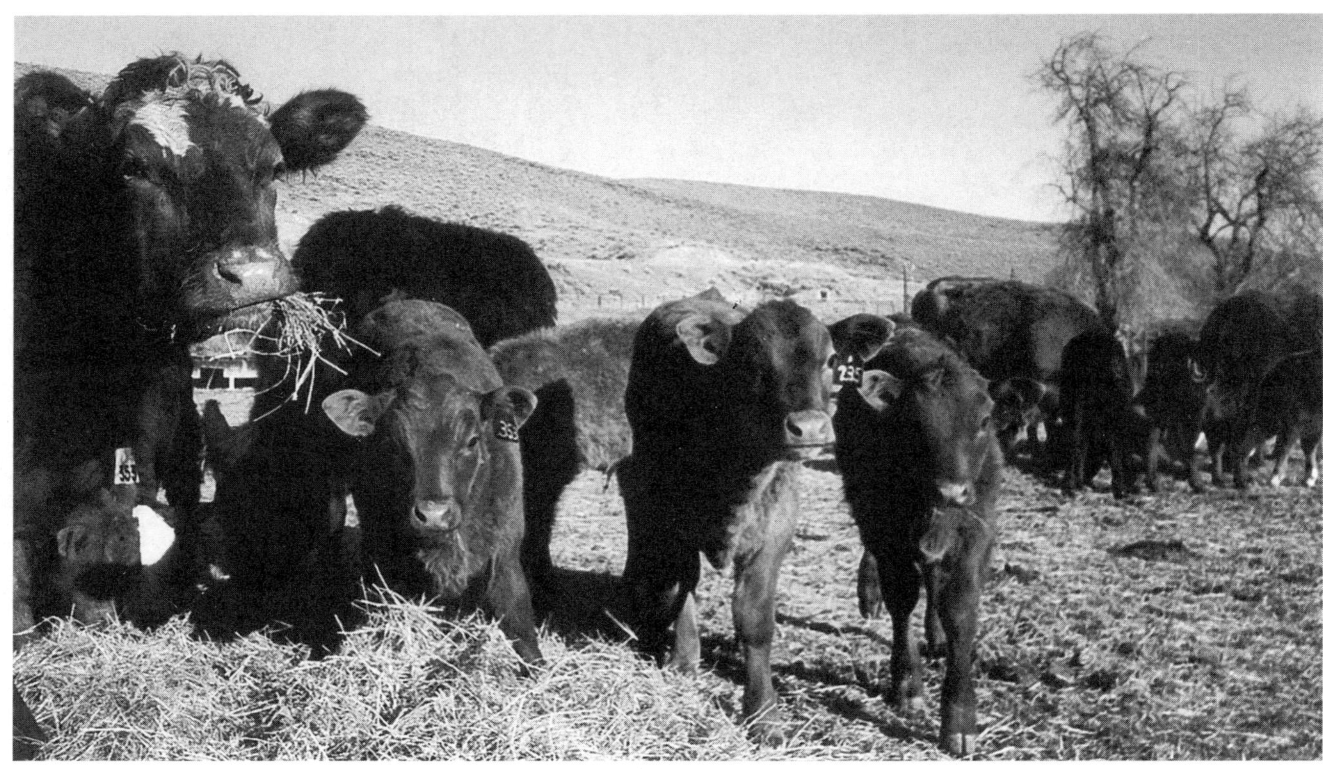

If cows are fed on the ground, using the same feed ground repeatedly (with fecal contamination of hay), there is much more risk for coccidiosis in baby calves.

Misunderstandings about Treatment

Since symptoms subside when the multiplication stage of protozoa is past, many treatments are credited with "curing" the diarrhea. The stockman gives the sick calf repeated doses of antibiotic or a drug to inhibit the protozoa and eventually the feces firm up again, giving the impression that the treatment worked. In many of these instances, however, the disease had run its course and the calf would have recovered anyway. Drugs commonly used for treatment have little effect on the late stages of coccidia, when damage to the intestine is already done and will take time to heal. Medication can help a calf that is being continually reinfected, however. The drugs will inhibit newly ingested coccidia and shorten the course of what would otherwise be a long illness. Most coccidiostatic drugs have a depressing effect on the early stages of the protozoa and can keep them from multiplying.

before the sick calf starts shedding oocysts. You may need to check again in a few days.

A fecal sample should be analyzed in light of a calf's history and symptoms. A single sample is not always an accurate diagnostic tool, especially just one sample from one calf in a group. Checking feces of several calves might give your vet a better idea as to whether coccidiosis is passing through the group. A fecal sample showing coccidia can also be confusing because they might be the nonpathogenic kind, which means the calf does not have coccidiosis.

Another drawback to relying on a fecal sample for diagnosis is that there's often more than one pathogen involved in diarrhea. A calf can have cryptosporidiosis (see page 260), which is even harder to diagnose with fecal samples, and also can be passing a few coccidia, leading to the misdiagnosis of coccidiosis. Treatment you'd give for coccidiosis won't help a calf with crypto, except for supportive care you might be giving, such as fluids. Crypto, more frequently seen in young calves, can affect baby calves as early as one week old, whereas coccidiosis can affect a calf at any age after three weeks.

Cryptosporidiosis Diarrhea in Calves

A protozoan that multiplies in the intestine, creating diarrhea in young calves, causes this disease. Earlier, it was a problem only in dairy cattle and was estimated to affect 70 percent of dairy calves one to three weeks of age, with a 100 percent infection rate on some farms. Now it is seen in beef herds as well. *Cryptosporidiosis* can also affect humans and other animals. Though the disease is often mild and self-limiting (the sick animal or person recovers without treatment), it can be life-threatening in any human or young animal with a compromised immune system.

Cryptosporidiosis can be deadly if young calves are challenged by the protozoan and several other pathogens at once, such as bacterial or viral scours. In many instances, calves with severe and hard-to-treat diarrhea have mixed infections, and crypto does not respond to antibiotics. Once you've had it on a farm, this disease is usually *endemic;* each new crop of calves may become infected.

The Disease

The protozoa attach to the intestinal lining but do not penetrate it; the parasites sit on the lining. The calf's body reacts to this and mounts a strong response to fight off the organism. White blood cells migrate to the site of infection and there is intense inflammation; the intestinal lining sloughs off. The damage is not due to protozoa disrupting the lining but to the calf's trying to get rid of the organism — and the only way he can do that is to get rid of the cell it's attached to, so the lining is shed. Thus, the gut loses ability to absorb fluid, electrolytes, and nutrients. Everything shoots on through, in a watery diarrhea. Peak diarrhea is three to five days after a calf ingests the organism. During the following three to five days he usually rids himself of it.

One reason some calves are very ill and some die is that they have not only crypto but also rotavirus infection (see chapter 11). This virus acts the same way as crypto in the intestine, creating inflammation of the lining. It sloughs off, leaving the calf with a reduced ability to absorb anything. The calf may become so compromised that it's hard to save him without extensive support treatment and IV fluids.

After a calf has lost his gut lining, it takes three to five days to heal enough to start functioning again, a period during which he's very compromised and may die from severe dehydration. Once he hits the peak period of diarrhea, several days after he ingests protozoa, it will take three to five more days to get things back to normal. Very young calves, younger than three weeks old, usually take longer to regenerate their damaged gut lining than an older calf, because they are more compromised and cannot heal nearly as fast.

Just as in coccidiosis, after a calf gets over the infection, he has some resistance to reinfection. Even though he encounters the protozoa again, he's less likely to become sick with diarrhea. He may, however, continue to shed a few oocysts in feces. Adult cattle serve as a source of infection for calves, just as they do with coccidiosis. Some types of crypto are not host-specific and are spread to calves by wildlife, rodents, or farm cats.

The life cycle of *cryptosporidia* is a little different from that of coccidia. In the latter, calves don't show signs of diarrhea until they're at least three weeks old; it takes longer for coccidia to get to the point of multiplying in the gut and damaging the lining. By contrast a calf can break with crypto scours as young as four days of age if he picked up the organism right after birth. He is infected when he is born in a dirty corral or in contaminated manure, when

Life Cycle of Cryptosporidia

Following the calf's ingestion of an oocyst, it attaches to the intestinal lining to sporulate and multiply, similarly to multiplication stages of coccidia, but the period between ingestion and the calf's breaking with diarrhea is only two to seven days. Thousands of new occysts are then passed in the feces for three to twelve days. The infection persists until the calf develops an immune response to eliminate the parasite.

he gets some in his mouth, or when he sucks a dirty udder. Most commonly, calves develop diarrhea by about seven to ten days of age, after ingesting immature-stage protozoa. If calves get diarrhea in the first one to three days of life, it is generally something else — *E. coli,* rotavirus, or coronavirus. Crypto affects calves later, and the diarrhea tends to last longer.

Calves are usually 5 to 15 days old when they get sick with crypto, with mild to moderate diarrhea, which persists for several days even if treated. Young calves 1 to 3 weeks of age are also likely to pick up rotavirus or salmonella. If they have several infections at the same time, this is more difficult to treat. To save these calves, it takes intensive nursing care (see pages 259 and 263) to try to keep them alive long enough for the gut to start to heal.

There is a rotavirus vaccine you can give the cow ahead of calving (see chapter 11) to create antibodies in her colostrum; this may help reduce the number of fatal cases of scours on some farms, minimizing risk for rotavirus infection along with crypto. There's been research on a vaccine against cryptosporidiosis, but it has not yet become commercially available. The best preventive measure against crypto diarrhea is a clean environment.

Symptoms

Calves with crypto usually have watery diarrhea — pale green, yellow, cream-colored or gray. By contrast, coccidiosis produces red or brown bloody feces. In cryptosporidiosis the gut lining is shed (mucus or shreds of tissue appear in the feces) but is not damaged so deeply that it bleeds. The calf may be dull and not nursing. Persistent diarrhea results in loss of weight and emaciation in some cases.

Glutamine Solution in the Works

Various oral rehydration solutions have been tested to see if anything might be more effectively absorbed than standard salt solutions with *glucose.* Glucose is often added to electrolyte solutions, not only to give energy but also to aid absorption of salts; transporters on the cells in the gut lining need a sugar molecule before they'll take in a salt solution.

This fact was discovered many years ago in human cholera patients in developing nations. Doctors found that if they gave dehydrated patients a salt solution, it had some benefit, but that if they put sugar in it, patients absorbed a lot more. Today, most electrolyte solutions given to help combat dehydration contain *dextrose* or some other type of simple sugar, along with electrolyte salts (sodium, chlorine, potassium).

The problem in treating calves with diarrhea caused by cryptosporidia, however, is that transporter cells on the intestinal lining that have glucose and sodium transport ability are the cells that are severely damaged when the gut lining is shed by the calf. So research was done on other nutrients, such as *glutamine,* that could stimulate uptake of salts. Glutamine is an amino acid, a protein nutrient. It is transported in exactly the same way as glucose, except that during a crypto infection there are more cells left in the gut that can transport glutamine. The small intestine uses glutamine rather than glucose as a nutrient for itself and prefers to absorb it, so whatever cells are left are more able to absorb glutamine than glucose.

Researchers compared glutamine-containing salt solutions with glucose-containing salt solutions and found glutamine solutions more effective; calves had more fluid absorption and didn't get as dehydrated. Eventually there may be an electrolyte product that contains glutamine rather than glucose that would be more beneficial for calves with crypto.

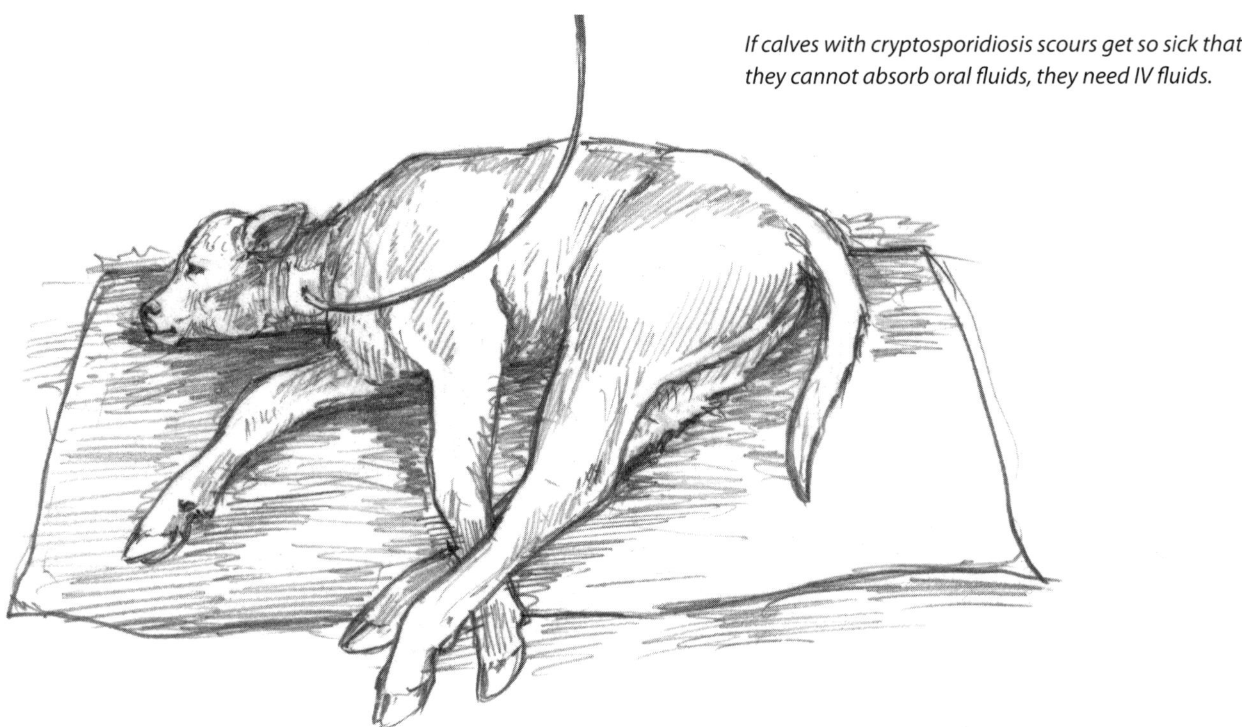

If calves with cryptosporidiosis scours get so sick that they cannot absorb oral fluids, they need IV fluids.

Treatment

To date, there are no commercially available drugs that have much affect on these protozoa. Supportive care is very important; calves need nutrition, fluid, and electrolytes to replace what they are losing. Success depends on how early you spot the problem and start treatment.

Do not withhold milk, or the calf may become extremely weak. If you feed only electrolyte fluids, he may collapse and be hard to save because of persistent diarrhea and malnutrition. These calves are losing fluid and not able to absorb more, so they get into trouble very fast. They cannot be saved with antibiotics, as some stockmen try to do, because antibiotics do not affect the protozoa. The calves need good nursing care to keep them hydrated. If they get to the point at which the gut cannot absorb oral fluids, they need IV fluids (see chapter 11).

Calves with diarrhea should be given fluid by stomach tube or esophageal feeder several times a day. For a seriously dehydrated calf, give fluids every six hours, or more often if the calf is only a week old or less. If he's not nursing the cow, add milk replacer to the solution. Whole milk or milk replacer should be given in small quantities several times a day, to optimize what might be absorbed and to minimize loss of body weight. It's very important to keep up

Checking Blood pH

If a calf goes too long before you start treatment, his blood pH, an indirect measure of how hydrated or dehydrated he is, drops and becomes more acidic, and his whole body suffers from acidosis; organs start shutting down, he becomes too weak to stand, and eventually he slips into a coma. If you start diligent treatment before blood pH gets down to about seven, you can usually save the calf. Blood pH can be measured by your vet. If it gets down to seven or below, you are usually out of luck, no matter how diligently you treat the calf.

When calves are already too far gone with diarrhea and dehydration, you can't save them even with massive amounts of fluid given intravenously. You may pour a lot of fluid, time, money, and energy into them, and they still die. In an epidemic of crypto scours, when treating a number of calves, blood tests could help you focus on those with a better chance of survival. The veterinarian can also check antibody levels in the calves' blood to see how much colostrum they absorbed, and check their systemic conditions to evaluate whether you might be able to save them.

When Crypto Strikes

If you do bring home crypto, ideally you isolated the calf and can clean the area where you kept him while he was sick. Crypto oocysts are resistant to all disinfectants except hydrogen peroxide, chlorine dioxide, ammonium hydroxide, and a few others, and will survive for months in cool, moist conditions, but their infective activity can be destroyed by drying or freezing. Don't let other cattle have access to that area for several weeks (longer in damp weather), so that it can thoroughly dry out. Infectivity of oocysts in calf feces is reduced after several days of complete drying.

the calf's food intake in spite of his diarrhea, if he's able to receive oral feedings and is not so down-and-out that he needs IV fluids, or he will become very weak. It may take several days of intensive care and tube feedings if he's not nursing.

Banamine also helps. One of the things that happens during inflammation associated with crypto is release of prostaglandins (hormones produced during inflammatory processes) in the sick calf's body. These inflammatory products inhibit absorption of salt and fluids. This negative effect is blocked by Banamine, which reduces inflammation and hinders the action of prostaglandins. Banamine also reduces pain and fever, so the calf feels better and is more likely to nurse his mother. Some veterinarians don't like to use Banamine because it can lead to digestive-tract ulcers, but research at North Carolina State University showed that if Banamine is used at the regular dosage rate for the weight of the calf, in conjunction with oral rehydration solutions, it makes a big difference in swifter recovery.

The calf will get rid of the protozoa by himself if you help him to fight the battle, but you need to catch it early and to keep him from getting weak and dehydrated, especially if the problem is complicated by multiple infections. If you start early enough with oral fluids, medication to slow down the diarrhea (Kaopectate), and Banamine injections, the calf won't get so dehydrated that he needs IV fluids.

Prevention

The best prevention? Never introduce this disease to your farm. If you don't already have it, don't buy questionable cattle. Since it's a common problem in dairy calves, do not buy dairy calves to raise on bottles or graft onto beef cows that lose their calves, unless you're absolutely sure that they are healthy. Even if they look healthy, isolate them for three to five days to make sure they've not been exposed to crypto. A healthy-looking calf could get diarrhea a few days after you bring him home if he was exposed before you got him.

The best prevention? Never introduce this disease to your farm.

If you already have crypto on your farm, use diligent management to keep calving cows and young calves in a clean environment (see chapter 10), so that calves won't be exposed early in life by ingesting protozoa. Some of the same precautions should be taken as for prevention of coccidiosis (see page 257). Isolate any calf with diarrhea in a "sick pen" so that the calf won't spread the organisms and infect other calves. Continue to keep him separated from other calves for several days after recovery. Make sure that you don't inadvertently spread the disease after handling or treating a sick one — change clothes, wash hands, and don't track feces from the sick pen to other locations. Use different footwear or rinse your boots in disinfectant solution before going somewhere else on the farm. Be aware that crypto can also affect lambs, young goats, piglets, foals, and humans (see page 265).

CLEANLINESS AND COMPOSTING

Even though we've never had crypto, we try to minimize spread of all pathogens. All the manure and straw from cleaning our barns goes into a large composting area, where it sits for several years and breaks down; the heat of fermentation kills any pathogens before this material is put out on the fields as fertilizer.

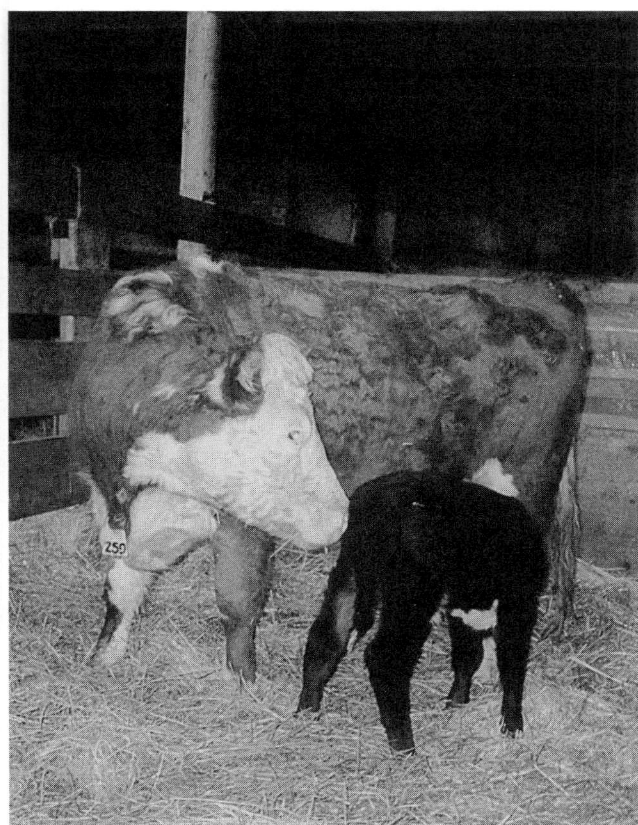

A recent North Carolina State University study showed that calves that did not receive antibodies from nursing colostrum were more readily infected with cryptosporidiosis.

Caution: Humans Can Get Cryptosporidiosis

Unlike coccidiosis, which is host specific, cryptosporidiosis can be spread from cattle or wildlife to people. When handling sick calves, protect yourself and members of your family. Wear gloves and protective clothing, and wash your hands afterward. The organism can be spread to people if ingested. This disease is not seen very often in humans, except in developing countries, because in the United States we try to prevent contamination of water supplies by human or animal fecal material. There are some strains of crypto that specifically affect humans, but people can also get diarrhea from the type that infects cattle, wildlife, birds, and fish.

If you've never been exposed to crypto and have no immunity, you may be at risk of getting it from a sick calf. Veterinary students, for instance, often get it from handling calves with crypto diarrhea, unless they wear protective gloves and clothing. A person who gets the disease develops severe diarrhea within three to five days of being exposed, but it usually runs its course, and no treatment is needed to cure it. Humans or animals in good health can usually handle the infection, but it can be devastating to the very young, the elderly, or any individual — calf or human — with a poor immune system. If you have young children in your household, be sure you don't bring crypto infection to them from the barnyard, and never let them interact with calves that might be sick.

Colostrum, Colostrum, Colostrum

Make sure every calf gets an adequate amount of colostrum soon after birth (see chapter 7). Though cows don't create many antibodies against cryptosporidia, they do produce some if they've been exposed to this organism. Also, various antibodies in colostrum, those against other pathogens, are important in assuring that a calf has adequate defenses against other diseases that could compromise his health. If he has a high antibody level, he has more resistance and is better equipped to fight off any invaders.

In all studies done at NCSU on cryptosporidiosis, colostrum was found to be an important factor, giving calves some antibody protection. In trials to evaluate various groups of calves using different treatments, some calves were purposely infected with crypto. When trying to get all calves "on the same playing field" for tests before infecting some of them to study, the researchers found that calves who didn't get adequate colostrum were most vulnerable, and that they shed higher levels of oocysts in feces.

Calves without antibodies from colostrum were more readily infected and much harder to treat successfully. The researchers concluded that if calves have good colostrum absorption, this will protect most of them from infection with cryptosporidia, and that the ones that do get infections will recover from them much more quickly, with good supportive treatment, than a calf with no colostrum protection. This is one more reason to make sure calves nurse quickly and get a full amount of colostrum — at least 2 to 3 quarts (1.9 to 2.8 L), depending on the size of the calf, immediately after birth.

Chapter 13

Respiratory Ailments

YOUNG CALVES ARE VULNERABLE to respiratory infections if stressed by cold or wet weather or subjected to a dirty environment or respiratory irritants such as dust, smoke, or ammonia fumes in a barn stall. They are especially vulnerable if they did not receive adequate antibodies from colostrum immediately after birth. Maternal antibodies are a calf's best prevention against pathogens he will soon encounter, including those that cause pneumonia and diphtheria, the most common respiratory diseases in young calves.

Pneumonia

Depending on the causative pathogen, stresses, and immune status of the calf, *pneumonia* can be mild, or swift and deadly. Many cases take a day or more to severely affect the lung tissue, giving you a chance to treat and save the calf if you can detect the problem early.

Pathogens that cause pneumonia are always present in the environment, but a calf with strong immunity, bolstered by maternal antibodies when he's young and later by vaccinations or exposure that triggers a sufficient antibody response, is often able to fight them off. Illness occurs when immunity is poor or the immune system is hindered by viral infections such as BVD or IBR, or stress. Pneumonia often follows a bad case of scours in a young calf, especially if the weather is wet, cold, or windy. Diarrhea wears him down and lowers his resistance. A young calf exposed to dusty bedding or ammonia fumes from dirty bedding in a humid barn with poor ventilation is another prime candidate for pneumonia. Amniotic fluid inhaled at birth can settle in any calf's lungs and make it easier for pathogens to invade.

Viral Pneumonia

Pneumonia can be bacterial or viral. Virus infections don't generally kill a calf; he is sick until he mounts an immune response. The initial illness in many cases of pneumonia is a viral infection such as *infectious bovine rhinotracheitis* (*IBR*), *bovine virus diarrhea* (*BVD*), *parainfluenza 3* (*PI3*), *bovine respiratory syncytial virus* (*BRSV*), etc. A calf with viral respiratory illness often has a snotty nose and a fever. Calves affected by respiratory viruses often run high temperatures of 104 to 108°F (40 to 42.2°C).

Viral pneumonia is often complicated by secondary bacterial infection, however, making illness much more severe; if a calf dies of pneumonia, the actual killer is usually a bacterium that moves in after the lungs are damaged by the virus. Pneumonia severe enough to cause the death of a calf is almost always bacterial; the actual killer is usually *streptococcus, pasteurella,* or other bacteria that take advantage of the calf's vulnerability.

Young calves are most susceptible to viral pneumonia between two weeks and two months of age, when temporary immunity from colostrum declines but before they develop their own immune system. Calves are most protected against viral respiratory

Treat Immediately

By the time the calf is obviously sick, there is already some lung damage, especially if infection is due to Pasteurella. Damage can become permanent within eight hours or less of the start of the illness. At that point, there can be scarring in the lungs even if you treat the calf and clear up the infection. Depending on the type of bacteria involved, the calf may develop lung abscesses or may relapse following treatment. Once abscesses form, or if there's too much damage, antibiotics may not be effective. The amount of scarring determines the length of the calf's life. Once the lungs are damaged and filling with fluid, a calf may be hard to save. He'll need aggressive treatment and good intensive care.

infection when their dams' vaccinations are up-to-date, providing adequate antibody levels in colostrum, and the calves are vaccinated at about six to eight weeks of age so that they can build their own immunity. Newborn calves are very susceptible to IBR, for instance, if antibody levels in colostrum are low or the calf did not get enough colostrum and is stressed by bad weather or overcrowding.

A calf's windpipe is lined with tiny hairlike structures that are always moving, like ocean waves, in a continual upward sweep. They constantly move dirt, mucus, fluid, and bacteria out of the windpipe to the back of the throat to be coughed out or swallowed. But viral respiratory infections damage these *cilia*; they no longer protect the lungs from foreign material or pathogens moving down the windpipe.

Some viruses make calves very sick, even without bacterial complications. Antibiotic treatment won't hinder the virus, but a secondary bacterial infection usually responds. Relapses are common, however, if the viral infection is extensive. Some calves with acute viral pneumonia die within a few hours, but many cases of uncomplicated viral pneumonia (that is, with no bacteria involved) recover in four to seven days. If bacteria are involved, the fever, difficult breathing, and *toxemia* (toxins from bacteria entering the bloodstream) are worse.

Bacterial Pneumonia

Many different bacteria cause pneumonia in calves, but one of the most common is *Pasteurella hemolyticum.* This bacterium is almost always present in the noses and sinuses of normal, healthy cattle, ready to move down into the windpipe if the cilia are damaged. As soon as bacteria move down into the lungs, they create pneumonia. Unlike a viral infection, *Pasteurella* pneumonia is likely to kill the calf unless treatment is begun promptly.

Even if the calf survives, resultant lung damage may hinder his ability to grow. As our vet once told us, if lung damage exceeds 15 to 20 percent of the lung capacity, the calf will not grow properly. Even if he seems healthy for several months, he may suddenly die when his body outgrows his lung capacity. The best defense against permanent lung damage is aggressive treatment with antibiotics as soon as you notice a calf is sick, and until he's fully recovered.

Signs of Pneumonia

A calf with pneumonia usually exhibits some or all of the following signs of illness:

- He stops nursing.
- He acts dull instead of lively.
- He spends most of his time lying down or standing with his back humped up and his head down.
- His ears droop instead of being perky and alert.
- He is less apt to run off if you approach.
- He moves slowly because he's in pain.
- He doesn't care about what's going on around him but focuses on his own discomfort.
- He pants or has labored breath, sometimes with his mouth open.
- He coughs.
- He has a thin and clear or thick and snotty nasal discharge.
- He makes grunting sounds as he forces air out of his lungs.
- He has a temperature of 103°F (39.4°C) or higher.

Treatment

It is important to detect early warning signs. Pneumonia can come on swiftly and kill a calf within a few hours unless you halt the infection. If you detect that a calf has a case of pneumonia starting and you start treatment immediately, the infection is much easier to clear up, and you won't have to treat him for such an extended period of time. If you wait too long before beginning treatment, however, lungs may be too damaged to recover. Early treatment can help to prevent complications like abscesses in the lungs, inflammation in the lung lining, scar tissue, and chronic dilation of the bronchial tubes.

Even if the initial infection is due to a virus and the calf is not very ill, antibiotics are usually given to protect the calf from bacterial pneumonia that might develop. Some viral infections can make a calf very ill, and he'll need supportive care and antibiotics to make sure that the stress of this illness does not set him up for a fatal bacterial infection.

Taking Temperatures

Sometimes you can test for fever by feeling a calf's nose or the inside of his mouth, but in cold weather neither respiration rate nor how his mouth or nose feels are sure tests of illness.

Use an animal thermometer or human rectal thermometer, and tie or tape a string to the end so that you won't lose it in the rectum. Keep it in a thermometer case so that it won't get broken. Shake it down before use. Lubricate it with a bit of saliva so that it slips easily into the rectum without friction and discomfort. Leave it in for two or three minutes to get an accurate reading.

Normal temperature in a young calf is 101 to 102°F (38.3 to 38.8°C); anything over 102.5°F (39.2°C) means that he's sick. If his temperature is subnormal, he is either very chilled or has been sick for a while and is going into shock or dying. Taking his temperature helps you to monitor illness and recovery. Treat him until his temperature has been normal for at least two days in a row.

Your veterinarian can advise you on appropriate antibiotics for pneumonia. For decades, penicillin or oxytetracycline were used. Penicillin is generally not as effective anymore because some bacteria have become resistant, but an oxytetracycline product, such as LA-200, still works well for pneumonia on many farms, especially if given in conjunction with a sustained-release sulfa, such as boluses that release for two or three days. You may have better results using an injectable sulfa for a very young calf instead of a bolus, though the injection may need to be given more often.

Pneumonia can come on swiftly and kill a calf in a few hours unless you halt the infection.

Tips for Choosing Medication

- If combinations of LA-200 and sulfa work well for pneumonia on your farm, there's no need to change to more expensive drugs.
- If you use sulfa, and the calf is not nursing enough, give supportive fluids via tube or esophageal feeder; otherwise, a dehydrated calf may suffer kidney damage. Sulfa use requires sufficient fluid in the animal's body to keep up adequate urine flow, or it will crystalize in the kidneys.
- If pneumonia does not respond to oxytetracycline and sulfa, there are newer, more expensive, sometimes more effective drugs that can be given, such as Naxcel and Micotil, both effective against Pasteurella pneumonia. Micotil can be deadly if you accidentally inject yourself and should be given by a veterinarian, unless he or she has instructed you on how to use it and what precautions to take.
- Some vets may prescribe Baytril or Nuflor in certain cases, or one of the newer drugs like Draxxin, which concentrates in lung tissue, or Excede. Work with your vet to determine the most helpful course of antibiotic treatment for each case of pneumonia.

Special Care

Good supportive treatment makes the difference between life and death for the calf. Keep him warm and dry in a barn, under a heat lamp, or in the house if necessary. If weather is hot, he needs shade and a cool place or a fan in a barn stall. A young calf can't handle heat, especially if he's sick. A barn stall, for shelter or for shade in hot weather, is better than an outdoor pen. If possible, keep him with his mama, even if he needs intensive care. Partition off a corner of the barn so that the calf can be under a heater if necessary and still have the comfort and security of being with Mama. He'll be more stressed if he's separated from her.

A calf with a fever may not nurse, and fever also causes him to dehydrate. He needs 1 to 2 quarts (.95 to 1.89 L) of fluid every four to eight hours, depending upon the severity of the illness and the outside temperature, just to combat dehydration from fever. Force-feed him if he's not nursing. Banamine is helpful to reduce pain, fever, and inflammation, and to ease difficult breathing, and it also prevents some of the scarring in the lungs. For a young calf, inject about 1 cc into muscle. If you catch pneumonia early and administer antibiotics and Banamine, calves recover faster. Don't give Banamine alone to a dehydrated calf, or there is risk of kidney damage. Use it only in conjunction with fluid therapy if the calf isn't nursing.

If a calf starts to feel better, he may nurse. If he doesn't, give him regular feedings, or supplemental feedings if he's only nursing a little, of milk or milk replacer. In serious cases, the calf needs IV fluids; if he is unable to stand or is comatose, his gut won't be working.

Be diligent with treatment. Use antibiotics immediately upon discovering the problem, and continue for two full days after all symptoms are gone. If treatment is halted too soon, he may relapse, and then your chances of saving the calf are greatly reduced.

Respiratory System Compromised during Birth

Environmental factors can predispose a newborn calf to pneumonia. A calf with a lot of fluid in his air passages at birth may have trouble getting rid of it quickly. Even though he coughs to clear his airways,

Use the Drug That Works

About 60 percent of bacteria are now resistant to tetracyclines, but these are cheaper than many of the newer drugs; if they work on your farm, there's no reason not to use them. Some people start with LA-200 and switch to another drug if it doesn't work. Others prefer to use a more expensive drug first because they feel that a calf will have had two more days of lung damage if the first antibiotic didn't work.

With any drug, the calf should be closely monitored; if he's not showing improvement in two or three days, change to something different. Find what works best by trial and error.

QUICK PNEUMONIA

ONE SUNDAY MORNING in early April 1972, a month-old calf, Duchess, was missing at feeding time. It hd been a cold, windy night and we were afraid that she might be sick. Lynn and I searched the brush at the edges of the field where our cattle often take shelter. We finally found her lying in the bushes, very ill — a victim of quick pneumonia. She had been lively and healthy the evening before and now was nearly dead the next morning.

She was too weak to walk, so we lifted her onto the tailgate of the pickup, which was still full of hay because we hadn't finished feeding yet. Duchess was so sick that she just lay there as I walked behind the pickup to make sure that she didn't fall off the tailgate. Lynn drove from the field to the barn, with the cow following.

We put Duchess in the barn under a heat lamp and treated her round the clock for more than two weeks with fluids, antibiotics, and medication to help her breathe. She had a fever of 105.6°F (40.8°C). We saved her, but if we'd found her an hour or two later, she would have been dead.

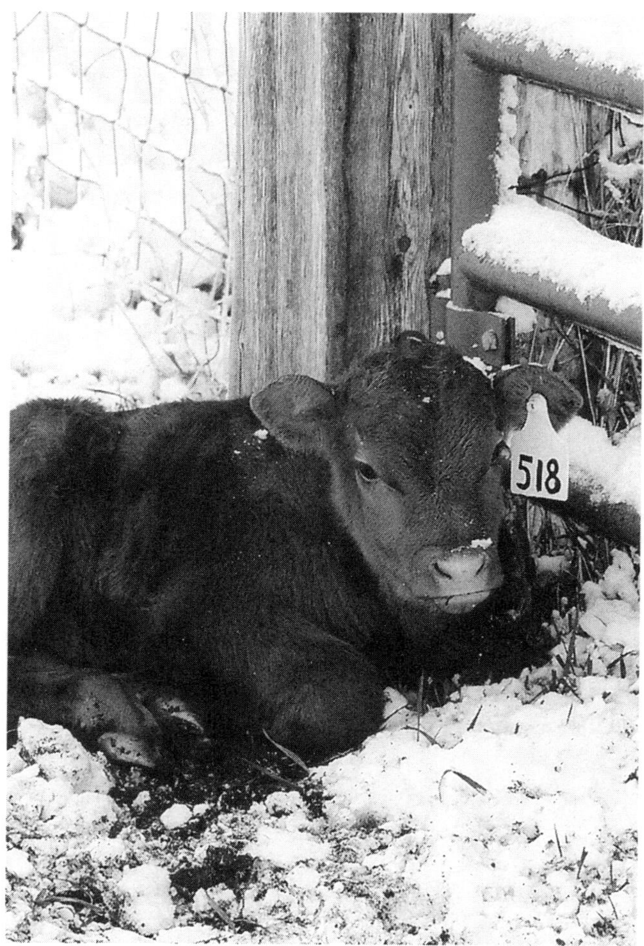

Cold, wet, weather-stressed calves are more vulnerable to pneumonia.

DMSO to Treat Pneumonia

Some vets prescribe dimethyl sulfoxide (DMSO), but others don't. DMSO helps to reduce swelling and inflammation in the airways and fluid buildup in the lungs, helping the calf to breathe more easily and aiding recovery. One of our vets recommends 1 cc per hundred pounds (45.4 kg) of body weight (usually 1 to 2 cc for a young calf) intravenously or mixed with a little warm water and squirted into the back of the mouth. It is absorbed immediately into body tissues when taken orally and is carried through the body and into the lungs. If you are not experienced in giving IV injections, giving it orally is nearly as effective.

he may "rattle" for several hours, and some fluid may get down into the lungs. Calves that breathe in fluid seem more vulnerable to early pneumonia. Symptoms appear in the first 24 hours of life, especially if the weather is cold or if the calf fails to nurse promptly, thereby delaying intake of antibodies.

Studies have shown that chilled calves don't absorb antibodies efficiently; the "openness" of a newborn's gut lining that allows passage of large antibody molecules closes much more quickly in a cold, stressed calf. If the calf's airways are compromised by fluid, he is less apt to nurse enough colostrum. A chilled calf that struggles to breathe and nurse at the same time provides a perfect setup for pneumonia: He's cold, he has a little fluid in the lungs, and he can't get enough antibodies to protect him.

Weather Stress

Pneumonia is likely to strike calves that are wet and cold for too long, if they don't have shelter in the first weeks of life. A calf sleeping in the snow or rain or lying in a puddle of rainwater or melting snow is vulnerable. And if he's a little sick and dull from scours, he's not as likely to seek shelter.

In summer, hot weather can stress calves and make them vulnerable to pneumonia. A young calf has very little body reserves; he dehydrates quickly in hot weather, just from panting and sweating. If it's so hot that he doesn't feel like nursing, the problem is greatly aggravated.

Other warm-weather stressors include dust when it's dry and windy, and smoke during a bad fire season; they irritate a calf's airway and damage the lining of the trachea. If the lining and cilia are compromised by dust or smoke, this may allow bacteria to gain entrance to the tissues, even without the help of a virus.

Sudden changes in temperature can also be a factor in onset of pneumonia. Whenever day-to-night temperature variations exceed 40 to 50°F (roughly 22 to 27°C), a calf is vulnerable to pneumonia. If nighttime temperature drops to 30 or 40°F (–1 or 4.4°C) and it gets up to 80 or 90°F (26.6 or 32.2°C) in the afternoon, or 20°F (–6.6°C) at night and 60°F (15.5°C) in the afternoon in early spring, these extremes are very stressful for young calves.

DOWDY'S DODIE: A CHALLENGING CASE

DOWDY CALVED ON A FRIGID NIGHT in February. The birth was easy, but her little black calf Dodie didn't get up. It was cold in the barn, so my daughter Andrea and I dried him with towels. We always make sure a calf nurses by the time he's an hour old, so we fed him part of a bottle of fresh colostrum while he was still lying down. Andrea milked one of Dowdy's front teats into a bottle as the gentle young cow lay in the straw beside her calf. Then we got them both up and tried to help the calf nurse his mother. Usually, once a calf gets a taste of colostrum, he becomes eager for more, but this calf was weak.

It took all of his effort to stand, and he would not nurse. Andrea milked more colostrum from Dowdy, and we tried to bottle-feed the calf again. He refused to suck this time; we finally fed it to him by stomach tube. He was still cold, but we thought he'd be okay, since he had a tummy full of colostrum and Dowdy was vigorously licking him. We misjudged this situation; we should have brought him into the house for complete warming and drying.

When we checked him a few hours later, he was up but still cold, weak, and lethargic, and he had not nursed the cow. Again, we milked Dowdy and fed Dodie by tube. The young cow was very patient; she stood still for milking if her calf was close by. By morning we knew that he had a serious problem. Dowdy had finally shed her placenta, and it was grey and unhealthy- looking. Her calf had been deprived of part of his blood supply before birth, which might be why he was so weak, listless, unable to nurse, and unable to keep warm.

Stress and cold had taken a toll. Dodie had pneumonia and a high fever. His breathing was fast and shallow. We started him on antibiotics (LA-200 and sulfa) and oral DMSO, but he still would not take a teat or a bottle, so we milked Dowdy every six hours and fed him by tube. We can usually halt pneumonia with LA-200 and sulfa, but this calf showed no improvement by the second day, so our vet recommended Naxcel. After three more days of treatment, we were still losing the battle, so we changed to Nuflor, and upon the advice of our vet, we gave the calf 5 cc of DMSO, injected into the jugular vein. As our vet told us, this "blast" of DMSO would go directly into the lungs, which is a little more effective than giving it orally, and would break up congestion better, clearing out the fluid buildup.

Dodie started breathing more easily within 24 hours and seemed normal by his second dose of Nuflor, 48 hours later. After being fed by tube every six hours for the first week of life, he was finally nursing his mother. We didn't continue antibiotics because his breathing and temperature were normal. After seeming normal for four days, he relapsed. His temperature rose, and breathing became impaired again. We put him back on medication, and it was a long, slow recovery. He had to be encouraged to nurse, and there were times when we had to milk Dowdy and tube him.

He lost part of his hair. This often happens after a fever. Every place we rubbed him, his hair came off, and he had a bald spot on the top of his head. He and Dowdy lived in a barn for five weeks, and we continued treating him. Finally he started feeling better and nursing more regularly, so we put them in a nearby pen for sunshine and exercise, and back in the barn when the weather turned bad.

They were able to go to pasture with the other cows on April 5, when Dodie was two months old! He took off running and bucking, excited and happy to have so much room. Dowdy bucked around after him. She'd been very patient, living in the barn and small pen for so long, but now she was glad to be free. With our diligence, Dodie survived and grew up. He was stunted for a while; perhaps it took all his energy to stay alive and there wasn't much left for growing. But by fall he was as large and healthy as the other calves.

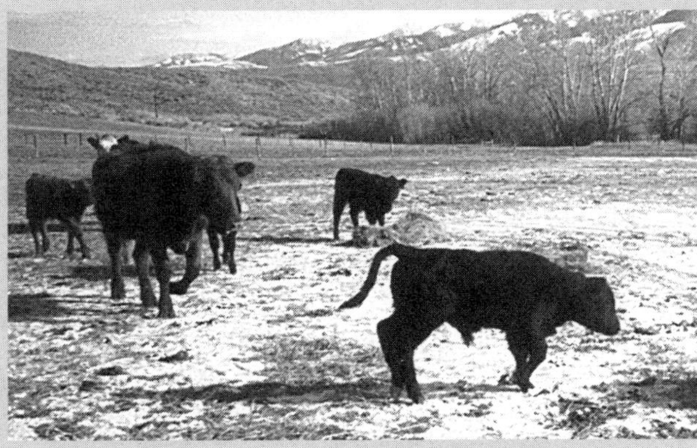

When we finally put Dodie and his mama out in the big wide world, Dodie ran and bucked happily. Here he checks out the hay being fed, while his worried mother follows him around, trying to keep track of him.

Lack of Ventilation in Barns

Barns provide shelter for calving in inclement weather, but unless the barn has good ventilation, it can cause respiratory illness in newborn calves. Dust from straw, and ammonia fumes from urine and manure buildup in wet bedding are irritating to a young calf's respiratory passages and can open the way for opportunistic pathogens. If you can detect an ammonia smell in the barn, it's too concentrated to be healthy for baby calves. Sit or lie on the barn floor, at calf level. If you smell ammonia fumes, you will probably notice a stinging in your nose and lungs. This type of irritation to the airways can open the way for pathogens. The barn needs better ventilation or a more thorough cleaning. Open the doors and get some fresh air in there.

Even if you have cold nights and cows need to be in the barn to calve, get them out before the next afternoon, or open barn doors if temperatures rise. Spring weather is fickle, and on warm afternoons the barn may get too hot unless you can open doors and windows to let air flow through. Newborn calves subjected to extremes in temperature, as well as overheated cows in a closed barn with their winter coats on, may become more vulnerable to pneumonia.

LOSING TRICKIE WOO

THE ONLY CALF WE LOST to pneumonia was a month-old heifer in 1975. Trickie Woo had scours for a couple of days, and we should have brought her and her mama in from the field to an isolated pen and shelter. Instead, we captured her and gave her an electrolyte solution out in the field. Her defenses were compromised by scours and warm days and cold nights. One night she got chilled. The antibiotic we'd used in earlier years for pneumonia, one that concentrated in lung tissue, had been taken off the market. We had to make do with some that weren't as effective, and we weren't able to save her. Since then, we have learned techniques like using DMSO in conjunction with antibiotics, and have used better drugs that have become available, making it possible for us to save all calves that subsequently became ill with pneumonia.

Aspiration Pneumonia

If a calf gets fluid in the windpipe and lungs, he is at risk for *aspiration pneumonia.* This can happen if you force-feed a calf with a bottle and he's not swallowing properly or if you *drench* a calf with medication, squirting or pouring it down his throat instead of administering it by stomach tube. If there is foreign material in the lungs that can't be worked out and coughed up, the calf will die — no matter how aggressively you treat the resultant infection.

Preventing Pneumonia

Making sure that cows have strong immunity by establishing a herd-health program that includes timely vaccinations and ensuring that each calf gets adequate colostrum are the best measures for preventing pneumonia. Keep in mind, however, that this protection wanes by the time most calves are three weeks old, and many cows don't have a strong immunity to *Pasteurella,* so they don't have high levels of antibodies in their colostrum. If you have spring and summer pneumonia in calves, vaccinate calves at about a month or so of age against *Pasteurella* infections.

Make sure that there are no underlying problems affecting herd health. If calves are getting pneumonia when they are less than three weeks old, it's usually the cows' fault. Cows may be short on protein, energy, selenium, copper, or some other crucial nutrient and may need a more nutritious diet to produce good colostrum.

Diphtheria

Diphtheria is an infection in the mouth and throat, sometimes mistaken for pneumonia if a calf has trouble breathing. The proper term for this disease is *necrotic laryngitis,* and it is caused by a gram-negative bacterium *(Fusobacterium necrophorum),* the same bug that causes foot rot in cattle and navel ill in calves. It is an opportunistic pathogen, causing illness whenever conditions are right, such as when stress or injury to membranes of the mouth and throat give bacteria access to the tissues.

As long as the lining of the calf's mouth or throat are intact, bacteria, which may be present in the feed or material the calf chews on, cause no problems. But if he gets a scratch in his mouth or throat when eating coarse forage or sharp seeds of cheatgrass, foxtail, and the like, the bacteria can cause infection. Diphtheria is not contagious from animal to animal; infection is most likely to develop if a calf has a compromised immune system due to stress or inadequate colostrum antibodies and most commonly follows a sore mouth or throat. When a calf gets diphtheria, the infection may settle in the *larynx* (voice box) and *pharynx* at the back of the throat or may be restricted to the mouth. In the latter instance, the calf is usually not as sick.

Infection in the Mouth

If the infection is confined to the mouth tissues, the calf may have a mild fever or go off feed, slobber, and drool, with swelling in the cheek area. He may have deep ulcers in membranes lining the cheeks and sometimes the tongue, causing swelling and protrusion of the tongue. His breath may smell foul.

Treatment

Ulcers in the mouth will usually heal in a few days if you swab them regularly with tincture of iodine and treat the calf with broad-spectrum antibiotics. Your veterinarian can recommend an appropriate antibiotic for treatment.

Throat Infection

If the larynx (the voice box) and the pharynx (the cavity behind the nose and mouth connecting them to the esophagus) in the back of the throat become swollen and infected, the windpipe is constricted and the calf is often quite ill with diphtheria. Look for the following possible signs:

- Coughing and drooling saliva
- Difficulty swallowing
- Appetite loss
- High fever
- Nasal discharge (thin, not thick, unless there's a secondary illness)
- Foul breath
- Labored breathing
- Wheezing

Mouth Ulcers

The only case we ever had was a bull calf that slobbered and had trouble eating. We gave him antibiotics and swabbed his mouth several times a day with iodine, which was not an easy task because he was a big, strong calf and didn't like it. He healed quickly, however, and was much less sick than the many other calves we've had to treat for diphtheria.

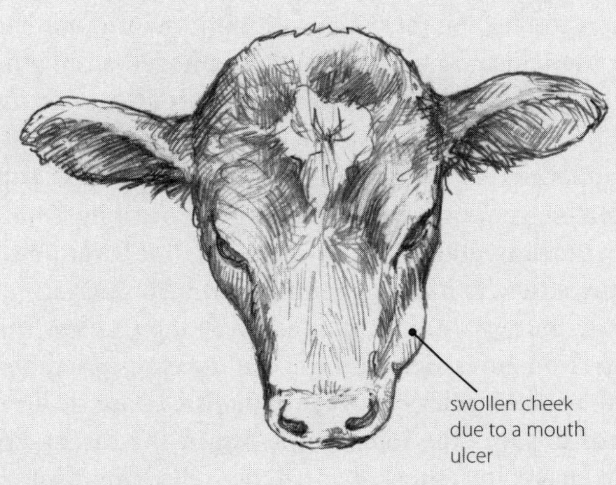

A calf with mouth ulcers has localized pain and may have swelling in the cheek area.

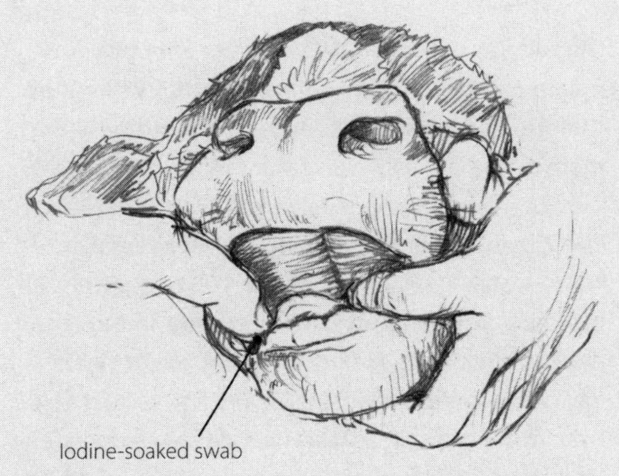

To swab the mouth or throat, hold open the calf's mouth and use one finger to reach back alongside the inside of the mouth with an iodine-soaked piece of cotton or gauze.

At first glance, the calf will seem to have pneumonia because breathing is difficult, sometimes with wheezing due to constricted air passages. But a closer look will show the difference between pneumonia and diphtheria. A calf with pneumonia is dull, with head and ears drooping, and he sometimes has nasal discharge. With diphtheria, the calf is usually alert, with head and neck often extended and parallel to the ground or higher. There's usually no evidence of thick nasal mucus expelled through the nose.

The most typical sign of diphtheria is difficulty drawing air *into* the lungs, due to obstruction in the throat. By contrast, a calf with pneumonia has trouble pushing air *out,* due to damaged and compromised lungs. Calves with pneumonia may grunt as they attempt to push air out of the lungs, due to trapped air within the lungs. If you watch the calf breathe, you can tell which phase of breathing is taking the most effort — in or out — and this is your best clue as to whether it's pneumonia or diphtheria.

Diphtheria does not affect the lungs, unless the infection gets worse and the calf develops pneumonia as a secondary problem, in which case he'll be hard to save. The infection is just in the throat. As the larynx becomes inflamed, it swells. The result is like soaking a donut; the outside gets bigger and the hole in the center becomes smaller.

As the larynx swells and the opening through it shrinks, breathing becomes difficult and is often quite audible. You may hear the calf wheezing from some distance away, especially if he's been exerting and is breathing hard.

If the throat is infected, the calf may have a high fever. He quits eating; he's spending all of his time and energy just trying to breathe. Toxemia, a general infection in the body due to bacterial toxins circulating through the bloodstream, may kill him, unless treatment is begun early, or he may die of suffocation due to obstruction of the passages. Calves with diphtheria may die two to seven days after onset of the illness unless treated. Spread of the infection to the lungs may cause a severe bronchopneumonia.

Treatment

A calf with infection in the throat needs diligent treatment with injectable antibiotics and medication to reduce the swelling. Treatment must start as soon as you notice the calf is sick to combat the infection quickly, because this condition can become life-threatening if the airway closes up, and because

DMSO Gargle

Dimethyl sulfoxide (DMSO) is an effective anti-inflammatory and can greatly reduce swelling in the throat. You can't safely use dexamethasone for more than a few days but can continue using DMSO for as long as needed. For a calf with diphtheria, DMSO can be given as a "gargle": Mix several cc of warm water with 1 or 2 cc of DMSO to squirt into the back of the mouth with a syringe (minus the needle, of course). Doing this a couple of times a day can help shrink swollen tissues. If the weather is cold, make sure the DMSO is added to warm water to keep it from "freezing" in your syringe; it solidifies at a higher temperature than water does.

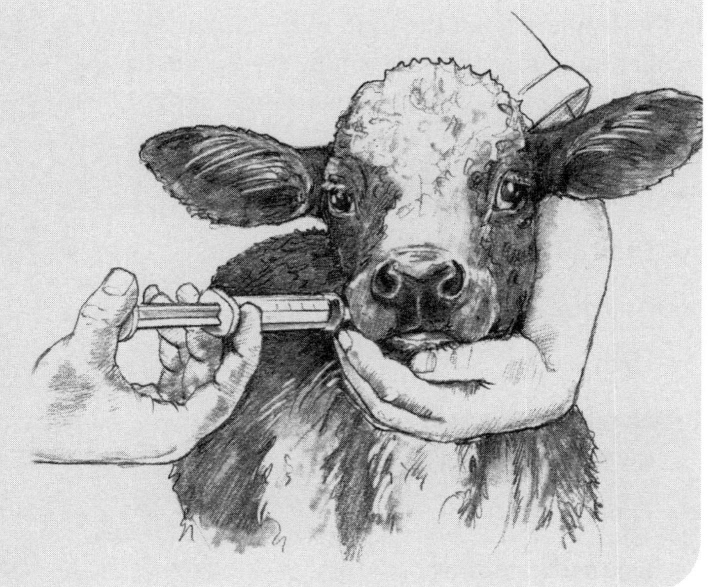

DILIGENCE PAYS OFF

WE LEARNED ABOUT DIPHTHERIA very early in our cattle-raising venture. The first year Lynn and I were married, we managed a dairy on our leased farm in southern Idaho. When we moved to our present ranch in 1967, we brought a few dairy heifers and two young milk cows with us. We wanted to raise some extra calves on the milk cows to make a little more money to help pay the bills. Since there was no cattle auction in our valley, we asked our local cattle buyer to pick us up some young dairy calves when he went to a sale in Montana. He brought us four nice calves, but within a few days they all got sick with severe scours and one of them also developed respiratory symptoms including coughing, wheezing, and drooling.

We consulted our veterinarian, who told us that the calf had diphtheria, and advised us in our treatment. We worked very hard to save those four calves, especially the one with diphtheria, and we never again bought any calves from an auction yard. The one good thing about that terrible experience was learning more about how to doctor calves and how to treat a calf for diphtheria.

Since then, we've treated many serious cases of diphtheria, and most have taken at least a week or 10 days to clear up. Cactus Pete's was probably the longest. We had to keep him and his mother, Desert Bloom, in the barn a long time. When the weather warmed up, they stayed in an outdoor pen where we could catch him easily for his treatments. By that time, all the other cattle were dispersed to breeding groups, so to make sure Desert Bloom got bred, we let her out every day into the pasture next to her pen, until she came into heat and was bred by the bull in the pasture. We had to keep Cactus Pete in that small, nearby pen so that we could treat him without stressing him. He was on antibiotics for nearly two months, but he finally recovered. The key was daily diligence and not ending treatments too soon. A relapse might have made it impossible to save him.

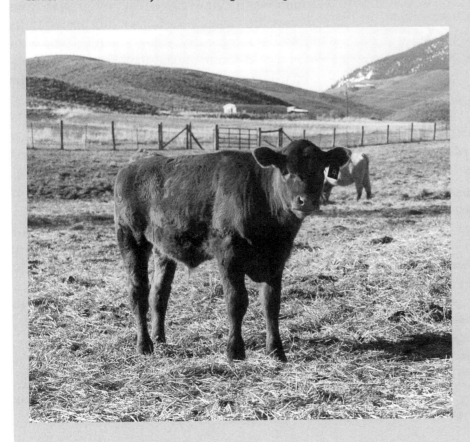

Cactus Pete finally recovered after a long ordeal with diphtheria.

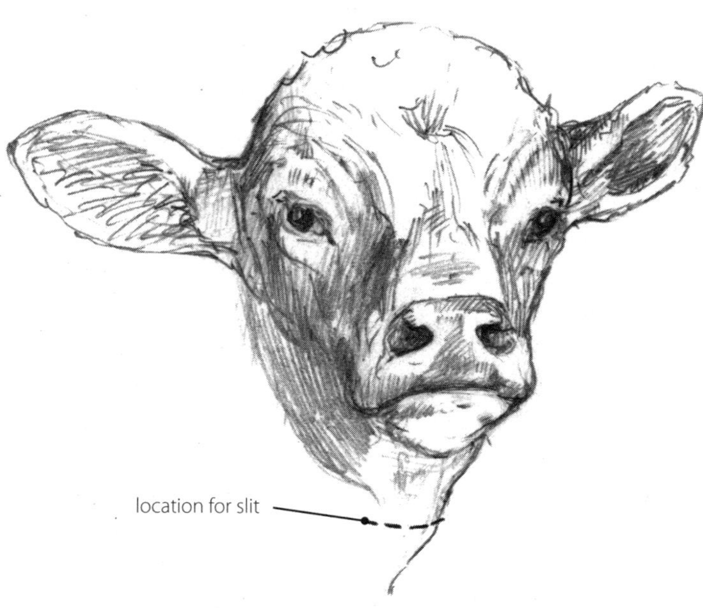

EMERGENCY TRACHEOSTOMY

Carefully cut between the firm cartilage ribs at the front of the windpipe — a few inches below the jaw — using a very clean, sharp knife. The cartilage ribs will feel like the ribs in a vacuum-cleaner hose.

Throat Problems May Affect Moo

Adult cattle occasionally develop infection in the throat, but it's not as serious as infection in a calf's throat. Cows have more resistance, and the throat and air passages are so much larger that infections don't hinder breathing. If an adult isn't very sick and does not quit eating, you might not even know that it has the infection. The main symptom is loss of voice. The cow can't bawl very loudly, since the infection may affect the larynx (the voice box). Some adults eventually regain their voice, but many remain voiceless or have an impaired ability to moo.

scar-tissue formation may make the restriction in the throat permanent even after the infection has been eliminated.

A broad-spectrum antibiotic should be given systemically — injected, not as a bolus, since putting pills down the calf's throat may cause more irritation and make swelling worse. Several antibiotics are effective, including oxytetracycline (LA-200, Bio-Mycin 200, Agrimycin 200, Oxy-tet, etc.), Naxcel and others. Injectable sulfa used in conjunction with oxytetracycline is often effective. Consult your vet. Antibiotic treatment should continue until the calf is fully recovered; this may take several weeks.

No matter what antibiotic you use, also give anti-inflammatory medication to reduce swelling in the throat and prevent formation of scar tissue. A corticosteroid like dexamethasone works, and our vet recommends giving it at least twice a day for the first three to five days to make sure swelling doesn't shut off the airway. Steroids tend to suppress the immune system, however, if given for more than a few days, but are safe to give at the beginning of treatment, especially if the calf is on antibiotics. The anti-inflammatory effects of dexamethasone can help if the calf is having trouble swallowing or breathing.

For best results, start treatment early, before swelling is extensive and before complications such as pneumonia and scar tissue develop. Treat a serious case twice a day with anti-inflammatory medication and feed him by esophageal feeder or tube if he's not nursing. Force-feeding a calf can be tricky, however, since putting a tube down his throat will irritate the swollen, inflamed area. It's better if you can keep swelling down and keep him feeling well enough to nurse his mother.

Treat the calf for however long it takes to get him fully over the infection. Even after he is breathing normally again, take his temperature, and don't halt treatment until his temperature is back to normal and he's eating and drinking well, and no longer slobbering or rattling or wheezing in his breathing.

Emergency Tracheostomy

If a calf gets short of breath and collapses because swelling in the throat shuts off air passages, an emergency *tracheostomy* can be performed to save him. There may not be time to call your vet — this is a case in which an attempt to save his life is better than being afraid to try, because he will certainly die if you don't make an opening through which he can breathe.

A tracheostomy involves slitting the windpipe at the front, a few inches below the jaw. Use a clean, sharp knife and cut horizontally, being careful to cut just through the soft tissue, between the firm ribs of the windpipe — like cutting between the ribs of a vacuum-cleaner hose. Air can then be drawn in by the calf; he can breathe in and out through this opening, bypassing the throat obstruction that is pressing the windpipe shut. If there is not time to have a vet come to your place, you can perform this procedure yourself, to keep the animal alive and breathing.

The slit in the windpipe should be kept open with some kind of tube, or even your fingers, until the vet arrives to put a tracheal tube in place. Then the calf can breathe until the swelling in the throat decreases and he can breathe normally again. Once the swelling goes down, the opening into the windpipe can be stitched shut by your vet, so that it can heal. The calf must be in a clean place, and separated from his mother so that she won't try to lick the tube out of his throat, until the hole can be closed back up again. If the calf is quite ill and not eating or drinking, he may need IV fluids.

Diphtheria is a serious situation, but with diligent care almost all these calves can be saved without having to resort to a tracheostomy or ending up with fatal pneumonia. The key is early treatment — and sticking with it until the calf recovers.

LOSING GOOSIE WOBBLES

THE ONE CALF WE LOST TO DIPHTHERIA was a heifer with a skeletal birth defect that made her walk crooked — Goosie Wobbles. We were raising her to butcher. That fall we had a weaned calf with foot rot that needed to be confined for treatment, and since we were short on pens, we put that heifer with Goosie Wobbles. Goosie contracted diphtheria because the bacteria that result in foot rot can also attack the throat. We started treating her, but swelling in her throat closed off her windpipe. A tracheostomy might have saved her, but we were not quick enough. She suffocated before we could perform it.

Chapter 14

Umbilical Health, Navel Ill, and Septicemia

PATHOGENS THAT ENTER A NEWBORN CALF via the moist umbilical stump can cause local infections or can gain access to the body via the bloodstream, making a calf very ill with septicemia. A bloodborne infection may be immediately life-threatening, as bacteria or their toxins damage vital organs, or it may localize, creating abscesses in various organs. Septicemia also can lead to painful *arthritis* and lameness in the joints. This chapter covers these problems involving the calf's umbilicus and surrounding area, infections that enter by this route, and other systemic infections with similar effects.

Navel Infections

Calves born on clean pasture or clean bedding are least likely to develop navel infection, though on rare occasions a calf becomes infected before birth due to uterine infection in the cow that creates septicemia and subsequent joint problems in the calf. Most cases are caused by contact with bacteria in a dirty environment; the infection enters the moist navel area soon after birth. In the southern part of the United States, bacteria can also be spread by screwworm flies from animal to animal and infect the moist navel in this way.

Swollen joints and lameness are common signs of infection without systemic illness, but abscesses may be present in liver, kidneys, spleen, or lungs, once bacteria invade the bloodstream. Infection may localize in joints, causing arthritis, or infect the eye tissues, heart valves, or membranes around the brain, causing *meningitis*. If septicemia occurs, the calf has fever and is very sick and will die without diligent treatment.

The navel is an ideal portal of entry for disease. There is always risk for infection until the stump dries up and seals off. A variety of bacteria may be involved. Pathogens entering the moist umbilical stump may cause inflammation of the navel cord and create swelling or a pus-producing abscess, inflammation of the umbilical veins or arteries, or infection of the *urachus* (the tube between navel and bladder). In serious cases of the latter, the infection may extend up to the bladder.

The umbilical cord consists of *amniotic membrane* surrounding the umbilical veins and arteries, vessels that carried blood back and forth between the placenta and the developing fetus. The cord also contains the urachus, which connects the fetus's bladder with the allantois of the placenta. This tube served as passageway for urine from the fetal kidneys and bladder, excreted via the urachus into the allantoic fluids in the water bag surrounding the smaller amniotic sac enclosing the fetus.

At birth the amniotic membrane (the outer cover of the umbilical cord) is torn as the calf comes out of the birth canal. It may remain intact for a few minutes if the cow and calf lie there with the calf's hind legs still in the birth canal, but it breaks as the cow gets up or the calf tries to get up. As the umbilical cord breaks, the torn arteries retract back into the

FETUS'S URINARY SYSTEM

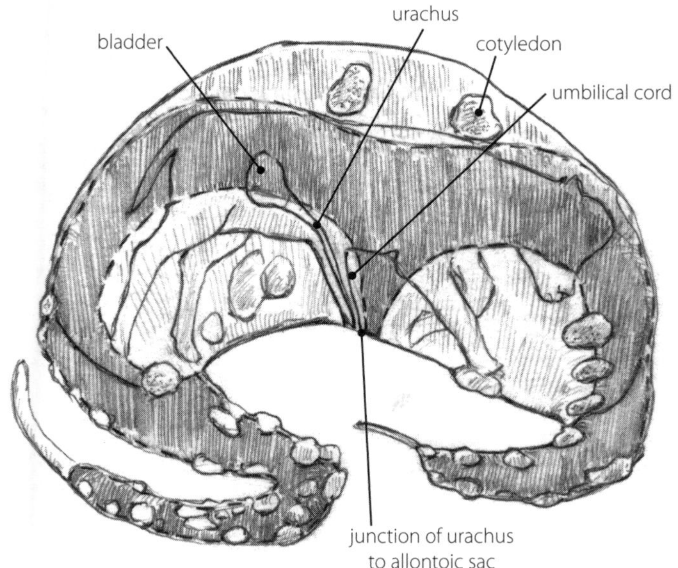

calf's abdomen, sometimes as far back as the top of the bladder. They seal off quickly with very little bleeding. The umbilical veins and urachus close up but remain temporarily outside of the abdomen until the cord stump dries and falls off. Occasionally a blood vessel will not close properly and bleeds from the torn cord, and must be tied off for an hour or so. In a few instances, a firm white-colored tube remains outside the abdomen and must be carefully cut off.

A heifer calf's navel cord usually dries in 24 hours or less, but a bull calf's may take longer.

Umbilical Stump Care

If umbilical tissues (the remains of the amniotic membrane covering and veins) hanging down from the calf's navel do not become infected, they dry up within a few days. A navel stump that does not dry quickly is usually infected. A heifer calf's navel cord usually dries in 24 hours or less, but a bull calf's may take longer. The navel stump is close to the penis and sheath in a bull calf, and if he urinates while lying down, as many bull calves do during the first days of life, the cord may become repeatedly dampened with urine and slow to dry and seal off.

Disinfecting the Navel Stump

If newborn calves come into contact with bacteria on the ground, bedding with a cow's birthing discharges, or discharges from infections such as foot rot, calves are at high risk for navel infection. To dry and disinfect a calf's umbilicus, you must dip the stump at birth.

- Immediately dip and fully saturate the umbilical stump with a good disinfectant (see chapter 7). Tincture of iodine has traditionally been used because it's also an astringent that helps the stump dry and seal off quickly.
- One dip immediately after birth is often adequate for a heifer calf, but for a bull calf or any calf with a thick cord with extra membrane, it may take several dips during the first 24 hours.
- On farms where navel ill or joint ill is a problem, multiple applications of iodine are necessary during the first day of life to prevent infection.
- Completely dip the entire length of the stump; dabbing disinfectant is not adequate.
- Some stockmen squirt iodine up inside the cord, but the caustic liquid can burn the inner tissues next to the abdomen and may keep them irritated and raw longer, delaying healing.
- If a calf has some extra or thick membrane or if it hangs nearly to the ground when he's standing, carefully break off some of the extra (without pulling on the abdomen) so that there's only 3 or 4 inches (7.6 to 10.2 cm) hanging down. These outer umbilical tissues are thick and dense in some calves, while in others they are thin and dry more readily. If the tissues are filled with clotted blood, it prolongs the drying period; carefully squeeze the blood from the tissues so that there's just membrane to dip.
- If calves are born in a clean stall with clean bedding added between cows or on clean grassy pasture, they're less likely to pick up infection, especially with dipped navels. But if calves are taken out of the stall and put into pens or contaminated pastures before the stump has dried and sealed off, they may still become infected.

Swollen Navel

Inflammation of the external portion of the umbilicus occurs commonly in calves and happens most often within two to five days of birth. The navel is enlarged and painful to the calf if pressed with your fingers. It may be a closed swelling, or it may be open and draining. The affected umbilical cord — palpable with your fingers, inside the navel area — may be large, like an apple core. The calf may be depressed, feverish, and not nursing as much as he should. Infection may persist for several weeks, even with antibiotic treatment, both systemically and with local flushing of the abscess. The most effective treatment is surgical removal of the infected umbilical tissue. After removal of the abscess, it may be necessary to leave a temporary drainage channel open for repeated flushing with an antiseptic solution.

If a calf develops a large, painful navel during his first week of life, have your veterinarian examine the calf. He or she can advise you on treatment or follow-up treatment to flush the wound if surgery is required. This surgery is quite simple and can be performed at the veterinary clinic or on the farm.

Inflammation of the Blood Vessels

An infection may stay localized in the umbilicus, the portion of the cord outside the abdominal wall that you can feel through the skin, or it may spread internally, traveling up the blood vessels that served the umbilicus. If it affects the arteries, the infection may ascend all the way to the iliac artery in the pelvic and hip area. More commonly, the umbilical veins are affected. This infection may involve only the lower portion of the veins near the navel or may travel to the liver.

Large abscesses may develop anywhere along the vein and spread to the liver, creating a large abscess that may take up as much as half of the organ. A swollen navel should be checked by your vet to determine whether the infection has spread internally. Often, by the time you notice that there's a problem, the infection has been quietly spreading through the calf's body for several weeks. Affected calves are usually one to three months old by the time illness is obvious to you. They become dull and unthrifty due to chronic toxemia (toxins in the bloodstream).

NAVEL SWELLING MAY BE MORE THAN MEETS THE EYE

ANY ENLARGEMENT AT THE NAVEL should be checked. Years ago, we had a bull calf with an abscess that we lanced and drained, but the infection did not clear up. We treated him with injected antibiotics and caught him daily to flush the draining area with an antiseptic solution squirted into the opening, but even after 10 days of flushing, the drainage still contained pus. Our vet had to surgically remove the labyrinth of infected and necrotic tissue up inside the abdomen. After that, the calf healed with no ill effects. It was a long ordeal, but at least the calf was nicely halter-trained from all the handling.

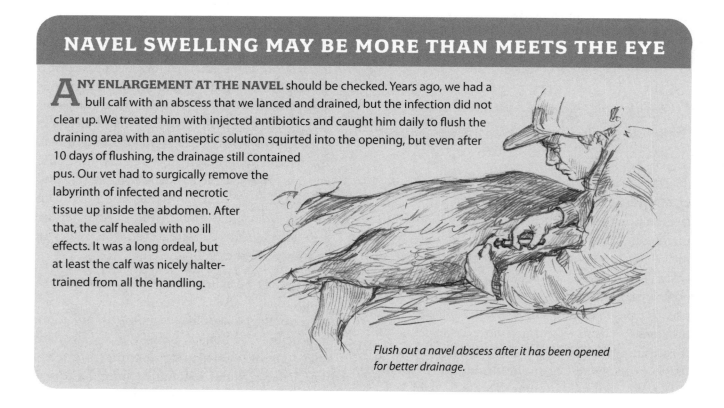

Flush out a navel abscess after it has been opened for better drainage.

TETANUS

In some areas, tetanus is a threat, since this clostridial soil-borne infection can enter via the moist navel if the calf is born on bare ground. Discuss this with your vet, to find out whether you need to worry. Cattle can be vaccinated, and calves can be given tetanus antitoxin at birth, but this is usually not necessary except in high-risk regions or situations.

The navel is often enlarged and abscessed, but in some cases there is no external swelling. Placing the calf on his back and palpating the abdomen by feeling beneath the navel area in the direction of the liver may reveal a firm abscess. You need your vet's help with diagnosis and treatment; antibiotics alone are usually ineffective. The liver abscess must be surgically removed to save the calf, and if the abscess is large, there may be no hope. The risk of this type of navel-infection complication emphasizes the importance of dipping navels and watching for infection.

Infection of the Urachus

Another complication that can occur is infection of the urachus, the tube that goes from navel to bladder. The navel is usually enlarged and draining, but not always. Deep palpation of the calf's abdomen by a vet may reveal an abscess. If the infection extends to the bladder, it too may be infected, with pus in the urine. Surgical removal of this abscess usually results in complete recovery. This condition should be diagnosed and taken care of by your vet.

HANDLING NAVEL ILL

AFTER NEARLY A HUNDRED YEARS of cattle use, our holding pastures and pens were very contaminated by the time we came to our ranch. We had several cases of navel ill in calves born in outdoor pens and pastures, in spite of diligently dipping naval stumps in iodine, because we sometimes were not there at birth to disinfect the navel immediately.

After changing to winter calving to get away from scours in March, we reduced incidence of navel ill. With barn calving, we could provide clean bedding for every cow and new calf, and we were there to dip every navel at every birth. We try to have the navel dry before a calf leaves the barn, but sometimes bull calves are not completely dry, and we've had some infection. A few calves have suffered from joint stiffness or joint tenderness with knees and fetlock joints cocked forward. We treated these with antibiotics and anti-inflammatories and they all recovered quickly.

One of the worst cases was Pipsy, one of our son's calves, born on another ranch (she came here as a weanling). She was born in mud in a barn lot and required extensive treatment for several weeks to save her life after she developed septicemia from navel infection. She recovered but has permanent enlargements in knees, hocks, stifles, and fetlocks. She got over her lameness by the time she was weaned, and she's now a six-year-old cow with big joints. They kept her because they could not sell her; the buyer wouldn't take a calf with big joints.

Bacteremia and Septicemia

Bacteremia simply means the presence of bacteria in the bloodstream that enter through a wound or opening, such as the navel stump in a new calf, and circulate through the bloodstream. Bacteria can localize anywhere in the body and cause problems in organs and joints. Septicemia (sepsis) is systemic disease associated with the presence and persistence of pathogenic bacteria and/or their toxins in the bloodstream. This may occur with certain types of bacterial infections and can be fatal in young animals.

A bloodborne infection may start anywhere in the calf's body, but the most common sites are the intestinal tract, where certain pathogens are ingested and enter the bloodstream through the compromised gut lining (see chapter 11), the respiratory tract, when pneumonia becomes septicemia (see chapter 13), and the moist navel of a new calf. Puncture wounds are another route, but these cases are not as common.

JOINT ILL AS A SECONDARY PROBLEM

WITSI, our month-old calf who survived acute gut infection and endotoxic shock due to colicky bloat (see chapter 11), ended up with sore joints. We noticed joint soreness the second day that she was back with her mother in the barn, after she had spent 24 hours in intensive care in our house and at the vet clinic, receiving IV fluids. Bacteria circulating in her blood during her acute illness settled in her leg joints. We discussed this with our vet and he confirmed our suspicions that Witsi had developed septic arthritis, known to herdsmen as joint ill.

For a couple of weeks, she didn't walk around or stand up for very long, and she walked stiffly. We kept her on a broad-spectrum antibiotic (LA-200, as recommended by our vet) for as long as she had joint pain, giving injections every 3 days for 42 days to prevent permanent joint damage; it took that long before she was walking without lameness. We rubbed DMSO on her fetlock joints, knees, and hocks every day for the first week, to increase circulation in those joints and reduce pain and stiffness. She was a big, strong calf and might have been a challenge to handle. But even though she did not like the daily application of DMSO, she stood patiently for it because she was so accustomed to us.

When Witsi started walking better, we put her and her mother outside, but cold weather made her stiff and lame again, so we put them back into the barn until the weather warmed up. That cow and calf hold the record for longest residence in the barn, and it took a lot of bedding! Fortunately, by the time Witsi had to live in the barn in early February, we were done calving, so we gave the pair several stalls' worth of space, which kept it cleaner.

We still had to perform a major clean-out job when Witsi and her mother could finally live outdoors. After cleaning out all the old bedding, we washed down the walls with disinfectant. We have a rule about never putting sick calves into our calving barn, but it was our warmest barn and it helped save Witsi's life. Technically, she wasn't "sick" by the time we put her in there; she was past the gut infection and just needed a warm, dry place to convalesce. But we washed the walls to make sure that the barn would be clean enough for newborn calves to reside there the following year.

When bacteria and their toxins spread throughout the body and the infection is no longer localized, the toxins are likely to kill the calf. A simple bacteremia, without toxins, is not as life-threatening but may create abscesses somewhere in the body or settle in the joints to cause *joint ill. Septic arthritis* (abscesses in joints) may develop, particularly in leg joints because they are stressed from weight bearing. If the calf survives septic arthritis, he may have enlarged, stiff, and painful joints.

A calf with septicemia from navel infection may show symptoms soon after birth, becoming lethargic, weak, and reluctant to get up. Infection may spread and cause acute and fatal septicemia, or the disease may become chronic after localizing in various organs, joints, or the eyes. Eye inflammation may develop soon after birth. In some cases the calf may die within 12 hours, but many have lingering illness and die after several weeks. At one or two weeks of age, the sick calf has an enlarged navel (umbilical abscess) or sore and swollen joints. At this point, diligent treatment may save him. If neglected, infection will kill the calf.

Broad-spectrum antibiotics are usually effective if given soon enough. There's always a chance for recovery if there's no permanent damage yet to joints or internal organs. If arthritis is already present or there's a navel abscess, the calf may need antibiotics for two weeks or longer, and the abscess should be surgically drained and flushed. Continue antibiotics for several days after he seems fully recovered, or the calf may relapse and be very difficult to save.

Since the intestinal tract and umbilicus are the most common sites of entry, it is important to keep calving areas clean and disinfect the calf's navel cord immediately after birth. Even if you dip the navel in iodine, infection may start if you did it after the stump became dirty as the calf floundered around on the ground or dirty bedding trying to get up.

Effects of Septicemia

If bacteria gain entrance to the body, some types start releasing toxins, causing circulatory dysfunction. Blood pressure drops; the calf goes into septic shock. The body does several things to try to protect itself, but some of these are damaging. Heart rate increases and temperature rises as the calf tries to fight the infection. Respiration rate rises at first, due to fever. The body uses a lot of energy, and the calf is weakened.

The sick calf becomes acidotic because he can't get proper blood flow to organs and muscles. Inadequate blood flow creates lactic acidosis, as it does in an athlete who has been running hard, pushing his or her body to the limit. The combination of decreased blood flow to the calf's body, the shortage of oxygen supply to the muscles, and the increase in lactic acid result in acidosis, which causes muscle weakness and abnormalities in heart rate and intestinal function. The calf can't get enough oxygen to the body tissues. There is poor blood circulation to the gut, so it shuts down. The calf stops nursing. Bacterial toxins affect the liver, and eventually other organs of the body. There is multiorgan failure as the calf goes into shock, unless effects of septicemia are quickly reversed.

LEARNING THE HARD WAY

THE CALF THAT TAUGHT US about diligence in treating navel infection was Esmerelda. She was born in an outdoor pen in the spring of 1968, and we didn't realize that she had an infected navel until she developed signs of septicemia and an enlarged navel at six weeks of age. She had a high fever, was dull, and was not nursing. We brought her home from summer pasture in the back of our Jeep, with her mother following, and treated her for 10 days. Her fever came down, she started nursing again, and we stopped treatment.

A few days later she relapsed with a high fever. Renewed intensive treatment could not save her. Within several days, she went into a coma and died. From then on, we became more careful when tending navels of newborns and never quit treatment of any calf with a navel problem until well after full recovery. Since Esmerelda, we've never lost another calf to navel infection.

Treatment for Septicemia

No matter what route bacteria take when they invade the bloodstream — the umbilicus, the intestines, the lungs — treatment is the same. In all cases the calf needs systemic antibiotics immediately. If septicemia has occurred with lung infection, the calf needs an antibiotic that is effective in lung tissue. If the entry route was the navel, there may also be an abscess in that location, and it must be surgically removed. But antibiotics specific to the case are a must.

Your vet can tell you which antibiotic might be most beneficial and how often to give it. Blood serum may be cultured from a blood sample taken before the calf is treated to find out which pathogen the calf is fighting and which antibiotics would be most effective against it, but growing a culture will take a couple of days, and the calf can't wait that long for treatment. The vet will usually recommend a broad-spectrum antibiotic to start treatment and use it until results of the culture are available. Antibiotics should be continued until the calf is completely recovered, with normal vital signs, for several days, with no more heat, swelling, or pain in the joints if the infection has localized there. This may take two weeks or longer.

If a calf is too sick to nurse, then supportive fluids and nutrients should be given orally or by IV, depending on whether the gut is functional. If the gut shuts down, the calf must be fed by IV. Fluids will help to prevent or reverse shock. Sometimes additional medications are needed to help increase blood pressure. Treating a calf with septicemia is an intensive-care emergency — a round-the-clock job.

Antibiotics and good supportive care are crucial to keep the calf alive until his body can fight the infection. If the infection has a head start before treatment is undertaken, it may be a losing battle.

Prevention

Prevention for any type of septicemia is a clean environment (see chapter 10). It's also crucial to make sure every newborn calf nurses colostrum within the first hour or two of birth to get the antibodies he'll need, to fight common infections. Have an emergency supply of frozen colostrum at the ready (see chapter 7). A number of studies have shown that calves receiving adequate levels of antibodies from colostrum have less incidence of septicemia and are less at risk for fatal infections.

Umbilical Hernia

This problem is sometimes mistaken for a navel abscess, because there's an enlargement in that area. An *umbilical hernia* is a hole or separation in the outer wall of the abdomen that allows fluid or tissue to bulge through and creates an enlargement under the skin. The hole may be small, just enough to allow passage of one or two fingers, and all that protrudes is a bulge of fluid-filled tissue that you can press back in. This enlargement may be the size of a marble or a golf ball. If it's larger than that, allowing passage of several fingers, have your veterinarian check it.

If the hole is small, it will generally close up as the calf grows. If it's large enough to allow a loop of intestine to slip through, it may be dangerous to the calf. If a piece of small intestine gets caught in the hole, it may strangulate (impair the blood supply to the intestine) and cause fatal complications. Your vet can assess the risk and decide whether the opening will close as the calf grows or whether it needs to be surgically corrected.

Surgical correction is simple and can be done at the clinic or farm. With the calf on his back, to keep him from struggling and to make sure intestines stay inside the opening, the area is anesthetized, the skin is slit, the opening in the abdominal wall is stitched closed, and the skin is sewed up again.

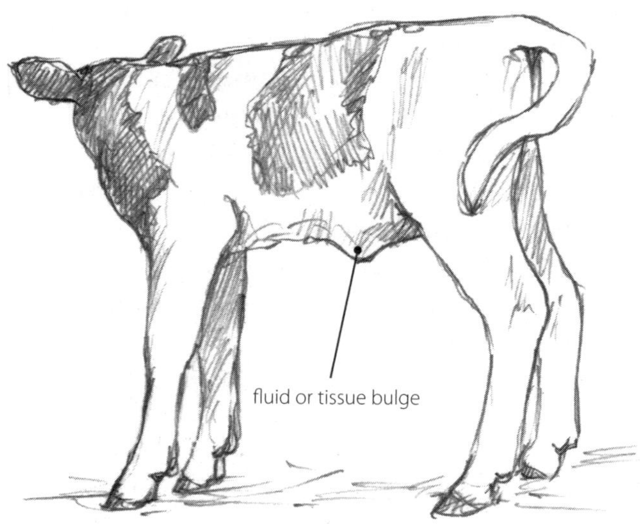

A loop of intestine is contained within the skin of the belly in the most common umbilical hernia types.

HERNIA CORRECTION

OVER THE PAST 40 YEARS, we've had two calves that had surgical corrections of hernias. Both the surgeries were performed here on the ranch in a clean barn stall, one on a month-old heifer. After monitoring her hernia, it was determined that it wasn't closing up well enough and needed help. The other calf was a bull born with a huge hole at the navel that the vet stitched up.

We had another hernia case that did not require surgery but was immediately life-threatening. Loops of intestine prolapsed down into the umbilical membranes of the navel cord on a newborn calf after he got up to nurse, creating a bulging "cord" about 6 inches long and 3 inches in diameter. It looked like a big sausage. We called our vet and he showed us how to correct it by simply pushing and squeezing the intestine back up into the abdomen. We then placed an elastrator band over the umbilical membranes at the belly to hold them closed and so that the intestines could not drop down again. The hole was then able to close up and heal.

Umbilical hernias occur most often in heifers, and there may be a genetic tendency. A cow with an umbilical hernia as a calf is more likely to have calves that have this problem. There may be more incidence of umbilical hernia in some breeds than others. Because of the tendency for this problem to be inherited, it is not wise to keep a heifer for breeding if she had a hernia.

CORRECTING A HERNIA

If a loop of intestine drops down into the umbilical cord membranes of a newborn calf, it's a serious emergency and must be treated as soon as it is observed. This type of hernia can be corrected without surgery, however. If you have an elastrator banding tool and band, you can deal with this problem yourself, without having to take the calf to a veterinarian.

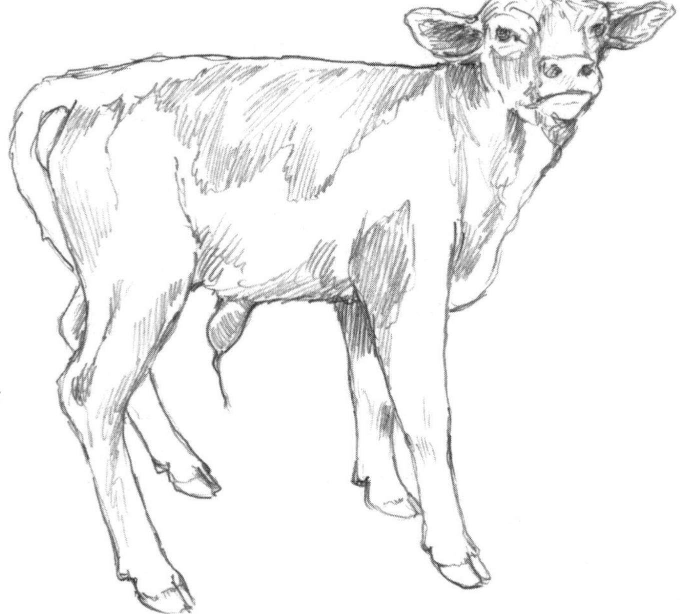

A loop of intestine protrudes through an opening in the skin but is still contained within the umbilical membranes, the cord stump tissue, of a newborn calf. While this sort of umbilical hernia is uncommon, it is more life-threatening, because the thin membranes may rupture.

To Correct an Umbilical Hernia

1. Gently push or squeeze the intestines back up into the abdomen and out of the umbilical cord.

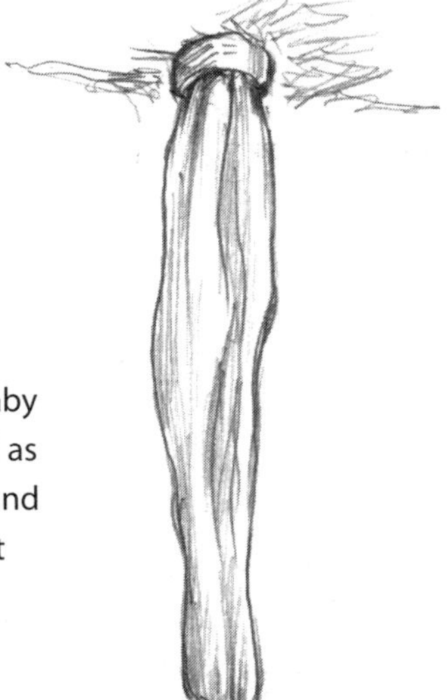

2. Place a rubber elastrator band, used for banding and castrating baby bull calves, over the now empty umbilical cord and push the band as high as possible on the umbilical stump before releasing it. The band will then hold the cord closed so that the loops of intestine cannot come back down. With the band in place, the navel area will have time to heal and grow together, closing the hole in the belly wall.

Chapter 15

Miscellaneous Calfhood Problems

In the first months of a calf's life, the animal can be plagued by any number of possible ills. Some problems can be prevented with proper feeding and good management, but others are accidents or caused by environmental situations that are hard to anticipate or prevent. It helps to know what some of the possible problems are; if you can suspect or recognize a certain situation, you may be able to save the calf.

White Muscle Disease

White muscle disease is a degeneration of muscle tissue in calves whose dams are deficient in selenium during pregnancy. In certain geographic areas, soils contain little of this important trace element, and feeds grown in these areas are also deficient. If a cow's diet is low in selenium during pregnancy, her calf is at risk unless he's given an injection of selenium soon after birth. This is often given with vitamin E, since these two essential micronutrients work together.

A calf that has inadequate selenium usually appears to be normal at birth, but he may die suddenly within a few weeks during exercise or may be found lying down, unable to get up. If he can stand when you try to get him up, he may be weak and trembling and may collapse. He walks with a rotating movement of the hocks if he's strong enough to walk. Nursing is difficult, and he spends most of his time lying down. Muscles of the diaphragm and chest are also affected, which makes it hard for him to breathe. If treated at this point with an injection of vitamin E and selenium, he may recover within a few days. But if he develops the condition after he's several months old, he may die suddenly of heart failure.

Postmortem examination of a calf that dies will show obvious muscle degeneration. Large areas are white or streaked with white (hence the name of white muscle disease) rather than normal red. The damaged muscles are inactive and have less *myoglobin,* the red iron-containing protein pigment of normal muscles. Calcium salts deposited in the damaged muscle tissue add to the whiteness.

Certain internal organs are affected more than others. Scar tissue may build up in the heart, reducing its elasticity. A fast-growing calf may suddenly die of heart failure by the time he reaches three hundred to four hundred pounds. Even if he survives after treatment with selenium, he may not do well, since scarred tissue cannot regenerate.

Prevention

If you live in a selenium-deficient area, supplement your cattle with this trace mineral, using salt or mineral blocks or mixes that contain selenium. If there's a question as to the dams' nutritional status regarding selenium, calves can be given an injection soon after birth to prevent muscle degeneration. Find out from your vet if your area is deficient. Discuss whether or not you should give supplemental doses, and if so, how much. The vet can also tell you what products to use.

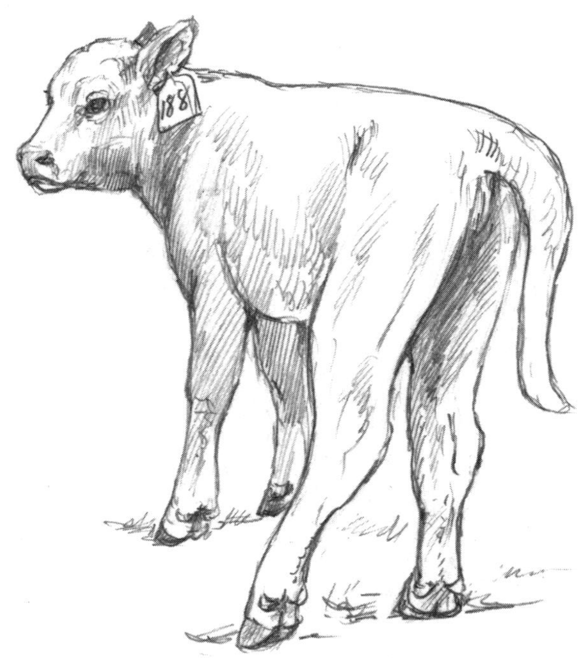

Some calves are born with crooked "windswept" hind legs due to lack of room in the uterus. The legs often straighten within a few weeks.

LEARNING ABOUT COPPER DEFICIENCY

IN EARLIER DAYS, the ranchers in our valley didn't know about copper deficiency. Signs are often subtle. Looking back, we realize that some problems in calves may have been due to copper deficiency.

In 1975, a calf named Huckle had contracted tendons with knees and fetlock joints poking forward so much that it was hard for her to walk. She could not be sold with the other calves that fall, so we kept her through winter to get her big enough to butcher. One day, we noticed that she was missing. We searched that evening with flashlights and found her lying partly on her back in a dry ditch. She had fallen and couldn't get out.

Cattle cannot survive for very long on their backs. Abdominal pressure against the lungs reduces air capacity, and because they can't belch, they tend to bloat, which puts even more pressure on the lungs. Fortunately, we rescued Huckle before she suffocated.

Crooked Legs and Other Deformities

Some calves are born with crooked legs due to *contracted tendons.* Others have curved limbs due to inadequate space in the uterus or a placenta deficiency. A long-legged calf may have *"windswept"* hind legs, with both legs curving the same direction, shaped like double parentheses. Windswept legs usually straighten in the first weeks of life. Contracted tendons may not correct, however. The leg or legs may be cocked forward at the knees and fetlocks. This can be due to a number of causes, including nutritional deficiencies. In some cases, the deformity is temporary and may be helped by exercise or by injections of vitamin A or by copper supplementation, which can be given as an oral time-release bolus, by injection, or in a salt-mineral mix. In other cases, the deformity is permanent, depending on the cause.

Many regions in the United States and Canada have problems with copper deficiency because of excess of certain other minerals. Molybdenum, iron, zinc, lead, or calcium carbonate can tie up copper so that it can't be utilized by the animal's body. When molybdenum levels in soil are high, or there is too much molybdenum relative to the amount of copper, this type of copper deficiency can create weak and brittle bones in calves and increased incidence of broken legs.

If you have instances of contracted tendons or broken bones in calves, talk to your vet. He or she can take blood samples or liver biopsies of cattle in your herd, or liver samples from an aborted fetus or any animal that dies or is butchered on your place, to see if there is a deficiency problem. If so, it can be corrected with proper mineral supplements or injections recommended by your vet.

Signs and Symptoms of Copper Deficiency

Look for the following subtle signs of copper deficiency in young calves:

- Skeletal problems
- Poor hair coat
- Impaired immune system: poor response to vaccinations, more susceptibility to illness

- Reduced weight gain
- Change in hair color: black animals have a red or gray tint to the hair, and red animals become more bleached and light-colored; hair is dull instead of shiny.
- Possible diarrhea, anemia, brittle bones, or lameness
- Stiffness in the gait
- Ends of cannon bones enlarged and painful (sore fetlock joints)
- Pasterns very upright
- Contracted flexor tendons at the back of the leg
- Calf walking on his toes

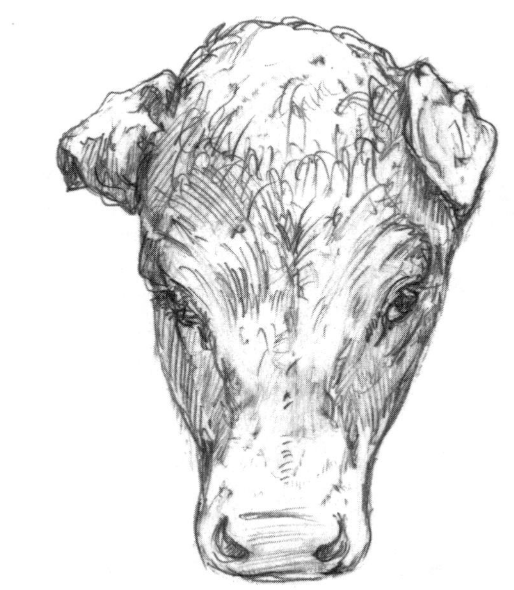

Birth defects may be minor — unsightly but not serious. A calf may be born with abnormal ears . . .

Birth Defects

Some common birth defects are covered in chapter 2 of this book. Many defects result in death or humane destruction of a calf if it can't survive outside of the uterus. Some defects are less crippling (moderately crooked legs, cleft palate, blindness, etc.), and the calf can be raised for butchering. Others do not significantly hinder the calf, such as malformed ears, no tail, etc., or can be corrected with minor surgery. For instance, we had one calf born with extra eyelid tissue, which had to be removed because the eyelashes were digging into his eyeball.

When an abnormal calf is born, evaluate the problem and determine whether he can be raised, or consult with your vet to see if there is hope for the calf to lead a normal life. Some skeletal problems are only mildly crippling, and the calf can still get around, while other defects severely impair mobility. Some internal problems interfere with function of vital systems, such as incomplete formation of the intestines. When in doubt, have your vet examine the calf.

Some defects are inherited as a *dominant gene* passed on by one parent, or a *recessive gene,* the trait hidden in each parent, only showing up in the offspring because it's doubled up. This is good reason to pay attention to genetics. Do not breed cows with known recessive defects to bulls with the same undesirable recessive traits evident in their offspring. *Inbreeding* should be avoided, since undesirable hidden traits not evident in the parents can show up in the calves. Some defects, like dwarfism, show up only if both parents carry the recessive gene, as when breeding father to daughter or siblings to one another.

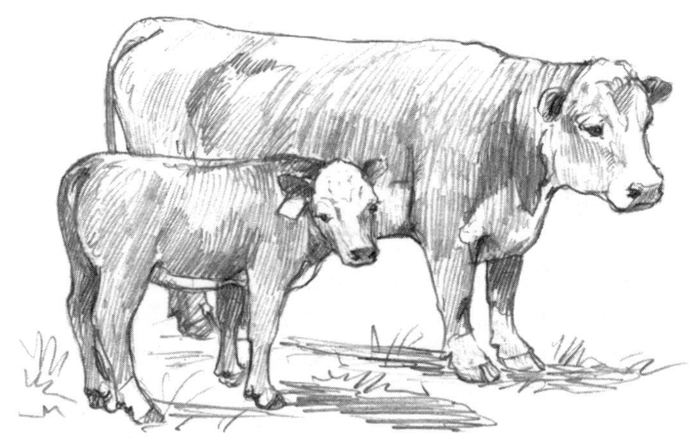

. . . or with no tail at all.

Scrotal Hernia

Although scrotal hernia tends to be an inherited defect, and you can usually trace it back to a certain sire, you might not even notice it until you go to put a rubber band on a bull calf or prepare to castrate him with a knife. On the other hand, it may be so large that you can see a bulge of tissue in the scrotal area; the scrotal sac may be so distended that you might think the calf has extremely large testicles. With this defect, the small opening in the abdominal wall that

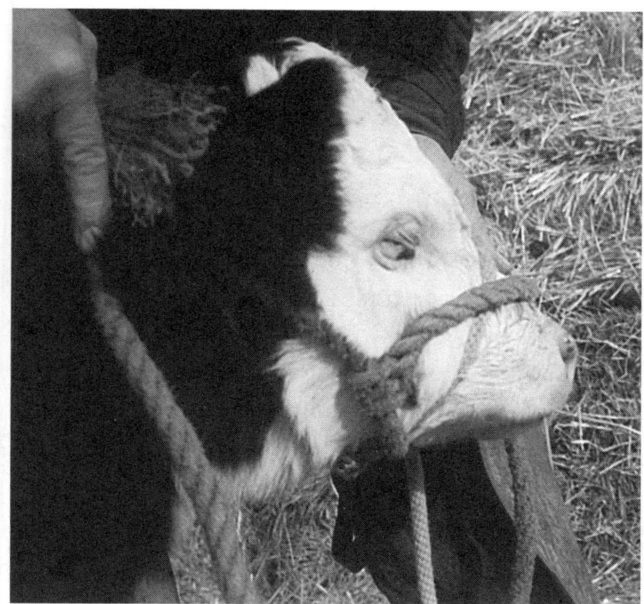

This calf was born with an extra piece of tissue on one lower eyelid, with the eyelashes slanting into the eye and irritating the eyeball.

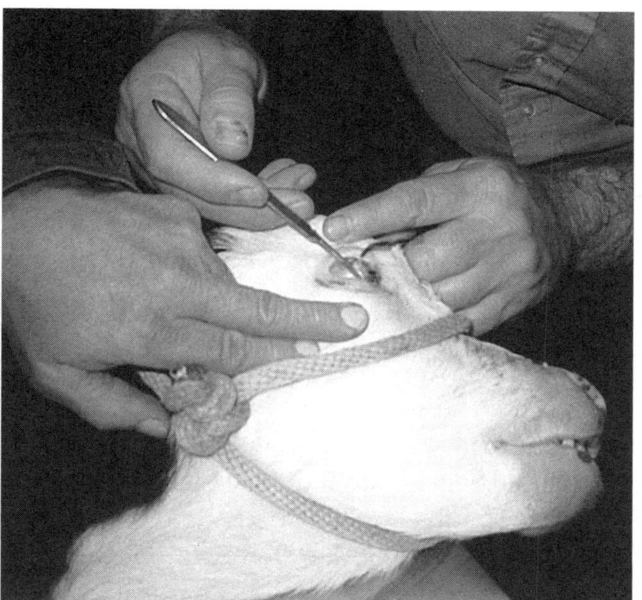

Removing the extra tissue, with the calf sedated

BLOODLINE DEBACLE

IN THE EARLY 1970s, we discovered that the expensive bull that we bought in 1969 carried a defective gene. We used him for several years, and he had such good calves that we kept many of his daughters, and three of his sons as bulls. We had enough cows and separate breeding pastures for different bull groups, so we could avoid inbreeding by selecting an unrelated sire for each cow. But back then, we were not yet to the point where we could breed all our cows at home in a chosen breeding group. We were still turning bulls on the range to finish the breeding season — and on the range all cattle run in the same big pasture.

We made the mistake of turning out on the range one of the sons of our expensive bull. He bred two of his half sisters, and both had defective calves the next year. We knew their calves were sired by their half brother because of the dates of birth, which showed that they were range-bred, born later than the calves sired in the fields in selected breeding groups. The calves looked normal, except for slightly rounded foreheads, but neither had a normal suck reflex. The first one was born small and seemed a little premature and impaired. She was unable to get up and nurse her mother, so we brought her into the house and fed her colostrum by stomach tube. We named her Bitty Baby Belle and kept her in the house in a box for three weeks as I tried to get her to nurse a bottle, but I always ended up feeding her by tube. If she struggled and bumped her head on the side of the wooden box, she went into convulsions.

The second calf was proper size and got right up after birth but seemed retarded and wouldn't nurse her mother. We tried to feed her a bottle, and she refused to suck. While fighting our attempts to feed her, she'd throw herself down or bump into the stall wall. After bumping her head several times and going into a spastic fit each time, we recognized the similarity between the two calves and admitted defeat. We were dealing with an inherited defect. Because our efforts were futile, we humanely destroyed them both. From then on, we made sure that we never doubled up those bloodlines, and we had no more retarded calves.

We were able to continue on with all the daughters of our expensive bull, including the two that had defective calves, by making sure always to breed them to unrelated bulls. We kept no more bull calves from that bloodline, and this eliminated the chance of doubling up the recessive gene that caused the problem.

allows for tubes and blood vessels serving the testicles is too big, allowing loops of intestine to fall through. If the opening is only slightly larger than it should be, intestines won't come down through it and you'll probably never know it's there.

If you castrate little bulls by putting a rubber band above the testicles, this resolves the problem, because nothing can come down into the scrotum and the tissue grows together after the testicles die and fall off. If you castrate surgically, however, cutting off the end of the scrotum to remove the testicles, the calf may herniate. Loops of intestine fall through the hole in the abdomen. If he struggles as you are castrating him, his straining to get free may push a big pile of intestines right out into your lap. If this happens, the best thing to do is place the calf on his back, try to keep him from struggling, and put gentle pressure over the mass of intestines with a clean, wet towel to protect them and to prevent more loops from coming out of the hole. If the calf is small and easy to transport, rush him to your vet clinic if you have a couple of people to hold him still in a vehicle. Otherwise, call your vet and try to hold the calf still and keep the intestines contained until the vet gets there to disinfect them, push them back in, and stitch up the abdominal hole.

Hairballs

Over the past 40 years raising cattle, we've had several calves suffer gut blockage from ingesting wads of hair. Cattle often swallow some hair when licking themselves, especially when shedding winter coats in the spring, and this is usually not a problem. Curious calves, however, often chew on and lick everything and may ingest clumps of hair rubbed off on a fence, tree stump, or some other itching spot, or a clump of hair hanging from their mothers' udders when cows are shedding. Usually the hair goes on through the tract and is sometimes seen in manure, but occasionally a large clump will lodge in a narrow place in the tract, such as the valve between stomach and small intestine. If not resolved, this blockage will kill the calf.

If the hairball or clump creates blockage in the intestines, fluid and food cannot go through. Material in the gut builds up at that spot, creating pressure and pain. The calf is usually dull or uncomfortable, goes off feed, and has no bowel movements. When faced with a dull calf that's not nursing, you might be inclined to treat for diarrhea, but it would be a mistake to fill him with fluid that can't go through, or a gut soother like Kaopectate. If there is no evidence of diarrhea, or if fecal material is scanty or absent, suspect a blockage or shut-down gut. The calf may pass manure for a while, material that was in the "rear end" of the tract, but soon the large intestine is empty. He may eventually go into shock if there is trauma to the gut. If he doesn't die of shock, then sooner or later the gut ruptures, and he dies swiftly.

Treatment

If you suspect blockage from dirt or a hairball, the best "home" treatment is castor oil, a laxative that lubricates the gut contents and stimulates the gut to move. If the hairball is small, castor oil may help the calf move it past the narrow spot; we've found wads of hair in the manure of treated calves after the gut started working again. Castor oil works better than mineral oil. The latter is a good lubricant but does not stimulate the gut to contract and move. A large dose of castor oil is more effective and will work unless the hairball is too large to come through.

Surgery

In a couple of cases that we could not resolve with castor oil, we saved the calves by taking them to our vet for surgery to remove the hairball. If surgery is done soon, before the calf's condition deteriorates too much, after being blocked for several days, he has a good chance for recovery.

HAIRBALL BLOCKAGE

OUR FIRST CASE, a month-old calf named Spud, was dull and off feed for two days, and we couldn't figure out what the problem was. He did not improve with antibiotics and supportive treatment, and he died. When we cut him open to investigate the cause of death, we discovered that he'd ruptured internally, and we found a big wad of hair.

Hairballs Can Be Fatal

One morning during the spring of 2003, we discovered that a month-old calf was dull, bloated, and not nursing. We brought Bingo and his young mama in from the field and gave him an oral antibiotic and a big dose of castor oil. We put the pair in our sick barn, out of the wet weather. Bingo did not improve, however, even after several days of castor oil, fluids (both oral and IV), and enemas; he did not pass any manure. We suspected a hairball blockage, since the cows were shedding and rubbing off wads of hair on the trees and fences. Even though we gathered up a lot of it, the calves were nibbling on some of the hair they found.

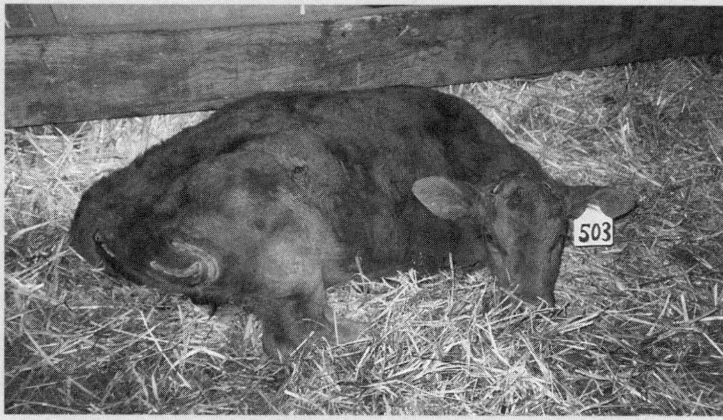

A dull calf has total gut blockage by a hairball. If the blockage is not resolved, a calf with a hairball will eventually go into shock, or the gut will rupture, and he will die. In this particular calf, we suspected a hairball and wanted our vet to do surgery, but the vet didn't think it was a hairball and didn't want to perform the surgery. The calf died several days later, in spite of all our efforts at intensive care (IV and oral fluids, castor oil, etc.).

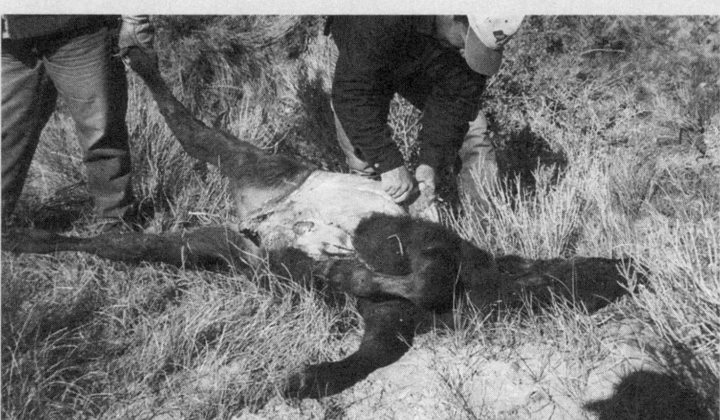

Our son skinned the abdominal area in preparation to open the calf up to confirm the cause of death.

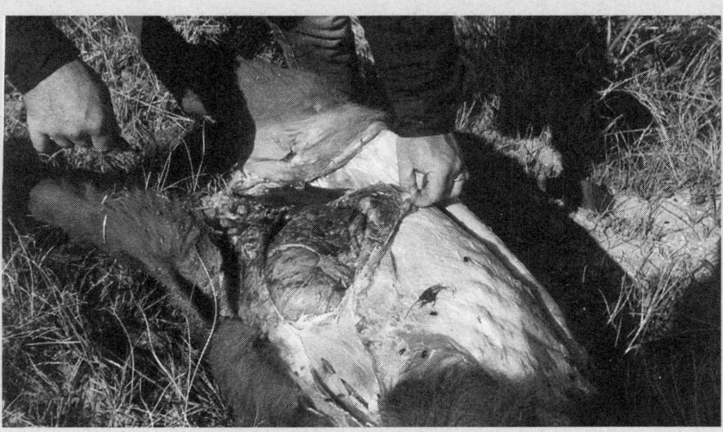

With the calf cut open, we discovered that the gut had ruptured, and that there were big wads of hair all through the abdominal cavity and in the fluid that had escaped from the ruptured intestine. This confirmed our suspicions that blockage was due to a hairball and that surgery to remove it was the only action that might have saved this calf.

Other Types of Gut Blockage

Calves may develop fatal blockage from eating plastic bags, baling twine, or anything that gets caught in a narrow part of the tract and can't go through. A wad of twine can plug the valve between stomach and intestine, for instance. Cattle often eat baling twine left in the hay, and a calf will chew on twine out of curiosity. Twine should never be left lying around where calves can find it. A cow generally won't die from eating twine; she has a larger tract, and it tends to pass through or is eventually broken down by digestive action. A calf, though, is always at risk for fatal blockage.

Calves can also die from eating dirt that plugs up the valve that leads out of the stomach. Young calves often nibble dirt or mud, just to sample it. In some instances they eat a lot of dirt, especially if they're short on salt or certain minerals. Even if you supplement with minerals, however, calves born in winter or early spring, with no green grass and lots of mud to sample, tend to consume a lot of mud and dirt, partly just as something to do. Usually dirt will go on through, and you often see it in the feces. Problems arise when calves consume a lot, creating blockage, or eat small rocks or gravel with the dirt. In some situations sharp rocks can puncture the stomach or gravel can irritate, create ulcerations, or wear a hole through the lining, resulting in fatal peritonitis. If calves are eating dirt, work with your vet or extension agent to see if your feeds are short on certain minerals and you need to provide a mineral supplement. Meanwhile, keep calves away from their favorite dirt banks with fencing, if possible.

Gut blockage can also be due to bruising of the stomach or intestines. Sometimes the damaged part no longer functions properly, and nothing can pass through. If it heals soon enough, things start working again, unless there's impaction of food material at that spot. But if damage is severe and blood supply to the intestine too compromised, that section of intestine may die, with no hope for spontaneous resolution.

Sometimes these cases can be resolved with exploratory surgery to find the problem and remove the damaged part. Your vet can assess the situation and determine whether there might be a chance for the calf with supportive treatment and laxatives or surgery. We were able to save one calf (Dixie — see chapter 9) with surgical removal of a section of dead intestine.

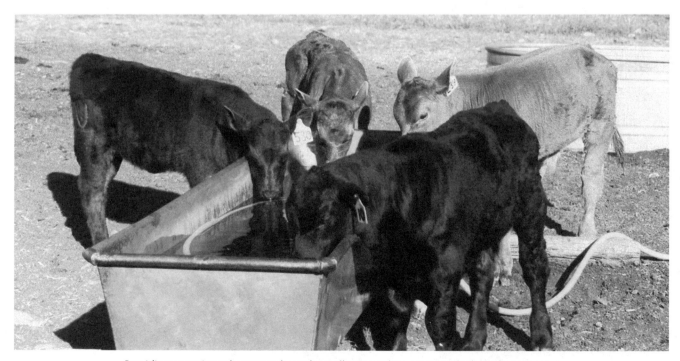

Providing water in tanks or troughs and not allowing calves access to ditch banks or streams where there is lots of dirt, sand, or gravel to nibble can help reduce dirt-eating.

WASH THAT DIRT RIGHT OUT OF THE GUT

WE'VE ALWAYS HAD PROBLEMS with winter-born calves eating dirt and on two occasions plugging up their digestive tract, despite the availability of mineral supplements. A calf that's off feed for any number of reasons will often nibble on strange things rather than nursing his mama. Dirt is one of their favorite things to sample.

Our first vet, who taught us how to use a nasogastric tube for giving fluids to sick calves, also showed us how to wash dirt out of a calf's stomach. The idea is to put water into the calf's stomach through the tube and then let the water drain back out of the calf. If the calf is standing and you have someone to help hold him still, it's not hard to lower your end of the tube (and the calf's head and neck) when you siphon the water back out. If the calf is lying down, it's more difficult to get your end of the tube below stomach level unless you elevate the calf. When flushing dirt out of calves brought to his clinic, our vet usually laid the patient on a table so he could lower the funnel end of the tube below the calf's body to drain the stomach.

When we discovered that our month-old calf Jillie was plugged with dirt, bloated, and not passing manure, we noticed that she had dirt on her muzzle — telltale evidence that she had been eating dirt. Some calves will actually still have dirt in their mouths when you realize that they're sick, because they continue to eat it even after their digestive tract is upset or blocked.

We used the flushing technique to save Jillie. We backed her into a corner and inserted the tube to put water into her stomach, then lowered one end below stomach level so the water would come back out the tube, bringing some of the dirt with it. We repeated this flushing several times, until fluid came back out clear, rather than full of dirt. After getting as much dirt out as possible, we gave Jillie 7 ounces (207 mL) of castor oil to help work any residual dirt on through, and this resolved her problem. Her bloat disappeared, and the next day she passed large quantities of feces, full of dirt. We told our vet about it; he chuckled and said he was glad that it was Jillie, not he, receiving that much castor oil! But it worked; she survived and had 11 calves of her own.

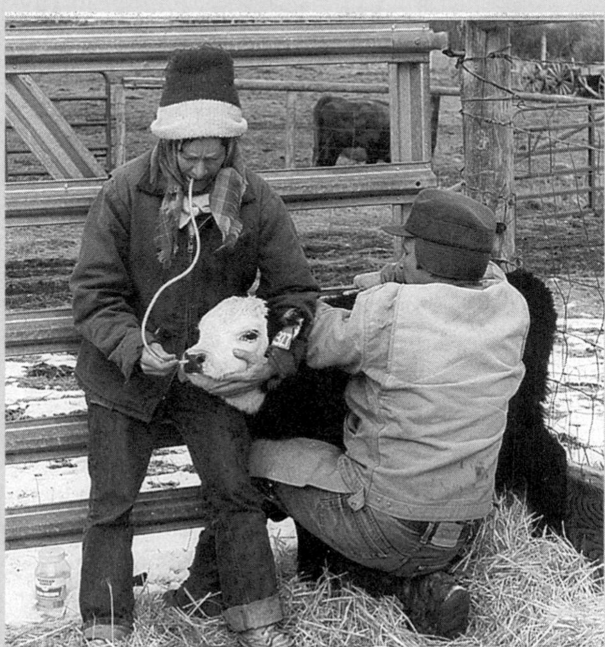

We inserted a stomach tube into a calf that was plugged with dirt.

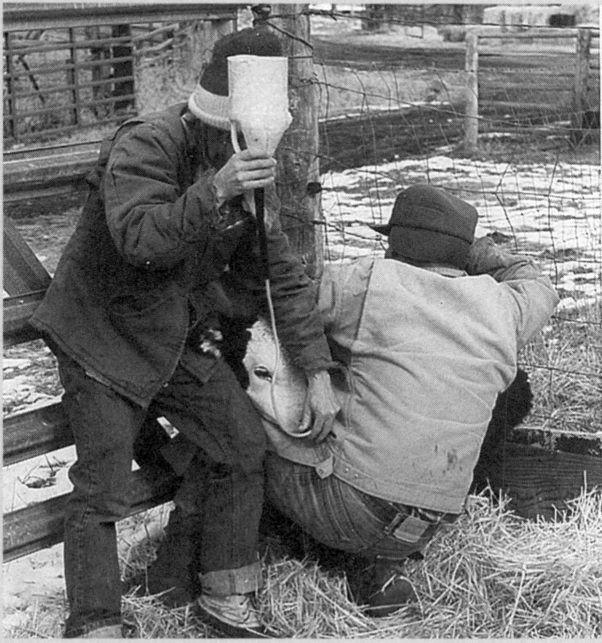

We then ran water into the stomach, so that we could siphon it back out the tube and bring some of the dirt with it.

Digestive-Tract Ulcers

This problem occasionally occurs in calves and can be due to infection that damages the intestinal lining (see chapter 11), stress, or certain types of nutritional deficiency. Ulcers can be serious, causing discomfort and pain. The calf goes off feed and is dull, often grinding his teeth (a grating sound). He may drool from all the teeth-grinding. The ulcers usually heal if you force-feed him when he won't nurse and sooth the raw gut lining with mineral oil or other gut soothers, like Kaopectate or bismuth subsalicylate, to coat and buffer the ulcerated tissue. If the calf is passing scanty, firm bowel movements, mineral oil is better than Kaopectate, because you don't want to make him more constipated.

A calf with signs of ulcers should always be treated and force-fed if he's not nursing. Otherwise, he may become emaciated and vulnerable to illness because of his run-down condition. If an ulcer becomes too severe and deep, it may go clear through the stomach or intestinal wall and lead to fatal peritonitis. If you have a high number of calves with ulcers, work with your vet to find the cause. If it's due to gut irritation from eating dirt because of mineral deficiency, you might be able to correct the deficiency.

Bloat

Bloat in adults, or older calves with functional rumens, is generally caused by fermentable feeds. Gas produced by the fermentation process of digestion is excessive in certain instances, and belching can't get rid of it fast enough, so it distends the rumen. Serious bloat in a large animal can often be relieved by passing a tube down the throat into the rumen to let out gas or by sticking the rumen with a sharp tool such as a trocar, which is designed for this task, or even a pocketknife.

Bloat in a young calf is more often due to gut infection than fermentable feeds; a young calf doesn't overeat on forage or grain. Most of his nutrients come from milk. He relies at first on his simple stomach to digest milk; at birth his rumen is small. He starts nibbling grass or hay at an early age, following his mother's example, and may start chewing his cud at 10 to 12 days of age, but it takes several weeks before his rumen is fully functional and capable of digesting much roughage. You typically don't see bloat caused by fermentable feeds in a calf younger than four weeks.

Sometimes a young calf will develop bloat, however, due to digestive-tract infection and bacterial toxins that produce gas. This can happen as young as two weeks of age and up to several months of age. Depending on the type of bacteria involved, the infection may simply hinder proper digestion for a while or it may shut down the gut, as some toxin-forming bacteria can do, and create serious bloating. The infection itself can kill the calf unless treated, but the bloat may be so severe that the calf is in danger of immediate suffocation. It must be relieved.

A bloated calf will have a very large abdomen. Viewed from front or rear, he looks like a balloon with legs. If his rumen is distended, it will be sticking up higher, protruding upward and outward on his left side.

Signs and Syptoms

A bloated calf will have a very large abdomen. Viewed from front or rear, he looks like a balloon with legs. If his rumen is distended, it will be sticking up higher, protruding upward and outward on his left side. After the distended rumen or digestive tract becomes so full that it encroaches on space needed for lung expansion, he'll be breathing very shallowly; he cannot take a deep breath. Abdominal movements from breathing are reduced, often accompanied by grunting sounds. He stands with head and neck extended and mouth open, trying to breathe. Unless he is very ill and unable to stand, he will be standing, since lying down puts more pressure on his lungs, making it harder to breathe. By that point, when he starts gasping for air, he has only a short time left, unless you immediately relieve the bloat. If he staggers and goes down, only swift action can save his life.

Treatment

In a calf up to two or three weeks of age, the rumen is not large enough to be the main area of gas accumulation. Gas distension may be in the intestines and difficult to relieve except by giving a large dose of castor oil by tube. Castor oil works better than mineral oil for this sort of bloat (see chapter 11) because it not only breaks up foamy gas bubbles but also stimulates the shut-down gut to start moving again, thus getting toxin-forming contents out of there, and it binds up some of the bacterial toxins to inactivate them.

The large volume of gas in a calf with a distended rumen puts so much pressure on the calf's lungs that he has little space to breathe. He needs castor oil to start moving the digestive tract again and halt bloating, but first he needs to get rid of the gas that's causing immediate danger to his life — before he suffocates. A severely bloated calf has no room in his tract for anything else (such as castor oil) and is apt to die before you get the oil into him; if he struggles while you're treating him, his need for extra oxygen will kill him even faster. Release the gas with a needle before giving him oil (see box).

If the calf is not severely bloated, and you've decided that your first course of action is to tube him with oil (mineral oil for simple bloat from fermented feeds, castor oil if gas is due to a gut infection and toxins), you may hit a pocket of gas when inserting a nasogastric tube. In those instances, gas will come rushing out your end of the tube (an esophageal feeder probe doesn't go far enough into the stomach to release gas). If you begin to give him oil via the tube and you see that he's struggling to breathe and starts to collapse, discontinue the oil treatment and stick him with the needle.

IF YOU'VE GOT TO LUBE IT, TUBE IT

Always give oil by tube; never try to "drench" a calf by putting it in the mouth to make him swallow it, or some may get into his windpipe. If oil gets into the lungs, it stays there — it can't be coughed up, like water — and will cause aspiration pneumonia.

Pass the Gas with a Needle

If gas distension is in the rumen rather than spread throughout the intestines, follow these steps to release it:

1. Have a helper restrain the calf, or hold him against a fence or backed into a corner so he won't move away — unless he is on the ground and about to suffocate, in which case he won't try to get away from you.
2. Stick the rumen with a 2- to 3-inch (5 to 7.6 cm)-long sterile hypodermic needle, 16-gauge or larger.
3. Thrust it forcefully into the distended area on the calf's left side, in the middle of the triangular area between hip bone, backbone, and last rib. In a normal calf, this area is soft and hollow; in a bloated calf it bulges like a balloon, higher than the backbone. If the rumen is distended, there is no danger of hitting anything vital if you aim for the middle or highest area of that "balloon."
4. Jab through the skin, on through the abdominal lining and into the rumen. All these tissues are pressed tightly together on a bloated calf; the needle goes right into the rumen. Gas should immediately come rushing out through the puncturing needle.
5. Hold the needle in place while the gas releases.
6. If the needle plugs before the gas is all out, wiggle it around or attach a small syringe, and blow the plug out with back pressure from a little air in the syringe.
7. Continue holding the needle in place until all gas is out, the rumen is deflated and no longer bulging upward, and the calf is breathing normally again. The last bit of gas to come out may be foamy with some fluid in it, which can plug the needle.
8. If the calf bloats again later, stick him again if necessary. Repeat as many times as needed to keep him from suffocating until the medication you give him — oil or oil and antibiotics if it's a gut infection rather than a feed problem — has time to correct the condition creating the bloat.

Seizures

On rare occasion you may have a calf that suffers from seizures or *convulsions.* He may stagger around and fall to the ground, and his muscles may go into spasm. While he's lying there, his legs may make paddling movements. His neck stiffens, and his head arches upward and back. He may stop breathing and pass out; then, as the muscles gradually relax, he starts breathing again. In some instances the seizures don't let up and become almost continuous, as in the end stages of encephalitis or poisoning, when the calf is dying.

Convulsions may be due to a number of factors, such as injury to the brain; infection that affects the brain, such as meningitis or encephalitis; shortage of oxygen to the brain; poisoning from certain plants or chemicals; and inherited or congenital defects. Brain injury or shortage of oxygen during birth can also lead to seizures. Heredity; malnutrition in the dam, such as vitamin A deficiency; and virus infection or exposure to certain toxins in early pregnancy can be factors that lead to seizures in newborn calves.

There are a few inherited defects in cattle that cause mild or complete paralysis of calves, including a spinal defect in Angus and Charolais calves. An inherited defect can cause convulsions and lack of coordination in Angus calves soon after birth, and an inherited spastic condition is sometimes seen in Jersey and Hereford calves by the time the calf is between two to five days old. There is a type of inherited epilepsy found in some Brown Swiss calves. Over the years we've had three otherwise normal calves that suffered periodic convulsions, with seizure episodes starting several days to a week after birth. Though one lived to be a month old, none survived. They all eventually suffocated during one of their seizures.

Sometimes you never know the cause of a seizure problem or the best way to deal with it. In many instances the calf's chances are poor, especially if the problem is due to infection, poison, brain damage or an inherited defect in the brain, but in others there may be hope for him to outgrow the problem if he can be helped to survive his seizure episodes. There is medication that may help some calves. This is something to discuss with your veterinarian.

Lupine Calves

Range pastures in the West and Midwest are habitat for several species of *lupine,* a hardy wildflower that blooms early in spring, with blooms staying on for many weeks. Some are harmless if eaten, but other types contain alkaloids that cause deformities in unborn calves when eaten by cows in early pregnancy. On our ranch, over a span of 40 calving seasons, we have had 11 "crooked calves" with one or both front legs cocked forward with deformed or fused joints. They were able to walk around, however, and we raised them. Another lupine calf, Prue, was born with a cleft palate (see chapter 9).

Until 2003 we had only one calf so deformed, with twisted spine and legs that it could not function and had to be destroyed at birth. That calf was so abnormal that it was a wonder the cow was able to give birth without surgery. We were not so lucky in 2003, when our son and his wife, who pasture their cows on part of our place, our range, and the neighboring ranch, had five malformed calves, three of which were so deformed that they had to be delivered by c-section.

A cow is most at risk for fetal defects if she eats lupine between day 30 and day 70 of gestation. The poisonous species are dangerous from the time they start growing in spring until they dry up in the fall, and the pods shatter and the toxic seeds have dropped. Cool, wet weather is ideal for lupine growth. Incidence of crooked calves can be reduced by keeping cows out of lupine patches, but if rangeland is the only pasture you have during summer, it's hard to avoid the risk.

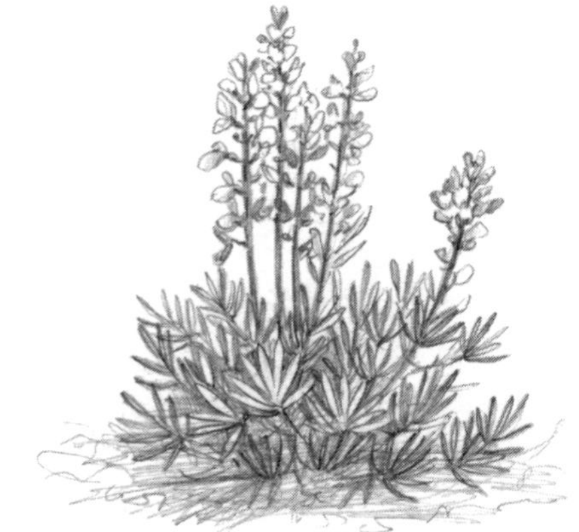

Several types of lupine, some of which are toxic to cows, are common in range pastures in many areas of North America.

THE LUPINE LADY

QUEENIE WAS A LUPINE CALF that became our daughter's pet. Andrea had a few cows of her own, and one of them, a crossbreed named Zimbobbee, had trouble giving birth to her second calf. We had to pull it, and it was a very hard pull, even though the calf was not large. Andrea named the calf African Queen, but we soon called her Queenie. The calf did not get up, so we helped her to stand and discovered that her front legs were crooked.

Zimbobbee was upset with our handling her calf when we held her up to nurse her but stood still for nursing. Andrea helped Queenie nurse again six hours later and in the evening. Zimbobbee seemed to know that there was something wrong with her baby and became more patient. Andrea noticed that the calf was very abnormal; her legs were not only bent but came out of her shoulders at an odd angle, as on a preying mantis, making it hard for her to stand. Her head and jaw were not quite right, and her eyes didn't track properly.

Zimbobbee and Queenie stayed in the barn for two weeks, and Andrea helped the calf to nurse every eight hours. She was determined that this baby would live. Queenie's legs got stronger, and she'd stand briefly to nurse. She couldn't hold herself up very long, yet she tried to buck and play when Andrea was in the barn. She finally got strong enough to nurse without help, and we put the pair outside. They lived in a large pen next to a field, and in April, when bulls were with cows in various breeding groups, we put Zimbobbee in that field so that she'd be bred, letting her back into the pen twice a day to suckle her calf. Queenie was too handicapped to live with a group of cows. Zimbobbee didn't like confinement but loved her baby and resigned herself to her circumstance. We let them out in a bigger field after the other cows went to the range and there were no extra cattle to pester Queenie.

The calf grew fast, but the heavier she got, the harder it became for her to get around. She often crawled on her knees because her bent front legs couldn't hold her up. She spent most of her time lying down except when nursing her mother. We knew we'd have to butcher her, but Andrea wanted her to have as long a life as possible.

Andrea finally made the decision to end Queenie's life when she suspected that she was starting to have joint pain. She did the butchering herself because she was curious about her crippled joints. They were very abnormal, and the leg bones were quite twisted. The hind leg joints were not formed properly either; there were no hip sockets, and the cartilage on the bone ends had worn through.

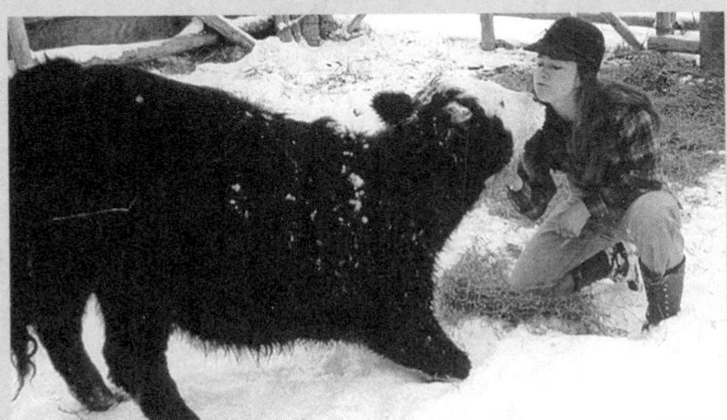

At ten months of age, Queenie is big and heavy, making it harder for her to get around on her crooked legs and malformed joints. Andrea is preparing to say good-bye to her special friend.

The calf was very handicapped, and most people would not have taken the extra effort to raise her, but she enjoyed interacting with her mama and with Andrea. Queenie had a good life, albeit short, and was very special to Andrea.

When you are raising cattle, there are occasional heartbreakers. We are in this vocation not just as a business but also because we love it and have a deep sense of caring and respect for the animals we raise. It may not have been cost-effective to raise Queenie, though she did provide meat for our table. But the time spent caring for her was not wasted time. Our lives are intricately tied to those of our animals, and we cannot really separate our paths from theirs. Helping vulnerable animals is part of the reason we're involved with livestock, part of our responsibility as ranchers. It's not just a job; it's a way of life.

Even though it was sad to have a calf as crippled as Queenie, to realize she had no future as a cow, our personal relationship with her, her trust and appreciation for us, and the communication between us gave us all a lot of satisfaction. There was a sense that we had come a little closer to our purpose as stewards of the land and the animals in our care. We are richer for these experiences, for the tasks that did not come easily.

Zimbobbee is now 14 years old and has given us 13 calves, but Queenie is the one we will always remember.

Epilogue

THE LONGER YOU RAISE CATTLE, and the more calves you come to know in the first moments of their lives, the greater the chances of encountering odd and difficult things. Some situations can't be bettered no matter what you do, but most can be managed and have positive outcomes if your efforts to resolve them are diligent and innovative. The challenge of raising cattle, and part of the satisfaction, comes with the understanding that you can often make a difference in the life of an animal. When you see a recovered calf running around bucking and playing with herd mates, it does your heart good to know that you were instrumental in saving his life and making such joyous exuberance possible.

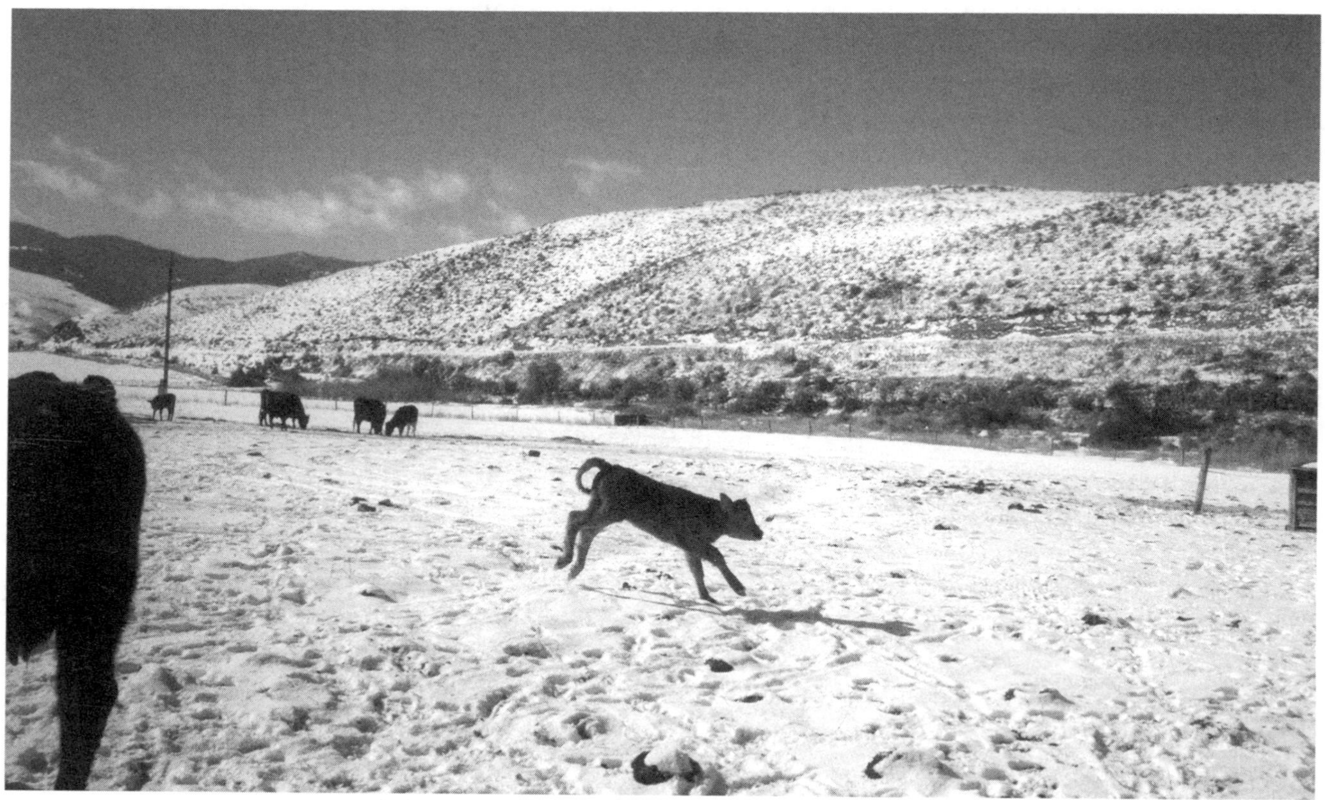

Appendix

Vital Signs

Normal Adult Cow

Temperature: 101.5°F (38.61°C)
Critical point: 103°F (39.44°C)
Pulse: 60 to 80 heartbeats per minute
Respiration: Variable, depending on ambient temperature, but usually about 10 to 30 breaths per minute on a cool day. In hot weather the respiration rate will be much higher, since cattle will pant to help cool themselves.

Normal Newborn Calf

Temperature: 101.5°F (38.61°C)
Critical Point: 102.5°F (39.17°C) to 103°F (39.44°C)
Pulse: 100 to 120 heartbeats per minute
Respiration: Variable. A calf will have a faster respiration rate than an adult, because of smaller body size, but as in an adult, the actual rate will vary with ambient temperature. The calf will breathe much more rapidly on a hot day than on a cool day.

CONVERSION TABLE
1 pound = 16 ounces = 453.6 grams = 0.454 kg
1 ounce = 28.35 grams
1 gram = 1000 milligrams
1 kg = 1000 grams = 2.2046 pounds
1 gallon = 4 quarts = 128 fluid ounces = 3.785 liters
1 quart = 2 pints = 0.946 liters = 32 fluid ounces
1 pint = 16 fluid ounces = 2 cups = 473 ml (cc)
1 cup = 16 tablespoons = 8 fluid ounces = 236.6 ml (cc)
1 fluid ounce = 30 ml (cc) = 2 tablespoons
1 tablespoon = ½ fluid ounce = 15 ml (cc) = 3 teaspoons
1 teaspoon = ⅙ fluid ounce = 5 ml (cc)

ANATOMY OF THE COW (LEFT SIDE)

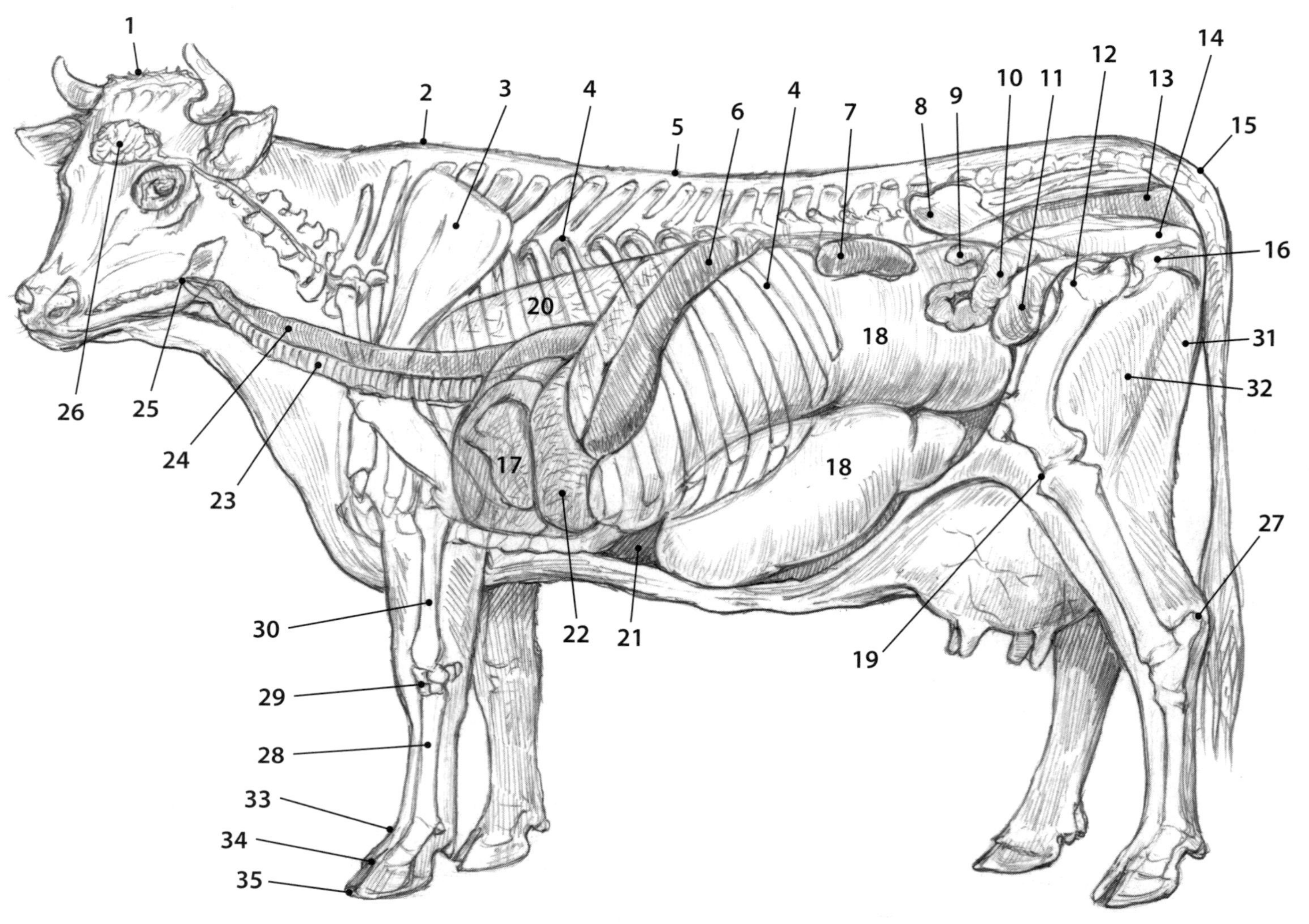

1 poll
2 withers
3 shoulder
4 ribs
5 back
6 spleen
7 kidney
8 hipbone
9 left ovary
10 uterus
11 bladder
12 hip joint
13 rectum
14 vagina
15 tail head
16 pin bone
17 heart
18 rumen
19 stifle joint
20 left lung
21 abomasum
22 recticulum
23 trachea (windpipe)
24 esophagus
25 larynx and pharynx
26 brain
27 point of hock
28 cannon bone
29 knee
30 forearm
31 buttocks
32 thigh
33 pastern
34 coronary band
35 toe (claw)

ANATOMY OF THE COW (RIGHT SIDE WITH INTERNAL ORGANS)

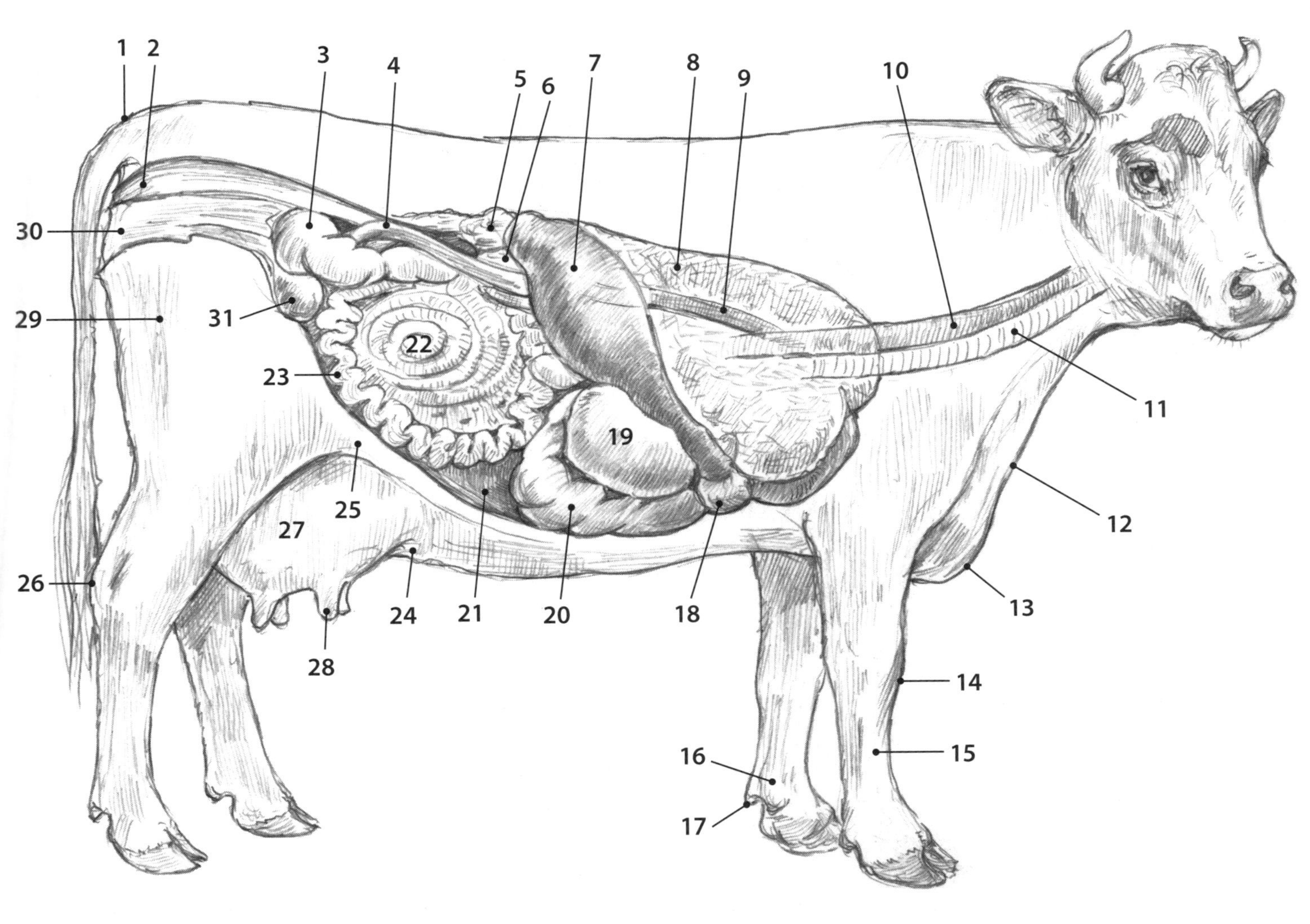

1 tail head
2 rectum
3 cecum
4 duodenum
5 right kidney
6 pancreas
7 liver
8 right lung
9 aorta
10 esophagus
11 trachea
12 brisket
13 dewlap
14 knee
15 cannon bone
16 fetlock joint
17 dewclaw
18 reticulum
19 omasum
20 abomasum
21 rumen
22 colon
23 intestines
24 milk vein
25 flank
26 hock
27 udder
28 teat
29 buttock
30 vagina
31 bladder

Common Bovine Medications

Adrenalin
Synthetic preparation of epinephrine (adrenaline), the hormone released in response to stress and to trigger labor. This drug is given to help reverse the effects of shock.

ampicillin
A broad-spectrum antibiotic that combats both gram-positive and gram-negative bacteria.

amprolium (Corid)
Drug used against coccidiosis.

antibiotics
Compounds produced by living organisms that impede the growth of other organisms. Antimicrobial drugs include antibiotics as well as synthetic and semi-synthetic compounds that have the same effects. Bacteria can often be killed or inhibited by these drugs, but viruses are not.

anti-inflammatory
Medication given to reduce pain, fever, swelling, inflammation. Steroids (like dexamethasone) and non-steroidal anti-inflammatories (bute, Banamine, aspirin, etc.) are used for this purpose.

Banamine (flunixin meglumine)
Non-steroidal anti-inflammatory drug that reduces pain, fever, and inflammation.

Baytil (enrofloxacin)
Broad-spectrum antibiotic (cephalosporin).

Betadine (trademark for povidone iodine)
"Tamed" iodine; a compound used as a disinfectant that is not as harsh as iodine.

bicarbonate
Alkalizing agent used in electrolyte solutions for sick calves, to help reverse acidosis.

bismuth
Ingredient in antidiarrhea medication to soothe and slow the gut.

broad-spectrum antibiotic
Antibiotic effective against both gram-positive and gram-negative bacteria.

castor oil
Laxative that stimulates the intestine to contract and move the contents through; also relieves bloat.

cephalosporin
Group of broad-spectrum antibiotics.

cocciostat
Drug that inhibits the multiplication of coccidia.

Corid
See amprolium.

Deccox
See decoquinate.

decoquinate
Drug that inhibits coccidia.

dexamethasone
Synthetic steroid used for reducing pain, inflammation, swelling, and fever.

DMSO (dimethyl sulfoxide)
Solvent with medicinal value as a linament and an anti-inflammatory, swelling-reducing drug.

Draxxin (tulathronmycin)
Broad-spectrum antibiotic that tends to concentrate in lung tissue; used for treating pneumonia.

Epinephrine
See Adrenalin.

Excede (ceftiofur)
Semi-synthetic broad-spectrum cephalosporin antibiotic.

iodine (tincture)
Chemical disinfectant.

ionophores
Antibiotics used in low levels in ruminant feeds to promote better growth by reducing acidosis, and also used to inhibit coccidia and to prevent coccidiosis.

keolin/pectin
Ingredients in products for diarrhea that coat, soothe, and slow the gut.

Keopectate
Antidiarrhea product that contains keolin and pectin.

Lasalocid
An ionophore.

Micotil (tilmicosin)
Antibiotic used in cattle but not safe for humans.

mineral oil
Laxative and gut soother, coating the intestinal lining and lubricating the gut contents for easier passage. Also reduces bloat.

monensin
Ionophore sometimes used to prevent coccidiosis in older calves.

Naxcel
See cephalosporin.

Neomycin
Broad-spectrum antibiotic.

neomycin sulfate solution
Oral liquid antibiotic that works well against most bacterial infections in the digestive tract.

Nolvasan (chlorhexadine)
All-purpose disinfectant.

Nuflor (florfenicol)
Broad-spectrum antibiotic.

oxytetracycline
Broad-spectrum antibiotic; brand names Biomycin, Liquimycin, LA-200, Oxy-tet, etc.

oxytocin
Hormone drug used to trigger labor and stimulate uterine contractions (to help a cow clean) and milk let-down.

penicillin
Broad-spectrum antibiotic.

Pepto-Bismol (bismuth subsalicylate)
Antidiarrheal medication.

probiotic
Products containing micro-organisms needed for proper digestion; given to sick calves to restore gut function.

steroid
Group of organic compounds that includes many hormones. Synthetic steroids like dexamethasone are often used for reducing pain, swelling, inflammation, and fever.

sulfa
Broad-spectrum antibiotic.

tetracycline
Broad-spectrum antibiotic.

trimethoprim
Broad-spectrum antibiotic.

Glossary

A

abdominal hernia. Rupture or muscle separation in the lower part of the abdominal wall, perhaps due to a severe blow, such as being horned in the belly, or a weakness in the abdominal muscles.

abomasum. Fourth or true stomach.

abortion. Expulsion of an embryo or fetus before it is mature enough to be viable outside of the uterus.

abscess. Accumulation of pus in infected tissue.

acardiac monster. Fetal mole; deformed "twin" that's a mass of connective tissue attached to the membranes of the normal twin.

acetate. Alkalizing agent used in calves to help reverse acidosis.

acidosis. pH imbalance in the body due to accumulation of acid or depletion of bicarbonate content in blood and body tissues, as a result of such things as shock, lack of blood oxygen, dehydration, and septicemia.

adrenaline. Hormone released in response to stress; synthetic preparations are given to help reverse effects of shock. Also called epinephrine.

afterbirth. See placenta.

alkaloid. A compound of plant origin with druglike properties.

allantoic fluid. The "water" in the outer water bag (allantoic sac or allantochorion) surrounding the fetus.

ammonia. Caustic, irritating gas produced by the breakdown of urine and manure; irritating to lungs of animals that breathe it.

amnion sac. Fluid-filled membrane around the fetus.

amniotic fluid. Thick, clear fluid surrounding the fetus.

amniotic membrane. The outer cover of the umbilical cord; also the membrane around the fetus.

anemic. Having low levels of red blood cells.

anestrus. Period after calving in which the cow does not cycle.

anovulatory heat. Heat without ovulation.

anterior presentation. Front; calf coming front-first through the birth canal.

antibiotic. Drug used to combat bacterial infection.

antibodies. Protein molecules in the blood that fight a specific disease.

antigen. Any foreign substance invading the body that stimulates creation of protective antibodies.

antitoxin. An antibody that counteracts a bacterial toxin.

anti-inflammatory. Medication to relieve pain, swelling, inflammation, and fever.

anus. Rectal opening through which feces pass.

arthritis. Inflammation of a joint. See also septic arthritis.

artificial insemination (AI). Inserting semen from a bull into the cow's uterus to create pregnancy.

artificial respiration. Blowing air into the calf's nostril (while holding mouth and other nostril shut) until the calf can begin to breathe on his own.

aspergillus. A type of mold that can cause abortion when eaten.

aspiration pneumonia. Pneumonia caused by irritation from foreign material or fluid in the lungs, setting up conditions for infection.

B

bacteremia. The presence of bacteria in the bloodstream.

bacteria. Tiny one-celled organisms.

Bang's disease. See brucellosis.

Betadine. Trademark for povidone iodine; "tamed" iodine, a compound used as a disinfectant that is not as harsh as iodine.

bicarbonate. Alkalizing agent, often used in electrolyte solutions for sick calves to help reverse acidosis.

biopsy. Tissue sample taken to examine for diagnosis.

birth canal. Vagina; passage through which the calf is born when he is expelled from the uterus during labor.

blackleg. Disease caused by Clostridium chauvoei, a soil-borne bacterium, resulting in muscle inflammation and death.

blind tube vagina. An abnormality in which the vagina is not connected to the uterus.

bloat. Distension of the rumen by gas. See also colicky bloat.

boluses. Large, oblong pills.

bony lump jaw. An infection that settles in the jawbone.

bovine respiratory syncytial virus (BRSV). A serious respiratory viral infection.

bovine virus diarrhea (BVD). A viral disease that causes abortion, birth of diseased calves, respiratory or digestive-tract illness, and suppression of the immune system.

breech. Posterior presentation in which the hind legs do not enter the birth canal; the rump (and sometimes hocks) are pressed against the cervix but can't come through.

brisket. The area between the front legs; tissue covering the front of the breastbone; dewlap.

broad spectrum antibiotic. Drug effective against gram-negative and gram-positive bacteria.

bronchial tubes. The two main branches of the trachea (windpipe) that each enter a lung and then split into smaller branches.

bronchopneumonia. Pneumonia caused by infection descending into the lungs from the bronchial tubes.

broom snakeweed. A low-growing, sticky-leaved shrub brush that grows in great abundance in the southwestern United States; it may cause abortions in cattle that eat it.

BRSV. See bovine respiratory syncytial virus (BRSV).

brucellosis (Bang's disease). A bacterial disease that causes abortion.

bunt. To hit with the head.

buttons. See cotyledons.

BVD. See bovine virus diarrhea.

C

cake. Hard swelling in the udder before calving; most common in first calvers.

calf puller. Mechanical device used to put traction on the calf with chains on his legs, via a winch or ratchet and positional leverage.

campylobacteriosis. See vibriosis.

cannon bones. Bones between knee and fetlock joint, or hock and fetlock joint, on the hind leg.

carrier. An animal that appears healthy but harbors pathogens or parasites that can be shed or passed to other animals.

caruncles. Bumps on the lining of the uterus that attach to the cotyledons of the placenta.

castor oil. Laxative that stimulates the intestine to contract and move the contents through.

cervix. Opening between uterus and vagina. It is tightly closed except during estrus and calving.

cesarean section. Surgical delivery of a calf; c-section.

chlamydia. Pathogen similar to a virus that can cause abortion.

chorion. "Water sac"; the larger, most external fluid-filled membrane surrounding the amnion sac and the fetus.

cilia. Hairlike structures that line the windpipe and move in waves to sweep pathogens and foreign material to the back of the throat.

CL. See corpus luteum.

clean. To shed the placenta, after the calf is born.

cleanup bull. Bull used after AI breeding to breed any cows that did not settle with an AI service.

cleft palate. Hole in the roof of the mouth and the bottom of the nostril due to an accident in gestation such as exposure to toxic alkaloids in lupine ingested by the dam in early pregnancy.

clinical signs. Evidence of illness; obvious symptoms.

clitoris. Small organ at external lower portion of vulva.

clostridial bacteria. Bacteria that cause diseases, including blackleg, tetanus, and enterotoxemia, that produce powerful toxins, causing sudden illness that is usually fatal.

coccidia. Pathogenic protozoa that cause coccidiosis.

coccidiosis. Intestinal disease and diarrhea caused by a certain type of pathogenic protozoa.

coccidiostat. Drug that inhibits multiplication of coccidian.

colic. Acute abdominal pain.

colicky bloat. Acute gut infection that can kill a calf within 3 to 12 hours if not discovered and treated.

colostrum. First milk after a cow calves, containing high-energy fat and antibodies that give temporary protection against diseases.

conception. Fertilization of an egg by a sperm cell, beginning at pregnancy.

conceptus. Fertilized egg, at any stage after the egg and sperm meet, including embryonic or fetal stages.

congenital. Acquired before birth, such as a birth defect.

contracted tendons. Tendons that are too "tight," pulling the joints out of line, such as when knees or fetlock joints are cocked forward.

contracture. Limbs of fetus cannot be straightened enough to come through the birth canal.

convulsion. Seizure; violent, involuntary spasms or contraction of the muscles.

coronavirus. A highly contagious viral disease that causes diarrhea in newborn calves and lambs.

corpus luteum (CL). Structure that forms in the ovary in the spot where a follicle ovulated, producing progesterone.

cortisol. Hormonal steroid produced by the body during stress, regulating the immune system and affecting metabolism of glucose, fats, and proteins; also one of the hormones important in labor.

cotyledons. Lumpy red "buttons" that attach the placenta to the uterine lining.

cow. Bovine female that has had a calf.

creep. Small area in a pen or field, usually made with panels, into which a calf can enter to eat but cows cannot.

cryptosporidia. Pathogenic protozoa that cause cryptosporidiosis.

cryptosporidiosis. Protozoal disease that causes diarrhea in calves and humans.

culture. To grow microorganisms in the laboratory.

cycle. To have a heat period. See estrous cycle.

cystic ovary. Malfunctioning ovary due to imbalance of hormones; the cow may not show heat or may seem to be in heat all the time.

cytopathic. Viral strain of bovine viral diarrhea that can alter tissue cells in the body.

D

dam. The mother of a calf.

dehydration. Shortage of fluid in body tissues.

dewclaws. Horny protuberances at the back of the lower leg.

dewlap. See brisket.

dexamethasone. Steroidal anti-inflammatory drug.

dextrose. Simple sugar, often added to an intravenous electrolyte solution to give a calf energy and to oral solutions to aid uptake of salts by the cells in the intestinal lining.

diarrhea. Watery feces.

diestrus. One of the four stages of the estrous cycle; period of time between heats in which the cow is not receptive to being bred.

diphtheria. Bacterial disease causing swelling in mouth or throat; necrotic laryngitis.

dominant gene. The trait expressed when more than one gene for a certain trait is present.

double monster. Two-headed calf.

double muscling. Recessive trait inherited from both parents in which the muscles have extra fibers; results in calving problems due to extra muscle mass of the calf. Also called hypertrophy.

drench. To administer fluid or medication via the mouth, forcing the animal to swallow it.

dry cow. Cow that has weaned or lost her calf; not lactating.

dwarfism. Recessive trait in which the skeleton is small, the legs and head are too short, and the forehead bulges.

dysmature. Full term in length of time but immature (similar to a premature calf), due to uterine or placental insufficiency.

dystocia. Delayed or difficult birth.

E

early embryonic death. Loss of a pregnancy occurring before 45 days of gestation.

edema. Swelling.

ejaculate. Act of the male depositing semen into the female.

electrolytes. Important body salts that must be replaced when an animal is dehydrated.

embryo. The conceptus, during its rapid early development when all major structures are formed (in bovines, the first 45 days).

endemic. Always present in a population or geographic area.

endometritis. Inflammation or infection of the uterine lining.

endotoxin. A toxin produced by the outer covering of certain gram-negative bacteria as they die, including various enterobacteria that produce severe diarrhea and sometimes shock. See exotoxin.

enterotoxemia. Serious bacterial gut infection in calves caused by Clostridium perfringens, in which toxins leak into the bloodstream.

enterotoxigenic. Producing or containing a toxin that affects the cells of the intestinal lining.

enterotoxin. A toxin that specifically affects the cells of the intestinal lining, making it incapable of absorbing fluid and nutrients, causing diarrhea.

enzootic bovine abortion. See foothill abortion.

epidemic. Sudden outbreak of disease, with the number of cases much higher than what would normally be expected.

epidural. Injection of anesthetic into the spinal column near the base of the tail to keep the cow from straining; spinal block.

epinephrine. Hormone (adrenaline) released in response to stress; synthetic preparations are given to help reverse effects of shock.

epithelial cells. Cells that form a covering layer.

Escherichia coli. Gram-negative bacteria, some of which cause serious intestinal infection in calves; *E. coli.*

esophageal feeder. Tube put down a calf's throat to the stomach inlet to force-feed fluids from a feeder bag.

esophageal groove. Fold of tissue that routes milk directly to the true stomach, bypassing the rumen, when a calf nurses.

esophagus. Tube/passage between the mouth and the stomach.

estrogen. Hormone secreted by a follicle on the ovary; brings a cow into heat.

estrous cycle. Recurring hormonally controlled reproductive cycle that includes estrus, metestrus, diestrus, and proestrus, and is marked by a period of sexual activity, ovulation, and changes in the uterine lining and in behavior of the cow.

estrus. heat period (part of the heat cycle) when a cow will accept a bull to be bred.

exotoxin. Toxin created while bacteria are still alive and produced as they multiply. See also endotoxin.

F

fecal sample. Sample of manure to test for presence of pathogens.

feces. Manure.

fertile. Capable of reproducing.

fetal mole. See acardiac monster.

fetlock joint. Joint at the end of the lower leg bone, just above the pastern, with horny protuberances (dewclaws) at the rear.

fetotomy. When the fetus is cut apart to bring it out through the birth canal in pieces.

fetus. The developing calf, after 45 days of gestation.

fever. Body temperature above normal.

flank. Rear part of the abdomen and belly, just ahead of the hind leg and above the udder.

follicle. Pouchlike depression on the ovary, containing a cell that becomes a mature egg if that follicle ovulates.

follicle stimulating hormone (FSH). Hormone that triggers growth and development of follicles on the ovary.

foothill abortion. Enzootic bovine abortion; disease, possibly spread by ticks in certain areas of the West, which causes abortion in cows.

foot rot. Acute infection causing severe pain, swelling, and lameness in the foot, caused by Fusobacterium necrophorum, the same bacteria that can cause navel ill and diphtheria.

foreskin. Fold of skin over the penis.

founder. Inflammation of the sensitive hoof-producing part of the foot most often caused by ruminal acidosis due to high-concentrate feeding; laminitis.

freemartin. Infertile heifer, born twin to a bull, with abnormalities of the reproductive tract.

fungi. Group of organisms that include molds and yeasts and which live on dead organic matter or living tissue; some are toxic and cause disease or abortions in cows or heifers.

G

gene. Part of a chromosome that determines the inherited traits of an individual.

genitalia. Internal and external organs pertaining to reproduction.

germ cell. Egg or sperm; contains half the chromosomes needed to become a new individual.

gestation. Length of pregnancy; average for cows is 283 days.

glucose. A simple sugar, often added to electrolyte mixes.

glutamine. Protein that helps stimulate uptake of salts by cells in the intestinal lining.

gluteal nerve. The main nerve that serves the gluteal muscles, the large muscles of the buttocks.

gonads. Sex organs; ovaries and testes.

graft. To convince a cow to accept and raise a substitute calf in place of her own.

gram-negative bacteria. Bacteria with thin cell walls; some of these types are associated with serious intestinal illness.

gram-positive bacteria. Bacteria with a thick cell wall.

grass tetany. Muscle and nervous system malfunction due to low levels of magnesium in the body.

gut. Digestive tract.

H

Haemophilus somnus. Bacterial infection that causes abortion and infertility.

hairball. Wad or clump of hair in the stomach or intestine that may block the tract.

hardware disease. Peritonitis (infection in the abdomen) caused by a sharp foreign object penetrating the stomach wall.

head snare. A loop of stiff cable, sometimes used to try to direct a calf's head into the birth canal if it's turned to the side.

heat. See estrus.

heifer. Young female bovine before she's had a calf.

hernia. Protrusion of tissue through an abdominal opening. See abdominal hernia; umbilical hernia.

hiplock. Calf stuck in the birth canal because his hips are too wide to come through the cow's pelvic opening.

hock. Large joint halfway up the hind leg.

hormone. Chemical substance produced in the body, having a specific regulatory effect on the activity of an organ or organs.

horn, uterine. See uterine horn.

hydramnios. Too much fluid in the amnion sac around the calf.

hydroallantois. Too much fluid in the outer "water bag" (allantoic sac) surrounding the fetus.

hydrocephalic calf. Calf with large head or forehead due to accumulation of fluid ("water on the brain").

hypertrophy. Enlargement or overgrowth of a body part. See double muscling.

hypocalcemia. Low calcium levels in the body.

I

IBR. See infectious bovine rhinotracheitis.

IgA. Antibody from colostrum that remains in the gut, rather than being absorbed into the bloodstream, to fight diarrhea-causing pathogens.

IgG. Antibody from colostrum that can be absorbed through the gut lining immediately after birth, to give the calf passive immunity to diseases.

immersion reflex. Instinct to refrain from breathing while the face/nose is covered, as in a newborn calf encased in the fluid-filled amnion sac.

immune system. Important network of defense systems within the body that fights pathogens and creates antibodies.

immunity. Ability to resist a certain disease.

immunoglobulins. Antibody proteins.

inbreeding. Breeding closely related animals such as father to daughter, mother to son, brother to sister, etc.

incisors. Front teeth.

incubation period. Time elapsing between when a pathogen enters the body and when the animal shows signs of disease.

infectious bovine rhinotracheitis (IBR). Respiratory virus that can also cause abortion in cows; red nose.

intravenously (IV). Into a vein.

involution. Shrinking up of the uterus after calving.

iodine. Trace mineral; also a chemical disinfectant.

ionophores. A group of antibiotics (monensin, lasalocid, salinomycin) used in low levels in ruminant feeds to help prevent acidosis of the rumen. They also inhibit coccidia and help prevent coccidiosis.

isotonic. Electrolyte (salt) concentration the same as that of body tissues/fluids.

J

joint ill. See navel ill.

jugular vein. Major vein in the neck; one of the easiest veins to use when giving an intravenous injection.

K

ketosis. Pregnancy toxemia due to changes in the liver.

killed-virus vaccine. See modified live-virus vaccine.

K99. Strain of *E. coli* bacteria that causes diarrhea in baby calves.

L

labor. Birth process. Early (first stage) labor: uterine contractions to position calf for birth; active (second stage) labor: cow adds abdominal straining to uterine contractions, to expel calf through birth canal; third-stage labor: placenta is shed.

lactating. Producing milk.

laminitis. See founder.

larynx. Voice box at the back of the throat, between the nasal passages and the windpipe.

leptospirosis. Bacterial disease that can cause abortion; also called "lepto."

libido. Sex drive.

listeriosis. Bacterial disease that can cause abortion.

locoweed. Poisonous plant that can cause abortion.

lupine. Wildflower that can cause birth defects in calves if cows eat it during early gestation (between the 30th and 70th days).

luteinizing hormone (LH). Hormone produced by the pituitary, causing a follicle on the ovary to ovulate and develop a corpus luteum (CL).

lymphocyte. White blood cell.

M

maceration. Rotting of the soft tissues of a dead fetus, due to bacteria in the uterus.

malignant edema. Acute and usually fatal wound infection caused by Clostridium septicum.

malpresentation. Faulty or abnormal fetal presentation that usually must be corrected in order for birth to proceed.

mammary tissue. Milk-producing glands in the udder.

mastitis. Infection and inflammation in the udder.

meconium. Dark, sticky first bowel movements of a newborn calf.

meningitis. Inflammation and infection of tissues around the brain.

metestrus. One of the four stages of the estrous cycle, in which about 12 hours after the end of standing heat, ovulation occurs and the CL forms and secretes progesterone.

metritis. Inflammation and infection of the uterus.

milk fever. Inability of a cow to get up, due to acute lack of calcium in the body as a result of sudden high production of milk at calving time.

mineral oil. Often given by stomach tube to cattle to relieve bloat caused by fermented feed or to soothe raw, ulcerated gut lining, or to lubricate its contents if a calf is constipated.

modified live-virus vaccine. Vaccine created by using live virus that has been altered or inactivated so that it stimulates immunity but won't cause disease, as opposed to killed virus vaccines that are safer but not as effective in producing strong immunity.

molybdenum. Element in soil that can tie up copper and make it inaccessible to the body, producing symptoms of copper deficiency.

mortality rate. Percentage of animals that die from a disease.

mount. To rear up over the back of a cow to "ride" her, as a bull does when breeding the cow.

mucous membranes. Moist tissues lining many body cavities that secrete or are covered with mucus, such as gums and mouth tissue.

mucus. Slimy lubricating substance secreted by mucous membranes.

multiplier effect. The passage of pathogens through an animal, creating many more times the numbers of pathogens than what originally entered the animal.

mummification. The process by which a dead fetus that was retained in the uterus instead of being expelled when it died is turned into a mummylike object.

myoglobin. Red pigment in the iron-containing protein of muscles.

N

nasogastric tube. Long, flexible tube put into the nostril to the back of the throat, down the esophagus, and into the stomach.

navel ill. Infection entering via the navel stump at birth, often causing problems elsewhere in the body, such as joints (joint ill).

necropsy. Postmortem examination to determine cause of death or cause of infection.

necrotic. Dead.

necrotic laryngitis. See diphtheria.

neosporosis. Protozoal infection that can cause abortion in cows; spread by canine feces that contaminate cattle feed.

Nolvasan. All-purpose disinfectant; chlorhexidine.

nurse. Suckle.

O

obstetrical. Having to do with pregnancy and birth.

obturator nerve. Nerve that runs along each side of the pelvic cavity to serve the thigh muscles; if it's stretched or compressed during calving, the cow's hind legs may be temporarily paralyzed.

omasum. Third stomach.

oocysts. Immature encapsulated "eggs" of protozoa.

oocyte. Egg cell.

open cows. Cows that have not been impregnated.

oral. By mouth.

otter calves. Calves with no legs.

ovary. Oval-shaped organ that produces reproductive hormones and eggs that have the potential to be fertilized and become calves.

overeating disease. In calves whose mothers are good milk producers, sudden milk overload creates ideal conditions for toxic bacteria to multiply.

oviduct. Tiny tube leading from the ovary to the uterus.

ovulation. Ripening and discharge of an egg from a mature follicle on the ovary for possible fertilization.

oxytocin. Hormone that stimulates uterine contractions, labor, and milk let-down.

P

palpate. Feel with the fingers, as through a wall of tissue.

parainfluenza 3 (PI3). Serious respiratory viral infection.

parasite. Organism (plant or animal) that lives on or within another organism, depending on the host for its nutrients.

parturition. Act of giving birth.

passive transfer. Temporary protection against disease, given to the calf when he absorbs antibodies from his dam's colostrum.

pastern. Area between the hoof and fetlock joint.

Pasteurella hemolyticum. Bacterium that often causes pneumonia.

pathogen. Harmful invader of the body, such as a virus or certain bacteria, protozoa, or fungi.

pelvic ligaments. Connect the pin bones (point of buttock) to the spine; these ligaments relax and become soft a few hours before calving, to allow more stretching of the birth canal.

pelvis. Bony circle to which the hind legs attach and through which the calf is expelled via the birth canal.

peritoneum. Inner lining of the abdominal cavity.

peritonitis. Infection in the abdominal cavity.

persistent hymen. Tight rings of tissue just inside the vulva in a heifer, constricting the circumference of the vagina.

persistently infected (PI) animals. Calves infected in utero with BVD during the first three to four months of gestation and carrying the virus for the rest of their lives.

pH. Measure of acidity or alkalinity on a scale of 1 to 14; 7 is neutral, 1 is most acidic, and 14 is most alkaline.

pharynx. Throat; passage between the mouth and rear part of the nasal passages and the larynx and esophagus.

pilli. Minute appendages of certain bacteria that are associated with antigenic properties and that can stick to the small intestine. Once there, the antigen can be destructive, but if it can't bind, it is harmless.

pine needle abortion. Abortion caused by the cow eating ponderosa pine needles.

pinocytosis. Process by which movement of antibodies through the intestinal wall of a newborn calf is aided by creation of tiny fluid pockets.

pipette. Long narrow tube used to insert semen into the cow's uterus through the open cervix for artificial insemination.

pituitary gland. Small gland at the base of the brain that secretes various hormones that regulate body functions.

placenta. Tissue attached to the uterus during pregnancy, as a buffer around the fetus, and the portal through which oxygen and nutrients from the dam's bloodstream are exchanged with waste products from the fetus; afterbirth.

placentitis. Inflammation of the placenta.

placentomes. Places of attachment where the cotyledons of the placenta hook into the caruncles of the uterus.

pneumonia. Infection in the lungs.

polled. Genetically hornless.

posterior presentation. Calf coming backward through the birth canal, hind feet first.

post-legged. An animal that is too straight in stifles and hocks.

postpartum. After calving.

potassium. One of the crucial elements of the body, included in electrolyte "salts."

premature. A calf born before full term but alive and possibly able to survive, if given appropriate care.

probiotics. Products containing the microorganisms needed for proper digestion.

proestrus. One of the four stages of the estrous cycle, in which the follicles attain final growth and secrete estrogen, causing the cow to come into standing heat.

progesterone. Hormone responsible for continuation of pregnancy and the predominant hormone in the cow's body between heat periods.

prolapse. Protrusion of inverted organ (vagina, uterus, rectum).

prostaglandins. Hormones secreted by the uterus that influence the estrous cycle; also produced in the body during inflammatory processes.

protozoa. One-celled animals, some of which cause disease.

puberty. Age at which an animal matures sexually.

pyometra. Pus in the uterus.

Q

quarters of the udder. The four compartments of the bovine udder.

quiet heat. See silent heat.

R

recessive gene. Gene that must be received from both parents before the trait can be expressed (seen) in offspring.

rectum. Final portion of the large intestine.

red nose. See IBR.

repeat breeders. Cows that continually return to heat and do not settle when bred.

resorbed. Broken down and assimilated, as when a dead fetus is resorbed by the uterus.

respiratory system. Consists of nasal passages, windpipe, bronchial tubes and lungs.

retained placenta. Failure to shed the placenta after calving.

reticulum. The second stomach compartment.

rotavirus. Highly contagious virus spread by feces, causing acute diarrhea in young calves.

rumen. Largest stomach compartment, where roughage is digested with the aid of microorganisms in a fermentation process.

S

salmonellosis. Severe illness and diarrhea caused by salmonella bacteria.

sarcocystosis. Protozoan infection spread to cattle by predatory animals, sometimes causing abortion in cows.

schistosoma reflexus. Fetal "monster" with an acute bend in the backbone and internal organs or intestines exposed.

scours. Diarrhea (watery, fluid feces).

scrotal circumference. Measure of testicle size (distance around the scrotum at widest part), related to semen-producing capacity and age at puberty.

scrotal hernia. Hole in the abdominal wall at the scrotum that allows loops of intestine to fall into the scrotum.

scrotum. Sac enclosing the testicles of a bull.

secondary infection. Another pathogen moving in, taking advantage of an animal's lowered resistance due to the original disease.

selenium. Mineral needed in very small amounts in the diet; too much or too little can be harmful to health.

self-limiting. A disease that runs a definite limited course with no need for treatment; the animal throws off infection and recovers.

semen. Thick, whitish secretion of male reproductive organs; contains sperm.

seminal fluid. A secretion containing sperm.

septic arthritis. Abscesses in joints caused by bacteremia.

septicemia. Generalized infection throughout the body, when bacteria and their toxins travel through the bloodstream; sepsis.

serotype. The type of microorganism, as determined by the antigens present within it.

settle. Become pregnant; to impregnate.

sheath. Tube-shaped fold of skin into which the penis retracts.

sheep hook. Long handled hook used for catching sheep or calves by a hind leg; shepherd's crook.

shepherd's crook. See sheep hook.

shock. Extreme circulatory and metabolic disturbance in the body, characterized by failure of the circulatory system to maintain adequate blood supply to vital organs.

sickle hocked. Describes an animal that has too much angle in the hock joints.

silent heat. Ovulation with no signs of heat; quiet heat.

sire. To father a calf; father of a calf.

snare. See head snare.

sodium. Combines with chloride to produce table salt; one of the crucial elements needed by the body.

sperm. Germ cells from the bull that swim to meet the egg in the cow's reproductive tract to fertilize the egg and create an embryo.

spermatogenic cycle. The amount of time (about 60 days) it takes from when the sperm cell is produced until it is mature and ready to be ejaculated.

spinal block. See epidural.

spore. Reproductive element of fungi, protozoa, and algae.

sporozoite. Mobile, infective stage of coccidian protozoa.

sporulation. Formation or liberation of spores (multiplication process of protozoa).

standing heat. Estrus; time during heat period when the cow allows the bull to mount and breed her.

steroid. Hormone or hormonelike substance. Cortisol is a steroid produced by the adrenal glands; gonadal steroids (estrogen and testosterone) are produced by the ovaries and testes; dexamethasone is a synthetic steroid used as a drug.

stifle. Large joint high on the hind leg, by the flank.

stillborn. Born dead.

stomach tube. See nasogastric tube.

streptococcus. Common bacteria that cause a variety of serious conditions if they enter the body.

subclinical. Showing no signs; not obvious.

subcutaneous. Under the skin.

suckling. Nursing.

supplement. Feed additive that supplies something missing in the diet.

suture. Stitch to sew up incision.

systemic. The whole body, as opposed to localized (pertaining to infection, treatment, etc.).

T

teratogens. Any factors or agents that cause abnormality in a developing embryo or fetus.

testicles (testes). Male gonads, situated in the scrotum, which produce sperm cells and testosterone.

testosterone. Male hormone.

tetanus. Acute, fatal, infectious disease caused by clostridial bacterium C. tetani, which produces deadly neurotoxins; usually enters through a wound or the navel stump or postpartum uterus.

tetany. Powerful muscle spasms.

torsion. Twist.

torsion of the uterus. A turning over of the uterus and its contents, putting a twist in the cervix; the calf can't be born.

toxemia. Condition in which bacterial toxins invade the bloodstream and poison the body.

toxins. Poisons; usually refers to proteins produced by plants and certain pathogenic bacteria.

toxoid. Modified or inactivated bacterial toxin; used in a vaccine to stimulate immunity against that bacterium and its toxins.

trachea. See windpipe.

tracheostomy. Cutting into the windpipe to create an opening through which the animal can breathe when upper air passages are blocked or constricted.

trichomoniasis. Disease spread by infected bulls during the act of breeding, caused by protozoal infection and resulting in abortion.

tuberculosis (TB). Infectious disease caused by mycobacterium and characterized by formation of tubercles in various organs, such as the lungs; can cause abortion in cattle.

U

udder. Mammary glands and teats.

umbilical cord. Tissue containing blood vessels and urachus, attaching the developing fetus to the placenta, for exchange of blood and nutrients with fetal waste products. When the calf is born, this "lifeline" breaks, and he must start to breathe.

umbilical hernia. A hole or separation in the outer wall of the abdomen that allows fluid or tissue to bulge through, creating an enlargement under the skin at the navel.

umbilical tape. Wide, strong cotton "string" ideal for stitching across an opening (rectal or vaginal) to prevent prolapses.

umbilicus. Navel.

undulant fever. The form of brucellosis (Bang's disease) acquired by humans.

urachus. Tube between the calf's bladder and navel, and through the umbilical cord while he is still in the uterus.

urethra. Tube from the urinary bladder to the external opening just inside the vulva (in a female) and through which urine passes.

uterine horns. Two separate portions of the bovine uterus.

uterine inertia. Insufficient uterine contractions (weak or absent) when the cow is in labor. Primary uterine inertia in early labor may be due to hormonal or mineral imbalances. Secondary inertia occurs after hard labor in a difficult birth, when the cow becomes exhausted and contractions become weaker or cease.

uterine milk. Yellow-white thick fluid secreted by the uterine glands; it seeps through the chorion and amnion to nourish the developing embryo during early gestation.

uterus. Womb; in the cow it is divided into two segments (horns), joined together for a short distance in the main body of the uterus.

V

vaccine. Fluid containing killed or modified live germs or the antigenic proteins obtained from them, injected or sprayed into the body to stimulate production of antibodies and create immunity.

vagina. Passageway between uterus and vulva; birth canal.

vaginitis. Irritation and inflammation of the vaginal tissues.

vibriosis. Venereal disease of cattle that causes abortion; campylobacteriosis.

viruses. Group of very tiny infectious agents that can multiply only in a living host.

vulva. External opening of the cow's reproductive tract.

W

water bag. Fluid-filled membrane that often comes through the birth canal ahead of the calf, spilling a large quantity of amber-colored fluid when it breaks.

white blood cells. Cells in the bloodstream that devour bacteria, produce antibodies, and fight infection.

white muscle disease. A fatal condition in calves in which some of the heart muscle fibers are replaced with connective tissue, due to selenium deficiency.

wind chill factor. Cooling effect of wind on exposed skin producing the equivalent of a much lower temperature.

windpipe. The tube between the larynx at the back of the throat and the lungs; trachea.

windswept legs. Both legs (front or hind) bent abnormally in the same direction, such as both bowed to the left or to the right.

Resources

Cooperative State Research, Education, and Extension Service

A nationwide, noncredit educational network overseen by the United States Department of Agriculture. Each U.S. state and territory has an office at its land-grant university and a network of local or regional offices. Experts provide useful, practical, and research-based information to agricultural producers and small business owners and others in rural areas and communities of all sizes. **Contact to find nearest cooperative extension office:**

Cooperative State Research, Education, and Extension Service
United States Department of Agriculture
Washington, D.C.
202-720-7441
www.csrees.usda.gov/Extension

Livestock and Veterinary Supply Companies

American Livestock Supply
Madison, Wisconsin
800-356-0700
www.americanlivestock.com
Vaccines, medications, and other supplies

Jeffers Livestock Supply
Dothan, Alabama
800-533-3377
www.jefferslivestock.com
Vaccines, etc.

Koehn Marketing
Watertown, South Dakota
800-658-3998
www.koehnmarketing.com
Unique livestock equipment, including calf sleds, calf carriers, calf pullers, calf catchers, calf jackets, etc.

Nasco Farm and Ranch Supplies
Fort Atkinson, Wisconsin
800-558-9595
www.enasco.com
Vaccines, tags, and other cattle equipment

Valley Vet Supply
Marysville, Kansas
800-468-0059
www.valleyvet.com
Vaccines, medications, and other cattle supplies

Western Ranch Supply
Great Falls, Montana
800-548-5855
www.westernranchsupply.com
Vaccines, medications, tags, calving supplies, etc.

Index

Page numbers in *italic* indicate illustrations; those in **bold** indicate tables.

C

D

E

N

O

P

T

Other Storey Titles You Will Enjoy

The Family Cow, by Dirk van Loon.
Essential details, complete with illustrations, for the family that decides to keep a cow.
272 pages. Paper. ISBN 978-0-88266-066-7.

Getting Started with Beef & Dairy Cattle, by Heather Smith Thomas.
The first-time farmer's guide to the basics of raising a small herd of cattle.
288 pages. Paper. ISBN 978-1-58017-596-8.
Hardcover with jacket. ISBN 978-1-58017-604-0.

Grass-Fed Cattle, by Julius Ruechel.
The first complete manual in raising, caring for, and marketing grass-fed cattle.
384 pages. Paper. ISBN 978-1-58017-605-7.

Oxen: A Teamster's Guide, by Drew Conroy.
The definitive guide to selecting, training, and caring for the mighty ox.
304 pages. Paper. ISBN 978-1-58017-692-7.
Hardcover. ISBN 978-1-58017-693-4.

Raising a Calf for Beef, by Phyllis Hobson.
A no-nonsense guide to choosing a calf, providing housing and nutrition, and finally butchering.
128 pages. Paper. ISBN 978-0-88266-095-0.

Small-Scale Livestock Farming, by Carol Ekarius.
A natural, organic approach to livestock management to produce healthier animals, reduce feed and health care costs, and maximize profit.
224 pages. Paper. ISBN 978-1-58017-162-5.

Starting & Running Your Own Small Farm Business, by Sarah Beth Aubrey.
A business-savvy reference that covers everything from writing a business plan and applying for loans to marketing your farm-fresh goods.
176 pages. Paper. ISBN 978-1-58017-697-2.

Storey's Guide to Raising Series.
Everything you need to know to keep your livestock and your profits healthy. Latest title is Meat Goats. Other titles in the series are Rabbits, Ducks, Turkeys, Poultry, Chickens, Dairy Goats, Llamas, Pigs, Sheep, and Beef Cattle.
Paper. Learn more about each title by visiting *www.storey.com.*

These and other books from Storey Publishing are available wherever quality books are sold or by calling 1-800-441-5700.
Visit us at *www.storey.com.*